"To beloved
our beloved
Geo.

May this book bring
to you, the great pleasure
you have brought to us always.
May you achieve also, the success
you so richly deserve.

Mum & Dad

December 1961.

113/-

Obstetric and
Gynecologic Milestones

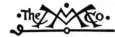

THE MACMILLAN COMPANY
NEW YORK • CHICAGO
DALLAS • ATLANTA • SAN FRANCISCO
LONDON • MANILA

IN CANADA
BRETT-MACMILLAN LTD.
GALT, ONTARIO

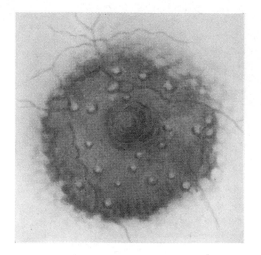

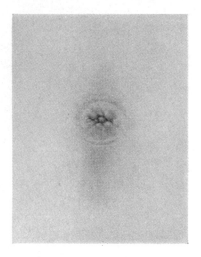

The mammary areola in the sixth month of pregnancy (Montgomery's tubercles; see pp. 213–16). (Reproduced from Montgomery, W. F.: *An Exposition of the Signs and Symptoms of Pregnancy, the Period of Human Gestation, and the Signs of Delivery*. Sherwood, Gilbert, & Piper, London, 1837.)

Discoloration of the umbilicus in ruptured extrauterine pregnancy (Cullen's sign; see pp. 260–61). (Reproduced from Cullen, T. S.: In *Contributions to Medical and Biological Research*. Paul B. Hoeber, Inc., New York, 1919.)

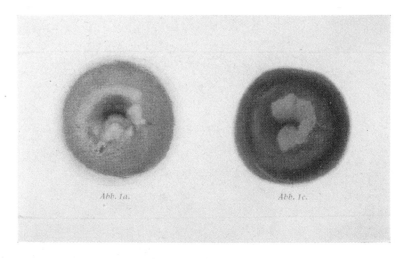

Iodine staining of the cervix (the Schiller test; see pp. 291–94). *Left:* Unstained cervix with leucoplakia. *Right:* The same cervix after iodine application, revealing extent of carcinoma. (Reproduced from Schiller, W.: Zur klinischen Frühdiagnose des Portiokarzinoms. *Zentralbl. f. Gynäk.*, **52**:1886, 1928.)

ESSAYS IN EPONYMY

Obstetric and Gynecologic Milestones

HAROLD SPEERT, M.D.

Assistant Professor of Clinical Obstetrics and Gynecology,
Columbia University College of Physicians and Surgeons;
Assistant Attending Obstetrician and Gynecologist,
The Presbyterian Hospital, New York

New York, 1958
THE MACMILLAN COMPANY

First printing, November, 1958

Printed in the United States of America

Library of Congress catalog card number: 58–10472

Preface

Human names embellish the terminology of every science and art, identifying man's major discoveries, inventions, and creations, and perpetuating the fame of the pioneers who advance civilization's frontiers. Newton's laws, the Strait of Magellan, Mount Everest, the Ferris wheel, Hudson Bay, the Monroe Doctrine, Halley's comet, the Geiger counter, Malthus' theory, the Eiffel Tower—these and countless other eponymic terms have become part and parcel of our language.

In some of the biologic sciences, notably botany and bacteriology, eponyms are accepted as indispensable to nomenclature. The use of proper names in anatomy, on the other hand, has long been disputed. The commission of experts who compiled the *Basle Nomina Anatomica* in 1895, unable to agree on the acceptability of eponyms in standard anatomic terms, compromised by allowing their retention in brackets after the objective Latin names. The fate of proper names in anatomic terminology was to be decided by time and general usage. Despite the resolute resistance of some authorities, the eponymic forms for many anatomic structures, such as eustachian tube, Glisson's capsule, and circle of Willis, have become too deeply entrenched to permit uprooting by fiat. Clinical medicine likewise boasts a rich and colorful vocabulary of eponymics, shunned by some but constantly growing, nonetheless, as the contributions to medicine continue. Behind each of these terms lies a story, the narration of which is the history of medicine.

This volume tells the stories, some for the first time, others long forgotten, behind the eponymic nomenclature of obstetrics and gynecology. In a sense, therefore, it is a record of the specialty's development. It differs from the usual history, however, in being written by and for the practicing obstetrician and gynecologist, whose primary interest lies in specific diseases, instruments, and techniques. I have sought to provide the background for recent and current clinical practices and terminology, and to point out the paths that have led to the obstetrics and gynecology of the mid-twentieth century. Knowledge of these paths cannot fail to increase our appreciation of our tremendous scientific heritage. It may also spare us the needless retracing of steps, if we are to believe with Santayana that "he who is disposed to ignore history must be prepared to repeat it."

The chapters are separate essays, independent of one another. They have been grouped into what has seemed the most logical of several possible arrangements; still a certain overlap proved unavoidable because a few chapters encompass more than one topic. Treatment of each has included a description of related earlier work, excerpts from original sources, biographic sketches, portraits, and original illustrations. Gathered from the four corners of the earth, this material has never before been collected in one volume or even under one roof. Some of the biographic data and a number of portraits, obtained from surviving relatives and other private sources, have never been published before. Included are many of the classic contributions to the literature of obstetrics and gynecology—dealing with the female anatomic parts; clinical signs, tests, and rules; physiologic phenomena; bacteria of gynecologic significance; ovarian tumors; syndromes; positions; obstetric and gynecologic instruments; and operations and therapeutic procedures. A high degree of selection has been necessary, however, to keep this work within the bounds of one volume, for the eponymically named instruments alone are almost without number.

In Trevelyan's essay on Clio, the muse of history, we are reminded that "only the documents can tell us the truth." The original authors have therefore been allowed to speak for themselves through extensive quotations from their own writings, many of which are herein translated into English for the first time. Some of the Latin works have never before been translated into any modern language. In the translations I have enjoyed the valuable assistance of Mrs. Marion Slain for the Latin, Dr. Mario Petrini for the Italian, and Miss Kira Kalichevsky for the Russian. I have held myself completely accountable, however, for the accuracy of all the translations, as well as for their style and wording, trying always to avoid the pitfall pointed out by the French wag who compared translations with women: "Lorsqu'elles sont belles, elles ne sont pas fidèles."

Special thanks are due Miss Kalichevsky and Mrs. Emilienne Lopat of the Columbia University Medical Library for their bibliographic assistance; to my wife, Kathryn H. Speert, for deciphering my notes, typing the manuscript, and offering many helpful suggestions; and to Miss Joan C. Zulch of The Macmillan Company, for supervising the countless editorial details involved in transforming a manuscript into a book. Permission to reproduce my essays previously published—in *The American Journal of Clinical Pathology;* the *Bulletin of the Sloane Hospital for Women; Cancer; Fertility and Sterility; The Journal of the Mount Sinai Hospital; The Journal of Obstetrics and Gynaecology of the British Empire; Medical History; Obstetrics and Gynecology;* and *Surgery, Gynecology and Obstetrics*—is gratefully acknowledged. I record with deep appreciation my gratitude to Professor Howard C. Taylor, Jr., for his encouragement in these studies and for the support provided by the Department of Obstetrics and Gynecology of Columbia University.

September, 1958

Harold Speert

Contents

PART III. *Phenomena of Pregnancy and Labor*

PART IV. *Bacteria*

PART V. *Ovarian Tumors*

PART VI. *Syndromes*

PART VII. *Positions*

PART VIII. *Instruments*

CONTENTS

PART IX. *Operations and Therapeutic Procedures*

Anatomic Parts,
Landmarks, and
Measurements

PART I

Gabriele Falloppio and the Fallopian Tubes*

The uterine tubes, or oviducts, are inseparably linked with one of the most famous of all medical eponyms. The term *fallopian tube* has been incorporated into the nontechnical vocabulary of practically all modern languages; and in medical and anatomic literature it is usually spelled with a small *f*, the acme of eponymic acceptance.

The writings of Galen suggest that the uterine tubes were known to Herophilus (335–280 B.C.),[9] † but none of the latter's works remain extant. Ruphus of Ephesus, of later date (end of the first century A.D.), described briefly the oviducts of the ewe, picturing them as varicose and tortuous vessels passing from the testes, as the ovaries were then called, to the cavity of the uterus, and comparing them to the spermatic ducts. Ruphus also noted the presence of the tubes in women but made no reference to their function and seems to have regarded the tubes, like the round ligaments, as suspensory structures.[12]

THE DARK AGES OF ANATOMY

Very little advance in anatomic knowledge was made between the second and sixteenth centuries, for corpses for dissection were hard to obtain and the conditions for anatomic dissection and demonstration were rigidly prescribed by the civil authorities. In Bologna it was the students' responsibility

---

* This chapter originally published in *Obst. & Gynec.*, 6:467–70, 1955; reprinted by permission. Copyright © 1955, by the American Academy of Obstetrics and Gynecology.

† Superscript numbers indicate references at the end of each chapter.

3

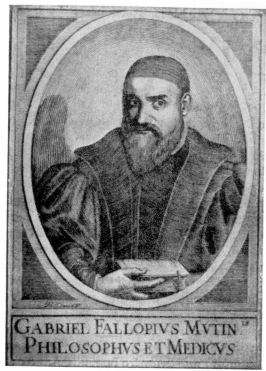

Fig. 1-1. Gabriele Falloppio (1523[?]–1562).

both to procure the cadavers and to stand the expense of the demonstrations, until 1442, when the city assumed this burden. Even then, however, only the bodies of executed criminals who had been born at least 30 miles distant could be used.[6] As a result, only one or two dissections were performed each year, and dissections of female cadavers were very rare. There is little, if any, evidence to support the commonly stated charge that dissection of the human body was prohibited in Italy by religious prejudice.[1] On the rare occasions when dissections were carried out in conjunction with courses in anatomy at the universities, the professor read aloud from Galen, whose authority remained beyond question, while assistants performed the dissections. For 1500 years the grossest errors were thus perpetuated, until the anatomic renaissance ushered in by the famous quintet of the sixteenth century: Sylvius, Vesalius, Fabricius, Eustachius, and Gabriele Falloppio.[4]

FALLOPPIO'S DESCRIPTION OF THE OVIDUCT

The first accurate description of the human oviduct was made by Falloppio in his *Observationes Anatomicae* (Fig. 1-3), published in Venice in 1561. In this work he called the tube the *uteri tuba,* or trumpet of the uterus: [7]

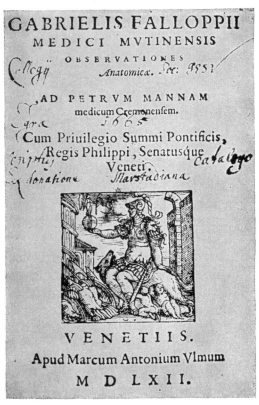

Fig. 1-2. Title page of *Observationes Anatomicae* (second printing, 1562).

That slender and narrow seminal duct rises, fibrous and pale, from the horns of the uterus itself; becomes, when it has gone a little bit away, appreciably broader, and curls like a branch until it comes near the end, then losing the horn-like curl, and becomes very broad, has a distinct extremity which appears fibrous and fleshy through its red color, and its end is torn and ragged like the fringe of well-worn garments, and it has a wide orifice which lies always closed through the ends of the fringe falling together; and if these be carefully separated and opened out, they resemble the orifice of a brass trumpet. Wherefore since the seminal duct from its beginning to its end has a likeness to the bent-parts of this classic instrument, separate or attached, therefore it has been called by me the Uteri Tuba. These are present not only in the human body, but also in the sheep, cows and all other animals which I have dissected.*

It was not long before the oviducts became known universally as the fallopian tubes.

* From: *Eternal Eve. The History of Gynaecology and Obstetrics* by H. Graham, reprinted by permission of Doubleday & Co., Inc., New York, and William Heinemann, Ltd., London.

Meatus ueró iſte ſeminarius gra-
cilis & anguſtus admodum oritur
nerueus ac candidus à cornu ipſius
uteri, cumque parum recefferit ab
eo latior ſenſim redditur, & capreo
li modo criſpat ſe donec ueniat pro
pè finem, tunc dimiſſis capreolari-
bus rugis, atque ualde latus reditus
finit in extremum quodam, quod
membranoſum carneumque ob co
lorem rubrum videtur, extremum-
que lacerum ualde & attritum eſt,
ueluti ſunt pannorum attritorum
fimbriæ, & foramen amplum habet,
quod ſemper clauſum iacet conci-
detibus fimbriis illis extremis, quæ
tamen ſi diligenter aperiantur, ac di
latentur tubæ cuiuſdam æneæ extre
mum orificium exprimunt. Quare
cum huius claſſici organi demptis
capreolis, uel etiam iiſdem additis
meatus ſeminarius à principio uſq;
ad extremum ſpeciem gerat, ideò à
me uteri tuba uocatus eſt. Ita ſe hæc
habent in omnibus non ſolùm hu-
manis, ſed etiam ouinis, ac uacinis
cadaueribus, reliquiſque brutorum
omnium, quæ ego ſecui.

Fig. 1-3. Excerpt from Falloppio's description of the human oviduct. From *Observationes Anatomicae.*

FALLOPPIO'S LIFE AND WORK

Gabriele Falloppio, descended from a noble Italian family,* was born in Modena, Italy, about 1523, there being some question as to his precise date of birth, certain historians giving a date 33 years earlier.[5]

* The origin of the family name is shown in its coat of arms, which contains three *falloppe,* or imperfect silk cocoons. The original Italian spelling of the name was probably *Falloppia;* the Latin, *Fallopius* or *Falloppius.* It has since been written in several other forms: *Falloppio, Fallopio,* and *Faloppio.*[3]

Before he undertook the study of medicine, Falloppio held an ecclesiastic appointment in the cathedral of his native town,[2] but the details of his early life remain unknown.

He later studied medicine at Ferrara, under Antonio Musa Brasarola, and soon achieved renown as a surgeon. As a pupil of Vesalius, some of whose erroneous views he subsequently corrected, Falloppio attained, through his anatomic discoveries, the most illustrious name in Italian medicine. In 1548 he was appointed professor of anatomy at the University of Pisa, at the instance of Cosimo I de' Medici, the Grand Duke of Tuscany, but relinquished this post three years later in response to a call by the Senate of Venice to the chair of surgery, anatomy, and botany at Padua, where he succeeded Vesalius and Realdus Columbus. Here Falloppio remained, conducting his most important researches, until his death from pleurisy, October 9, 1562. An attempt was thereupon made by the Venetian Senate to recall Vesalius from his pilgrimage to the Holy Land to the chair he had previously held at Padua. His return voyage was rough and prolonged, however, resulting finally in shipwreck on the desolate island of Zante, where Vesalius is believed to have died of typhus in October, 1564.[8] The chair at Padua was then filled by Falloppio's favorite pupil, Fabricius ab Aquapendente.

The collected works of Falloppio, published in Venice in 1606 in three folio volumes, embrace 24 treatises containing a total of more than 1500 pages. Because of the variations in style, however, some authorities maintain that these works, with the exception of the *Observationes Anatomicae,* were not published from Falloppio's manuscripts, but rather from the notes of the students who attended his lectures.

Although best known for the uterine tubes, with which his name has since been associated, Falloppio made many other important contributions to the knowledge of anatomy. He gave the first precise description of the clitoris, the skeletal system of the fetus, and the epiphyses of the long bones; introduced the anatomic use of the word *vagina,* and was the first to use the word *luteum* in describing the ovary.[11] Falloppio is credited by some historians with having originated the name *placenta,* but this term also appears in the writing of Realdus Columbus, and there is some question as to who actually invented it. Falloppio first described the villi conniventes of the small intestine, the ileocecal valve, and the inguinal ligament, later erroneously named after Poupart. He introduced the terms *hard* and *soft palate,* and first described the muscles of the latter. His description of the ear was more minute than any previously published, calling attention for the first time to the semicircular canals, the chorda tympani, the fenestrae rotunda and ovalis, and the communication of the mastoid cells with the tympanic cavity. He was also the first to describe the ethmoid and sphenoid bones; the trigeminal, auditory, and glossopharyngeal nerves; and the canal (which bears his name) for the facial nerve.[10]

In addition to his anatomic researches, Falloppio maintained an active interest in horticulture and for several years served as superintendent of the botanical gardens at Padua, in recognition of which a genus of plants (*Fallopia*) was named after him. Little wonder that he has been referred to as the "Aesculapius of his century." [13]

REFERENCES

1. Alston, M. N.: The attitude of the Church toward dissection before 1500. *Bull. Hist. Med.,* **16**:221–38, 1944.

2. Baily, H., and Bishop, W. J.: *Notable Names in Medicine and Surgery.* H. K. Lewis & Co., Ltd., London, 1946.

3. Castiglioni, A.: Fallopius and Vesalius. In Cushing, H.: *A Bio-Bibliography of Andreas Vesalius.* Henry Schuman, Inc., New York, 1943, p. 182.

4. Effler, L. R.: *The Eponyms of Anatomy.* McManus-Troup Co., Toledo, Ohio, 1935, p. 93.

5. Fisher, G. J.: Historical and biographical notes: V. Gabriello Fallopio, 1523–1562. *Ann. Anat. & Surg. Soc.,* **2**:200–204, 1880.

6. Gnudi, M. T., and Webster, J. P.: *The Life and Times of Gaspare Tagliacozzi.* Herbert Reichner, New York, 1950, pp. 59–60.

7. Graham, H.: *Eternal Eve. The History of Gynaecology and Obstetrics.* Doubleday & Co., Inc., New York, 1951, pp. 160–61.

8. Leonardo, R. A.: *A History of Gynecology.* Froben Press, Inc., New York, 1944, pp. 191–93.

9. Marx, K. F. H.: *Herophilus: Ein Beitrag zur Geschichte der Medicin.* Carlsruhe & Baden, 1838, p. 31.

10. Mettler, C. C., and Mettler, F. A.: *History of Medicine.* Blakiston Co., Philadelphia, 1947, pp. 46–47.

11. Ricci, J. V.: *The Genealogy of Gynaecology.* Blakiston Co., Philadelphia, 1943.

12. Ruphus of Ephesus: *Oeuvres de Ruphus d'Éphèse.* Ed. by C. Daremberg and C. Emile Ruelle. Paris, 1879.

13. Sampson, J. A.: Little biographies: VII. Fallopius, 1523–1563. *Albany M. Ann.,* **27**:496–98, 1906.

Reinier de Graaf and the Graafian Follicles *

The *graafian follicle*, like *fallopian tube*, belongs to that select group of eponymics which, through long usage and universal acceptance, are no longer capitalized in spelling. The story of the graafian follicle comprises an exciting chapter in man's long search for the mammalian egg, an effort that engaged his attention for two millennia. The high lights of this search have been narrated with charm and authority by George Corner in one of his delightful essays on the history of medicine.[2]

According to the views of Aristotle, long accepted by succeeding generations, the mammalian egg was formed in the uterus as the result of activation of the menstrual blood by the male semen. This theory was seriously disputed for the first time by Galen, who thought that the female semen, like the male semen, was made in the blood vessels supplying the gonad, in which organ the semen was strained and purified. The semen elaborated by the ovary, according to Galen, was then transmitted via the tubes to the uterus, where admixture with the male semen produced a coagulum from which the embryo evolved.

The presence of vesicles in the female testes was mentioned in the sixteenth-century writings of Vesalius and his disciple, Falloppio, but these Paduan anatomists had no thought of the true function of the fluid-filled structures. Falloppio's successor, Fabricius ab Aquapendente, described the

* This chapter originally published in *Obst. & Gynec.*, **7**:582–88, 1956; reprinted by permission. Copyright © 1956, by the American Academy of Obstetrics and Gynecology.

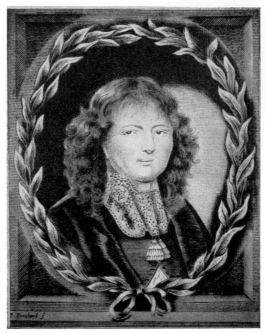

Fig. 2-1. Reinier de Graaf (1641–1673).

hen's ovary and even gave it the name *ovarium,* recognizing it as the organ of egg formation. But so strongly entrenched was the Aristotelian teaching that the egg was formed in the uterus that Fabricius naturally believed the ovary to be simply a part of the brood chamber. According to La Torre, Gian Matteo de Gradi of Milan, also known as Ferrari d'Agrate (died 1480), had long before applied the name *ovary* to the female testis and, by analogy with the hen, assumed its egg-producing function in other species.[5]

OVARIAN FUNCTION OF THE FEMALE TESTIS

The latter part of the seventeenth century witnessed a resurgence of the idea that the mammalian female testes, like the ovaries of birds, are the site of egg formation. Swammerdam and Van Horne, working together in Leyden in 1666, and the Danish anatomist Stensen in 1667, independently developed this theory in relation to the human and exchanged letters concerning their views. Stensen, "for friendship's sake," acceded to Swammerdam's brazen request that he and Van Horne be permitted to publish a proposed book on the subject, in preparation by Van Horne, before Stensen; but Van Horne never completed it and died in 1670, the book remaining unpublished.

Two years later there appeared a brilliant volume by Reinier de Graaf, his third, entitled *De Mulierum Organis Generationi Inservientibus* (Figs.

2-2, 2-3), Chapter XII of which was devoted to the female testes.[4] Here, with due credit to Van Horne, de Graaf advanced the evidence that this organ is indeed an ovary and in it he described the follicles which have ever since been associated with his name.

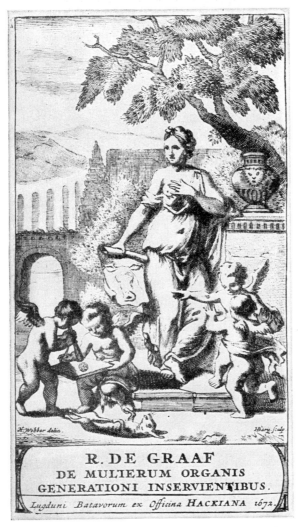

R. DE GRAAF
DE MULIERUM ORGANIS
GENERATIONI INSERVIENTIBUS.
Lugduni Batavorum ex Officina HACKIANA *1672.*

Fig. 2-2. Frontispiece from *De Mulierum Organis.*

After describing the gross morphologic characteristics and anatomic relations of the female testes and contrasting them with the male, de Graaf proceeded to the internal structure of the organ, illustrating the chapter with drawings of the bisected ovaries of the cow, sheep, and human (Fig. 2-4). Of the follicles, he wrote:

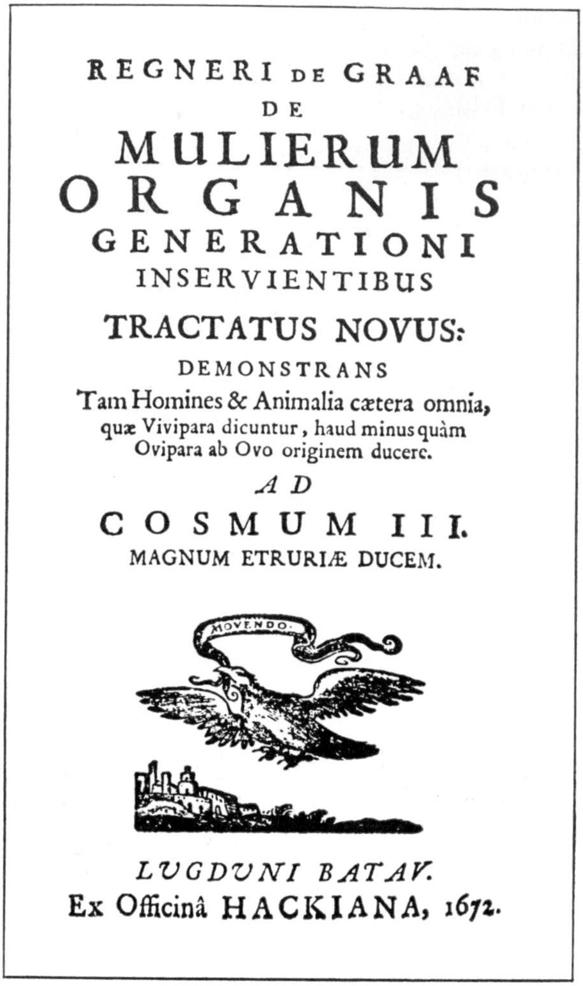

REGNERI DE GRAAF
DE
MULIERUM
ORGANIS
GENERATIONI
INSERVIENTIBUS

TRACTATUS NOVUS:
DEMONSTRANS
Tam Homines & Animalia cætera omnia,
quæ Vivipara dicuntur, haud minus quàm
Ovipara ab Ovo originem ducere.

AD
COSMUM III.
MAGNUM ETRURIÆ DUCEM.

LVGDVNI BATAV.
Ex Officinâ HACKIANA, 1672.

Fig. 2-3. Title page of *De Mulierum Organis.*

The normal structures, regularly found in the membranous substance of the testicles just described, are vesicles full of liquor, nerves, and nutritive vessels, which run to the testes in almost the same way as in males . . . and course throughout the whole of their substance, and enter the vesicles, within whose tunics many branches end after free division, in just the same way as we have seen happening in the ovaries of fowls composed of clustered egg yolks. . . .

These vesicles have been described under various names by Vesalius, Fallopius . . . and others, whose accounts it would be too tedious to repeat here in full. . . . Some call these vesicles hydatids, but the celebrated Dr. Van Horne in his *Prodromum* preferred to call them *ova,* a term which, since it seems to me more convenient than the others, we shall in the future use, and we shall call these vesicles *ova* as does that distinguished man, on account of the exact similitude which they exhibit to the eggs contained in the ovaries of birds; for these, while

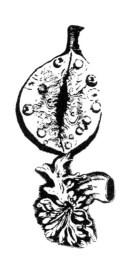

Zaɟ. **XVI**

192 REGNERUS DE GRAAF

TABULA DECIMA-SEXTA

Exhibet Tefticulum feu Ovarium
Mulieris cum annexo Tubarum
extremo.

A. *Tefticulus fecundùm longitudinem in infe-
riori parte apertus.*
BB. *Ova diverfæ magnitudinis in membranofâ
Teftium fubftantiâ contenta.*
CC. *Vafa fanguinea in medio Teftium ab ejus
fuperiori parte copiosè provenientia,
prout ad Ova excurrunt.*
DD. *Ligamentum Tefticulorum, quo Utero anne-
ctuntur, abfciffum.*
E. *Tubæ Fallopianæ pars abfciffa.*
F. *Tubæ abfciffæ cavitas.*
GG. *Foramen in extremo Tubarum exiftens.*
H. *Foliaceum Tubarum ornamentum.*
I. *Foliaceum Tubarum ornamentum Teftibus
annexum.*

Fig. 2-4.   Illustration of bisected human ovary from *De Mulierum Organis.*

they are still small, contain nothing but a thin liquor like albumen. That albumen
is actually contained in the ova of women will be beautifully demonstrated if
the ova are boiled, for the liquor contained in the ova of the testicles acquires
upon cooking the same color, the same taste and consistence as the albumen
contained in the eggs of birds.

It is of no importance that the ova of women are not, like those of fowls,
enveloped in a hard shell, for the latter are incubated outside the body in order
to hatch the chickens, but the former remain within the female body during
development, and are protected as thoroughly from all external injuries by the
uterus as by a shell. . . .

These ova arise and are developed in the testes in exactly the same way as the
eggs in the ovaries of birds, inasmuch as the blood flowing to the testes through
the nutritive arteries deposits in their membranous substance materials suitable
for the formation and nourishment of the ova, and the residual humors are carried
back to the heart through the nutritive veins or lymphatic vessels. . . .

Thus, the general function of the female testicles is to generate the ova, to
nourish them, and to bring them to maturity, so that they serve the same purpose
in women as the ovaries of birds. Hence, they should rather be called ovaries than
testes because they show no similarity, either in form or contents, with the male
testes. . . .*

* Excerpts from the English translation of Chapter XII of *De Mulierum Organis*
by G. W. Corner.[3] An earlier English translation, by R. Knox, is to be found in *The
British Record of Obstetric Medicine and Surgery,* Vol. I, 1848.

De Graaf's great mistake, now obvious, but one which can scarcely fail to arouse our sympathy as a natural conclusion in a premicroscopic era, was his assumption that the entire follicle was the ovum. We can only surmise how many troubled hours he must have spent in an unsuccessful effort to reconcile this concept with his observations on early rabbit embryos. Examining the contents of the doe's genital tract at different time intervals after mating, he recovered nothing in animals killed during the first two days; on the third day after coitus he found only tiny spherical masses in the fallopian tubes, and only slightly larger spheres in the uterus on the following day. De Graaf had unwittingly made the first discovery of tubal ova and supplied the potential, crucial evidence that the embryo begins to develop before reaching the uterus.

Only a few weeks after the publication of de Graaf's book the irate Swammerdam, whose priority of publication had been thwarted by the procrastination of his erstwhile collaborator, Van Horne, issued a bitterly worded pamphlet impugning de Graaf's personal integrity as well as the scientific accuracy of his observations and claiming for himself the credit for discovery of the ovarian function of the female testis. Diemerbroeck, professor of anatomy at Utrecht, who knew both contestants, remarked that Swammerdam had "smeared the ovary, not with honey, but with the bitterest gall." Swammerdam had made his bid too late; and de Graaf was rewarded with eponymic immortality.

More original than his thoughts concerning the ovarian follicles were de Graaf's observations on the corpus luteum, of which he gave the first detailed description, calling it the *substantia glandulosa*. He believed that each egg (follicle) was surrounded by this glandular substance which, as it ripened and moved toward the surface of the ovary, forced the egg out. His erroneous assumption that the presence of a corpus luteum implies impregnation was doubtless based on his study of rabbits, in which species ovulation normally occurs only after coital stimulation. He wrote:

These structures [corpora lutea] which, though normal, are only at certain times found in the testes of women, are globular bodies in the form of conglomerate glandulae which are composed of many particles, extending from the center to the circumference in straight rows, and are enveloped by a special membrane. We assert that these globules do not exist at all times in the testicles of females; on the contrary, they are only detected in them after coitus, [being one] or more in number, according as the animal brings forth one or more foetuses from that congress. Nor are these always of the same nature in all animals, or in the same kind of animal; for in cows they exhibit a yellow color, in sheep red, in others ashen; because a few days after coitus they are composed of a thinner substance and contain in their interior a limpid liquor enclosed in a membrane, which when ejected with the membrane leaves only a small space within the body which gradually disappears, so that in the latter months of gestation they seem to be composed of a solid substance; but when the foetus is delivered these globular bodies again diminish and finally disappear.

De Graaf and his contemporary scientific world thought that the mammalian ovum and its ovarian origin had been demonstrated; yet a century and a half later, in 1821, a contest was sponsored by the Göttingen Academy of Sciences offering a prize for the discovery of its site of formation. The prize was awarded, three years later, to the author of a paper proving that the ovum is formed in the uterus!

The search for the mammalian ovum concluded about the first of May, 1827. Karl Ernst von Baer, studying the embryology of the dog, had departed slightly from the usual procedure of examining the embryos in sequential stages of development and was working backward instead, taking the later stages first. After he had studied the free blastocysts in the fallopian tubes, as others had done before him in other species, he stated: [1]

The next step was to learn the state of the ova in the ovary, for it is very clear that such minute eggs cannot be the graafian follicles themselves expelled from the ovary, nor does it seem likely that such solid corpuscles as we find the tubal ova to be are formed by coagulation of the follicular fluid. Examining the ovaries before making any incision I saw plainly in almost every follicle a yellowish-white point. . . . Led by curiosity rather than by any thought that I had seen the ovules in the ovaries through all the layers of the graafian follicle, I opened one of the follicles and took up the minute object on the point of my knife, finding that I could see it very distinctly and that it was surrounded by mucus. When I placed it under the microscope I was utterly astonished, for I saw an ovule just as I had already seen them in the tubes, and so clearly that a blind man could hardly deny it. It is truly wonderful and surprising to be able to demonstrate to the eye, by so simple a procedure, a thing which has been sought so persistently, and discussed *ad nauseam* in every textbook of physiology, as insoluble!

DE GRAAF'S LIFE

Reinier de Graaf * was born in Schoonhaven, Holland, July 30, 1641. After completing his early studies in Delft, he continued his training in France under de la Boë, then returned to Delft where he entered the private practice of medicine. When only 23 years old, and while still a student, he published his famous *De Natura et Usu Succi Pancreatici,* which reported his pancreatic-fistula experiments and established the digestive function of the pancreatic juice. He subsequently studied the functions of the bile by the same method. Four years later, in 1668, his *De Virorum Organis Generationi Inservientibus* appeared, dealing with the anatomy of the male genital organs and giving

* The first name is variously spelled *Regner, Regnier, Reinier,* and *Reijnier,* and on the title page of his publications, written in Latin, *Regnerus.*

especially good descriptions of the vasa deferentia and the spermatic tubules of the testicle.

It was his *De Mulierum Organis,* however, published in 1672, which achieved for de Graaf his greatest renown. This volume contains a full and remarkably accurate account of the female reproductive organs, including certain gynecologic disorders, and is beautifully illustrated with detailed drawings. In it he described the pelvic blood supply, the lymphatic system of the uterus, and the crura of the clitoris, in addition to the ovaries and their function. He also reported on prolapse, myoma, and closure of the fallopian tubes, illustrating the last condition with excellent drawings (Fig. 2-5), prob-

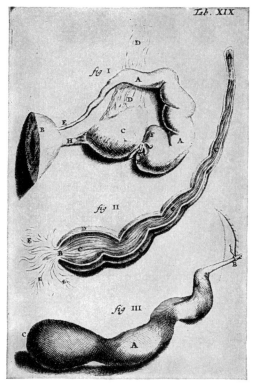

Fig. 2-5. Probably the first illustration of closure of the fallopian tubes. From *De Mulierum Organis.*

ably the first recorded of this common affliction, with the titles *Oviductus Extremum Testibus Naturam Agglutinatum* and *Oviductus Extremitas Praeter Naturam Clausa.* Gonorrhea was not mentioned by de Graaf as the cause of tubal closure, but he clearly recognized the para-urethral ducts as a focus of this disease.

De Graaf had been deeply aggrieved by Swammerdam's reckless and damaging charges against him; and although de Graaf published a pamphlet in his own defense which convincingly absolved him of all taint of plagiarism or dishonor, he continued to brood over the affair. Some believe that his continuing preoccupation with this unpleasant incident was a factor in his premature death on August 17, 1673, at the age of only 32 years.

REFERENCES

1. Baer, K. E. von: *De Ovi Mammalium et Hominis Genesi.* L. Voss, Leipzig, 1827.

2. Corner, G. W.: The discovery of the mammalian ovum. In *Lectures on the History of Medicine: A Series of Lectures at the Mayo Foundation, 1926–1932.* W. B. Saunders Co., Philadelphia, 1933, pp. 401–26.

3. Corner, G. W.: On the female testes or ovaries. By Regner de Graaf. In *Essays in Biology, in Honor of Herbert M. Evans.* University of California Press, Berkeley, 1943, pp. 121–37.

4. Graaf, R. de: *De Mulierum Organis Generationi Inservientibus.* Hackiana, Leyden, 1672.

5. Leonardo, R. A.: *History of Gynecology.* Froben Press, Inc., New York, 1944, p. 183.

Caspar Friedrich Wolff, Johann Christian Rosenmüller, Hermann Treschow Gartner, and the Mesonephric Remnants of the Female Genital Tract

The female genital tract, from the ovary to the hymen, contains a mine of embryonic remnants, vestiges of the primitive urogenital system, which produces a yield of never-ending interest to the clinical gynecologist as well as the student of embryology. The parovarium, epoophoron, or organ of Rosenmüller (residuum of the fetal mesonephros) lies between the leaves of the mesosalpinx, consisting of a series of small tubules, up to 20 in number and grouped in the general shape of a trapezoid, each tubule opening at one end into the common excretory duct of the mesonephros, the Wolffian duct of the fetus and Gartner's duct of the adult, the other end of each tubule ending blindly near the ovarian hilus. These tubular structures, homologues of the epididymis and vas deferens in the male, rarely undergo complete involution in the developing female fetus, leaving discontinuous, functionless rudiments from which parovarian, cervical, and vaginal cysts and tumors may develop in later life.

THE WOLFFIAN BODY AND DUCT

The elongated abdominal masses that comprise the mesonephros of the early vertebrate embryo were named the Wolffian bodies by the nineteenth-century embryologist Rathke, in recognition of Caspar Wolff's discovery of these primitive kidneys, reported in 1759 in his *Theoria Generationis*.[10] This work, published as Wolff's doctoral dissertation when he was only 26

18

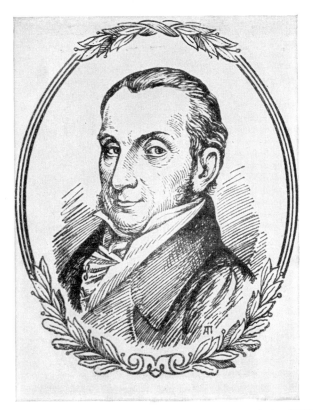

Fig. 3-1. Caspar Friedrich Wolff (1733–1794). (Courtesy of the USSR Ministry of Health.)

years old, is generally regarded as the introduction to modern embryology. Copies of the original have become exceedingly rare. The pages illustrated in Figures 3-2, 3-3, and 3-4 were reproduced from a copy graciously loaned by the Yale Historical Collection, from the library of the late Harvey Cushing.

Describing the development of the kidney in the chick embryo, Wolff wrote:

It is neither rare nor difficult to see embryos that show no trace of kidneys. . . . On the third or fourth day, in the regions between the extremities but somewhat cephalad, from which the cell substance had previously disappeared, there arises a new cell substance, which is somewhat tougher and bound together in little round masses and which partly joins together all the parts of the fetus, the head, heart, and extremities, with the dorsal spine, and thus provides a sort of fixed point, restraining the embryo itself in its expansion; but this cell substance, which is rather transparent and whose contents can easily be seen, still contains no trace of an organ.

On the fourth and fifth days this cell substance (*b, d*) proceeds caudad into the

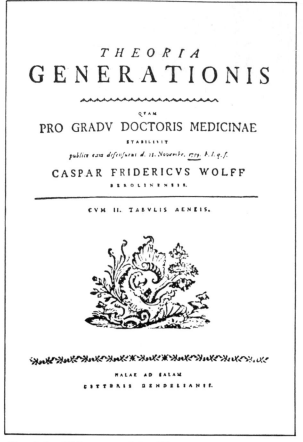

Fig. 3-2.   Title page of Wolff's *Theoria Generationis.*

region of the lower extremities and into the allantois (*e*), which is filled with a more transparent liquid, while cephalad, because of the extremities, the heart, and the head, it appears too opaque to permit sufficiently clear visualization of its contents. If one removes its covering with a knife, in order to expose its contents, he then discovers a homogeneous cell mass densely adherent to the anterior surface of the spinal column (*b*), occupying most of the space between the two lower extremities and with nothing present between them and the drawn-up tail (*d*).

After a few more days the abdomen of the embryo is closed (except for the large umbilicus). If it is made opaque with spirits of wine and then cut open, it reveals the stomach, hind-gut and cecum, identified by little nodules, and the duodenum, which connects with the stomach. The remaining delicate parts cannot yet be differentiated from the surrounding cell tissue, which becomes the mesentery. The rest of the abdominal cavity caudad, around the rectum and slightly above it, is filled by a remarkable and characteristic cell mass (*b.b.c.c.*) which demarcates a channel from the intestine, somewhat compressing the latter

§. 218.

Prima rudimenta. Fig.5. In perfectiori vero embryone tum in capite oculorum, cerebri, cerebelli, medullæ oblongatæ, tum in spina vertebrarum dorsalium delineationes (f) & lumbarium levissimæ (d) in conspectum prodeant; Et corpusculo ita efformato, excepto capite, circumflua levis deprehenditur substantia (c.c.c.) (quam, licet improprie, cellulosam vocavi,) aliqua globulorum cohæsione nisa, largissima circa extremitatem, inde adscendens utrinque, magis magisque coarctata, donec circa cordis & medullæ oblongatæ regionem evanescat, condensata magis proxime ad embryonem, indeque diffusa rarior.

§. 219.

Eorum ulterior elaboratio. Fig.9. Fig.11. Hæc deinceps coarctatur in substantiam solidiorem. æqualibem ubique & æque largam, & distinctioribus limitibus terminatam (b.b.). Tandem incipit restringi sensim sensimque omnis ad duo utrinque loca determinata, inferius nempe ad vertebras lumborum (r), & superius ad regionem cordis. Donec sic ab intermedia spinæ parte, vertebris dorsalibus (e), & reliquo extremitatis osse coccygis omnis cellulosa subtracta (Fig.11. g.g.) & in dictis locis in proubeantias (r.r.) coacta sit. Hæ proubeantiæ deinde in extremitates extendantur, harumque vera prima flamina exhibent, quæ falsæ a NALPIGHIO in forma crucis ad truncum delineata sunt, quippe ne sub ullo quidem perfectionis gradu ita apparent.

§. 220.

Historia eorum. Videre embryonem, qui renum nulla vestigia monstrat, non difficile est, neque rarum. Figuræ enim omnes hactenus citatæ tales offerunt. Die vero tertio vel quarto in illis regionibus, ubi extracta prior cellulosa fuit, inter extremitates nempe sed antrorsum nova talis cellulosa, paulo tenacior in globulorum cohæsione, suboritur, conglutinans quasi omnes sœtus partes, caput, cor & extremitates cum spina dorsali, tanquam puncto fixo, ipsiusque embryonem in suo sinu laterali detinens, absque tamen ullo viscerum rudimento, quippe diaphana satis est hæc cellulosa, & permittit, quæcunque continet, perspicere.

§. 221.

Fig.15. Die quarto & quinto hæc ipsa cellulosa (b.d.), inferius circa extre-

---

extremitatum inferiorum regionem in allantoidem (e) **Prima statum,** continuata, pellucidissimo liquido repletam, superius extremitates, & cor, & **mine.** caput complicans, nimis opaca, cujus contenta satis distincte perspiciantur, si caute removeatur ope cultelli, ut, quæ continet, appareant; Præter sui reliquias, cellulosam nempe mere confusam, spinæ anteriori faciei pertinaciter adhærentem (b), præfertim interstitia replentem inter duas extremitates inferiores, & inter has & caudam contractam (d), nihil plane offert.

§. 222.

Eorum augmentum. Fig.15. Post aliquot abhinc dies embryoni abdomen clausum est, (ex cepto peramplo umbilico) & ille, si spiritu vini opacus reddatur, dein secetur, monstrat ventriculum & intestinum rectum cum cæcis, tubercula referentibus, nec non duodenum, ventriculo appendicem. Reliqua tenuia a vinciente cellulosa, mesenterium exhibitura, nondum distingui possunt. Reliquum vero cavum abdominale inferius circa rectum, & paulo supra hoc ipsum, notabilis singularis massa cellulosæ (b.b.c.c.) confusa tamen, totum replet, reliquens pro intestino fossam, quasi ab hoc impressam (f), longitudinaliter per medium inferius abdomen decurrentem, terminatam circa infimam intestini partem, ubi cum hac utrinque cellulosa substantia decurrens connectitur, conspicuam, si intestinum removetur.

§. 223.

Deinceps sensim sensimque hæc cellulosa substantia, utrinque **Uterior elaboratio.** circa intestinum rectum posita, contrahit se in cumulos, aliquis par tibus magis separatos, deorsum in longas appendices, infimæ intestini parti innexas, excurrentes utrinque; deinde in glomeres, magis magisque minores (fig.16.) in relatione ad reliquas partes, sed adhuc inæquali villosa superficie gaudentes, tandem in corpuscula ovalia (fig. **Fig.16.** 17.), exacte determinata, polita superficie, & tenuibus filis, deorsum **Fig.17.** in intestinum decurrentibus, ornata.

§. 224.

Protuberantias (§. 219. fig. u. r.) extremitatem prima rudimenta. Extremitata, tubercula (§. cit. fig. 12. r.), levius a continuata cellulosa reliqua **tum modus** eminentia, illarum protuberantiarum incoeamenta, & cellulosam sub- **vegetatio-** stantiam, spinæ adversius circumposium (§. cit. fig. 9. b.), nec non **nis** latius

N

Fig. 3-3. Pages from Wolff's *Theoria Generationis* [10] describing the embryogenesis of the chick's kidney.

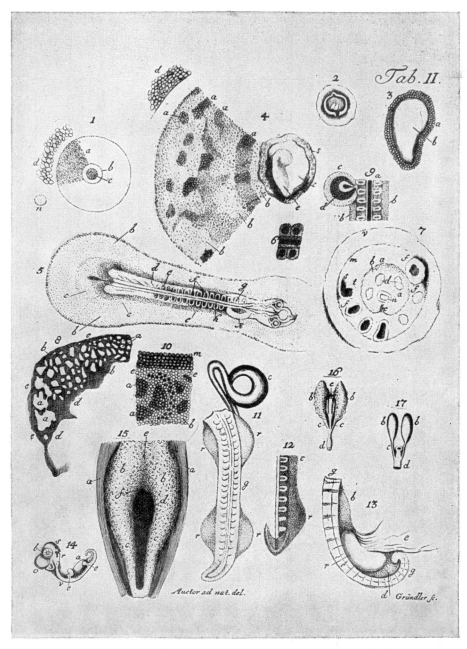

Fig. 3-4. Plate from Wolff's *Theoria Generationis* [10] containing his illustrations of the development of the kidney (*13, 15, 16, 17*).

(*f*); and extending longitudinally in the middle of the lower abdomen, it ends near the hindmost part of the intestine, where the cell masses on either side come together, as is readily seen if the intestine is removed.

This cell substance on either side of the hind-gut gradually collects into mounds which are more or less separate from the other parts and extend posteriorly in long appendages alongside the gut; on them small elevations are present, which become smaller and smaller (Fig. 16) in relation to the other parts but still result in an uneven, shaggy surface. Finally, small, sharply circumscribed, oval bodies (Fig. 17) arise, with a smooth surface, and supplied with filaments coursing from the kidneys back to the intestine.

Wolff summarized in a later paragraph:

The cell substance that first appears along the surface of the spine on the third day and proceeds into the allantois on the fourth and fifth days, represents the first material that is destined to be transformed later into the kidneys.

Thus was described, for the first time, the embryonic mesonephros, known also, since the early part of the nineteenth century, as the Wolffian body, its excretory duct as the Wolffian duct.

WOLFF'S LIFE

Caspar Friedrich Wolff was born in Berlin, Germany, in 1733, the son of a tailor.[5,7,9] He obtained his early scientific education in his native city, but in the midst of his medical studies transferred to Halle, where his famous essay on the theory of generation was published. Two years later, in 1761, Wolff received a teaching appointment in anatomy in Breslau, carrying out his duties there with such distinction that when he returned to Berlin at the conclusion of the Seven Years' War, in 1763, he encountered the immediate and unrestrained hostility of a large segment of the university faculty, who, it is said, feared for their own status. Failing to achieve a professorship in Berlin and smarting under the constant assault of his colleagues, Wolff forsook Berlin in 1769 for St. Petersburg, Russia, where he spent the rest of his life as a member of the academy. Religious opposition to his radical scientific views probably also played a part in Wolff's decision to leave Germany. It is interesting that Darwin's *Origin of Species,* published exactly 100 years after Wolff's *Theoria Generationis,* met with the same ecclesiastic attack.

In 1768 and 1769, at about the time of his departure from Berlin, Wolff published his work on the development of the chick's intestinal tract, *De Formatione Intestinorum,* referred to by the embryologist von Baer as "the greatest masterpiece of scientific observation." For many years, however, this important contribution lay dormant, virtually unnoticed until translated from the Latin into German by J. F. Meckel in 1812.

Practically all that is known of the remainder of Wolff's life is contained in a letter from his assistant, Mursinna, to Goethe, which was published in the latter's *Morphologie* in 1820. "He taught logic," according to Mursinna, "probably better than it had ever been taught before, and applied it in particular to medicine, thereby creating, so to speak, a new spirit in his hearers, so that they were enabled to understand and assimilate his other teachings more easily." Wolff died suddenly on March 6, 1794.

Embryogenesis in Wolff's time was explained by the theory of *emboîtement,* or preformation, which visualized the embryo as a miniature adult, invisible but completely formed within the ovary. According to this doctrine Eve's ovaries must have contained the compressed forms of all mankind, each generation encased within the gonads of the preceding, development of the individual consisting of a mere unshelling and growth. Not only was this theory of generation grievously in error but it guarded the secrets of embryology by discouraging investigation in the field. Harvey had questioned the theory of *emboîtement* earlier in the seventeenth century, espousing in its stead the doctrine of epigenesis—that the organism develops through the process of accretion, with gradual building up of its constituent parts—but Harvey's theoretic speculations failed to gain support until revised by Wolff. The latter's microscopic observations of growing plants and chick embryos convinced him of the fanciful nature of *emboîtement,* and most of his scientific efforts were henceforth directed at replacing this myth with the doctrine of epigenesis, his greatest contribution. He wrote:

The particles which constitute all animal organs in their earliest inception are little globules, which can always be distinguished under the microscope. . . . How, then, can it be maintained that a body is invisible because it is too small, when the *parts* of which it is composed are easily distinguishable?

Some insight into Wolff's personality may be gleaned from one of his letters, written in 1766 to the influential Haller, who continued to oppose the theory of epigenesis. Wrote Wolff:

I thank you for wishing me well, for loving me, sublime man, although you have never seen me, and know me and my character only from my letters. May God reward you for this, since I can never hope in all my life to attain to such distinction, that I may show you worthy acknowledgment of your goodness, if you will not receive in lieu of it my everlasting veneration of your intellect. And as to the matter of contention between us, I think thus: For me, no more than for you, glorious man, is truth of the very greatest concern. Whether it chance that organic bodies emerge from an invisible condition, or form themselves out of the air, there is no reason why I should wish that the one were truer than the other, or wish the one and not the other. And this is your view also, glorious man. We are investigating for truth only; *we seek that which is true.* Why then should I contend with you? Why should I withstand you, when you are pressing toward the

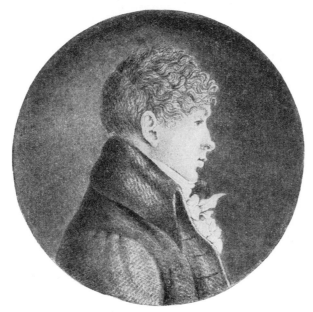

Fig. 3-5. Johann Christian Rosenmüller (1771–1820).

same goal as myself? I would rather confide my epigenesis to your protection, for you to defend and elaborate, if it is true; but if it is false, it shall be a detestable monster to me also. I will admire evolution, if it is true, and worship the adorable Author of Nature as a divinity past human comprehension; but if it is false, you too, even if I remain silent, will cast it from you without hesitation.

THE ORGAN OF ROSENMÜLLER

In the human the mesonephric remnant, or Wolffian body, was first described in 1802 by Johann Christian Rosenmüller, in a pamphlet of 12 pages [6] on the development of the fetal ovary. The vestigial tubules were well pictured in a fetus of 12 weeks. Rosenmüller wrote:

The ovaries are as in the fetus, except that they are somewhat larger and rounder. The form of the tubal fimbriae is much more complex. Seen between the ovary and tube are innumerable vessels, which branch from a stem behind the round ligament of the uterus and course toward the ovary between the peritoneal folds, having a relation to the tube similar to that of the mesenteric vessels to the intestine. For, connected to one another, they form an arc, and the veins accompany the arteries in the same duct.

Most noteworthy but hitherto unknown to me is the fact that the observed structure appeared conical in the cadavers of all the born fetuses I have seen. In an infant of 12 weeks I found that it consisted of many little canals, extensively convoluted at the base of the conical structure, these canals merging toward

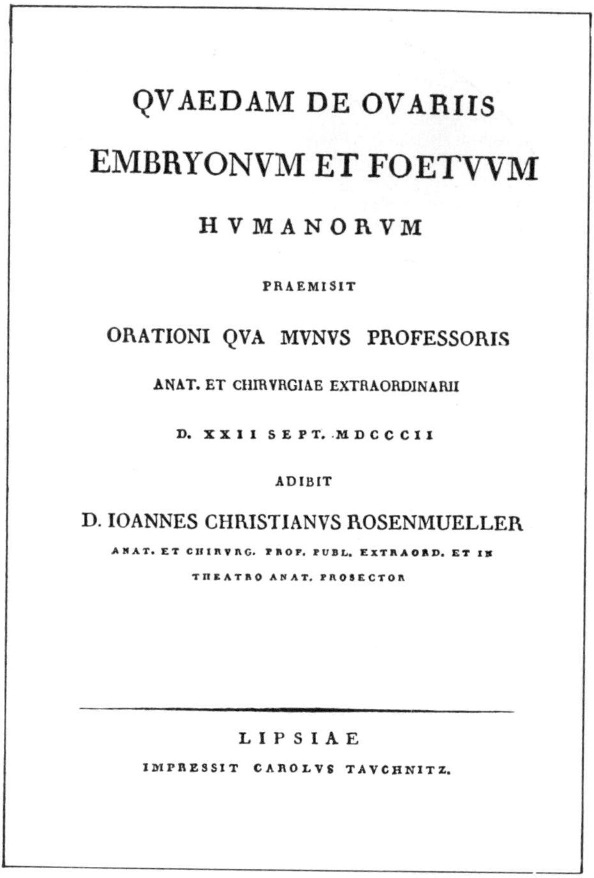

QVAEDAM DE OVARIIS

EMBRYONVM ET FOETVVM

H V M A N O R V M

PRAEMISIT

ORATIONI QVA MVNVS PROFESSORIS

ANAT. ET CHIRVRGIAE EXTRAORDINARII

D. XXII SEPT. MDCCCII

ADIBIT

D. IOANNES CHRISTIANVS ROSENMUELLER

ANAT. ET CHIRVRG. PROF. PVBL. EXTRAORD. ET IN

THEATRO ANAT. PROSECTOR

LIPSIAE

IMPRESSIT CAROLVS TAVCHNITZ.

Fig. 3-6. Title page of Rosenmüller's pamphlet in which the epoophoron is first described.

the upper extremity of the ovary where, after narrowing and coming closer together, they united and disappeared. I counted about 20 of these little canals. At first I took them to be lymphatic vessels, but when I examined them with an armed eye [lens] I was overjoyed by the most beautiful sight. For in addition to the very bright little canals already described, I observed, included among those running from the base of the conical body, other much thinner ducts, convoluted among themselves with a serpentine flexibility. Proceeding thus, they show the form of circles intimately joined together. Toward the ovary they become less curved and then disappear in straight lines. Indeed, the apex of the cone is actually attached to the ovary, but since the little canals and ducts in it are so very narrow, nothing can be seen, except in a certain small area in the fold of the peritoneum, which is at the end of the cone. I do not wish to state with certainty whether the similarity between this conical body and its duct [on the one hand] and the vas deferens and epididymis of the male body [on the other] arises by

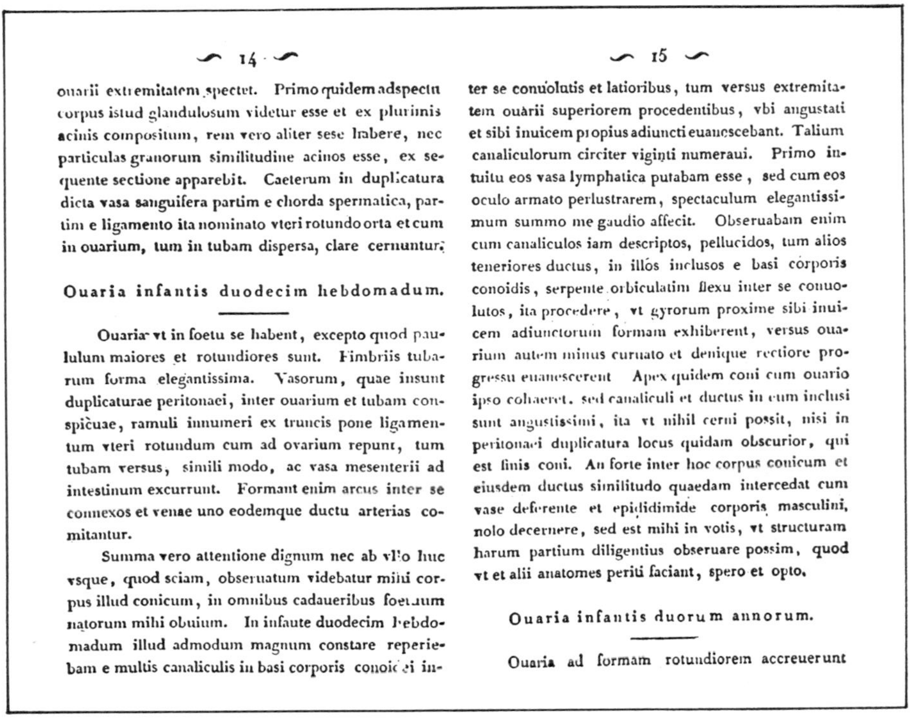

～ 14 ～

ouarii extremitatem spectet. Primo quidem adspectu corpus istud glandulosum videtur esse et ex plurimis acinis compositum, rem vero aliter sese habere, nec particulas granorum similitudine acinos esse, ex sequente sectione apparebit. Caeterum in duplicatura dicta vasa sanguifera partim e chorda spermatica, partim e ligamento ita nominato vteri rotundo orta et cum in ouarium, tum in tubam dispersa, clare cernuntur;

Ouaria infantis duodecim hebdomadum.

Ouaria vt in foetu se habent, excepto quod paululum maiores et rotundiores sunt. Fimbriis tubarum forma elegantissima. Vasorum, quae insunt duplicaturae peritonaei, inter ouarium et tubam conspicuae, ramuli innumeri ex truncis pone ligamentum vteri rotundum cum ad ovarium repunt, tum tubam versus, simili modo, ac vasa mesenterii ad intestinum excurrunt. Formant enim arcus inter se connexos et venae uno eodemque ductu arterias comitantur.

Summa vero attentione dignum nec ab vllo huc vsque, quod sciam, obseruatum videbatur mihi corpus illud conicum, in omnibus cadaueribus foetuum natorum mihi obuium. In infante duodecim hebdomadum illud admodum magnum constare reperiebam e multis canaliculis in basi corporis conoidei in-

～ 15 ～

ter se conuolutis et latioribus, tum versus extremitatem ouarii superiorem procedentibus, vbi angustati et sibi inuicem propius adiuncti euanescebant. Talium canaliculorum circiter viginti numeraui. Primo intuitu eos vasa lymphatica putabam esse, sed cum eos oculo armato perlustrarem, spectaculum elegantissimum summo me gaudio affecit. Obseruabam enim cum canaliculos iam descriptos, pellucidos, tum alios teneriores ductus, in illos inclusos e basi corporis conoidis, serpente orbiculatim flexu inter se conuolutos, ita procedere, vt gyrorum proxime sibi inuicem adiunctorum formam exhiberent, versus ouarium autem minus curuato et denique rectiore progressu euanescerent Apex quidem coni cum ouario ipso cohaeret, sed canaliculi et ductus in eum inclusi sunt angustissimi, ita vt nihil cerni possit, nisi in peritonaei duplicatura locus quidam obscurior, qui est finis coni. An forte inter hoc corpus conicum et eiusdem ductus similitudo quaedam intercedat cum vase deferente et epididimide corporis masculini, nolo decernere, sed est mihi in votis, vt structuram harum partium diligentius obseruare possim, quod vt et alii anatomes periti faciant, spero et opto.

Ouaria infantis duorum annorum.

Ouaria ad formam rotundiorem accreuerunt

Fig. 3-7. Rosenmüller's description[6] of the epoophoron in a human fetus of 12 weeks.

chance, but I hope and pray that I might be able to observe the structure of these parts more carefully than other experienced anatomists have been doing.

This "conical body" was soon to become known as *the organ of Rosenmüller.*

Subsequent anatomists suggested the names epoophoron and parovarium for the remnant of the Wolffian body in the female; and the individual tubules are often designated as the *tubules of Kobelt,* after George L. Kobelt, who described them in detail in 1847. Eponymic priority, however, belongs to Rosenmüller.

ROSENMÜLLER'S LIFE

Johann Christian Rosenmüller was born in Hessberg, Germany, May 25, 1771.[2,8] He entered the University of Leipzig in 1786, where he received his master's degree in 1792 and his doctorate five years later. In 1794 he was made prosector in anatomy; and from 1802 until his death, served as professor of anatomy and surgery. From 1804 to 1809 he also held the administrative position of *Physikus* in the university. He died on February 28, 1820. Rosenmüller is known primarily for his anatomic works, his principal con-

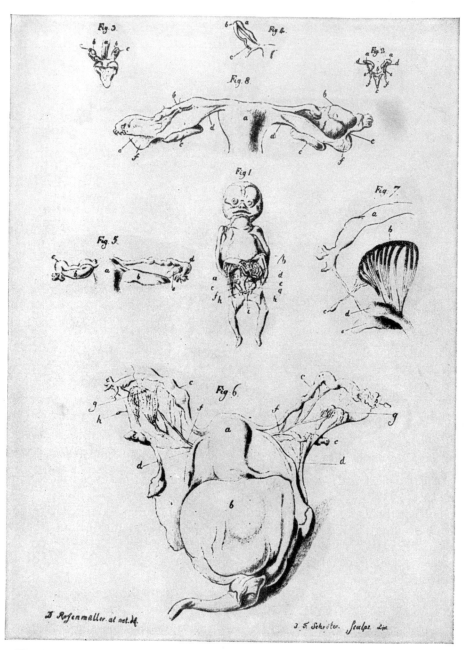

Fig. 3-8. Plate of illustrations from Rosenmüller's paper.[6] The epoophoron is shown in his Figures 6(*g*) and 7(*b*).

tributions comprising, in addition to his description of the fetal ovary, an anatomic study of the lacrimal apparatus, a handbook of anatomy, a surgical atlas profusely illustrated with colored plates, a monograph on the obturator nerve, and a number of papers on fossil bones. He is known particularly for his use of art in the teaching of anatomy. In addition to the epoophoron, Rosenmüller's name is also associated eponymically with the pharyngeal recess, or Rosenmüller's fossa, the lacrimal gland, and a lymph node in the femoral ring.

GARTNER'S DUCT

The mesonephric, or Wolffian, duct begins to involute in the female human fetus at about the 55-mm stage of development, ultimately becoming discontinuous, with long breaks intervening among the tubular remnants identifiable at birth. These vestiges lie along bilateral paths more or less parallel to the fallopian tube, within the leaves of the broad ligament, entering the substance of the cervix at the level of the internal os, continuing caudad just beneath the cervical mucosa and in the lateral wall of the vagina, and ending with a sharp turn into the hymen. Embryonic remains of the mesonephric duct have been reported in the cervix of up to 40 per cent of newborn infants and young children, and are readily recognized in fully 1 per cent of routine histologic sections of the adult cervix. The vestigial epithelium is distinguishable from that of the endocervix by the low cuboidal or flat character of the former and its failure to take the mucicarmine stain. It has been suggested that some adenocarcinomas of the cervix may take their origin in these remnants of the primitive urogenital duct.

This structure was probably recognized first in the calf, by Marcello Malpighi in 1681. Not until almost a century and a half later, however, was it illustrated and described in detail. In 1822 the Danish anatomist and physician Hermann Gartner [4] redirected attention to this delicate tube in the cow and described for the first time its homologue in the sow. It was immediately given the name of Gartner's duct, by which it is still known. For his discovery Gartner was awarded an honorary medal from the Royal Society of Sciences of Copenhagen. The following account is taken from an abstract of Gartner's publication, which appeared in the *Edinburgh Medical and Surgical Journal* in 1824:

The author was engaged in an investigation of the lymphatics on the uterus of the cow, when, by accident, he discovered a canal full of a clear, yellowish fluid. From its appearance, he was convinced that it was neither a blood-vessel nor absorbent; and upon cutting into it, he found that he could inflate it both above and below the opening. Upon further investigation, he found that traces of the canal could be seen to within an inch of the ovary, and that, on following it downwards, it opened beside the orifice of the urethra. Having experienced some difficulty in fully developing the organ in the cow, he proceeded to search for a similar part in the sow. Here his researches were immediately crowned with success. . . .

The first uterus which the author examined, was that of a sow three years old. Upon the paries of the vagina, which adjoins the bladder, the author felt a round, hard body, somewhat like an artery to the touch. This he opened and dissected upwards, and for some inches he found it to be a single canal. By degrees, however, it branched out into a body that had the appearance of a gland, and resembled very much the pancreas. After giving out branches to this body for about two inches, it became again a single canal, though very minute, and stretched towards the uterus, or rather cornu of the uterus, as the uterus of the sow is destitute of a body. In order to see how this duct opened into the vagina, the author injected quicksilver through a part of it, which he had left unopened, and which lay hid under the muscle of the bladder. The mercury passed into the vagina, and he perceived that the duct terminated in a small opening close beside the orifice of the urethra.

"I have," says the author, "examined many uteri, in a pregnant as well as unimpregnated state, and the uteri of those animals that have been deprived of their ovaries, and I have generally found the same result, namely, a canal which begins on each side of the place, where the vagina terminates in the cornu uteri, passes through a glandular body in the middle of the vagina, goes under the sphincter vesicae, and perforates the vagina close beside the orifice of the urethra."

A similar duct was found on the other side of the vagina which followed exactly the same course as the one above mentioned.

Dr. Gartner was sometimes able to trace the duct much further than is here described; he has even succeeded in following it to within an inch or two of the ovaries. In general, however, it could not be distinctly traced further than the place where the vagina terminates in the uterus. In these cases, however, small knobs or glands were seen in the tract of the duct.

The author contrived, though not without difficulty, to inject the whole canal with quicksilver.

"Before the canal is injected with mercury, it has a white and compact appearance, and seems to be about as thick as the barrel of a pen. When filled with mercury, it appears less compact, and becomes twice as large in diameter. Upon cutting into it, it has somewhat the appearance of a *vas deferens,* though not quite so compact in substance, or if I may use the expression, so cartilaginous."

The organ is much more complicated in the cow, and the author accordingly experienced greater difficulty in developing it. . . . As far as we have been able to discover from the description before us, assisted by the plates, the organ in the cow consists of three parts.

1. A duct on each side of the vagina, which, beginning by a small orifice near the mouth of the urethra, immediately expands into a *capitulum* or sac, large enough to admit the point of the finger. This part differs altogether in structure from the rest of the canal, for its inner surface is smooth and polished, and its outer is fibrous and somewhat muscular while the inner surface of the rest of the

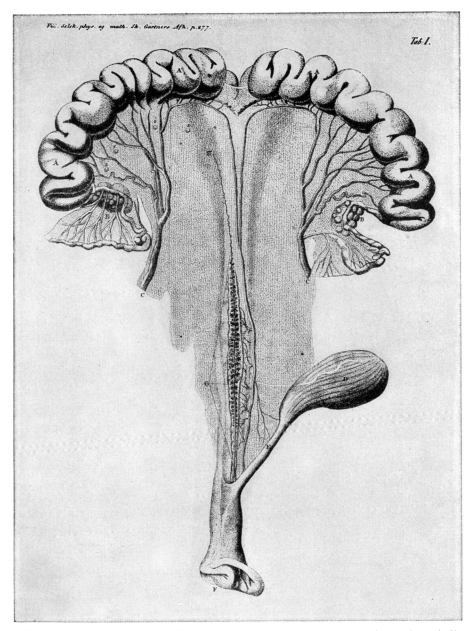

Fig. 3-9. Illustration from Gartner's paper,[4] showing the sow's internal genitalia with the mesonephric remains (*G, H*).

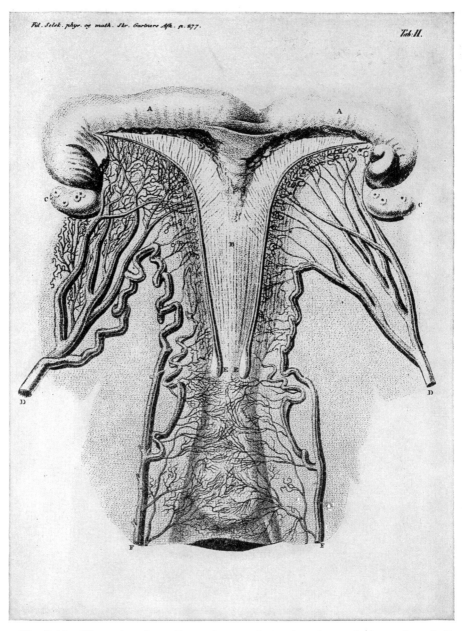

Fig. 3-10. Illustration from Gartner's paper,[4] showing the cow's internal genitalia (Gartner's ducts: *E, E*).

duct is composed of a mucous membrane, the outer consisting of the common cellular substance. From this part the canal runs on the paries of the vagina next the bladder, and terminates about an inch from the os uteri in a *cul de sac* which communicates by a valvular or cribriform opening, with the canal that begins at this part.

2. A number of follicles or cysts, on which numerous blood-vessels are ramified. These cells are generally full of a viscid fluid. Sometimes little glandular knobs are found mixed with them, and sometimes hydatids are found adhering. In a cow 16 years old, Dr. Gartner found on one side a canal of a spiral form, and on the other a number of cells, under and among which ran the duct. The cells were nearly as hard as cartilage, and large enough to admit the point of the finger.

3. Under and among the cells, a canal is observed, at first of a tortuous or spiral form, which, running along the neck of the uterus, follows the curve of its horn, upon which it extends to within an inch of the ovary. This canal in the cow is pervious, from its beginning, to the place where it turns towards the cornu uteri.

GARTNER'S LIFE

Hermann Treschow Gartner was born October 26, 1785, on the island of St. Thomas in the West Indies, where his father was employed as a governmental tax official.[1,3] When young Gartner was ten years old the family moved to Copenhagen, where he began his medical studies in 1803. In 1807 he was appointed intern in the Fredriks-Hospital and the following year received his certificate from the surgical academy. Following a year of service with the Norwegian Army and a medical administrative job in a rural community, Gartner resumed his medical studies for two years in London and Edinburgh. Returning to Copenhagen, he published his dissertation for his medical degree in 1815, based on studies of the surgical anatomy of inguinal and femoral hernias. Thereupon he settled down to practice. In 1824 he was made a surgeon to the Danish Army. Gartner died three years later, April 4, 1827. His grave is marked by a memorial stone in the Garnisons Kirkegaard in Copenhagen, but no portrait of Gartner is known.

REFERENCES

1. *Biographisches Lexikon der hervorragenden Ärzte aller Zeiten und Völker,* 2nd ed. Ed. by W. Haberling, F. Hübotter, and H. Vierordt. Urban & Schwarzenberg, Berlin & Vienna, 1930, Vol. 2, pp. 690–91; Supplement, 1935, p. 316.

2. *Biographisches Lexikon der hervorragenden Ärzte aller Zeiten und Völker,* 2nd ed. Ed. by W. Haberling, F. Hübotter, and H. Vierordt. Urban & Schwarzenberg, Berlin & Vienna, 1932, Vol. 4, pp. 880–81.

3. Erslew, T. H.: *Almindeligt Forfatter-Lexicon for Kongeriget Danmark med Tilhørende Bilande, fra 1814 til 1840.* Forlagsforeningens, Copenhagen, 1843, p. 488; Supplement 1, 1858, p. 546.

4. Gartner, H.: *Anatomisk Beskrivelse over et ved Nogle Dyr-Arters Uterus undersögt Glandulöst Organ. Det Kongelige Danske Videnskabernes Selskabs Naturvidenskabelige og Mathematiske Afhandlinger.* Förster Deel. Trykt I Hartv. Frid. Popps Bogtrykkerie, Copenhagen, 1824, pp. 277–317. Reprinted from an earlier publication in 1822. Abstract: An anatomical description of a glandular organ observed in the uterus of some of the lower animals. By H. Gartner, M.D., Military Surgeon, Member of the Royal Medical Societies of Copenhagen and Edinburgh. *Edinburgh M. & S. J.,* **21**:460–63; 1824.

5. Goethe, J. W.: *Sämmtliche Werke. Vollständige Ausgabe in zehn Bänden.* J. C. Cotta, Stuttgart, 1885, Vol. 9, pp. 374–78.

6. Rosenmueller, J. C.: *Quaedam de Ovariis Embryonum et Foetuum Humanorum.* C. Tauchnitz, Leipzig, 1802.

7. Samassa, P.: Caspar Friedrich Wolff's Leben und Werke. In Wolff, C. F.: *Theoria Generationis* (1759). Part 2. Translated into German by P. Samassa. Engelmann, Leipzig, 1896, pp. 96–98.

8. Wegner, R. N. von: *Das Anatomenbildnis. Seine Entwicklung im Zusammenhang mit der anatomischen Abbildung.* Schwabe, Basle, 1939, pp. 142–43.

9. Wheeler, W. M.: Caspar Friedrich Wolff and the *Theoria Generationis.* In *Biological Lectures from the Marine Biological Laboratory, Wood's Hole, Mass., 1898.* Ginn & Co., Boston, 1899, pp. 265–84.

10. Wolff, C. F.: *Theoria Generationis.* Hendel, Halle, 1759, pp. 96–97.

Johannes Müller and   CHAPTER

the Müllerian Ducts   4

The female genital tract is initially paired in all vertebrates. The varying extent of the subsequent fusion of the paired sexual ducts during their embryonic development results in the different forms of the uterovaginal canals that characterize the various species; errors in fusion, in some of the congenital malformations of the internal genitalia encountered in postnatal life. Intimately identified with the primitive paired sex tubes of the female is the name of Johannes Müller, not primarily because of his discoveries or original contributions to the subject, but because of the skill with which he synthesized the knowledge of his day and the new clarity and added meaning he succeeded in imparting to it. For more than a century the rudiments of the tubes and uterus have been known as the Müllerian ducts.

DESCRIPTION OF PARAMESONEPHRIC DUCTS

Müller's celebrated treatise on the embryology of the genitalia in verte-brates, his *Bildungsgeschichte der Genitalien* (1830),[3] encompassing his own observations as well as those of other distinguished embryologists, contained the clearest picture, to that time, of the development of the mammalian uterus. The following passage is characteristic of the skillful manner in which Müller wove his own observations together with those of his predecessors and contemporaries:

35

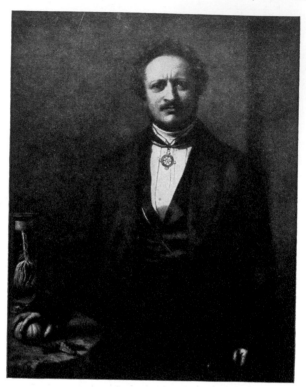

Fig. 4-1. Johannes Müller (1801–1858).

I have not actually seen evidence that the united, unpaired middle section [of the reproductive tract] is not yet present as an independent structure in the human, when the anlage of the tube is already present; but I have shown it in mammals, and Rathke noted the same in mammalian embryos. Both of these ducts empty quite separately into the common *sinus urogenitalis,* which leads below into the *fissura urogenitalis,* forward and above into the urachus. The middle unpaired part develops as the section of that common tube between the insertion site of both ducts is gradually drawn out, and elongates independently to the main part of both canals. This unpaired section, short at first but longer later, is however not itself the rudiment of the uterus, but the fundus of the uterus is formed in part from the lower part of the side ducts or tubes, as J. F. Meckel has very well shown.

In an embryo 1 inch long Meckel found no swelling yet that simulated the uterus at the site where both ducts or tubes united into a thin, unpaired, scarcely noticeable wider part; even less was there a difference between uterus and vagina. Distal to the short unpaired segment both ducts or tubes were still quite similar in their entire length. The boundary between uterus and tubes was only indicated by the insertion site of the round ligament, which was attached under the lower pole of the ovary to the duct, the lower part of which becomes the horn of the uterus, the upper part the tube. The lower part of this duct was shorter than the upper. Meckel concluded correctly from this that the human uterus is likewise two-horned at first, because the later insertion site of the round ligament is no longer the tubes but rather the upper part of the side wall of the uterus itself. There can be no objection to this view, which is proved by the approximation of the insertion sites of the round ligaments and the corresponding diminution in size of the horns, until their complete merging and disappearance in the fundus of the uterus. Meckel also found that the younger the embryo the longer the horns of the uterus and the more acute their angle of junction, the uterus being two-horned up until the end of the third month. At the end of the fourth month it widens out at its upper end for the first time as the horns, which are present originally, disappear, forming a single cavity. . . .

I actually see in a human fetus, which I have before me and which measures 3½ inches from crown to rump, the almost complete transition of the already shortened horns into a single fundus of the uterus. The fundus shows a shallow furrow in the middle, from either side of which a hornlike dilatation proceeds, and at the end of which the round ligament is attached . . . [Fig. 4-2].

In recording the special development of the lower end of the unpaired sexual duct and its adjacent structures, Müller was more than the descriptive morphologist; he was constantly seeking an embryologic interpretation of the

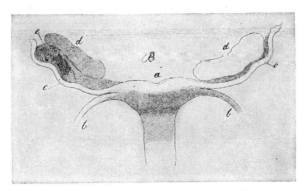

Fig. 4-2. Müller's drawing[3] of the internal genitalia of a 3½-in. human fetus, showing: *a,* uterus bicornis; *b,* round ligaments; *c,* tubes; *d,* ovaries; *e,* Wolffian body.

common malformations involving the distal ends of the genital tube, the urinary duct, and the intestinal canal. Wrote Müller:

That the allantois in the mammalian embryos is not originally separated from the end segment of the intestinal canal but instead flows into it as in the case of the birds, is an observation of Rathke. . . . The mammals thus possess originally a cloaca, the outer opening of which, as Tiedemann has also observed in the human embryo, is in the perineum and is common to the intestinal canal, the genitalia, and the urinary apparatus. According to Rathke, the side walls of the cloaca approximate each other and two longitudinal folds arise, later fusing into one and leading to a vaginal partition, which separates the anus from the other part of the tube. The communication of the anus with the urinary apparatus is thus [the result of] an arrest of development.

In regard to the next period of development I am following my own observations. The tube, separated from the end of the intestine, exists in common with several other parts; into it, from behind, flow the ureters and the excretory ducts of the genitalia; from in front, the urachus; it leads away into the common urogenital sinus. Still there appears no division of this duct from the various aforementioned parts; it is equally wide everywhere, and colored fluid, injected into the urogenital fissure, fills this tube, the excretory ducts of the sexual parts . . . and the urachus simultaneously. I shall name this common tube the *sinus urogenitalis,* the outer opening the *fissura urogenitalis.*

This common sinus now undergoes a further division.

In the female embryo a middle segment arises out of the most posterior part of the urogenital sinus, to which segment, the unpaired part of the uterus, the tubes attach. As this division of the genital and urinary parts proceeds downward, the distal part of the canal becomes the vagina in females.

The urachus likewise becomes disconnected from that part of the urogenital sinus into which the ureters enter, and as its lowermost part narrows, the middle however widening, the female urethra and bladder arise. But for a long time the bladder itself is only an elongated dilatation of the urachus, which only later becomes more delimited above and below, being transformed finally into the fibrous urachus.

In the male embryo the urinary meatus remains the main canal, into which the excretory ducts of the sexual parts run; the common part would be much better named *canalis urogenitalis* rather than *urethra.* In the female animals the *canalis genitalis* of the main canal becomes the vagina, and the separation of both canals gradually proceeds up to the vaginal opening. In several animal species the division progresses to a complete separation of the ureters from the opening of the sexual parts.

MÜLLER'S LIFE

Johannes Müller was born in Coblenz, Germany, July 4, 1801, the son of a cobbler and the eldest of five children.[1,2,4,5] During his 57 years he wrote 20 books, and about 250 scientific papers illustrated with 350 hand-drawn plates, contributing to almost all fields of basic medical research, and established himself as the foremost German physiologist of his day and one of the most illustrious of the nineteenth century. After completing his preliminary education at the local gymnasium, Müller spent a year in army training, in compliance with the Prussian military law. He hesitated long in deciding between a career of medicine and the priesthood; it is believed that he was strongly influenced in favor of the former by the writings of Goethe, for whom he had an intense and abiding admiration. Indeed, Goethe's influence seems to have been with Müller throughout his career, constantly directing him toward concrete values and ideas susceptible of experimental proof, and away from abstract thought and philosophy.

Müller received his doctorate at the University of Bonn in 1822, but while pursuing his medical studies there he managed to find time to attend lectures in poetry, rhetoric, Shakespeare, and Dante. His essay *De Respiratione Foetus,* written during his student days, was awarded first prize. His inaugural dissertation, *De Phoronomia Animalium,* dealing with the mechanism of locomotion of all classes of animals, was likewise judged outstanding, although Müller was only 21 years old when he wrote it. He then went to Berlin for his state examinations, but after meeting Rudolphi, the famous physiologist, remained for an additional half year, studying experimental physiology and the functions of the spinal nerves. In 1824 Müller returned to Bonn, where he had received an academic appointment, to begin his relentless succession of investigations and publications, with which he achieved prompt recognition and rapid ascent of the academic ladder. His early work was devoted chiefly to the phenomena of vision, and these studies were soon followed by investigations of the blood constituents and his classic publications on the development of the genitalia.

In 1830 Müller was made ordinary professor of medicine at Bonn, and three years later was recalled to Berlin to occupy the combined chair of anatomy, physiology, and pathology vacated by the death of Rudolphi. His scientific activity in Berlin was truly prodigious. He experimentally confirmed Bell's doctrine, which stated that the anterior roots of the spinal nerves carry centrifugal impulses, the posterior roots centripetal fibers. He studied the mechanism by which the voice tones are produced in the larynx. In Müller's youth there had been no knowledge of cells, no microtome, no histologic staining methods, no binocular microscope. Assisted by one of his students, Theodore Schwann, he established pathologic histology as a scientific discipline through his work on the minute anatomy of tumors, recognizing the cell as the principal element of morbid growth and cytologic differences in neoplasms as a diagnostic criterion for distinguishing tumor types among them. Schwann later became known as the founder of the cell theory, and Rudolph Virchow, another of his disciples, as the father of cellular pathology. Henle also was trained in Müller's laboratory. Through Müller's efforts the microscope, previously limited in its clinical application to the examination of the urinary sediment, became an instrument of increasing importance and ultimate indispensability for clinical practice. His *Lehrbuch der Physiologie* was a work of tremendous authority. Not only did it replace all other physiology texts in Germany, but, translated into most other European languages, it was used in other countries as well. Müller undertook the active direction of *Meckel's Archiv für Anatomie und Physiologie,* which came to be known popularly as *Müller's Archiv.*

With all this he found time to serve as director of three anatomy museums in Berlin, for which he was particularly well fitted because of his great interest in comparative anatomy, especially ichthyology. Müller was often referred to as the German Cuvier. His treatises on the metamorphosis of the echinoderms are still regarded as outstanding. To facilitate his researches on marine animals he spent his vacation each year at the seashore. In 1855, while on the return voyage from Norway, where he and an assistant had gone in pursuit of biologic specimens, their ship was sunk in a collision. Müller was rescued with great difficulty, but his assistant drowned. Greatly disturbed by this tragedy, Müller became melancholic, his health declined, and he died less than three years later, April 28, 1858. After his death his position at the university was divided, anatomy being taken over by Karl Reichert and physiology by Du Bois-Reymond. A fitting tribute was paid Müller in a commemorative address by Virchow:

> Thus he himself became, as he had remarked of his great predecessors, a priest of nature. The cult that he served bound his pupils to him in close ties, as by a religious bond; and the serious, priestly fashion of his speech and movements completed the veneration with which everyone regarded him. His mouth, with its tightly compressed lips, conveyed a notion of severity; around his eyes and forehead played an expression of profound thought; every furrow in his face stimulated the idea of a perfectly finished work—thus did this man stand before the altar of nature, freed by his own energy from the fetters of education and tradition, a living witness to personal independence!

REFERENCES

1. Bautzmann, H.: Johannes Müller und unsere Lehre von der organischen Gliederung und Entwicklung. *Anat. Anz.,* **94**:225–56, 1943.
2. Ebbecke, U.: *Johannes Müller, der grosse rheinische Physiologe.* Schmorl & von Seefeld, Hannover, 1951, pp. 7–41.
3. Müller, J.: *Bildungsgeschichte der Genitalien aus anatomischen Untersuchungen an Embryonen des Menschen und der Thiere, nebst einem Anhang über die chirurgische Behandlung der Hypospadia.* Düsseldorf, 1830.
4. Obituary. John Müller. *M. Times & Gazette,* **17**(n.s.):66–68, 1858.
5. Sigerist, H. E.: *The Great Doctors.* W. W. Norton & Co., Inc., New York, 1933, pp. 307–11.

Martin Naboth and Nabothian Cysts*

Mucous cysts of the cervix are seldom referred to by any other name than Nabothian cysts. This exceedingly common variant from the normal cervical structure was described, to be sure, by Martin Naboth; it is ironical, however, if not surprising, that not only was Naboth's interpretation of the cervical cysts erroneous but the structures had actually been described a quarter century earlier by the long-since-forgotten Desnoues.

DESNOUES' DESCRIPTION OF CERVICAL CYSTS

Guillaume Desnoues was a French surgeon who later became professor of anatomy in Genoa. Very little is known about him except for his studies of blood vessels by means of wax injections, a technique that he used before either Swammerdam or de Graaf.[1] His discovery of the cystic irregularities in the cervix was reported in February, 1681, in *Zodiacus Medico-Gallicus*,[3] a journal edited by Nicolas de Blegny and devoted to important current advances in medicine. Caspar Bartholin had already announced his discovery of the vulvovaginal glands as the source of the coital lubricant in women. Confusion still prevailed, however, over the female semen, its site of production, and its role in fecundation. From his dissections of three female cadavers, Desnoues thought he had at last discovered the female analogue of the male seminal apparatus. In his brief report (Fig. 5-1) trans-

---

* This chapter originally published under the title "Martin Naboth and Cervical Cysts" in *Fertil. & Steril.*, **7**:66–70, 1956; reprinted by permission. Copyright © 1956, by The American Society for the Study of Sterility.

lated herewith, Desnoues described, probably for the first time, the cysts later identified with the name of Naboth.

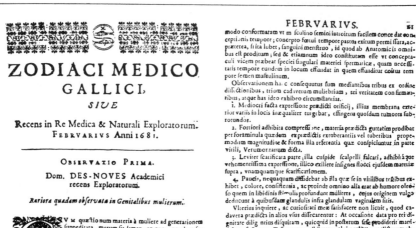

Fig. 5-1. Original paper by Guillaume Desnoues describing the cystic structures in the cervix.[3]

The question, which consists in knowing whether the material which a woman supplies for generation is a pure semen or eggs, still being unanswerable, and the two schools of thought that have formed on this subject having both been supported by sufficiently good reasons to permit uncertainty to remain in the minds of the most enlightened; I have had good reason for thinking that our ignorance was the cause of our doubts, and that by bringing more exactitude to the investigation of the true anatomy of the genital organs of woman, we could escape from an irksome uncertainty. This is what led me to examine them [the genital organs] anew in recent opportunities I have had, and this is what gave me the opportunity to make a few observations, which will be of very great use later on.

For I have observed that the part of the uterus that protrudes into the vagina, and that is called the internal orifice, is not only formed in a suitable manner to allow entrance of the male semen at the time of conception, to permit the exit of the conceptus at the time of delivery, and for the issue of menstrual blood, as all anatomists have thought, but that it is also arranged to serve as a reservoir for a sort of spermatic substance and to secrete it if necessary at the place where that of the male is deposited during coitus.

Three almost consecutive dissections of women have convinced me of this fact, and as a result of the following observations

1. In my pressing gently on this orifice, its external membrane was raised unevenly in several places, forming sorts of rounded elevations.

2. When the pressure was increased considerably, the substance that I have mentioned escaped from these elevations in small drops, by means of certain openings about the size and shape of those at the verumontanum in men.

3. Pricking the organ superficially with the point of a lancet and then pressing it very firmly resulted in the immediate appearance of large flecks of this same matter over each puncture site.

4. In a word, it was exactly similar in color and consistency to what is found in the male testicles, and thus quite different from the oily humor that is secreted by women in the throes of amorous emotion, which [humor] is believed to come from certain glands found under the vaginal membrane.

NABOTH'S DESCRIPTION OF CERVICAL CYSTS

Naboth, in 1707, when he took up the subject of these cystic structures in the cervix in his *De Sterilitate Mulierum* (Figs. 5-2 and 5-3),[4] acknowledged

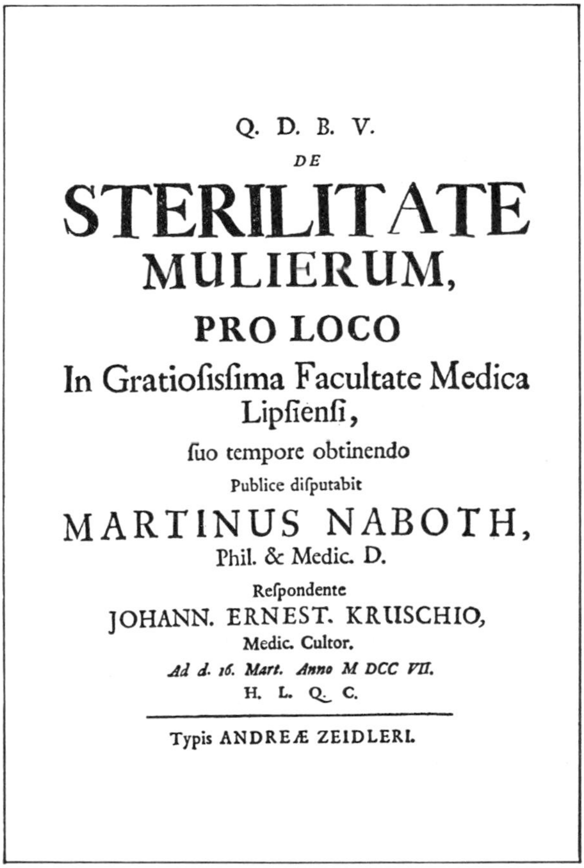

Q. D. B. V.

DE

STERILITATE
MULIERUM,
PRO LOCO

In Gratiosissima Facultate Medica
Lipsiensi,

suo tempore obtinendo

Publice disputabit

MARTINUS NABOTH,
Phil. & Medic. D.

Respondente

JOHANN. ERNEST. KRUSCHIO,
Medic. Cultor.

Ad d. 16. Mart. Anno M DCC VII.
H. L. Q. C.

Typis ANDREÆ ZEIDLERI.

Fig. 5-2. Title page of Martin Naboth's treatise on sterility in women.

the earlier publication of Desnoues; but in attempting to correct the latter's views Naboth himself erred, regarding the cervical cysts as eggs or ovisacs and referring in fact to the cystic cervix as an *ovarium* (see Fig. 5-3). In its literal translation this word means a keeper of eggs; but in an effort to convey Naboth's meaning, and at the same time to prevent confusion with the modern meaning of the word *ovary,* I have used the term "egg structure" in my English translation of Naboth's Latin:

> If now the egg structure itself is examined anew under favorable conditions . . . the lining of the cervical canal, which extends from the lowest part of the uterus up to the cavity of the fundus, is seen to be swollen with vesicles bulging with ripe semen. However, when one examines the vagina a few vesicles also

mentionem quippe earum *Regnerus de Graaf de Mulier; Organ, p. 237. A. 1672.* & *Des Noues* apud *Nicolaum de Blegny Zodiaci Medico-Gallici Ann 1681. p. 21. 77. 106.* fecerunt. Quia prior tamen easdem pro hydatidibus i. e. præternaturalibus, non semper, sed sæpenumero saltem occurrentibus, habuit, posterior autem ipsas magis in orificio interno consideravit, tanquam organa, materiam spermaticam asservantia, in coitu à fœminis excernendâ, à nemine autem alio tales, quantum quidem scio, pro veris ovulis adhuc assertæ fuerunt, nullus, spero, vitio mihi vertet, quod ejusmodi vesicularum, tanquam genuinorum ovulorum congestum ovarii novi titulo eadem libertate nunc velim insignitum, qua muliebres testes *Steno* quondam, *Hornius, Kerckringius. Swamerdam,* & *de Graaf* ovaria appellarunt. A quibus tamen præsens novum multum distat, quod in fœmellis semper sine discrimine temporis reperiatur, quod sit solitarium seu unicum, quod veris demum constet ovulis, quæ sperma virile contingere, eorumque unum vel alterum actuare sive fœcundare possit, absque eo, ut de via anxie prius disputandum veniat, per quam virile semen ad illud debeat pervenire.

XV.

Ovarium siquidem novum in commodo deprehenditur loco, in ipsa videlicet, prout jam indigitatum, cervicis uteri superficie interna, quam omnem fere, ad infimam usque cavitatis fundi uterini partem, ocupat, egregie imprimis vesiculis in fœmellis viro maturis, turgens. Aliquando tamen vesiculæ etiam nonnullæ limbum sive circulum orificii interni, quo cum vaginam respicit, excurrunt, interdum, licet rarius, in cavitate quoque fundi uterini una vel altera occurrit. Et licet ovarium tale sit simplex, subinde nihilominus in circumferentia cervicis interna fere instar binarum arbuscularum cum ramulis expansarum atque fructibus conspicitur. Cujus-

Cujuslibet vesiculæ, figuram rotundam seu ovalem quodammodo præ se ferentis, pars tertia circiter extra internam cervicis uterinæ superficiem prominet, duæ vero partes substantiæ cervicis immerguntur, cum eadem veluti continuatæ. Magnitudine non minus ac numero, vesiculæ dictæ satis variant, dum earum aliæ pisum majus, aliæ minus, nonnullæ semen cannabis, plures grana milii, magnitudine æmulantur; in subjectis junioribus vesiculas plures & minores, in natu majoribus majores & germen promtius, in senioribus easdem pauciores videre licuit. Propter vesicularum autem protuberantiam æque ac propter fibrosam sive cellulosam cervicis figuram, non potest non ovarium integrum apparere inæquale.

XV.

Ast quo constet, ovulorum nomen vesiculis istis merito decerni, exactius paulo vesicularum ejusmodi conformationem juvabit lustrare, ex Placenta nempe, Tunicis, Humore, Embryone atque Vasis i. e. tot partibus, quot ad fœtum producendum, tegendum & nutriendum requiruntur, resultantem. Quantum namque ovuli. i. e. duæ tertiæ substantiæ cervicis immersum, tantum placentæ uterinæ explet vicem, utpote ex meris vasculis sanguiferis æque contextum, ac placentæ alias structuram ex solis talibus vasculis conflatam *Casserius* & *Clariss. Ruyschius* evolvunt. Ideoque circa uterum nullibi quoque majores & copiosiores rami vasorum hypogastricorum & spermaticorum inseri videntur, quam circa cervicem, ubi ovarium interius locatur. Quæ autem ovuli pars à connexione libera, i.e. tertia, prominet membranosa, in ovulis majoribus haud difficulter in duas laminas discerpi valet, ita ut hæ rudimenta existant, chorii & Amnii, ceu duarum tunicarum fœtum involentium, quarum illa crassior, hæc subtilior habeatur; prout ovula immaturius exclusa & à *Celeberrrimo Ruyschio in Thesaur. Anat.*

Fig. 5-3. Section of Naboth's treatise[4] dealing with cervical cysts.

appear around the edge or rim of the cervical orifice, or more rarely they are present here and there in the uterine cavity as well. Thus in such a case the egg structure may be solitary, but nevertheless one sees in the internal circumference of the cervix something like two little bushes spreading out with fruit on their branches. The vesicles assume a round or oval form, two groups in fact projecting into the substance of the cervix as if continuous with it, while a third group is prominent about the exterior of the cervical lining. The vesicles vary somewhat in size as well as number; while some are as large as a pea, others are smaller, some being the size of a hemp seed, a greater number, though equal in size, resembling a grain of millet. In younger subjects a greater or lesser number of vesicles may be seen, in older subjects their number is greater and they develop more rapidly, but in the aged they are fewer. Because of the protuberance of the vesicles and also because of the fibrous and compound character of the cervix, the entire egg structure can appear uneven.

Naboth's dissertation on sterility in women, from which this excerpt is taken, achieved new prominence by its inclusion in von Haller's *Disputationum Anatomicarum Selectarum,* published in 1750, and the well-known mucous vesicles in the cervix have been designated ever since as Nabothian cysts.

NABOTH'S LIFE

Martin Naboth was born on January 16, 1675, in Kalau, Saxony.[2] He studied in Leipzig and Halle, receiving his doctorate in medicine in 1703. Very little information is available concerning Naboth or his life, and there is no known portrait of him in existence. His early years after graduation were devoted to general practice and anatomic research, which latter interest he continued to pursue even after his appointment as professor of chemistry in Leipzig in 1707. In addition to his *De Sterilitate Mulierum,* Naboth was the author of *De Organo Auditus,* published in 1703. He died in Leipzig, May 23, 1721.

REFERENCES

1. *Biographisches Lexikon der hervorragenden Ärzte aller Zeiten und Völker,* 2nd ed. Ed. by W. Haberling, F. Hübotter, and H. Vierordt. Urban & Schwarzenberg, Berlin & Vienna, 1930, Vol. 2, p. 242.

2. *Biographisches Lexikon der hervorragenden Ärzte aller Zeiten und Völker,* 2nd ed. Ed. by W. Haberling, F. Hübotter, and H. Vierordt. Urban & Schwarzenberg, Berlin & Vienna, 1932, Vol. 4, p. 315.

3. Desnoues, G.: Rariora quadam observata in genitalibus mulierum. *Zodiacus Medico-Gallicus, sive Miscellaneorum Medico-Physicorum Gallicorum.* Annus Tertius. Leonard Chouët, Geneva (Feb., 1681), 1682, pp. 20–21. Also published in French: Nouvelle découverte anatomique sur les parties génitales de la femme. *Journal des Nouvelles Découvertes, Concernant les Sciences et les Arts, qui sont parties de la Medicine,* Vol. 3, 1681.

4. Naboth, M.: *De Sterilitate Mulierum.* Leipzig, 1707. Also published in A. von Haller's *Disputationum Anatomicarum Selectarum.* Göttingen, 1750, Vol. 5, pp. 233–59.

Caspar Bartholin and the Bartholin Glands*

Female semen, the name once applied to the fluid that issues from the woman's genitals during coitus, was assumed for many years to originate in the female testes, as the ovaries were called. This fluid, regarded as essential to fecundation since the time of Aristotle, was thought to discharge into the urethra, as in the male. Herophilus, whose original writings are all lost, but some of which had been copied down by Galen and incorporated into the latter's writings, believed that he had traced the course of the seminal ducts from the female testes to the bladder. In Galen's *De Semine*, Herophilus is quoted as follows: "A very small seminal duct occurs on each side, arising from the uterus. The first part of this duct is much folded, and as in males it runs from the testicle to the fleshy part of the neck of the bladder." Corner [3] has suggested that this description is based on an examination of the genitalia of a sow with persistent Wolffian or Gartner ducts, not rare in this species. The true source of the female semen was not recognized until the latter part of the seventeenth century. Following the discovery of the .vulvovaginal glands in cattle by Duverney, one of his contemporaries, Caspar Bartholin, in 1677 first called attention to, and described the functions of, these glands in women.

---

* This chapter originally published under the title "Caspar Bartholinus and the Vulvo-vaginal Glands" in *M. Hist.*, 1:355–58, 1957; reprinted by permission.

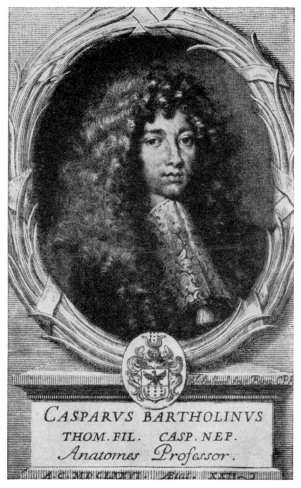

Fig. 6-1. Caspar Bartholin (1655–1738).

BARTHOLIN'S DESCRIPTION OF VULVOVAGINAL GLANDS

The para-urethral ducts had recently been described by de Graaf in his *De Mulierum Organis*[4] as the portal of exit of the fluid that lubricates the introitus and stimulates libido. Bartholin,[1] referring to the ducts through which the female semen was believed to empty into the urethra, wrote:

These I did not judge adequate for this function, but elsewhere in the vicinity of the urethral meatus and the vaginal orifice I saw larger openings [*] which, after

* Bartholin was apparently unaware of Francisco Plazzoni's earlier reference to the vulvovaginal ducts (*De Partibus Generationi Inservientibus Libro Duo*. F. Lopez de Haro, Leyden, 1664 [Book 2], p. 113; first ed. published in 1621).

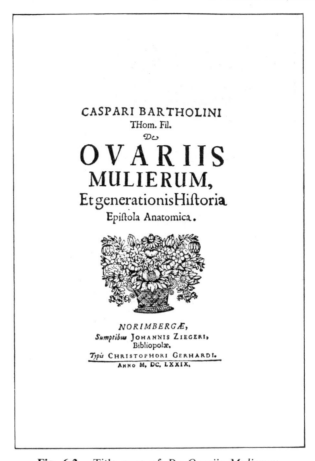

CASPARI BARTHOLINI
THom. Fil.
De
OVARIIS
MULIERUM,
Et generationisHiſtoria
Epiſtola Anatomica.

NORIMBERGÆ,
Sumptibus JOHANNIS ZIEGERI,
Bibliopolæ.
Typis CHRISTOPHORI GERHARDI.
ANNO M, DC, LXXIX,

Fig. 6-2.   Title page of *De Ovariis Mulierum.*

careful consideration, I judged to be better suited for carrying off the fluid from the gland that is nearly analogous to the male prostate, the ducts of which empty into the urethra, as described by Graaf. Examining these structures again more closely in cows, I discovered in these animals, near the walls of the vagina and not far from the urethral orifice, a prominent gland on both sides that drains into the vaginal canal; and when the gland is pressed, the protuberant ostium opens conspicuously in a nipple within the vulva. . . . It is composed of many glands and covered entirely with its own fleshy fibers; and the great secret of nature that I discovered is that this fluid does not flow freely except during coitus or masturbation, nor can the ostia be found except when the nipple protrudes. Therefore, since the fluid cannot be drained off unless the nipple protrudes, nature adds fleshy fibers that compress the glands during the venereal act so that the nipples protrude and the fluid may be discharged. The fleshy fibers are seen to arise near the vesical sphincter, as in the prostates of men, which are also covered by small muscle fibers that originate and spread out from the bladder sphincter, according to Graaf. This gland, which is to be seen on either side, is made up of many parts and excretions flow from it in large quantity into the nipple, which protrudes when the gland is compressed; otherwise it retracts, leaving hardly a trace of itself. One finds that these excretory ducts, where they discharge through their ostium, are distended when a catheter is inserted, and the ducts ramify into various branches to the periphery of the gland, as is observed in the excretory ducts of other glands; the ducts gradually decreasing in caliber in the various ramifications (which are of course in the substance of the gland) and ending. Moreover one might say that connected to the glands are vesicles or small elongated sacs in which the fluid secreted in the glands is stored and then discharged.

Since this description, Bartholin's name has become so intimately identified with the vulvovaginal glands that each of these structures is seldom called by any name other than Bartholin's gland, a term occasionally applied to a division of the sublingual gland as well. In recent years the tendency has grown to drop the word *gland* when referring to affections of the vulvovaginal gland, so that the terms "Bartholin cyst" and "Bartholin abscess" are now in common use; and inflammations of the organ, properly termed Bartholin adenitis, are now acceptably written as "bartholinitis," with a small *b*.[5]

BARTHOLIN'S LIFE

Caspar Bartholin, second, was born in Copenhagen, September 10, 1655, into a family of scientists of long-distinguished reputation (Table 6-1). It is probably his father, Thomas, to whom *Dissertatio de Cygni Anatomia* should properly be attributed, for Caspar was only 13 years old at the time of its publication in 1668.[2] Yet this treatise is believed to have paved the way for his appointment by King Christian V as professor of philosophy at age 19, only three years after he matriculated as a student in the University of Copenhagen. Following a three-year tour of various universities in Holland, France, Italy, and Germany, he returned to Copenhagen in 1677, when his famous *De Ovariis Mulierum* was published. As professor of physics he now proceeded to give lectures in anatomy while carrying on his own investigations, which were based largely on the previous work of his teachers—Ruysch, Swammerdam, and particularly Steno.

Bartholin was a man of wide interests and great versatility; and as a result of the many demands made upon him he found less and less time for teaching and research. By 1701 his active participation in the work of the medical faculty had practically ceased, while he found himself in such positions as assessor of the highest tribunal, later Procurer-General, and ultimately Deputy for Finance. In recognition of these efforts on behalf of the government he was given many decorations, and in 1731, together with his father and all his descendants, was elevated to the nobility. Even after the cessation of his medi-

cuïit, ut in pisce à *Stenonio* dissecto ex canum genere ; in aliis autem circa extrema interiora divisus manet, ut in muliere & quadrupedibus.

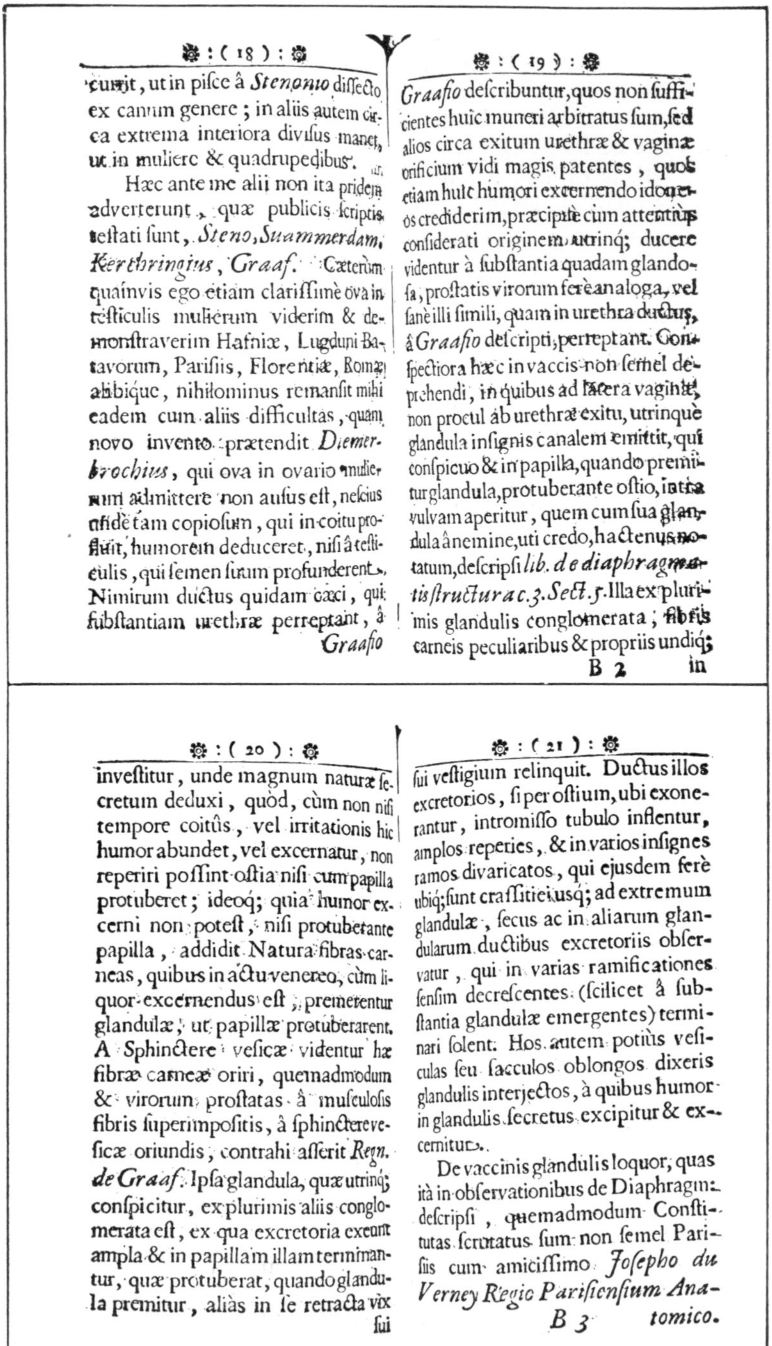

Hæc ante me alii non ita pridem adverterunt, quæ publicis scriptis testati sunt, *Steno, Suammerdam, Kerkringius, Graaf.* Cæterùm quamvis ego etiam clarissimè ova in testiculis mulierum viderim & demonstraverim Hafniæ, Lugduni Batavorum, Parisiis, Florentiæ, Romæ alibique, nihilominus remansit mihi eadem cum aliis difficultas, quam novo invento prætendit *Diemerbrochius*, qui ova in ovario mulierum admittere non ausus est, nescius cui dè tam copiosum, qui in coitu profluit, humorem deduceret, nisi à testiculis, qui semen suum profunderent. Nimirum ductus quidam cæci, qui substantiam urethræ perreptant, à

Graafio

19

Graafio describuntur, quos non sufficientes huic muneri arbitratus sum, sed alios circa exitum urethræ & vaginæ orificium vidi magis patentes, quos etiam huic humori excernendo idoneos crediderim, præcipuè cùm attentius considerati originem utrinq; ducere videntur à substantia quadam glandosa, prostatis virorum ferè analoga, vel sanè illi simili, quam in urethra ductus, à *Graafio* descripti, perreptant. Conspectiora hæc in vaccis non semel deprehendi, in quibus ad latera vaginæ non procul ab urethræ exitu, utrinque glandula insignis canalem emittit, qui conspicuo & in papilla, quando premitur glandula, protuberante ostio, intra vulvam aperitur, quem cum sua glandula à nemine, uti credo, hactenus notatum, descripsi *lib. de diaphragmatis structura c. 3. Sect. 5.* Illa ex plurimis glandulis conglomerata ; fibris carneis peculiaribus & propriis undiq;

B 2 in

investitur, unde magnum naturæ secretum deduxi, quòd, cùm non nisi tempore coitûs, vel irritationis hic humor abundet, vel excernatur, non reperiri possint ostia nisi cum papilla protuberet ; ideoq; quia humor excerni non potest, nisi protuberante papilla, addidit Natura fibras carneas, quibus in actu venereo, cùm liquor excernendus est, premerentur glandulæ, ut papillæ protuberarent. A Sphinctere vesicæ videntur hæ fibræ carneæ oriri, quemadmodum & virorum prostatas à musculosis fibris superimpositis, à sphinctere vesicæ oriundis, contrahi asserit *Regn. de Graaf.* Ipsa glandula, quæ utrinq; conspicitur, ex plurimis aliis conglomerata est, ex qua excretoria exeunt ampla & in papillam illam terminantur, quæ protuberat, quando glandula premitur, aliàs in se retracta vix

sui

sui vestigium relinquit. Ductus illos excretorios, si per ostium, ubi exonerantur, intromisso tubulo inflentur, amplos reperies, & in varios insignes ramos divaricatos, qui ejusdem ferè ubiq; sunt crassitiei usq; ad extremum glandulæ, secus ac in aliarum glandularum ductibus excretoriis observatur, qui in varias ramificationes sensim decrescentes (scilicet à substantia glandulæ emergentes) terminari solent. Hos autem potiùs vesiculas seu sacculos oblongos dixeris glandulis interjectos, à quibus humor in glandulis secretus excipitur & excernitur.

De vaccinis glandulis loquor, quas ità in observationibus de Diaphragmate descripsi, quemadmodum Constitutas scrutatus sum non semel Parisiis cum amicissimo *Josepho du Verney Regio Parisiensium Anatomico.*

B 3 tomico.

Fig. 6-3. Pages from *De Ovariis Mulierum*[1] containing Bartholin's description of the vulvovaginal glands. See text for translation.

50

Table 6-1

THE BARTHOLIN FAMILY *

Caspar, Primus (1585–1629) Theologian and Physician, married Anna, daughter of Thomas Finke (1561–1656), Mathematician and Physician.			

       :
       :
       :

(i) Jacob (–1653) Orientalist.	(ii) Thomas, Primus (1616–1680) Anatomist, originally Professor of Mathematics.	(iii) Erasmus (1625–1698) Physicist.	(iv) Albert Bibliographer.

       :
       :
       :

(i) Caspar, Secundus (1655–1738) Anatomist.	(ii) Thomas, Secundus (1659–1690) Distinguished for his literary works.	(iii) Margaret, Poetess.	Also three other dis- tinguished sons.

* From Dobson, J.: *Anatomical Eponyms*. Baillière, Tindall & Cox, London, 1946, p. 25.

cal and teaching activities and for the ensuing 37 years until his death, June 11, 1738, he retained both his professorial rank and salary, despite the envy and resentment of his medical colleagues, and continued to occupy a position second only to the dean of the medical faculty.

REFERENCES

1. Bartholin, C.: *De Ovariis Mulierum, et Generationis Historia*. Johann Zieger, Nuremberg, 1679, pp. 19–21 (first printing: Rome, 1677).
2. *Biographisches Lexikon der hervorragenden Ärzte aller Zeiten und Völker*, 2nd ed. Ed. by W. Haberling, F. Hübotter, and H. Vierordt. Urban & Schwarzenberg, Berlin & Vienna, 1929, Vol. 1, pp. 358–59.

3. Corner, G. W.: The discovery of the mammalian ovum. In *Lectures on the History of Medicine: A Series of Lectures at the Mayo Foundation, 1926–1932.* W. B. Saunders Co., Philadelphia, 1933, pp. 401–26.

4. Graaf, R. de: *De Mulierum Organis Generationi Inservientibus.* Hackiana, Leyden, 1672.

5. *Stedman's Medical Dictionary,* 18th ed. Williams & Wilkins Co., Baltimore, 1953, p. 159.

Alexander Skene and the Para-urethral Ducts*

CHAPTER

7

More than two centuries elapsed between the first description of the para-urethral ducts in women and their rediscovery by Alexander Skene, for whom these structures are now named. As early as 1672 Reinier de Graaf, in his *De Mulierum Organis,* had recorded his observations on the paired "lacunae situated at the termination of the urinary passage," which, by analogy with the male, he assumed to be the excretory ducts of the female prostate. According to de Graaf, these ducts were the source of the lubricating fluid discharged from the woman's parts when she is sexually stimulated, and also the focus of gonorrheal infection. In one of his dissections of a woman who had had gonorrhea, he described the diseased condition of "the glandular body embracing the urethra," while the uterus and vagina appeared normal. Purulent discharge from the para-urethral ducts was regarded by de Graaf as pathognomonic of gonorrhea, which he sharply distinguished from other causes of leucorrhea by this criterion.[3]

De Graaf's notion that the coital fluid secreted by women was discharged through the urethra by way of the para-urethral ducts was corrected by Caspar Bartholin in 1677, when he described the glands that now bear his name and explained their function.[2] The para-urethral ducts rapidly faded into temporary oblivion and were not heard of during the next 200 years.

* This chapter originally published in *J. Obst. & Gynaec. Brit. Emp.,* **63**:908–10, 1956; reprinted by permission.

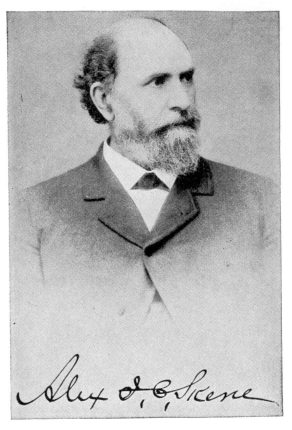

Fig. 7-1. Alexander Johnston Chalmers Skene (1838–1900). (Courtesy of American Gynecological Society.)

SKENE'S DESCRIPTION OF PARA-URETHRAL DUCTS

Skene was obviously unaware of the observations of the seventeenth-century anatomists, for, when he announced his own discovery of the para-urethral ducts in 1880,[5] he stated that he had been unable to find any reference to them in any of the textbooks of the day. "So far as I know," he wrote, "the anatomy of these glands has not been described, nor have the diseases to which they are subject been referred to by pathologists." Later in his paper Skene stated, "I know nothing about the physiology of these glands. They serve some purpose in the economy, no doubt, but what is their function is a question to be answered in the future."

The circumstances that led to Skene's discovery are related in graphic detail in this case report:

The patient was a married lady, 30 years of age. She was well developed, and had always enjoyed good general health. With the exception of a mild form of dysmenorrhea, she had had no disease of her sexual organs until one year before she came under my observation. At that time she was abruptly attacked with a profuse leucorrhea, and other symptoms of inflammation of the vulva and vagina, including painful urination. She placed herself at once under the care of her family physician, who treated her locally until she came to me. Her leucorrhea had, by that time, diminished and the painful urination had passed away, but otherwise she had not improved. At my first examination I found traces of the former inflammation of the vulva and vagina. The meatus urinarius was everted and surrounded by a number of papillary projections, of a deep-red color, and altogether presenting an appearance resembling that which is known as vascular tumor, or caruncle of the meatus. . . .

The diagnosis then made was subacute vaginitis, perhaps of gonorrheal origin, and inflamed papilloma of the meatus urinarius. The vaginitis was treated in the usual way, and soon it terminated in complete recovery, but the inflammation and tenderness of the meatus remained unchanged, and annoyed the patient exceedingly. She could not walk or sit without pain, and coitus had to be avoided entirely.

I presumed at first that the disease of the meatus was kept up by the irritating discharge from the vagina, and I hoped that when the one was removed, the other would get well, but such was not the case. I then thoroughly cauterized the elevated and tender points about the meatus with nitrate of silver. This caused very great pain at the time, and was followed by no improvement. Pure nitric acid was used in the same way, but with no better result, except to destroy elevations of the mucous membrane around the orifice. The same areola of inflammation around the meatus continued, and the symptoms remained the same. . . . Suffice it to say that for eight months I treated the disease with diligence and care, but at the end of that time she was very little better.

Caustics and cauteries being unsatisfactory, I tried sedatives and alteratives, including iodoform, iodine, mercury, and bismuth. At times the inflammation subsided slightly, and the elevated points became smaller, but in a short time fresh proliferations sprang up again, and the mucopurulent secretion continued to bathe the parts. Towards the end of this long period of treatment, and while making a critical examination, I observed that on each side of the meatus there were two depressions filled with a yellowish-gray matter, looking like minute ulcers, but upon probing them with a view to determine their depth, I found that they admitted the probe over half an inch. After withdrawing the probe, I made pressure upon the urethra from above downwards, and succeeded in expressing a purulent fluid which could be distinctly seen escaping from their orifices. Treatment was then directed to these canals; first they were injected with tincture of iodine, and subsequently they were cauterized by passing a probe, coated with nitrate of silver, along their entire depths. Prompt improvement followed this application. The inflammation around the meatus gradually subsided, and the pain and tenderness passed away. In less than two months from the time that a correct diagnosis was made, and appropriate treatment employed, the patient recovered completely. . . .

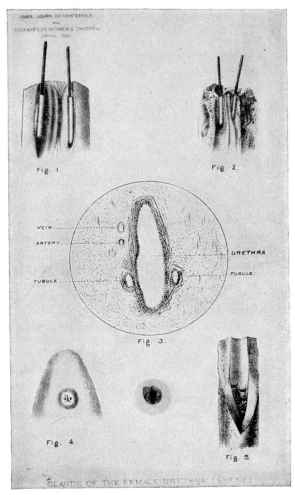

Fig. 7-2. Plate of illustrations from Skene's paper[5] showing the para-urethral ducts.

Stimulated by his experience with this patient and another in whom prompter response to treatment was obtained, Skene undertook a systematic investigation of the para-urethral ducts in the patients thereafter coming under his care. His studies were almost entirely clinical, however, supplemented by only an occasional histologic preparation; and he referred to the structures, promptly to be identified with his name, as glands rather than ducts. He stated:

I have called them glands because they differ in size and structure from the simple follicles found in abundance in the mucous membrane.
When I first discovered these glands I presumed that they were mucous follicles

that were accidentally of unusual size in the subject examined, but having investigated more than one hundred of these, in as many different subjects, and finding them constantly present, and so uniform in size and location, I became satisfied that they were worthy of a separate place in descriptive anatomy.

[The ducts] run parallel with the long axis of the urethra. They are located beneath the mucous membrane, in the muscular walls of the urethra. . . . The mouths of these tubules are found upon the free surface of the mucous membrane of the urethra, within the labia of the meatus urinarius. The location of the openings is subject to slight variation, according to the condition and form of the meatus. In some subjects, especially the young and very aged, and in those in whom the meatus is small and does not project above the plane of the vestibule, the orifices are found about an eighth of an inch within the outer border of the meatus.

Continuing with a consideration of the various pathologic conditions to which the para-urethal ducts are subject, Skene wrote:

When the mucous membrane of the urethra is thickened and relaxed, so as to become slightly prolapsed, or when the meatus is everted, conditions not uncommon among those who have borne children, the openings are exposed to view upon each side of the entrance to the urethra.

Gonorrheal inflammation was correctly regarded by Skene as the most important pathologic condition observed in these structures:

These glands may, I presume, become involved in any inflammation of the vulva, urethra or vagina, but from the history of the cases that have come under my observation I have been led to believe that the disease observed was caused by gonorrhea, and it persists in the glands long after all traces of the original disease had disappeared. Indeed, when this disease is once established, it has no natural tendency to recover.

SKENE'S LIFE

Alexander Johnston Chalmers Skene was born in Aberdeenshire, Scotland, June 17, 1838; [1,4] but like James Douglas, William Smellie, and our contemporary Benjamin Watson, he forsook the green hills of his native land to seek his fortunes elsewhere. After his early education in Aberdeen and King's College, Skene migrated to America at the age of 19. In 1860 he embarked upon the study of medicine, first at Toronto, and continuing at the University of Michigan and the Long Island College Hospital, from which he received his medical doctorate in 1863 and whose most famous alumnus he subsequently became. Skene spent the following year as assistant surgeon in the U.S. Army and is credited with formulating a plan for establishment of an army ambulance corps. He returned to Brooklyn and entered private practice in 1864, serving also as assistant to Austin Flint, Sr., while the latter was professor of practice at Long Island College Hospital. It is not clear at precisely what stage in his career Skene began to devote himself exclusively to gynecology, but he presumably elected this specialization sometime before 1870, for it was in this year that he was appointed professor of gynecology at the Long Island College Hospital, where he served as dean from 1886 to 1893 and as president for the following six years. In 1883 he was also made professor of gynecology at the New York Post-Graduate Medical School. Skene's practice was prodigious. In 1884, in partnership with William M. Thallon, he opened a private sanatorium on President Street near Prospect Park in Brooklyn, and five years later he incorporated Skene's Hospital for Self-Supporting Women. Skene was a founding member of the American Gynecological Society and served as its president in 1886–1887. A prolific writer, he explained the large volume of his literary output by his custom of writing at home in the early hours before breakfast, to avoid interruption. In addition to his many scientific articles, Skene was the author of five textbooks, of which his *Treatise on Diseases of Women* went into three editions, and his *Diseases of the Bladder and Urethra in Women* into two. He also invented or modified a number of surgical instruments, but his principal claim to fame lies in his rediscovery of the para-urethral ducts. Skene died in his summer home in the Catskills, July 4, 1900, at the age of 62. Brooklyn's traditional partisanship and pride in its own extend to its adopted sons as well as the native born. After Skene's death Schroeder wrote of him: "This is a distinction that has never come to any physician located on Long Island: to have his name connected with any part of the human body." De Graaf's priority still lay unrecognized.

REFERENCES

1. Alexander Johnston Chalmers Skene, M.D., LL.D. *Am. J. Obst.,* **42**:712–14, 1900.
2. Bartholin, C.: *De Ovariis Mulierum, et Generationis Historia.* Paolo Moneti, Rome, 1677.
3. Graaf, R. de: *De Mulierum Organis Generationi Inservientibus.* Hackiana, Leyden, 1672.
4. Schroeder, W.: Alexander Johnston Chalmers Skene, M.D., LL.D. *Brooklyn M. J.,* **14**:692–95, 704–12, 1900.
5. Skene, A. J. C.: The anatomy and pathology of two important glands of the female urethra. *Am. J. Obst.,* **13**:265–70, 1880.

Giovanni Battista Morgagni and the Hydatids of Morgagni*

CHAPTER

8

The word *hydatid* from the Greek, meaning a drop of water or a watery vesicle, has been adapted to two uses in gynecologic terminology, serving to designate a hydropic form of placental degeneration (hydatidiform mole) and the small fluid-filled cysts commonly attached to the fimbriae of the fallopian tubes (hydatids of Morgagni). The latter structures, usually only about 1 cm or less in diameter, rarely cause any clinical problems. Despite their frequency, the origin of these adnexal hydatids is still unsettled. They have been variously explained as pronephric or mesonephric remains, vesicular residua of the Wolffian duct and of the Müllerian duct, lymphangiectatic dilatations, elongated tubal fimbriae, and peritoneal inclusion cysts.[3,9]

Almost a hundred years before the publication in 1761 of Morgagni's celebrated *De Sedibus*[6] in which these and many other types of hydatids were described, de Graaf had recognized the difference between the follicles of the ovary and other small cystic structures in its vicinity, and described the criteria by which they could be distinguished. Wrote de Graaf in his classic description of the female testes or ovaries:[4]

Vesicles of the other kind, called *hydatids,* are usually formed with a double tunic. The interior layer, although very thin, is by no means difficult to separate

* This chapter originally published under the title "Giovanni Battista Morgagni and the Hydatids of the Broad Ligament" in *Am. J. Clin. Path.,* **25**:1341–48, 1955; reprinted by permission. Copyright, 1955, by The Williams & Wilkins Company.

59

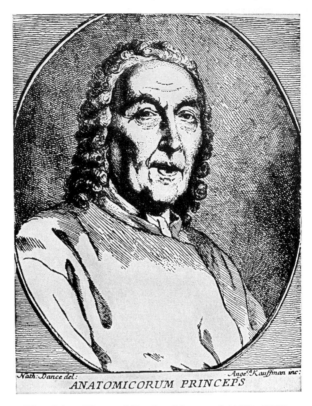

ANATOMICORUM PRINCEPS

Fig. 8-1. Giovanni Battista Morgagni (1682–1771).

from the exterior and the liquid content is not easily coagulated by boiling. On the contrary, the common coats of the ova are separated from each other with great difficulty and their liquid is coagulated by boiling; hence, whenever we have found in testes that have been boiled some vesicles filled with hardened substance and others with a liquid humor, we have considered the former ova, the latter hydatids. It must be added that the hydatids now and then are suspended from the membranes of the testicles as if by a peduncle, which as yet we have never found to be the case with true ova.

As recently as a century ago the term *hydatid* was applied to various types of cysts with watery contents. In Sir Astley Cooper's *Illustrations of the Diseases of the Breast*,[2] published in 1829, there appears, for example, a chapter on hydatid disease, in which four types of cystic swellings in this organ are described.

MORGAGNI'S DESCRIPTION OF HYDATIDS

Looking back to the time of Morgagni in the eighteenth century, we find a diverse assortment of pathologic entities characterized as hydatids, their only common tendency being the formation of encysted fluid. Although calling them by the same morphologically descriptive name, Morgagni was clearly aware of their varied nature and etiology when he wrote:

I think that the vesicles which are met with by anatomists, and are full of water, are not all of the same kind, and therefore, that the origins of different hydatids are to be differently explained: and the origin of some not, perhaps, in one way only, but in many joined together.

In his description, in a young girl, of what we would now assume to be tuberculous peritonitis, Morgagni spoke of the peritoneal vesicles as hydatids and ascribed the coexisting ascites to their rupture:

. . . the proximate cause of the dropsy . . . the ruptured hydatids seem to me to have been. For, as on the external surface of the intestines, and the spleen, some hydatids were prominent, which had not yet burst asunder; so I suppose that there had been almost innumerable others, both in these and in other parts, which, having been ruptured long before, had poured out their fluid into the cavity of the belly. And . . . the observations that I have very frequently made upon the tunica albuginea and vaginalis of the testicles, induce me to believe that the membranous laminae of the hydatids, or of the coats in which they are formed, after they have by rupture poured out the fluid that they contained, first contract themselves and their vessels into the form of a caruncle; and unless a fresh fluid continue to flow thither, are finally so indurated and dried up, as to represent those white and hard tubercles of a roundish figure, some larger in their size and some less, as the hydatids had been with which the internal surface of the peritoneum in the virgin described, and the production of it through the external surface of the spleen and intestines, were beset.

In some places Morgagni spoke of dropsy of the thorax and hydatids of the lung in the same patient, both almost surely of tuberculous origin; but elsewhere, in his references to animal dissections, he seems to have been describing parasitic cysts:

For he who, in brute animals, saw hydatids of the lungs . . . observed these appearances sometimes also in hydatids of the omentum, but more frequently that erosion which Galen required; and brought the water down from the neighboring liver, into the omentum . . . as Galen says, "to generate hydatids . . . the liver seems sometimes, even in animals that are killed without disease, to be full of them. . . ."

What Morgagni took to be a hydatid of the uterus may well have been a hydrosalpinx:

. . . the uterus has also its hydatids, sometimes . . . so large in their size that . . . Coiterus saw one "hanging from the side of the collum uteri, bigger

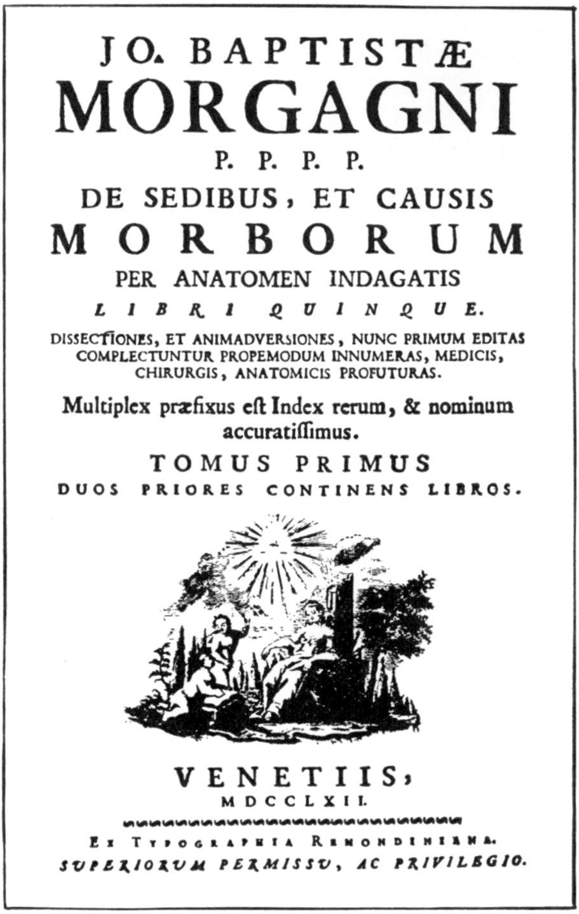

JO. BAPTISTÆ
MORGAGNI
P. P. P. P.

DE SEDIBUS, ET CAUSIS
MORBORUM
PER ANATOMEN INDAGATIS
L I B R I   Q U I N Q U E.
DISSECTIONES, ET ANIMADVERSIONES, NUNC PRIMUM EDITAS
COMPLECTUNTUR PROPEMODUM INNUMERAS, MEDICIS,
CHIRURGIS, ANATOMICIS PROFUTURAS.

Multiplex præfixus eft Index rerum, & nominum
accuratiffimus.

TOMUS PRIMUS
DUOS PRIORES CONTINENS LIBROS.

VENETIIS,
M D C C L X I I.

EX TYPOGRAPHIA REMONDINIANA.
SUPERIORUM PERMISSU, AC PRIVILEGIO.

Fig. 8-2.   Title page of Morgagni's *De Sedibus, et Causis Morborum per Anatomen Indagatis* (second printing).

to appearance than the natural bladder and very full of urine": or, as he says with more justice below, "full of thin and transparent water, and furnished like the natural bladder with two coats, but without any meatus whereby to collect or discharge its contents."

In another paragraph Morgagni seems to have been referring to cases of ovarian cancer and one of subphrenic or abdominal abscess, which he also characterized as a hydatid:

. . . those [hydatids] that are found in the ovaries of dropsical women, as they are made of enlarged vesicles . . . which are natural to these parts; and in like manner, those which he [Tyson] saw burst forth from the right side of a woman (who was laboring under disorder but afterwards perfectly cured) when opened a little below the spurious ribs; burst forth, I say, together with a great quantity of limpid water, to the number of five hundred; they being also turgid with a water of the same kind.

In similar manner, hydatids are mentioned in the kidney, in reference to either solitary cysts or polycystic disease.

The small adnexal cysts that now bear his name were described by Morgagni in his examination of a pigeon that had died from rupture of a blood vessel in the liver. He stated:

From the ovary, beside one pretty large egg, which was almost ready to fall off, some other hydatids were pendulous . . . and not connected immediately to the ovary, but by means of an intervening peduncle, or stalk, of a considerable length. Finally, there were some others, not larger than a very small bean, situated among these vitelli; but these much more white than the others, and full of a limpid water. Yet by boiling, neither this water nor the yellowish water of the others coagulated: and the eggs, which adhered to the extremity of that largest hydatid, as they had been less soft before boiling, were also more hardened than the others afterwards.

Morgagni's rancor, which he made no attempt to conceal, toward the servant who discarded the specimen, can be understood in view of the master's intense interest in hydatids. Continuing in the same paragraph, he wrote:

I intended to have examined internally the cells which I had seen through the coats of the larger hydatids, but being called away on some occasion, a servant unseasonably diligent, who supposed that I had examined every appearance to my satisfaction, threw them all away in the meanwhile, to a place from whence, though I was greatly chagrined at the accident, it was impossible for me to recover them.

Morgagni's discussion of the pathogenesis of hydatids is rather discursive, but it is clear that his critique did not permit his acceptance of any single theory as applicable to all hydatids. Exclaimed Morgagni:

. . . although I do not deny that hydatids may have their origin, in some certain way or other, at one time from a simple gland, and at another time from [lymphatic] interstices; yet I do not see how they can all be accounted for from thence. For it is long ago that Ruysch admonished us of a great number of hydatids being found in the placenta uteri sometimes, as I have also seen, and in other parts in like manner, wherein no lymph ducts are found. He therefore supposed "that hydatids were the extremities of sanguiferous vessels, which had changed their former nature and had degenerated into a diseased structure." There are some also who imagine that if a watery humor flow, not only from the injured parietes of the lymph ducts, but from any part whatever, among the surrounding membranes, they are consequently elevated and formed into hydatids.

In the next paragraph, in an effort to explain the slender-stalked hydatids of the female adnexa, he wrote:

And if hydatids that are pendulous by a long and slender stalk should chance to require an explanation, I mean such hydatids as . . . I have often seen particularly from the ovaries and the neighboring parts of women, and not only those that were pendulous from the ovary of that pigeon, the same person will be at liberty to suspect that the other cells of any hydatid, being broken off from the small sanguiferous trunk or being collapsed in consequence of having poured out the humor they contained, one of the extreme cells still remains connected and still retains its fluid. And indeed, I have sometimes very evidently seen a small sanguiferous vessel passing along with the filament, by which a hydatid of this kind was pendulous.

MORGAGNI'S LIFE

Giovanni Battista Morgagni, commonly referred to as the founder of pathologic anatomy, was born in Forli, Italy, February 25, 1682.[1,5,8] His aptitude for study became manifest at an early age, and when only 14 years old he began to compose poems and to engage publicly in philosophic discussions. While maintaining an active interest in classic literature and archaeology, he began the study of medicine in Bologna at the age of 16, where he later became assistant to his teacher, Antonio Maria Valsalva, before settling down to private practice.

Toward the end of the seventeenth century, quiet times had befallen the university at Padua and the medical faculty had lost much of its earlier luster; the Venetian government then made its brilliant decision to appoint Morgagni to the second chair of the theory of medicine at Padua in 1711, doubling the emolument on his account. Morgagni's first lecture, *Nova Institutionem Medicarum Idea,* outlined his teaching program and suggested that the students be instructed first in the principles of mathematics, then chemistry, botany, and zoology, followed finally by anatomy, "the indispensable premise for the clinician." Convinced that the understanding of nature is essential to the physician, he was almost constantly engaged in research and urged the experimental approach upon his students. Like Galileo, he insisted that nothing can be accepted as certain unless tested by experiment, and cautioned his students never to believe that the last words in science have been spoken by their masters or their books. Four years after coming to Padua, Morgagni was elevated to the position of professor of anatomy, occupying the chair held by a distinguished line of predecessors, including Vesalius and Falloppio. At this university Morgagni enjoyed the utmost in academic freedom and remained there for 60 years despite numerous invitations elsewhere. Many believe that he was the greatest of all the teachers who spread their knowledge from the old buildings at Padua, where the science of anatomy was born. It was here that he conceived the plan for his monumental work on pathologic anatomy, the first of its kind, which he published in 1761, when nearly 80 years old, under the title *De Sedibus, et Causis Morborum per Anatomen Indagatis.*

Various others before Morgagni had had experience in pathologic anatomy, and limited contributions to the subject had been made by a number of earlier investigators, such as Benivieni, Vesalius, Malpighi, Valsalva, Theophile Bonet, and Harvey. But it was Morgagni who for the first time collected, sifted, and analyzed the huge material that had become available, evaluating the data with the most searching and objective critique, correlating the observations on human beings with experiments on animals, and attempting to bridge the gaps between health and disease, between clinical phenomena and pathologic findings. His pathologic anatomy differed from that of his predecessors in the precision of reasoning he applied to the subject and in his steadfast attempt to correlate malfunction of an organ with specific pathologic change in it. The *De Sedibus* is the work of a serene old man who has collected the fruits of a long and active life of investigation and passed them on, in the form of letters, to his younger friends, in a kindly, mellow spirit. Among the outstanding descriptions in this treatise are the sections dealing with myocardial degeneration, postmortem clots in the heart, pulmonary tuberculosis, tumors of the pylorus, pathology of the appendix, alterations in the cerebral blood vessels and their relation to apoplexy and hemiplegia, and the clinical disorder later known as the Stokes-Adams syndrome. Osler regarded Morgagni's section on aneurysm of the aorta as one of the finest descriptions of this disorder ever written, combining to a rare degree clinical experience and careful anatomic observation. The *New Sydenham Society's Lexicon* [7] contains a list which, although incomplete, embraces 13 anatomic structures eponymically associated with the name of Morgagni.

Morgagni's fame spread over all of Europe, and in his later years his colleagues spoke of him as "his anatomic majesty" and "the prince of all European anatomists." It is said that a great many patients expressed the wish to have their bodies examined by Morgagni after their death. Despite the renown he had achieved, Morgagni continued to lead a rather secluded life, remote from the world of affairs, spending almost all of his time in study, teaching, and corresponding with his fellow scientists. A large proportion of the Italian anatomists of the eighteenth century, including Scarpa, were trained under him. When almost 90 years old, he was still teaching his course in anatomy, frequently in unheated buildings in the cold of winter. He died on December 5, 1771, of a ruptured ventricle. High tribute to his personal character is found in Sigerist's account [8] of his life:

From every physician we expect tact and moral earnestness, but we expect them from a pathologist in a supreme degree. It is the dead who are brought to the latter, persons whom medical practitioners have been powerless to save. All too often an autopsy demonstrates the insufficiency of human knowledge. In such cases the pathologist must not play the part of judge, but must be a helper and an exhorter. It is well that a man of such high character, a man so profoundly impressed with his mission, should have stood upon the threshold of the developing science of pathological anatomy.

REFERENCES

1. Castiglioni, A.: G. B. Morgagni, the founder of pathological anatomy, and the evolution of medical teaching. *Ciba Symposia,* **10**:986–91, 1948.

2. Cooper, A.: *Illustrations of the Diseases of the Breast.* Longman, Rees, Orme, Brown, & Green, London, 1829, Part I, pp. 20–50.

3. Frank, R. T.: *Gynecological and Obstetrical Pathology,* 2nd ed. D. Appleton & Co., New York, 1931, p. 331.

4. Graaf, R. de: *De Mulierum Organis Generationis Inservientibus.* Hackiana, Leyden, 1672, pp. 184–85.

5. Hutchinson, B.: *Biographia Medica.* J. Johnson, London, 1799, Vol. 2, pp. 161–62.

6. Morgagni, G. B.: *De Sedibus, et Causis Morborum per Anatomen Indagatis, Libri Quinque.* Venice, 1761. English translation from the Latin by B. Alexander: *The Seats and Causes of Diseases Investigated by Anatomy; in Five Books.* London, 1769, Vol. 2, Book III, Letter 38, Articles 35, 36, 37, 38, 42, 44.

7. Power, H., and Sedgwick, L. W. (eds.): *New Sydenham Society's Lexicon of Medicine and the Allied Sciences.* London, 1892, Vol. 4.

8. Sigerist, H. E.: *The Great Doctors.* W. W. Norton & Co., Inc., New York, 1933, pp. 229–36.

9. Watson, J. H.: Some observations on the origin and nature of the so-called hydatids of Morgagni found in men and women, with especial reference to the fate of the Müllerian duct in the epididymis. *J. Anat. & Physiol.,* **36**:147–61, 1902.

Eduard Pflüger and   CHAPTER

Pflüger's Ovarian Tubules   9

In their faltering but persistent efforts to understand certain pathologic changes in the ovary, especially the origins of neoplasms, gynecologists have turned repeatedly to the study of the organ's early development. The rapidly changing internal pattern of the ovary during its organogenesis has proved irresistibly tempting to the enterprising gynecologic pathologist, for the variety of forms encountered in the developing gonad and the adjacent mesonephros permit a wide range of speculation and theorizing by the imaginative mind.

The ovary, like the testis, begins as a thickening on the ventral surface of the mesonephros, or Wolffian body, resulting from a proliferation of the germinal epithelium. The closely packed, undifferentiated sex cells soon assume the form of columns, tubules, or cords, perpendicular to the surface of the mass and extending toward the hilum of the embryonic ovary, where they mingle and may even connect with the rete tubules or excurrent ducts of the mesonephros. These primary sex tubules or medullary cords, usually designated as Pflüger's cords or tubules, thus represent the homologue in the female of the testicular seminiferous tubules in the male.

In some species, such as the alligator [4] and hen,[2] the ovarian medullary cords persist into adult life. In the human ovary, by contrast, these cell columns normally appear as only transient structures in the fetus, although vestigial remains may be found occasionally in the ovaries of children and young adults. As a fresh wave of cellular proliferation emanates from the germinal epithelium, giving rise to the ovarian cortex, the primary sex cords

67

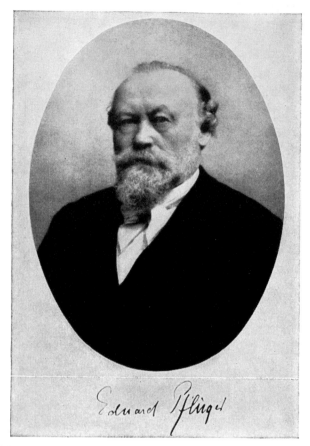

Fig. 9-1.   Eduard Friedrich Wilhelm Pflüger (1829–1910).

are crowded together in the medulla and ultimately disappear. Regression of the medullary cords begins when the fetal crown-rump length measures about 150 mm and is usually complete by the 280-mm stage.[5]

Lumens have been demonstrated in an occasional medullary column in the human ovary,[5,14] but some investigators [13] have insisted, nevertheless, that these structures should be designated only as "cords" rather than as "tubules." Gynecologic pathologists have, from time to time, traced to this source a variety of ovarian neoplasms, including dermoids, cystadenomas,[12] arrhenoblastomas,[6,7] and Brenner tumors.[1] Although their vestigial remains may be rich in pathologic potential in the human, the primitive sex cords make no contribution to the permanent structures of the ovary. The early descriptions of the medullary tubules in animals, on the other hand, ascribed to these cell columns an important role in follicle formation.

VALENTIN'S DESCRIPTION OF MEDULLARY CORDS

Medullary cords of the ovary were first described in 1838 by Valentin,[10] who called attention to tubular cell masses in the developing gonads of fetal calves and lambs. He wrote:

The peripheral part of the ovary is made up of ridges, while the central part remains solid. Through the process of exfoliation the ridges form into blind tubules, which radiate into the center. . . . In fetuses of the cow and sheep, of 3–5 inches crown-rump length, in which the follicles have already begun to develop, it is seen most clearly that the mammalian ovary consists of tubules that are blind at both ends, the distal end closing in a saccus coecus, the other end as a solid, elongated, round, centrally placed structure in the ovary. By means of fine perpendicular cuts or by teasing smaller fragments apart with a needle, one can often demonstrate here the very thin-walled and delicate tubules, which are paved with the greatest number of little epithelial balls. . . . In younger ovaries the smallness and softness of the tissues, and the numerous tiny masses everywhere present, pose almost insurmountable difficulties to observation; but I believe I have seen isolated tubules even here.

The greater the number of the follicles arising in these tubules, the better formed are the former, the larger the ovarian tubules become and the thinner their walls, and the smaller the solid central part of the ovary. Finally, after a group of follicles has developed to the size of significant vesicles the formation of tubules is suppressed and the individual tubules are displaced and compressed against one another by the proliferating follicles, so that demonstration of the tubules becomes progressively more difficult. . . . Nevertheless one can, with some patience, still clearly demonstrate and isolate the ovarian tubules, not only in the fetus but also in the newborn calf and lamb, as well as the cat and rabbit.

The tissue of the ovarian tubules consists of a very fine fibrillar membrane, on the inner surface of which round, somewhat granular epithelial balls are found. In both respects the tissues are very similar to those of the seminal vesicles of [male] fetuses or newborn of the same age. . . . If one succeeds in isolating a tubule he sees that the follicles are arranged in a row inside it. . . .

PFLÜGER'S DESCRIPTION OF MEDULLARY CORDS

Further understanding of the ovary's development had to await the application of the microscope to the study of embryology. No progress was made for a quarter century. Even the distinguished Johannes Müller, in his famous *Embryology,*[8] dismissed the subject with only one brief statement: "The ovarium of mammiferous animals, according to the observations of Valentin, is originally composed of tubes in which the graafian follicles are developed." Then, in 1863, after devoting almost all of the preceding two years to study of the problem, Eduard Pflüger published a monograph of 124 pages, *Ueber*

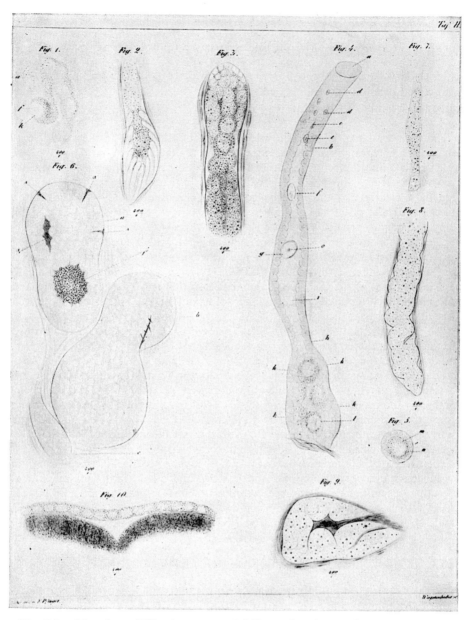

Fig. 9-2. Plate from Pflüger's monograph,[9] illustrating the ovarian tubules and ova in varying stages of development in the calf ovary.

die Eierstöcke der Säugethiere und des Menschen,[9] reporting his observations on ovarian development in the calf, cat, and dog. Pflüger's investigations extended Valentin's earlier studies, called attention for the first time to the origin of the medullary columns from the surface layer of cells, later to be designated as the germinal epithelium by Waldeyer,[11] and inspired the term *Pflüger's tubules.* Wrote Pflüger:

The mammalian ovary, consisting of a large number of tubules, belongs to the tubular glands, quite like its male analogue, the testis. The width of the tubules varies considerably in the same individual as well as in different animals . . . many being of colossal size, visible to the naked eye. The smaller tubules, which are most accessible to microscopic examination, permit the recognition of rather large-celled, nucleus-containing epithelium surrounding a light canal that courses down the center of the tubule. The individual epithelial cells often show markedly spherical projections into the canal of the tubules, while their external surfaces, the outer margin of the tubule, fuse in a straight line or a gentle curve. . . . In a considerable number of tubules I have also seen their contour as a dark line bordering the tubule, corresponding to the membrana propria, after the addition of acetic acid.

The graafian follicles develop inside these tubules: many alongside one another in the larger ones, and behind one another in simple sequence in the smaller ones. While the glandular epithelial tubule is still intact and not completely taken up by the growth of the follicles, the internal follicles already possess a single-layered membrana granulosa with a membrana propria folliculi, as can be seen with all reasonable certainty in isolated tubules, as well as the clear, nucleoli-containing germinal vesicle. . . . As the graafian follicles develop, one can see in isolated tubules how the follicles have already developed in this manner in one location, while progressively earlier stages are seen in more remote places, to the point where only a light, nucleus-containing vesicle is visible inside the tubule. Correspondingly, the tubule thus has greatly different widths at different places, since it enlarges according to the size and number of follicles developing within it. Each follicle, lying against the glandular wall of the tubule, corresponds to an outpouching of the latter. I have not drawn this conclusion from several preparations reconstructed into one, but rather this can actually be seen in a single, completely isolated, thin tubule. By repeatedly moving and rotating an isolated tubule one becomes more and more certain that follicle formation really takes place inside it.

These tubules can be demonstrated not only in young animals but also in adults. I have looked for them in very many different mammals and in none have I failed to find them.

In none, that is, except the human. Pflüger, in his description of the human ovary, made a number of interesting philosophic observations, but specifically noted his inability to demonstrate the tubules or cords that now bear his name. He reported:

I once obtained the ovary of a 17-year-old girl for examination without being able to demonstrate anything but young graafian follicles separated by rather abundant stroma. I must frankly note that at the time of this examination I did not possess the techniques best suited for the demonstration of the young glandular tissue. Nevertheless, reasoning from my observations in the cat, I concluded, because of the separation of the small follicles from one another, that the segmentation process as well as egg formation had long ceased before the time of my examination. . . . From my investigations on the human ovary I regard it as noteworthy that I could find no masses of similarly arranged cells [medullary cords]. The egg with its yolk, germinal vesicle, and nucleolus were always observed in the youngest follicles. The central cell of the young follicle was never formed like those of the membrana granulosa. The time interval for maturation of the follicle and egg, which lasts not quite a year in the cat, extends from the period of intrauterine life to the tenth, fifteenth, even twentieth year of life in the human. Nowhere do I find mention made of the incomparably wonderful fact that a human egg requires 14, even 20 years, from its first beginnings until it attains the state of maturity. The human egg, however, like that of mammals, is a structure that can be perceived by the naked eye only under the most favorable conditions and with the closest scrutiny. This fact appears all the more significant when one considers that the human body, with almost all its essential parts, has developed from the egg in perhaps less than four weeks after fertilization. It is now very difficult to determine whether the speed of development of eggs is any greater during adult life. In any case it appears somewhat paradoxical that the eggs of the human and of several animal species sometimes require decades to mature but do so quite rapidly at other times. Herein undoubtedly lies a great difference between the female and the male organisms, in that the sperm can be produced in an extraordinarily short time.

Pflüger failed to examine the human ovary during its fetal development, the only period in its life cycle when the ovarian cords named for him are normally demonstrable, but his observations in other species were confirmed in all essentials by Waldeyer [11] and subsequent investigators.

PFLÜGER'S LIFE

Eduard Friedrich Wilhelm Pflüger succeeded Johannes Müller as the leading figure among German physiologists. Born in Hanau, June 7, 1829,[3] he attended a mercantile school in Antwerp, where a rich uncle had a flourishing business, and remained there two years, long enough to learn French and English. Growing dissatisfied with the type of career his father had planned for him, Pflüger then returned home. After completing his preliminary education in the local gymnasium, he attended law classes at Heidelberg for two years, but this also failed to satisfy his restless, inquiring mind; and in 1849 he decided to study medicine, enrolling in the University of Berlin.

The Berlin medical faculty had reached full flower, and Pflüger quickly fell into the prevailing spirit of physiologic investigation that was to absorb his energies for the next 60 years. The first of his 200 publications, *Die sensorischen Functionen des Rückenmarks,* appeared in 1852; the last, *Ueber die Muttersubstanzen des Glykogenes,* in 1910. In 1860 he succeeded Helmholtz as professor of anatomy and physiology in Bonn, where he began a long series of embryologic and anatomic investigations. Physiology was growing rapidly, and Pflüger deprecated the efforts of his contemporaries to subdivide this expanding field into its component disciplines, such as chemistry, physics, anatomy, histology, and embryology. In an effort to stay this trend toward decentralization he founded the *Archiv für die gesamte Physiologie,* popularly known as *Pflüger's Archiv,* which soon attracted to his department a great increase in students and assistants and led to the development of a complete institute of physiology.

For more than 30 years Pflüger devoted himself to investigations of the problems of metabolism, concerning himself particularly with the vital functions of protein. In 1875 he published a paper suggesting that nitrogen exists in living tissue in the form of a cyanogen compound, which both results in the instability of the complex protein molecules and governs their ability to assimilate and convert dead protein material to living. The death of living substance, he further suggested, consists essentially of the absorption of water and the subsequent conversion of the cyanogen compound into an ammonia grouping.

Another of Pflüger's theories, widely heralded in its day but long since discarded, concerned the mechanism of menstruation. The ovarian distention resulting from the enlarging graafian follicle, Pflüger maintained, sends nerve impulses to the spinal cord, reflexly causing dilatation of the uterine and ovarian blood vessels and pelvic engorgement, this in turn leading to endometrial proliferation and ultimate menstruation. Regarded as the first integrated theory of menstruation, Pflüger's concept was generally accepted until disproved by the transplantation experiments of Knauer in 1896, to which the modern hormonal theories of menstruation trace their origin.

Pflüger's name is also intimately identified with the physiology of the nervous system. In a major contribution to neurophysiology, published in 1859 under the title *Untersuchungen über die Physiologie des Elektrotonus,* he formulated the principles governing the responses of nerve and muscle to electrical impulses, subsequently designated "Pflüger's law of contraction."

On the occasion of his eightieth birthday Pflüger was made an honorary citizen of Bonn, not quite a year before his death on March 16, 1910. Always a devout adherent to the Aristotelian doctrine of teleology, Pflüger had adopted the motto: "Gott und die Natur thun nichts vergeblich [God and Nature do nothing in vain]."

REFERENCES

1. Brenner, F.: Das Oophoroma folliculare. *Frankfurt. Ztschr. f. Path.,* 1:150–71, 1907.

2. Brode, M. D.: The significance of the asymmetry of the ovaries of the fowl. *J. Morphol. & Physiol.,* 46:1–57, 1928.

3. Cyon, E. von: Eduard Pflüger. Ein Nachruf. *Pflüger's Arch. f. d. ges. Physiol.,* 132:1–19, 1910.

4. Forbes, T. R.: Studies on the reproductive system of the alligator. VI. Further observations on heterosexual structures in the female alligator. *Anat. Rec.,* 77:343–65, 1940.

5. Forbes, T. R.: On the fate of the medullary cords of the human ovary. *Contrib. Embryol.,* 30 (No. 188):11–15, 1942 (Carnegie Inst. Wash. Pub. 541).

6. Meyer, R.: Über die Art der zur Vermännlichung führenden Ovarialtumoren. *Ztschr. f. Geburtsh. u. Gynäk.,* 98:149–67, 1930.

7. Meyer, R.: The pathology of some special ovarian tumors and their relation to sex characteristics. *Am. J. Obst. & Gynec.,* 22:697–713, 1931.

8. Müller, J.: *Embryology, with the Physiology of Generation.* Translated from the German by W. Baly. Taylor, Walton, & Maberly, London, 1848, p. 1639.

9. Pflüger, E. F. W.: *Ueber die Eierstöcke der Säugethiere und des Menschen.* Engelmann, Leipzig, 1863.

10. Valentin, G.: Ueber die Entwicklung der Follikel in dem Eierstocke der Säugethiere. *Arch. f. Anat. u. Physiol.,* 526–35, 1838.

11. Waldeyer, W.: *Eierstock und Ei.* Engelmann, Leipzig, 1870.

12. Waldeyer, W.: Die epithelialen Eierstocksgeschwülste, insbesondere die Kystoma. *Arch. f. Gynäk.,* 1:252–316, 1870.

13. Wendeler, P.: In Martin, A. (ed.): *Die Krankheiten der Eierstöcke und Nebeneierstöcke.* Arthur Georgi, Leipzig, 1899, p. 412.

14. Winiwarter, H. von: Recherches sur l'ovogenèse et l'organogenèse de l'ovaire des mammifères (lapin et homme). *Arch. biol., Paris,* 17:33–199, 1901.

Emma Call, Siegmund Exner, and the Call-Exner Bodies of the Ovarian Granulosa

CHAPTER

10

Tiny cystic spaces or vacuoles, which bear a superficial resemblance to ova, are commonly seen embedded among the ovarian granulosa cells. Initially described by Emma Call and Siegmund Exner, these distinctive ovarian structures are now known only as Call-Exner bodies or the bodies of Call and Exner; the eponyms are their only designation. Their presence furnishes strong presumptive evidence of the granulosal character of the surrounding tissue, for the Call-Exner bodies are often seen in granulosa cell tumors of the ovary as well as in the granulosa of the normal graafian follicles, but not in other tissues. Most pathologists now regard them as minute degeneration cysts.

DESCRIPTION BY CALL AND EXNER

The first description of these ovum-like structures in the follicular granulosa dates back to 1875. Emma Call, recently graduated in medicine, had just completed a period of postgraduate study in Vienna under the physiologist Siegmund Exner. She and her distinguished mentor reported their observations on the rabbit's ovary at the April 15 meeting of the section on mathematics and natural history of the Kaiserliche Akademie der Wissenschaften.[3] Discussing the possibility that the ova may arise from the epithelium of the graafian follicle as well as from the germinal epithelium, they wrote:

75

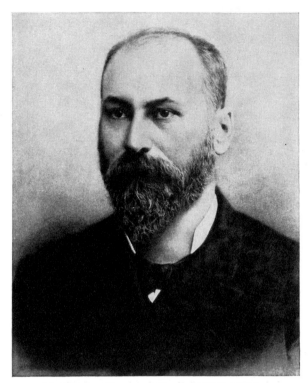

Fig. 10-1. Siegmund Exner (1846–1926).

This actually seems to occur:

If sections are made of the ovary of an adult rabbit one usually finds several large graafian follicles that are easily visible with the naked eye. Figure 1 [reproduced in upper part of Fig. 10-2] shows one of them drawn from nature.

At *a* there is a section of the follicular egg with its surrounding epithelial cells; the rest of the egg was present in the next section. The cavity is filled with coagulated fluid; in the follicle wall lies the oft-described layer of epithelial cells.

In this layer, round cells of varying size are usually found, as shown in *b* in the figure. Their relation to the epithelial cells is similar to that of the eggs. Figure 2 [reproduced in lower part of Fig. 10-2] shows such a cell with its surroundings, at higher magnification. The epithelial cells surround the round cells in a radial fashion and form a thick sheath around it, completely simulating the *discus oophorus*.

These cells are usually globular, like an egg. Only occasionally did we find irregular ones, flattened out by the epithelial cells. These were always relatively small, perhaps representing earlier stages of development. The size of these cells is usually about 0.03–0.04 mm, corresponding to the size of the follicular eggs, which are closely surrounded by a single layer of epithelium.

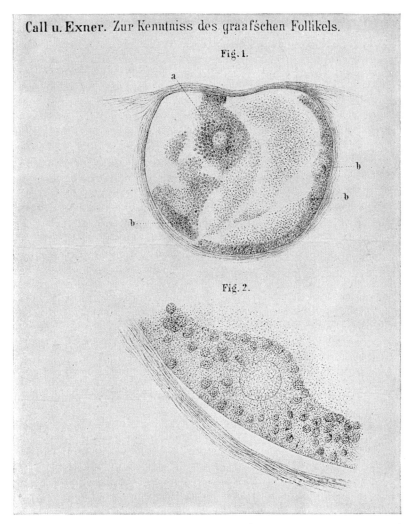

Call u. Exner. Zur Kenntniss des graafschen Follikels.

Fig. 1.

Fig. 2.

Fig. 10-2. Plate from paper by Call and Exner[3] illustrating the bodies now named for them. (Reproduced by permission of Österreichische Akademie der Wissenschaften.)

Speaking further of these newly found bodies, Call and Exner stated:

They are present at times in the graafian follicle in appreciable number, as can be seen in the section shown in Figure 1, in which three are visible. They are never seen in young follicles; only after a distinct cavity has developed in it does one find these cells in the follicle wall, never among the cells surrounding the follicular egg. Different sizes are found in the same follicle, as can also be seen in the figure. Follicles with such cells are not at all rare; almost every large

follicle of the rabbit contains them. We worked mostly on pregnant rabbits. . . .
The following significance can be attached to the cells under discussion.

The process of egg formation, having begun at the surface of the ovary and in the egg tubules, continues in the epithelium of the graafian follicle. New eggs form here, which attain maturity only long after the follicular egg is discharged. . . . A rapid increase in the epithelial cells of the follicle begins after the latter has ruptured, with the result that the *corpus luteum,* now present, is filled with the end products of this proliferation, that is, with normal ovarian substance. It is now possible for these eggs to be pushed into the *corpus luteum* by this proliferation. . . .

This in itself may be significant, in that it points to a new source of the large number of eggs that rabbits discharge from their small ovaries in their lifetime. A modification of this view would be necessary to permit agreement with the recently expressed opinion of Kölliker, that the follicular epithelium is, in the final analysis, a derivative of the Wolffian and not of the ovarian epithelium.

With commendable critique the authors questioned the tenability of their own suggested interpretation. They said:

The reason why we regard this view as a possibility only, and why we do not venture to speak of the aforementioned cells definitely as eggs, is twofold.

First, these cells do not look like the young ovarian eggs, which lie nearby in the stroma.

They are intensely granular (Fig. 2) and, perhaps because of this, show no nucleus; only occasionally did we believe that anything resembling a nucleus could be seen showing through. Obviously, therefore, there can be no discussion of nucleoli. We have treated ovaries of very young rabbits in the same manner and found that their youngest eggs appear essentially different from our cells.

Second, we have not succeeded in finding these cells again in early corpora lutea.

. . . Eggs already surrounded by epithelium are indeed present near the part of a *corpus luteum* pointing farthest away, toward the surface of the ovary, as we frequently saw; however, in these cases it was exactly here that the boundary of the corpus luteum was no longer sharp enough to exclude the suspicion that the egg had wandered in from the side.

These are the facts that restrain us from stating with certainty that a cell which, as shown in Figure 2, appears at first glance to be undoubtedly an egg, is actually one.

Everyone can easily apprise himself of the existence of such cells; skillful observations will perhaps clarify their significance.

We need scarcely mention that the above presentation has nothing to do with the recognized instances in which several eggs are present in one follicle, as is very common in rabbits. Here the eggs are always of approximately the same size and all are obviously ripe at the time of follicular rupture. We have also convinced ourselves repeatedly that the aforementioned cells actually lie near the normal ripe egg in the follicle.

The bodies of Call and Exner can be mimicked by artefacts of histologic preparation, as the authors were careful to point out:

Finally, let it be explicitly noted that a situation exists in which these cells can be simulated. If two follicles are half fused with each other, spurs of connective tissue project between them; if one of these is cut across, a picture of granular appearance is usually obtained, similar to that of the cells under discussion. Also, the epithelial cells of the follicle are then arranged radially in this transversely sectioned cord.

CALL'S LIFE

Emma Louise Call, one of the first women physicians in the United States, was born in Newburyport, Massachusetts, on August 1, 1847.[6] She attended the public schools of Boston, later studying medicine at the University of Michigan, where she received her degree in 1873. For further training she went to Vienna, here carrying out her studies on the rabbit's ovary under Exner's guidance. She then returned to Boston, where she practiced from 1875 to 1917, being associated with the New England Hospital for Women and Children for more than 40 years, ultimately with the title of attending physician and consultant in obstetrics. A founder of the New England Women's Medical Society, Dr. Call was the first woman elected to membership in the Massachusetts Medical Society, in 1884. She died on May 3, 1937, having achieved eponymic immortality through her sole contribution to medical literature.

EXNER'S LIFE

Siegmund Exner was born in Vienna on April 5, 1846, into a family of distinguished scholars.[1,2,4,5] His father had been professor of philosophy in Prague, and his three brothers also held important academic posts. He first studied under Ernst von Brücke in Vienna, where he published a paper on Brownian movement; then for a year in Heidelberg, where he was greatly influenced by the personality of Hermann von Helmholtz, famous for his physiologic investigations of the special senses. In 1871 Exner became assistant in von Brücke's laboratory. In 1875 he was made extraordinary professor at the Physiological Institute in Vienna, where he remained until called back to von Brücke's Institute, which he took over as ordinary professor in 1891. Exner's most important investigations were on the physiology of the eye and ear, nerve conduction, and the central nervous system, his outstanding contribution being *Die Localisation der Functionen in der Grosshirnrinde des Menschen,* published in 1881. His studies covered a wide range of other interests, however, including the structure and index of refraction of striated muscle, the innervation and musculature of the larynx, measurement of the width of the vocal cords by means of an instrument of his own invention, the physiology of flight in birds, the coloration of flowers, and the directional mechanism in carrier pigeons. From 1887 to 1893 he served as editor of the *Zentralblatt für Physiologie*. In his late years Exner became engrossed in the *Phonogrammarchiv,* with the idea of perpetuating the voices of important men. He died February 5, 1926, a few weeks before his eightieth birthday.

REFERENCES

1. *Biographisches Lexikon der hervorragenden Ärzte aller Zeiten und Völker,* 2nd ed. Ed. by W. Haberling, F. Hübotter, and H. Vierordt. Urban & Schwarzenberg, Berlin & Vienna, 1930, Vol. 2, p. 453.

2. Buess, H.: Sigmund Exner (1846–1926). *Schweiz. med. Wchnschr.,* **76**:284, 1946.

3. Call, E. L., and Exner, S.: Zur Kenntniss des Graafschen Follikels und des Corpus luteum beim Kaninchen. *Sitzungsb. d. k. Akad. d. Wissensch. Math.-naturw. Cl.,* **71**:321–28, 1875.

4. Durig, A.: Siegmund Exner. *Med. Klin.,* **22**:557–58, 1926.

5. Kreidl, A.: Sigm. Exner. *Ztschr. f. Psychol. u. Physiol. d. Sinnesorgane.* II. Abt. *Ztschr. f. Sinnesphysiol.,* **57**:281–87, 1926.

6. *New England J. Med.,* **216**:858, 999, 1937.

Max Walthard and the Walthard Cell Islands of the Broad Ligament

Tiny epithelial bodies with specific histologic characteristics are frequently encountered under the serosa of the broad ligament, in the wall of the fallopian tube, and, less commonly, within the substance of the ovary. Clearly demarcated from the surrounding tissues, these epithelial structures are usually composed of a cluster of flattened cells, sometimes with cavitation resulting from liquefaction of the center of the mass; glandlike formation is occasionaly seen; and not rarely ciliated columnar cells are present, which may produce a mucin-like secretion. These bodies are found most often in the genital tract of infants or young girls but may be seen also during sexual maturity and are by no means rare even in elderly women. Lacking only the dense fibromatous surrounding stroma of the Brenner tumor, the histologic similarity is otherwise so complete that most gynecologic pathologists now regard the tiny bodies as the site of origin of Brenner tumors of the ovary.

WALTHARD'S DESCRIPTION OF EPITHELIAL MASSES

The first description of these microscopic epithelial masses was recorded in 1887 by Werth,[3] in a study of extrauterine pregnancies. Several other authors, including Robert Meyer, called attention to them before they were redescribed in 1903 in the lengthy treatise on ovarian adenomas and inclusion cysts by Max Walthard,[2] whose name has since been eponymically associated with them, as Walthard islands, nests, or rests.

81

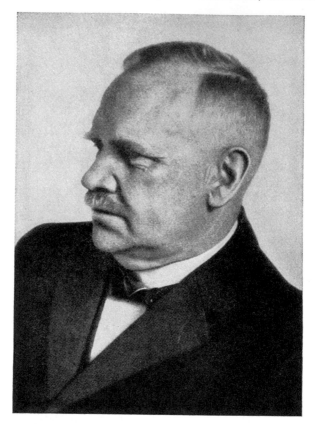

Fig. 11-1. Max Walthard (1867–1933). (Reproduced from *Zürcher Spitalgeschichte, 2:289, 1951.*)

Walthard's detailed description of the cell nests and his view concerning their origin appear in Chapter 4 of his monograph, accompanied by two illustrations (Fig. 11-2). Wrote Walthard:

While the granulosa masses partly disintegrate . . . and partly maintain a lumen in the larger masses and detach themselves from the ovarian epithelium and disappear after the first year of life, one still sees in later years, until after the menopause, cell rests of another sort, which bear a relation to the surface epithelium, projecting from it in fungoid fashion, or penetrating from the surface into the stroma, or lying more or less deep in the stroma, separated from the surface epithelium.

We see variations in the cell forms as well as in the relations of the cells to one another, depending upon the size of the masses.

In the smallest masses they are arranged so compactly, with elongated, flat, dark nuclei, pointed at one or both ends, that scarcely any space can be seen between two nuclei. Only among cells that lie in a looser relation to each other can one recognize that the nuclei lie in flat cells with scanty cytoplasm [Fig. 11-2].

In the larger masses the individual cells are also larger. Here the large, oval, pale nuclei lie a whole nuclear diameter and more apart. The individual cells are roundish in some places, oval in others, and polyhedral in still others, and contain a lightly granular, reddish cytoplasm. In the center of the mass they are usually less densely compressed than at the periphery, but here too without much intercellular substance [Fig. 11-2].

In many larger masses cavity formation occurs as a result of disintegration of the cells in the center. The lumens, which are sometimes oval but more often roundish, contain cellular debris and are lined by a smaller or greater number of foci of flat, densely crowded cells, depending on the intensity of the disintegration.

I observed one of these small cell nests in the middle third of the ovary of a 12-year-old girl, toward the front surface of which ovary, approximately halfway between the free cortex and the hilar margin, a plug of epithelium is penetrating into the substance of the ovary and is to be seen in constantly changing form in the next 24 sections.

At its site of origin [Fig. 11-2] the narrow strand, only four nuclei in diameter, penetrates into the stroma from the surface epithelium, forming a sharp angle with the ovarian surface, becoming gradually wider, and enlarging to a club-shaped field 0.105 mm long and 0.045 mm wide at its widest place. In the subsequent sections the field continues into the stroma, bending in a right angle and narrowing suddenly in the seventh section to a very thin strand containing only two nuclei in cross section.

After a distance of 0.1 mm the narrow strand again widens out suddenly, enlarging to an egg-shaped field 0.8 mm long and 1.05 mm wide in the subsequent sections. In the following sections the fields become smaller and smaller, with no significant changes in shape, finally disappearing in the twenty-fourth section.

In the thin strand as in the larger fields the oval, chromatin-rich nuclei, pointed at one or more often at both ends, lie only one fourth of a nuclear diameter apart and are thus very densely crowded together, so that in most of the sections the cell boundaries are not recognizable. Only in the second section of this mass, and in the later sections that contain the oval field, do the cells lie somewhat more loosely, and then a polyhedral cell form can be recognized in the dark cell margins.

Not all the cells are arranged with their nuclei parallel to their long axis. Just beneath the surface lies a group of nuclei that are all perpendicular to the field in view, so that the nuclei appear round and can only be recognized as elongated when one lowers and raises the microscope objective. The narrow end of the mass, adjacent to the surface epithelium, can only be seen in the second section of the mass, in which four oval, chromatin-rich nuclei lie directly next to each other and abut directly against the round, equally dark nuclei of the neighboring cuboidal ovarian epithelium. . . .

The connective tissue surrounding the cell mass is not so rich in nuclei as the connective tissue of the zona vasculosa, but contains just as many nuclei as many regions of the parenchymatous part of this ovary, which has a remarkably wide tunica albuginea amounting to more than half of the parenchymatous zone.

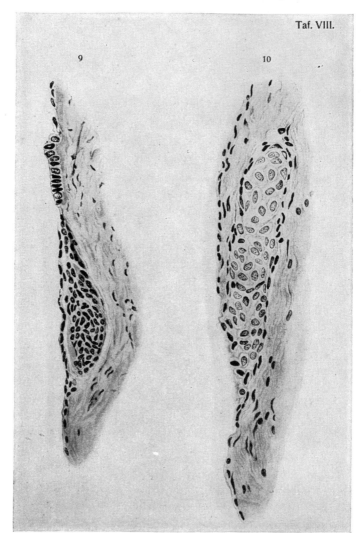

Fig. 11-2. Plate from Walthard's paper,[2] illustrating cell nests in the ovaries of two young girls. (Reproduced by permission of *Zeitschrift für Geburtshilfe und Gynä-kologie.*)

I observed a cell nest with larger cells [Fig. 11-2] in the ovary of a 14-year-old girl. In the middle third of this ovary . . . an epithelial strand 0.03 mm wide projected in a sharp angle toward the surface. In the cell nest large, oval, vesicular, pale nuclei lie widely separated from one another by a distance of a whole nuclear diameter and more, in the granular, reddish cytoplasm of large polyhedral cells. The nuclei are 0.009 mm long and 0.0045 mm wide. Near the surface the nuclei lie somewhat closer together; they appear somewhat darker and smaller than in the deeper regions. The end of the strand adjacent to the ovarian surface numbers five oval nuclei in clearly polyhedral cells, which directly adjoin the surface, denuded of epithelium. Immediately adjacent to the stroma the cell mass is bordered by a single row of small, flattened cells with narrow nuclei, 0.0066 mm long and 0.0015 mm wide; otherwise the connective tissue directly adjoining the cell mass does not differ from that of the remote areas.

Completely similar cell nests were found in another girl, also 14 years old, at different places among the normal germinal epithelium of both ovaries, penetrating from it into the stroma or directed toward the abdominal cavity as nodular aggregations perched on the surface of the ovary, as well as in relation to the peritoneal endothelium of the ovarian pedicle on the proximal side of the hilar cortex; also in an 18-year-old girl, in the middle of the parenchymatous zone, in the form of a round mass 0.225 mm in diameter.

. . . I have seen similar epithelial nests in the form of projections into the stroma or as nodules in the epithelium of the tubal fimbriae, as well as in the peritoneal endothelium of the tubal serosa, and also in the subserosa of the posterior surface of the ovarian ligament, in 1-year-old, 9-year-old, and 12-year-old girls.

Similar epithelial nests may still be found in mature and postmenopausal women also, always in relation to the surface epithelium. Changes in the epithelium, loosening of the cell relations, and cavity formation are seen, especially in the larger nests, as is shown by the following observation.

In the middle third of the ovary of a 65-year-old woman there was on the anterior surface of the hilus a structure, measuring 0.168 mm long and 0.042 mm wide at this point, which projects into the stroma in the next seven sections, and after five more sections is completely embedded in the stroma. Here the field attains its maximal size of 0.28 mm in length and 0.2 mm in width, diminishing in the following ten sections until it completely disappears. Large, clear, oval nuclei of 0.009-mm length and 0.005-mm breadth are seen in all the sections, separated from one another by half or even the whole length of a nucleus. In many cells, the cell borders take the form of reddish lines, which permit a polyhedral cell form to be recognized, and within which abundant granular cytoplasm surrounds the nucleus. Among these cells lie other individual cells with an irregular nucleus surrounded by a light, vacuolated halo, which compresses the reddish cytoplasm against the edges of the polyhedral cells. . . . A similar mass with abundant, irregular nuclei surrounded by a halo of light cytoplasm, is found nearby, likewise in relation to the peritoneal endothelium of the hilus. Its maximal length is 0.42 mm and its width approximately 0.04 mm. Nearby also, with a cavity formation in its interior, is a third cell mass in relation to the peritoneal endothelium of the hilus. The mass begins in the second section of the whole ovarian series and can be followed in 36 further sections. In sections 18, 19, and 20 its connection with the peritoneal endothelium can be shown and in section 26 the cavity inside the cell nest begins, ending with the mass in the last section, 37.

From section 2 to section 16 the aforementioned polyhedral cells with bright, oval nuclei lie next to one another without any intervening space, but in section 17 bright, clear spaces are to be seen between individual cells, which become progressively looser from there on, with the result that larger and larger, irregular, clear, empty crevices appear in the cell group. It is obvious that these spaces result only from shrinkage of the cells from each other and not from their displacement by secretion.

Arranged quite differently is the epithelium adjacent to the previously described cavity, which has an oval shape, attaining a maximal length of 0.49 mm and a maximal width of 0.28 mm in sections 27 and 28, and decreasing from here to the end of the cavity. Here the cavity is bounded by a row of concentrically arranged, flattened cells, which contain very dark, spindle-shaped nuclei up to 0.01 mm long within the eosin-red cytoplasm of their narrow cell bodies, [which range] up to 0.19 mm in length. The cavity contains eosin-red granular material, in which some cells with poorly stained nuclei may be seen. The cells of the mass adjacent to the flattened epithelium are arranged in two, three, or four layers closely adjoining each other; then the cell relations become looser, spaces develop, and only at the periphery of the nest are the cells again arranged with intervening spaces among them. The last row, bordering on the stroma, consists of cuboidal cells with bright, round, vesicular nuclei, and the adjacent connective tissue is indistinguishable from that located more remotely.

Similar masses of stratified squamous epithelium have been seen on the tubal serosa and on the undersurface of the mesovarium by v. Franqué, as well as by Schickele on the posterior leaf of the ala vespertilionis and on the broad ligament.

Stwitalski and Robert Meyer described similar structures, and Schickele saw them also on the surface of two ovaries and therefore regards the masses on the serosa of the broad ligament as resulting from the proliferation of the germinal epithelium from the surface of the ovary onto the broad ligament and the tubal serosa.

Since I pictured the fate of the germinal epithelial derivatives . . . in the ovary in Chapters 1 and 2, I cannot agree with Schickele's view.

In disagreement with Robert Meyer I maintain that I have seen the squamous epithelial masses not only in subserosal locations and in the peritoneal endothelium, but also in the ovary among the ovarian epithelium, and even deep in the ovarian stroma as well as superficially. Never did I observe any kind of inflammatory manifestations in the neighborhood of these masses and I can therefore not agree with Meyer's interpretation of the squamous epithelial masses in the ovary, but must regard them instead as congenital anlagen.

Gynecologic pathologists still disagree as to whether Walthard islands represent embryonic rests or the response to an inflammatory stimulus.[1]

WALTHARD'S LIFE

Max Walthard was born in Bern, Switzerland, April 7, 1867.[4] After concluding his schooling there he served for a brief period as assistant to Theodor Kocher, and then continued his studies in England, Germany, and France. In London he worked in experimental physiology under Horsley. In 1892 Walthard was appointed first assistant to Peter Müller at the Frauenspital in Bern, but soon quit to enter private practice. While in practice he maintained his interest in investigative work, carrying out a number of studies in pathologic anatomy and bacteriology. In 1908 he was appointed director of the State Frauenklinik in Frankfort-am-Main, and when the Universitäts-Frauenklinik opened in 1914 Walthard was made ordinary professor of obstetrics and gynecology. In 1920 he was called to Zürich, where he remained as head of the Universitäts-Frauenklinik until his death September 29, 1933, when he was succeeded by E. Anderes. Walthard contributed a section to the Veit-Stoeckel *Handbuch,* on the relation of the nervous system to functional gynecologic disorders, and was one of the first to recognize the importance of radiotherapy in gynecology. He is best known today for the cell islands to which his name is attached.

REFERENCES

1. Greene, R. R.; Peckham, B. M.; and Gardner, G. H.: Peritoneal bodies and cysts of the broad ligament. *Am. J. Obst. & Gynec.,* **57**:890–97, 1949.
2. Walthard, M.: Zur Aetiologie der Ovarialadenome. *Ztschr. f. Geburtsh. u. Gynäk.,* **49**:233–329, 1903. Ferdinand Enke, Stuttgart.
3. Werth: *Beiträge zur Anatomie und zur operativen Behandlung der Extrauterinschwangerschaft.* Ferdinand Enke, Stuttgart, 1887.
4. *Zürcher Spitalgeschichte.* Zürich, 1951, Vol. 2, pp. 289, 296–98.

James Douglas and the

Peritoneal Cul-de-Sac* | CHAPTER

12

The cul-de-sac is the rich domain of the gynecologist. Through its thin walls he palpates the pelvic viscera, ascertaining the size and position of the uterus and adnexa, outlining pelvic masses, and eliciting areas of tenderness, and plunges the culdescope for visualization of the pelvic contents; from its recess he drains pus in the treatment of pelvic abscess and aspirates blood in the diagnosis of ectopic pregnancy; he incises its trough in the performance of vaginal hysterectomy, and approximates its walls in the repair of enterocele.

Inseparably identified with this pouch of the peritoneum is the name of James Douglas, who first described it in 1730 in his famous treatise, *A Description of the Peritonaeum* (Figs. 12-1 and 12-2).[3] Less than a paragraph, however, was devoted by Douglas to the structure with which his name is now so constantly associated; little did he surmise the importance that subsequent generations would attach to it. Today many gynecologists, notably among the Germans, drop the word "pouch" in referring to the cul-de-sac and speak of it merely as "the Douglas."

Nowhere in Douglas' description are the terms pouch or cul-de-sac to be found. In fact, the French compound did not achieve its first use in the English language until 1737, seven years after the publication of Douglas' book, when Alexander Monro, professor of anatomy in the University of Edinburgh,

* This chapter originally published in *Surg., Gynec. & Obst.,* **101**:498–501, 1955; reprinted by permission. Copyright, 1955, by The Franklin H. Martin Memorial Foundation.

employed the term, in its present anatomic meaning, in describing the relations of the pelvic colon. Cul-de-sac is now used to denote any kind of blind alley or dead end. Wrote Monro: [6]

At the Part of the Mesocolon which connects the sigmoid Flexure of the Colon near the left Cavity of the Ilia, where in most adult Bodies there is an *Infundibiliform Cul de Sac,* or *Thimble-like* Cavity, I could never observe in Children more than one Part of the Mesocolon laid over the other, because of the great Flexure of the Gut at this Place; and therefore conclude the Cavity to be accidentally formed, by the growing together of the contiguous Parts of the *Mesocolon:* And that it is as needless to assign Uses to it, as it would be, to shew how useful the Concretion of the Lungs and *Pleura* is, which seldom misses to be observed greater or less in adult Bodies.

DOUGLAS' DESCRIPTION OF THE PERITONEAL CAVITY

The peritoneal cavity had been described as early as 3000 B.C., in the *Ebers Papyrus,* as a space in which the viscera are somehow suspended, but little was added to its understanding until Douglas' monumental work. Even then, Douglas' description received but scant attention, for abdominal surgery was still unknown, except for paracentesis and cutting for the stone. In his prefatory dedication of his book to Dr. Mead, Physician to His Majesty, Douglas stated:

It is now many Years since I first had the Honour to discourse with you concerning the Situation and Structure of the Peritonaeum; neither of which have, in my Judgment, been hitherto rightly described. When I began my Inquirys about this important Membrane, I had the Aetiology of several Diseases principally in view; among which were Dropsys, Hernia's, and some other accidents peculiar to Women.

Douglas' views on the anatomy of dropsy proved to be erroneous. He thought that the ascitic fluid collected in the "vesicular substance" lying between the anterior peritoneum and the transversalis fascia, and as it increased, pushed the peritoneum backward, thereby compressing the intestines against the vertebrae.

By contrast, his interpretation of umbilical hernia and omphalocele was remarkably accurate:

A fourth Production not always distinctly visible in Adults, reaching from the Navel of the Anteriour Point of the Bladder, contains the Urachus. So that in reality, all these Vessels are situated in the same manner with respect to the Peritonaeum, as the Viscera which are universally said to lie in its cavity. But what is still more observable about these Vessels is, that the Peritonaeum accompanys them through the Umbilicus out of the Abdomen of the Foetus, and thus

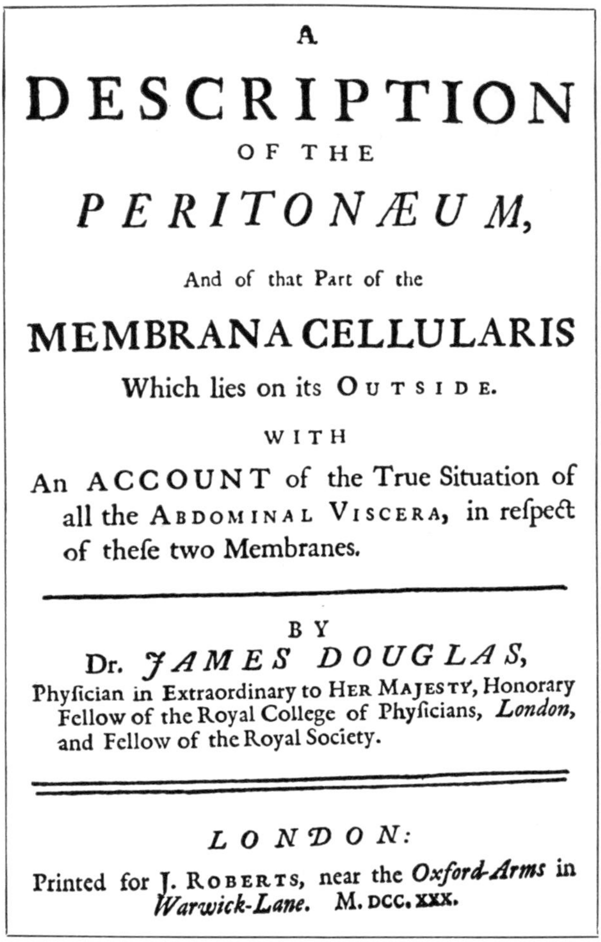

A

DESCRIPTION

OF THE

PERITONÆUM,

And of that Part of the

MEMBRANA CELLULARIS

Which lies on its O U T S I D E.

W I T H

An ACCOUNT of the True Situation of all the ABDOMINAL VISCERA, in refpect of thefe two Membranes.

B Y

Dr. *JAMES DOUGLAS*,

Phyfician in Extraordinary to HER MAJESTY, Honorary Fellow of the Royal College of Phyficians, *London*, and Fellow of the Royal Society.

LONDON:

Printed for J. ROBERTS, near the *Oxford-Arms* in *Warwick-Lane.* M. DCC. XXX.

Fig. 12-1. Title page of Douglas' book on the peritoneum.

becomes an Involucrum to the Funis Umbilicalis all the way to the Placenta. This may be easily exhibited to view in any proper Subject; but it became remarkably plain in a Child that I lately examined, in whom a Hernia Umbilicalis had been formed in Utero. Part of the Intestine was near two inches without the Navel, and the Peritonaeum which accompanied it, was evidently continuous with the Involucrum of the Funis.

Douglas' lucid explanation of the visceral and peritoneal relations has not been improved upon to this day:

. . . Concerning all the other viscera [except the omentum and part of the liver], it is to be observed, that no part of them immediately touches the Internal or concave smooth Surface of the Peritonaeum, and consequently they cannot be said

the two Incifions, the *Mefentery* forms a fort of longitudinal *Septum* going between the *Inteftines* and *Peritonæum*, and likewife another narrower Portion round the Edges of the fmall Guts, which is chiefly between the *Peritonæum* and *Colon*, being that part of the *Mefentery* termed *Mefo-Colon*. In this View of the *Peritonæum* we likewife perceive, that having reached as low down on the *Vertebræ* as the laft of the Loins, it ceafes to furround the *Inteftinum Rectum*, or, perhaps, the End of the *Colon* intirely, the pofteriour fide thereof being covered only by Veficular Subftance; and this bare fpace increafes in breadth as it defcends; the anteriour fide of the Inteftine remaining full covered by the *Peritonæum* all the way down to where it comes neareft to the *Veficulæ Seminales*: below this it is intirely furrounded by a thick Veficular Subftance, which here, if any where, deferves the Name of *Membrana Adipofa*, becaufe of the vaft Quantity of Fat contained in it. Where the *Peritonæum* leaves the forefide of the *Rectum*, it makes an Angle, and changes its Courfe upwards and forwards over the Bladder; and a little above this Angle, there is

is a remarkable tranfverfe Stricture or Semi-oval Fold of the *Peritonæum*, which I have conftantly obferved for many Years paft, efpecially in Women.

Spleen and Pancreas.

WHAT has been faid of the Stomach may likewife be applyed to the Spleen and *Pancreas*, both of them being involved by the *Peritonæum*, produced from where they are contiguous to it. The firft is feated in the left fide of the *Abdomen* nearly according to the length of the Body, reaching from the Diaphragm down below the Extremity of the twelfth Rib; the other lies almoft tranfverfely on the firft *Vertebra* of the Loins, above half of it being towards the left fide.

Liver.

The Liver has this peculiar to it, that a large Portion thereof is immediately joyned to the internal Surface of the *Peritonæum*, viz. all the fuperiour and back part of its convex Surface, which lies to the right of the *Ligamentum Latum*. This adheres clofely to part of the *Peritonæum* that lines the Diaphragm, the reft of it is involved in the fame manner as the other *Vifcera*, by means of feveral Folds which go from the *Peritonæum* in form of Ligaments, and are afterwards fpread on its

Fig. 12-2. Excerpt from *A Description of the Peritonæum* [3] containing Douglas' description of the cul-de-sac.

to be contained in its Cavity, as Liquor is in a Bottle, Money in a Purse, or in short, as any thing, whether Solid or Liquid, is in a Case, Bag, or Vessel, that simply surrounds it. To conceive therefore the Manner in which this is done, we must imagine the Peritonaeum as a Bag of a much larger Extent and Capacity than the Cavity of the Abdomen; and that the Viscera it contains being applyed to several Parts of its external Surface, thrust its yielding sides inwards, till at length the Edges of the Cavitys so formed by each Viscus, come to touch one another. Thus will the Capacity of the Peritonaeum be diminished in Proportion to the Number and Size of these Viscera; and each of them may be justly said to be contained in its Cavity, not only as they form particular Cavitys to themselves, where the Peritonaeum separately involves them, but as they all lie within the one common Cavity of the Abdomen lined by the Peritonaeum, considered as an uniform Membrane, without any regard to the particular Productions of it, which surround each viscus. From hence it is evident that the external Surface of the Peritonaeum alone is contiguous to the Surface of the Viscera contained herein. . . .

DOUGLAS' LIFE

James Douglas, brother of John Douglas the surgeon, was born in Scotland in 1675, but the details of his early life and training are little known.[1,4,7] There is not even a portrait of this important figure recorded in any of the great libraries or portrait galleries of Scotland, England, or the United States. After obtaining his medical degree in Rheims, Douglas settled in London, about 1700, where he developed a large and lucrative obstetric practice while carrying on his anatomic investigations. He ultimately achieved the position of personal physician to Queen Caroline.

In the winter of 1726 Douglas, together with Sir Richard Manningham, brought about the exposure of Mary Toft, a poor journeyman clothier's wife, who had achieved recent fame by professing to have borne large litters of rabbits. Of Mary the imposter's confession, Sir Richard later wrote: [5]

Accordingly on Wednesday December 7, in the Morning, in the Presence of . . . Dr. Douglas and myself, she began her Confession of the Fraud; and in her Confession she own'd, That upon her miscarrying she was seized with violent Floodings, and the womb was then . . . open as if she had been just deliver'd of a full-grown Child, she did verily believe one of her wicked Accomplices did then convey into her Womb part of the Monster . . . being the Claws and Body of a Cat and the Head of a Rabbet; this put her to much Pain: After that time she believed nothing was ever put into her Womb, but into the Passage only, by the Advice of a Woman Accomplice . . . who told her she had now no occasion to work for her Living as formerly, for she would put her in a Way of getting a very good Livelihood, and promised continually to supply her with Rabbets, and should therefore expect part of the Gain. . . . The Woman told her she must put up her Body so many pieces of Rabbets as would make up the Number of

Rabbets which a Doe Rabbet usually kindles at one time, otherwise she would be suspected. Mary Toft asked how many that was; the Woman told her, sometimes thirteen.

From that time Mary Toft did often, by the Assistance of that Woman, convey parts of Rabbets into her Body, till at last she could do it by herself, as she had an Opportunity to do so.

Douglas shortly thereafter published his own version [2] of the investigation, concluding with the statement:

I hope all breeding Women will depend on this as a certain Truth, that it is no less probable, that a Rabbit should conceive and be deliver'd of a Human Child, than that any Creature whatever, of an entirely different species, should be form'd in the Belly of a Woman.

Among Douglas' pupils were Albrecht von Haller and William Hunter. The latter came to live with Douglas in 1741, to assist in the dissections and supervise his son's education. Douglas died just 12 months later, on April 9, 1742, leaving also a daughter, Martha Jane, with whom Hunter had in the meantime fallen in love; but she too died two years after, at the age of 28.

In addition to his anatomic researches Douglas maintained a lively interest in botany, publishing papers "On the Flower of Crocus Autumnalis" and "On the Kinds of Ipecacuanha," a book entitled *Lilium Sarniense, or a Description of the Guernsey Lily,* and a full description of the coffee plant, including an account of the growth of the use of coffee as a beverage in England from its introduction during the reign of Charles I. Douglas was also noted as a bibliophile, his library containing the most complete collection of the editions of Horace in existence.

His reputation as an obstetrician was immortalized by Pope in *The Dunciad:*

> There all the Learn'd shall at the labour stand,
> And Douglas lend his soft, obstetric hand.

REFERENCES

1. *Dictionary of National Biography,* 4th ed. Ed. by L. Stephen and S. Lee. The Macmillan Co., New York, 1908, pp. 1234–36.
2. Douglas, J.: *An Advertisement Occasion'd by Some Passages in Sir R. Manningham's Diary Lately Publish'd.* J. Roberts, London, 1727.
3. Douglas, J.: *A Description of the Peritonaeum, and of that Part of the Membrana Cellularis Which lies on its Outside.* J. Roberts, London, 1730, pp. 37–38.
4. Graham, H.: *Eternal Eve. The History of Gynaecology and Obstetrics.* Doubleday & Co., Inc., New York, 1951, p. 308.

5. Manningham, R.: *An Exact Diary of What Was Observ'd During a Close Attendance upon Mary Toft, the Pretended Rabbet-Breeder of Godalming in Surrey From Monday Nov. 28, to Wednesday Dec. 7 Following. Together with An Account of Her Confession of the Fraud.* Fletcher Gyles, London, 1726.

6. Monro, A.: Miscellaneous remarks on the intestines. *Medical Essays and Observations,* rev. ed., **4**:76–92, 1737.

7. Oughterson, A. W.: James Douglas and the surgery of the peritoneum. *Yale J. Biol. & Med.,* **2**:331–39, 1930.

Anton Nuck and the Inguinal Canal

The inguinal canal in women, much narrower than in men, contains only the fanlike strands of the round ligament coursing through the abdominal wall to end in the upper part of the labium majus. The external inguinal ring is indeed so small in most cases as to be scarcely palpable. As the round ligament enters the inguinal canal during fetal development it is surrounded by a finger-like sheath of peritoneum, homologous with the processus vaginalis in the male. This diverticulum, known in the female as the canal of Nuck, usually becomes obliterated by the seventh month of intrauterine life but persists in some adults, variously estimated at 8 to 20 per cent, in whom it may provide a channel for subsequent hernia development or, if only a remnant of the canal remains, for later cyst formation.

According to Narbonne,[4] who included an excellent historic review of cysts of the canal of Nuck in his dissertation published in 1899, Aetius of Amida (500–575 A.D.) was the first to describe this tumor of the labium majus, based on the observations of the midwife Aspasia: "The aqueous hernia is a soft tumor occupying either or both of the labia majora and imparting a somewhat fluctuant sensation on palpation." Ambroise Paré, one thousand years later, cited the case of a girl of six or seven years with a collection of serous fluid in the inguinal region, which he treated by incision.

The female inguinal canal failed to attract the attention of anatomists, however, until the seventeenth century, when Swammerdam, in his *Miraculum Naturae*,[6] showed the round ligament encased in a membranous sheath of peritoneum, in his illustration of the female organs of reproduction.

95

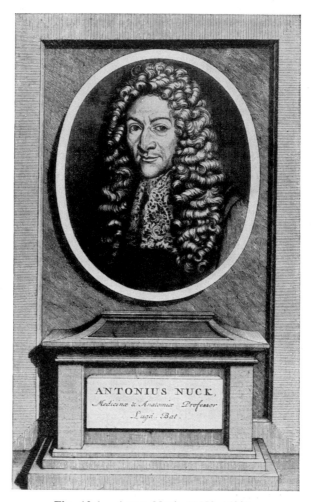

Fig. 13-1.   Anton Nuck (1650–1692).

NUCK'S DESCRIPTION OF THE INGUINAL CANAL

Nuck's interest in the inguinal canal developed from his efforts to explain the pathogenesis of inguinal hernia in women. His description of the canal that bears his name appears in Chapter 10 of the *Adenographia*,[5] published in Leyden in 1691:

It is most common among physicians, in dealing with hernias of the intestine or omentum, to attribute them to movement of the peritoneum, to excessive width or a tear or relaxation of the passages, so that part of the intestines or omentum escapes. In truth they should know that the same phenomenon occurs in

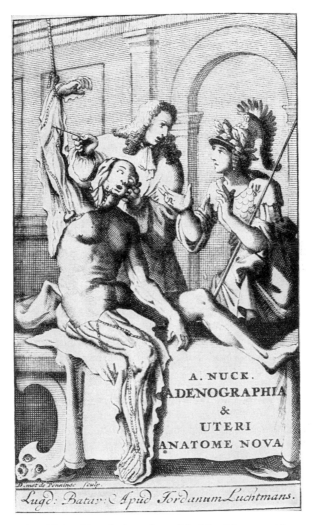

Fig. 13-2. Frontispiece from Nuck's *Adenographia.*

quadrupeds, even in marine animals, as in the human male, and that all hernias that I have examined in this sex have resulted from a forceful projection of the peritoneum, not actually from a dilated process but from a stretched part of the peritoneum, which is very pronounced in the inguinal region, alongside and in contact with the spermatic cord (lying under the peritoneum) and from pressure on the omentum, thus enveloping a more or less extensive saccular structure, according as a greater or smaller part of the intestines has been forced into it. The intestines or prolapsed omentum do not make such individuals uncomfortable, except from the pressure of the contents in the peritoneal sac, as long as the spermatic vessels remain undamaged and the pressure does not disturb the circulation of the blood. . . .

How do inguinal hernias arise in the female? This, in contrast to the hernias seen in the other sex . . . would seem difficult to explain. Indeed I have witnessed this many times, the intestines or the omentum slipping into the canal, either suddenly or gradually, and producing a swelling in the groin, from very violent motion of the body or from pregnancy, and often without the patient being at all aware of it. But our difficulty in this was that the peritoneum here has no accessible passage, and the tendinous parts of the abdominal muscles were not known to yield to the omentum or to the pressure of the intestines.

Indeed, so divergent were the opinions that I found among the anatomic and surgical authorities I first consulted, that I was unable to conclude anything definite from their writings. I therefore put my hand to the problem, and in the subject under investigation, the dog, I observed a sort of opening in the peritoneum, near the cornual fimbriae on either side and extending toward the inguinal region. Not knowing what it might be, I injected air through a tube into the orifice and immediately noticed a little vesicle arising from the peritoneum and extending obliquely through the tendinous parts of the abdominal muscles and toward the pubis. And I observed this many times afterwards, on one side or the other, whenever bitches were examined in our anatomy laboratory. Figure XXXIX [Fig. 13-4] shows the normal shape and size of these diverticuli.

Having discovered these spaces in animals, I worked with the greatest care in order to find the same in human female cadavers; but in no instance was this diverticulum demonstrated on both sides (in the same manner as it arises from the peritoneum in the animal). For I distinctly observed the round ligament, taking origin from the fundus of the uterus, ascending to the groin and approaching this opening, firmly attached to the side of the latter and of the whole diverticulum. Continuing, the part of the ligament going away from the fundus penetrates the tendons of the muscles obliquely, and after spreading out into fibers above the pubis, disappears in the region of the clitoris.

And although the diverticulum forms a continuous membrane with the peritoneum, the blood vessels of the former do not arise from the latter, but from the aforementioned ligament, which supplies very numerous blood vessels that produce exceedingly small branches dispersed through the diverticulum in every direction. Thus it is apparent that if one injects a colored solution into the blood vessels of the ligament he will see immediately that the membrane of the diverticulum shares in it.

When the form of these sacs is considered, we do not always find them of equal size, but their orifices, which are incorporated with the ligaments, are narrower, the ostium being about the width of a reed. The sacs themselves are actually a little wider, and we have often seen them admit the tip of the little finger. See Figure XL [Fig. 13-4].

And this is the reason why the intestine, having slipped into this diverticulum, is extricated from it with difficulty; for constricted as if by a noose, the intestine becomes inflamed and this leads to gangrene and death of the patient.

Occasionally, however, not only the orifice but the sac itself becomes sufficiently dilated in the course of time so that women may tolerate an inguinal hernia with-

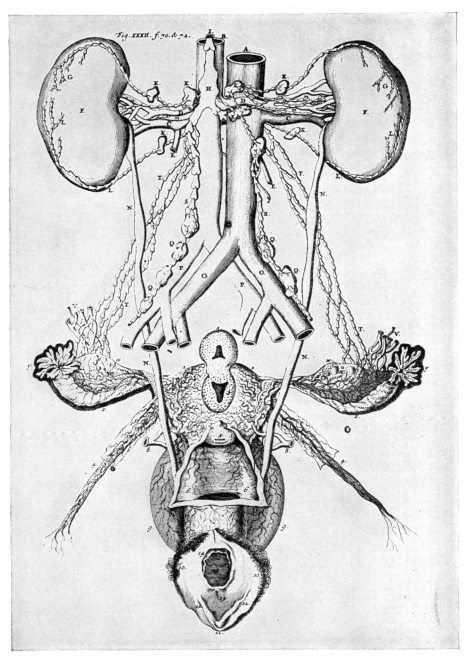

Fig. 13-3. Illustration from Nuck's *Adenographia*,[5] showing the lymphatics of the female internal genitalia.

out significant discomfort by pressing against the inguinal swelling and expelling
the prolapsed intestine from the diverticulum back into the abdominal cavity. But
soon thereafter, especially after strenuous exercise, if they move their body more
than usual, they fall again into the same condition.

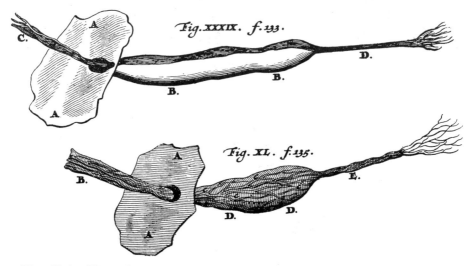

Fig. 13-4. Illustration from Nuck's *Adenographia*,[5] showing the round ligament
and its processus vaginalis in the dog (Fig. XXXIX) and human (Fig. XL).

The contents of inguinal hernial sacs in women, it was soon learned, are
not limited to the intestines and omentum. In August, 1706, only 15 years
after Nuck's publication, de Gouey[3] observed a rapidly growing pulsatile
tumor in the groin of a young woman. Upon incising the protruded peritoneum
he came upon a gestation sac harboring a live male fetus 6 in. long, probably
a herniated pregnant tube. The literature abounds with interesting, if less
spectacular, case reports of other viscera, including the bladder, herniated
into the canal of Nuck. The gynecologist must therefore be ever mindful of
such hernias, as well as hydroceles, of the canal of Nuck in his differential
diagnosis of inguinal masses.

NUCK'S LIFE

Anton Nuck was born in Harderwyck, the Netherlands, in 1650.[1,2] After
obtaining his medical degree in Leyden in 1677 he entered general practice
in Delft, but in 1683 moved to the Hague to accept a position as lecturer in
anatomy and surgery. Only four years later he was called to Leyden as professor of anatomy, where he remained until his death on August 5, 1692.
Here he established a great reputation as a teacher, soon took over the surgical
lectures as well, and made many noteworthy contributions to anatomic knowl-

edge and clinical science. Best known perhaps are his studies on the glands and the lymphatic system. Checking the earlier observations of Wharton and Steno, he redescribed the salivary glands on the basis of his own meticulous dissections in the human and carried out studies on the chemistry of the saliva and the factors influencing its secretion. He demonstrated the lymphatic vessels, nodes, and their connections by injections with air, mercury, wax, and a variety of colored solutions. Chapter 8 of his *Adenographia* contains the first description of the lymphatic network of the ovary. At first Nuck had the idea that the lymphatic vessels originated from the arterial capillaries and that the nodes consisted of conglomerates of tiny blood vessels, but his autopsy studies ultimately led him to a correction of this error. He also demonstrated the glandular structure of the female breast by injecting its ducts with mercury. He performed experiments on the artificial production of urinary calculi in the dog, and studied the spacing of the implantation sites in this species after ligation of one uterine horn. His clinical writings included instructions for the treatment of head wounds, nasal polyps, hydrocephalus, and deafness. He advised arterial ligation for aneurysms, paracentesis for ascites; described a technique for herniorrhaphy; and devised an original operation for cataracts. Much of his surgical teaching was recorded only in the form of incomplete notes, from which he gave his lectures. After his premature death at the age of 42, Nuck's surgical lectures were edited by one of his students and published under the title *Operationes et Experimenta Chirurgica*.

REFERENCES

1. Banga, J.: *Geschiedenis van de Geneeskunde en van hare beoefenaren in Neder-land*. W. Eekhoff, Leeuwarden, 1868, Vol. 2, pp. 645–54.

2. *Biographisches Lexikon der hervorragenden Ärzte aller Zeiten und Völker*, 2nd ed. Ed. by W. Haberling, F. Hübotter, and H. Vierordt. Urban & Schwarzenberg, Berlin & Vienna, 1932, Vol. 4, pp. 389–90.

3. Gouey, L. L. de: *La Veritable Chirurgie, établi sur l'experience et la raison. Avec des nouvelles découvertes sur l'Osteologie & sur la Myologie: des remarques necessaires sur les Maladies & sur la Pratique: Et un nouveau Sistéme sur la Generation du Fétus*. Pierre-Ph. Cabut, Paris, 1716, pp. 401–6.

4. Narbonne, P.: *Kystes du Canal de Nück*. Thesis, Paris, 1899.

5. Nuck, A.: *Adenographia Curiosa et Uteri Foeminei Anatome Nova. Cum Epistola ad Amicum de Inventis Novis*. Jordan Luchtmans, Leyden, 1691, pp. 130–38.

6. Swammerdam, J.: *Miraculum Naturae sive Uteri Muliebris Fabrica*. Severinus Matthaeus, Leyden, 1672, p. 34.

Alwin Mackenrodt,
Archibald Donald,
William Edward Fothergill,
and the Cause and Cure of
Uterine Prolapse

The unsatisfactory status of nineteenth-century treatment for uterine prolapse is well reflected in the multiplicity and character of the measures then in vogue.[13] These included local medication with astringents such as tannin and alum; cold sitz baths, surf bathing, and sea-water douches; postural exercises; "uterine gymnastics," which embodied anointing, massage, and manual replacement of the prolapsed parts; leeching; torsion of the uterus; intravaginal pessaries and uteroabdominal supporters; and attempts to produce fibrosis of the surrounding tissues by the introduction of gonorrheal exudate into the vagina, and even the deliberate induction of pelvic peritonitis. Surgical measures were equally numerous and varied, including shortening of the round ligaments through the inguinal canal; scarification of the vagina and chemical or thermal cauterization of the denuded areas; partial colpocleisis; infibulation, which consisted of union of the freshened surfaces of the labia majora; amputation of the cervix; perineorrhaphy; posterior colporrhaphy; anterior colporrhaphy; combined vaginal and abdominal operations, including ventrofixation of the uterus; posterior interposition of the fundus between the vagina and rectum; vaginal hysterectomy; and subtotal abdominal hysterectomy, combined either with colpoperineorrhaphy or with intra-abdominal support of the cervical stump.

The surgical approach to uterine descensus was greatly impeded during the first half of the century, of course, by the absence of anesthesia and the ignorance of asepsis; but even after these obstacles were removed, the

102

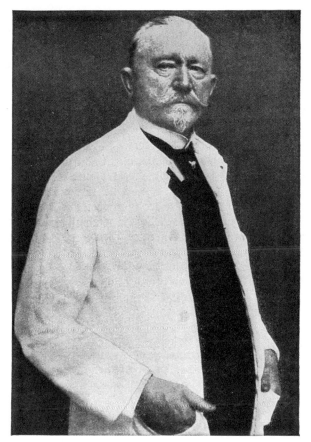

Fig. 14-1. Alwin Mackenrodt (1859–1925). (Reproduced from *Zentralbl. f. Gynäk.*, **50**:1041, 1926.)

rational, definitive treatment of prolapse remained handicapped by hazy knowledge and incomplete understanding of the uterine supports and the structures responsible for malposition. The position of the uterus was ascribed variously to the round ligaments, broad ligaments, uterosacral ligaments, uterovesical ligaments, intra-abdominal pressure, fullness of the bladder and bowel, the woman's posture, the pelvic peritoneum, the uterine muscle, the pelvic connective tissue, the elastic tissue of the pelvic blood vessels, the levator muscles, and the "vaginal tone."

THE CARDINAL LIGAMENTS

A significant contribution to the understanding of uterine retroversion was made by Bernhard Schultze [14] in 1872; but not until almost a quarter century later did Mackenrodt [8] publish his comprehensive and accurate description of the pelvic connective tissue, correlating uterine prolapse with specific anatomic deficiencies. In this paper Mackenrodt described the transverse cervical ligaments and stressed their significance for uterine support. These structures, usually known today as the cardinal ligaments, are also referred to as Mackenrodt's ligaments, in recognition of his demonstration of their anatomic relations and gynecologic importance. Wrote Mackenrodt:

Many gynecology textbooks assume a slit to be present in the apparatus that closes the inferior pelvic aperture, through which the urogenital canal and rectum make their exit. The idea persists that the inner genitalia, especially the uterus, close the genital opening like a sort of obturator. This assumption does not correspond at all with the facts.

The inferior pelvic aperture is closed by the visceral leaf of the pelvic fascia, a complex connective tissue plate containing muscular elements and elastic fibers, which should be regarded as a continuation of the iliac and transversalis fascia divided into several leaves that course in different directions. With the pelvic fascia we especially include the fascia of the small pelvis, whereas the iliac and transversalis fascias are part of the large pelvis and abdominal wall. While their course and relations in the male pelvis are delineated completely and very clearly, it is surprising that the textbooks of anatomy do not provide us with any satisfactory description of the important characteristics and variations of the pelvic closure in the female, especially concerning the role of the uterus.

The parietal pelvic fascia covers the obturator internus, the coccygeus, and the pyriformis muscles, forming the important obturator fascia in this region. More important to our present interest is the visceral layer, which takes its origin from the arcus tendineus, a thick tendinous band extending from the pubis to the ischial spine. It covers the levator ani (pelvic diaphragm), which likewise arises from the arcus tendineus.

If, in the pelvis of the newborn, one exposes this part of the pelvic fascia, which is readily accessible because it lies in large part directly under the pelvic peritoneum, then firm, bandlike, fibrous processes can be isolated, which attach directly to the uterine cervix, vagina, rectum, and bladder. These bands, arranged systematically, carry complex muscular elements as well as numerous bundles of elastic fibers, as shown by microscopic examination; they are very ductile, therefore. This whole ligamentous apparatus appears so excellent and extensive that it is quite surprising that it has not been recognized previously.

. . . Figure 6 [Fig. 14-2] is a median sagittal section through the pelvis of an eight-month fetus. . . . The dotted line on the corpus shows the line of attachment of the broad ligament. . . . Alongside the vertebrae the pelvic fascia is seen, with stout bundles of fibers emanating from it and inserting into the right side wall of the cervix. Above, this changes into a mass of fibers arranged in a flat band, which is bounded by the divided broad ligament of the uterine corpus. These masses of fibers extending from the pelvic fascia to the side of the cervix assume an important and independent position, so that we must sharply separate them generically from the broad ligament of the corpus. . . . The weak, chiefly perivascular con-

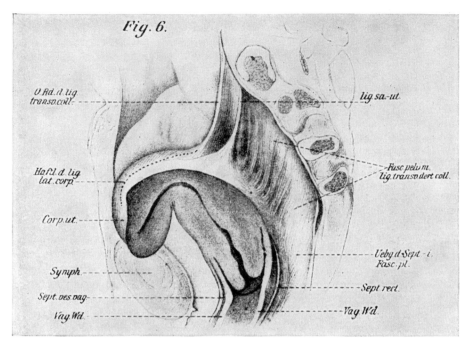

Fig. 6.

O.Rd.d.lig.
transo.coll.

lig.sa-ut.

Hafd.d.lig.
lat.corp.

Fasc.pelu.m.
lig.transo.dert.coll.

Corp.ut.

Ueby.d.Sept.-i.
Fasc.pl.

Symph.

Sept.rect.

Sept.oes.vag.

Sept.oes.vag.

Vag.Wd.

Vag.Wd.

Fig. 14-2. An illustration from Mackenrodt's paper,[8] showing the cardinal ligaments in a fetus of eight months. (Reproduced by permission of *Archiv für Gynäkologie*.)

nective tissue between the peritoneal leaves of the broad ligament, is sharply differentiated from the ligamentous structure beginning at the internal cervical os and continuing with the pelvic fascia, and presents only a loose connection with it. We are therefore justified in distinguishing the cervical ligament from the peritoneal fold of the corpus. Because of the anatomic and physiologic differences we no longer speak of the whole lateral ligamentous structure simply as the broad ligament, but only the peritoneal duplication attached to the corpus; while we designate the lateral ligamentous structure of the cervix as the transverse or lateral cervical ligament. . . . The purely connective tissue and muscular transverse cervical ligament is the principal means of support of the uterus, and in its upper edge it conducts the principal blood vessel of the uterus, the uterine artery.

The transverse cervical ligament has the following relations. In the fetus its upper edge extends inferiorly toward the midline to the side of the cervix, in the direction of the broad ligament, beginning near the last lumbar vertebra and inserting at the level of the internal os. Its fetal position changes in the course of later growth; the more the iliac fossae develop, the farther laterally is the origin of the ligament removed from the vertebrae, until it is moved into the transverse diameter of the pelvis when development is complete. . . .

At the level of the promontory, fiber bundles extend from the pelvic fascia and attach to the posterior wall of the cervix; likewise at the level of the internal os. These fiber bundles, of the same histologic composition as the transverse cervical ligament, are arranged at its upper edge into a rather stringlike band, the uterosacral ligament. Under this ligamentous thickening of the fibers, the latter are arranged in a very thin but still clearly fibrous plate, which forms a sharp angle with the mass of the transverse ligament.

Where the vagina is attached to the portio, fibrous processes, extending out from the transverse ligament, are arranged in a tubular membrane, which surrounds the vaginal wall and gives it a firm support all the way to the musculature of the perineum, there splitting into several layers. The posterior wall of this tube separates the vagina and rectum and is therefore called the rectovaginal septum; anteriorly it separates the vagina from the bladder and is called here the vesicovaginal septum. In addition to the fibers from the posterior pelvic wall, other special fibrous processes of the pelvic fascia attach to the rectum, giving the bowel firm support. The anterior wall of the tube of vaginal connective tissue, the vesicovaginal septum, proceeds anteriorly with the vagina and inserts directly on the arcus tendineus. This septum, pierced only by the urethra, thereby serves as a firm support for the bladder and the anterior corpus of the uterus that lies upon it.

At the level of the internal os still other fibrous processes extend from the transverse ligament, past the lateral wall of the bladder, and anterior to the part of the pelvic fascia that extends from the arcus tendineus to the posterior wall of the symphysis: the pubo-vesico-uterine ligament. . . .

Short fibrous bundles arise from the fascia of the levator ani, as a sort of inferior continuation of the transverse cervical ligament, and attach to the side of the connective tissue sheath surrounding the vagina, thus providing further support. These fibers disperse in front of the ischiorectal fossa. . . . This firm lateral attachment of the vaginal tube to the pelvic fascia results in a much smaller degree of mobility of the lateral vaginal walls than of the freer anterior and posterior walls, and results further in the fact that the side walls of the vagina never touch each other. The transverse diameter of the vagina is rather constant, while in the resting state the anterior and posterior walls remain in contact. The well-known H shape of the vagina finds its explanation herein. . . .

The closure of the inferior pelvic aperture of the female is thus pictured as a complex but extremely effectively arranged apparatus of ligaments and membranes, which extend from the pelvic fascia and come together at the uterus; this would therefore appear to be a very important part of the closure apparatus of the pelvis. The transverse cervical ligaments carry the brunt of the load, aided by the uterosacral and pubo-vesico-uterine ligaments. . . .

Applying his anatomic observations to an interpretation of normal uterine posture, Mackenrodt continued:

In the resting state, when the intra-abdominal pressure is least, the cervix is held, by its ligamentous apparatus, in its embryonic position, that is, in an arch concave anteriorly, and indeed in such a way that the uppermost quarter of the cervix is directed almost anteriorly, pointing toward the symphysis. The uterine corpus continues straight in this direction, its axis indeed directed toward the symphysis. . . .

Now the natural result of the typical anterior position of the cervix in its ligamentous apparatus is that with every increase of the intra-abdominal pressure the typical position of the uterus in anteversion-flexion is strengthened correspondingly. Even marked degrees of filling of the bladder and rectum can affect this position only within narrow limits, so long as the ligamentous apparatus remains intact.

Neither pregnancy, labor, nor the puerperium can produce any change in this position of the pelvic viscera, provided that nothing disturbs the involution of the organs. Not only can the birth process occur without producing serious lesions of the ligamentous apparatus, but the characteristic insertion of the genital canal in the closure apparatus of the external pelvic aperture makes it obvious that stretching of the cervical ligaments does not even occur in the course of labor. Dilatation of the centrally located cervical canal has just the opposite effect, displacing peripherally the ligaments inserting in its walls, with the result that the ligaments are shortened correspondingly. Stretching of these ligaments during labor is therefore out of the question. Only the vaginal tube undergoes any significant stretching, and this usually adjusts rapidly after delivery.

No definite stretching of the ligamentous apparatus occurs during the course of pregnancy either. The increase in volume of the ligamentous mass is simply attributable to the muscular elements and vessels, the later involution of which probably explains the diminution in size of the ligaments. The fact that prolapse occurs almost exclusively after an obstetric delivery does not militate against this concept, for descensus of the genitalia is attributable to atrophy of the ligaments or the internal pelvic musculature, which can develop during and after the puerperium. . . .

The mobility of the vagina is very slight, because of the tighter and shorter attachments of its side walls to the pelvic fascia. When the uterus is drawn down, the upper third of the vagina rolls or folds on itself so that, assuming normal relations, the uterus finds support in the natural resistance of the vagina below. If the ligamentous apparatus is relaxed or stretched, its physiologic elasticity is lost and the genitalia descend lower and retain this prolapsed position. The prognosis for spontaneous correction depends on the degree and duration of the attenuation of the ligaments. The prognosis is usually rather poor, therefore, because the tendency is not very great for reversal of the changes in the stretched ligaments and for strengthening of the relaxed ones.

Considering further the etiology of prolapse, Mackenrodt concluded:

The disposition is not infrequently an individual one, the basis of which is shown by evidence of a general nutritional disturbance in a certain number of cases, while the cause of atrophy of the uterine ligaments remains completely obscure in others. Although pathologic and normal births alike often cause descensus, one still occasionally finds complete prolapse in nulliparas who have been poorly fed while doing heavy work.

MACKENRODT'S LIFE

Alwin Mackenrodt was born near Nordhausen, Germany, November 12, 1859, the son of a country squire.[9] After his preliminary education in the gymnasiums of Nordhausen and Mülhausen, he entered Jena University in 1881 with the specific instructions of his strict father to study theology, as had his two elder brothers. So unsatisfying did he find this pursuit, however, that he soon abandoned it for medicine. He chose *Das Chloasma uterinum* as the subject for his doctoral dissertation, and after graduation served for a period as assistant in the surgical clinic of R. Volkmann before entering private practice in Strassfurt in 1886. A violent epidemic of diphtheria soon broke out in the region, claiming the lives of large numbers of infants. Mackenrodt's quick resort to tracheotomy, a little-known procedure in that community, soon won for him the reputation as the outstanding physician in the area, and his practice began to thrive. Becoming dissatisfied with the narrowly circumscribed opportunities of general practice in a small community, however, he gave it up in 1890 to enter the gynecology clinic of August Martin in Berlin as an unpaid volunteer. Within a few years Mackenrodt was one of the best-known gynecologists in Germany. In 1895 he founded his own clinic in Berlin, and in 1904 was given the title of professor in the university.

Mackenrodt's bibliography lists 73 titles, most of which relate to operative gynecology. He developed a technique for total abdominal hysterectomy for the myomatous uterus and also described a procedure for the vaginal removal of such tumors by morcellation. He devised an operation for the cure of bladder-neck fistulas with the aid of the interposed uterine fundus, and a vaginal approach for the cure of retroversion, which became known as the Mackenrodt operation. His procedure for the treatment of descensus and elongation of the cervix, described in 1894, was the forerunner of the Manchester operation. Patients were sent to him from all parts of Europe for the repair of urinary fistulas. Gynecologic cancer was the subject of Mackenrodt's greatest and most protracted interest, and he is said to have performed the radical abdominal operation for cervical carcinoma as early as 1894, but the results were so poor that he soon returned to the vaginal approach, using the cautery for the excision of the uterus and adnexa. He later returned to the abdominal operation, however, to permit access to the pelvic lymph nodes, and for the last 15 years of his life he employed a combined abdominal and vaginal approach. Mackenrodt died of pneumonia, December 29, 1925, in Berlin.

THE MANCHESTER OPERATION

Manchester lies at the hub of one of England's major industrial districts, whose chimneys belch forth their acrid smoke in large volume and without pause, polluting the atmosphere with bronchial irritants. Cough is endemic to the area. The wheels of Manchester's industry are turned in large part by women long inured to physical labor. This environment has continued to yield, year in and year out, a gynecologic clientele plethoric with cases of uterine prolapse. The treatment of this condition has consistently remained, therefore, a major interest of Manchester gynecologists; and it is only natural that the name of this center should have attained an honored position in the surgery of prolapse. Indeed, *the Manchester operation* is one of the rare medical eponymics associated with the name of a city rather than a person. The pre-eminence of the name of the community over that of its individuals can be explained also by the failure of historians to agree on the proper designee for the prolapse operation. What has come to be known, by default therefore, as the Manchester operation, is still referred to occasionally as the Donald or Fothergill procedure, in recognition of the roles of these Manchester gynecologists in the operation's development. The historically interesting question of priority remains beclouded by Donald's reticence to record his early surgical endeavors. As a result the Manchester operation is now credited to him by some,[12] while others [1] have named his contemporary, Fothergill, as the originator of the procedure.

Donald apparently acquired the germ of his operation for prolapse in 1888 while visiting Dührssen's clinic in Berlin. Until that time Donald had been using silver wire in his vaginal plastic work; but, observing the Germans' success with catgut, he switched to this material, which permitted the insertion of deep, buried sutures. He neglected to publish any account of his operation, however, until 1908, when a brief note [2] appeared, accompanied by diagrams drawn by Fothergill. In this, his only formal communication on the subject, Donald described his operation for complete prolapse as a very simple anterior and posterior colporrhaphy, including plastic repair of the cervix if the latter was lacerated or hypertrophied. Donald made no mention of utilizing the cardinal ligaments, although Fothergill, in the same year,[4] noted:

In the north of England several operators have for many years done anterior colporrhaphy in a way which enables them to bring together in the middle line in front of the cervix a good deal of the parametric tissue and a good deal of the paravaginal tissue of either side without endangering the uterus or the blood supply of the parts.

In a later paper [7] Fothergill added:

When I came to Manchester in 1895 I found that, owing to the initiative of my senior colleague, Professor A. Donald, the surgical treatment of genital prolapse was already highly evolved and most efficient. The anterior colporrhaphy incisions were larger than those I had seen, and the whole thickness of the vaginal wall was removed, not merely a superficial layer. Donald had also brilliantly combined the operation of posterior colporrhaphy and perineorrhaphy in a single operation done from above downwards. This was a great simplification and advance in the treatment of rectocele. For the last thirty years Donald has operated in Hospital four days a week and has cured an enormous number of cases of pro-

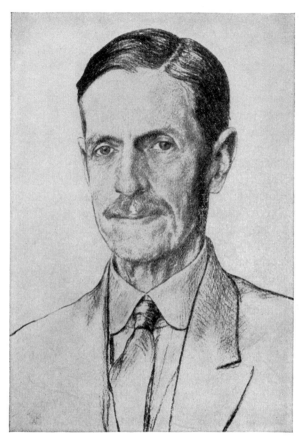

Fig. 14-3. Archibald Donald (1860–1937). (Reproduced from *J. Obst. & Gynaec. Brit. Emp.,* **44**:527, 1937.)

lapse by amputation of the cervix, extensive colporrhaphy and his own colpoperineorrhaphy.

DONALD'S LIFE

Archibald Donald was born in Edinburgh in May, 1860, and received his medical education in that city's university.[11,12,15] After a residency in the Royal Maternity Hospital he embarked on a voyage to India as ship's surgeon, resuming his obstetric training in 1885 at the St. Mary's Hospital in Manchester. Three years later he was appointed to the staff of that institution, one of the largest centers for obstetrics and gynecology in England. In 1895 he was elected surgeon to the Manchester Royal Infirmary, and in 1912 he was appointed professor of obstetrics and gynecology in the university, a position he held until his retirement in 1925. Until he withdrew from practice five years later, Donald remained the acknowledged leader in gynecologic surgery in the Manchester region; but for the dissemination of his surgical principles he relied largely on the direct instruction of those who came to watch him operate. "His modesty," wrote one of his followers, "so far as it concerned his own most valuable and original work was carried almost to the point of absurdity." His *Introduction to Midwifery*, written for students and nurses, went into eight editions and served as a standard text for midwives for many years. Donald died, at age 77, in April, 1937, probably on the seventeenth day of that month, although his date of death is variously recorded as the eighteenth and nineteenth in some of his obituaries.

FOTHERGILL'S WORK

In contrast to Donald's failure to describe the Manchester operation adequately in print, Fothergill wrote of the procedure repeatedly, with clarity, and at length. In his first paper on the treatment of prolapse,[4] published in 1908, the same year as Donald's meager note, Fothergill dismissed at once the theory, in vogue for over half a century, that cure of the condition depended upon narrowing of the vagina. Wrote Fothergill:

There is ample clinical evidence to show that inefficiency of the pelvic floor is quite a secondary and accidental factor. For we constantly see women whose perineums have been badly lacerated, but who present no symptoms of prolapse. Indeed, in cases of complete tearing into the rectum, prolapse is the rare exception and not the rule. . . . If the pelvic organs are loose, they will naturally descend more easily in a patient whose perineum has been torn than in one whose pelvic floor is sound; but inefficiency of the pelvic floor is a separable accident favourable to prolapse, not a cause of it.

In agreement with Mackenrodt's earlier observations, Fothergill recognized the cardinal ligaments as the key to the uterine supports, and his surgical application of this fact became the essence of his operation. He said:

The uterus itself is practically supported by the parametric tissue which lies below the free broad ligament, and above the vaginal fornices. This is the tissue which has been called the transverse ligament of the uterus.

The operation, as done by the writer, is begun by cutting across the vaginal wall between the cervix and the bladder. This transverse cut extends into the lateral fornices for about 1½ ins. on either side of the middle line. The bladder is then separated freely from the cervix and from the vaginal walls down to about 1½ ins. from the urethral aperture. The vaginal wall is then freely cut away. The portion removed is roughly triangular in shape, its base being at the vaginal roof and its apex 1½ ins. or so from the urethral aperture. The bladder, and with it the ureters, is pushed well up and out of harm's way. The uterus is also pushed up into the pelvis, and sutures are inserted so as to unite the parametric and paravaginal tissues to one another and to the anterior aspect of the cervix. These sutures may be buried, or they may be made to include the margins of the vaginal wall, so that when tied they bring together the portion of the original incision

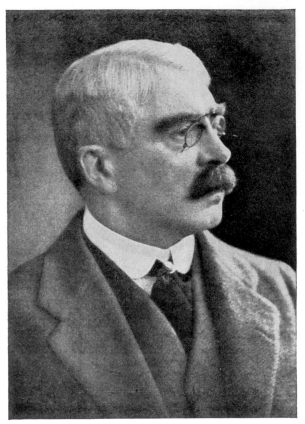

Fig. 14-4. William Edward Fothergill (1865–1926). (Reproduced from *J. Obst. & Gynaec. Brit. Emp.*, **34**:102, 1927.)

which is nearest to the cervix. In either case the result is to unite in front of the cervix certain portions of tissue which previously were widely separated and lay at the sides of the cervix and vagina. This effectively shortens the supports of the organs in question. As the lower part of the incision is closed, the sutures are made to penetrate the tissues underlying the vaginal wall, and thus the paravaginal tissue is drawn from the sides of the front of the vagina.

Despite Fothergill's exoneration of pelvic floor laceration as a cause of prolapse, he was equally insistent that posterior colporrhaphy be carried out as an adjunct to every prolapse repair.

It has been granted that relaxation or tearing of the pelvic diaphragm and of the perineum favours the prolapse of loose pelvic viscera by widening and straightening the canal through which they descend. Now, it is certain that the perivascular connective tissue, when once elongated, can never be perfectly repaired; and that pelvic organs which have once been loosened will always be loose. In every case, therefore, in which the operative treatment of prolapse is attempted, steps should be taken to improve the perineum and to narrow the vaginal canal, in order to check recurrence of the condition. In short, the operation of anterior colporrhaphy should always be reinforced by posterior colporrhaphy and perineorrhaphy.

Fothergill's view that ". . . unless the uterus is in such an unhealthy state that it is better away, it must be but rarely advisable to submit a patient to a hysterectomy in order to cure a prolapse" still represents the majority opinion among the gynecologists of northern England. Indeed, Fothergill's 1908 paper fails to advise amputation of even the prolapsed or hypertrophied cervix. Not until 1913 did he advocate cervical truncation as part of the procedure,[5] but this addition then remained a cardinal feature despite minor modifications of other details of the operation.[6,7] Of his combined procedure he now wrote: [6] "The operator who would secure success in operating for prolapsus must remove the cervix when it is ulcerated, badly lacerated, or hypertrophied, and when the uterus is more than three inches in length." In 1921 [7] Fothergill added the further improvement:

. . . that by carrying the colporrhaphy incision round behind the cervix instead of in front of it, anterior colporrhaphy and amputation of the cervix could be conveniently combined in a single operation instead of being done separately and seriatim. This not only saved time and trouble, but fully exposed the parametrium as well as the paracolpos. When the wound is closed, the stump of the cervix passes upwards and backwards so far that the uterus is left in a position of anteversion. This dispenses with the need for exaggerated narrowing of the vagina, a gain of some importance with a view to subsequent coitus and parturition.

Bickering still prevails over the relative contributions of Donald and Fothergill to the cure of uterine prolapse, but the principals themselves lusted not for priority. Indeed, Fothergill's writings make repeated and generous acknowledgment of Donald's role in the development of the operation. Sir William Fletcher Shaw, who lectured on this subject before an American audience in 1933 and discussed its historic aspects again in 1947,[16] sounded the note of compromise, in an effort to conciliate the partisans of both Donald and Fothergill, by suggesting that "rather than attach any individual operator's name . . . it was preferable to use one term to cover all such operations which include a double colporrhaphy with amputation of the cervix and suturing of the deep structures and, as the operation was developed in Manchester and has been continuously employed in that school for fifty-nine years, it seems reasonable to employ the generic term of 'The Manchester Operation.' " This has become its commonest designation.

FOTHERGILL'S LIFE

William Edward Fothergill was born in Southampton, October 4, 1865, descended from a brother of John Fothergill, the distinguished eighteenth-century physician.[1,3,10] William represented the sixth generation of his family boasting a doctor of medicine. He entered the University of Edinburgh at the age of 17 for the study of arts and sciences, continued into the medical curriculum, and graduated in 1893 with many prizes and honors, including a scholarship in obstetrics and gynecology. For the next two years he served as assistant to Professor Alexander R. Simpson in the gynecologic wards of the Royal Infirmary and at the Maternity Hospital. In 1895 he began practice in Manchester, exactly ten years after Donald had migrated to that city. The first of five editions of Fothergill's *Manual of Midwifery* was published the next year, followed in 1897 by his doctoral thesis, *The Ultimate Fate of Placental Tissue Retained in Utero,* for which he was awarded a gold medal. His *Manual of Diseases of Women,* which appeared in 1910, was regarded as a radical departure from the standard gynecology texts in its arrangement of material, the disorders being classified according to their pathologic basis rather than organ of involvement. During the period 1899 to 1905, while serving as director of the clinical laboratory in the Royal Infirmary, Fothergill introduced radiology to Manchester. In 1908 he was appointed assistant gynecologic surgeon to that hospital, where he ultimately advanced to the post of senior surgeon on Donald's retirement. In the University of Manchester, Fothergill rose through the academic ranks, from the position of lecturer in 1901 to professor of clinical obstetrics and gynecology in 1925. He died suddenly on November 4, 1926, following an after-dinner speech.

Fothergill was one of the founders of the *Journal of Obstetrics and Gynaecology of the British Empire,* and it is said that he did more than any other English physician to stress the unity of obstetrics and gynecology and bring about a coordination of their teaching. He maintained a special interest in athletics and loved after-hours relaxation with his students and house officers. One of the latter, at a house staff–faculty party, sang of Fothergill in the manner of Gilbert and Sullivan:

> A "Webster's-Sling" young man,
> A tongue-with-a-sting, young man,
> A man who glories in dubious stories,
> Colporrhaphy-King young man!

REFERENCES

1. Brentnall, C. P.: A note on Fothergill's colporrhaphy. *J. Obst. & Gynaec. Brit. Emp.,* **54**:164–71, 1947.
2. Donald, A.: Operation in cases of complete prolapse. *J. Obst. & Gynaec. Brit. Emp.,* **13**:195–96, 1908.

3. Fairbairn, J. S.: William Edward Fothergill. *J. Obst. & Gynaec. Brit. Emp.*, **34**:102–6, 1927.

4. Fothergill, W. E.: On the operative treatment of displacements of the pelvic viscera. *Tr. Edinburgh Obst. Soc.*, **33**:129–45, 1908.

5. Fothergill, W. E.: Clinical demonstration of an operation for prolapsus uteri complicated by hypertrophy of the cervix. *Brit. M. J.*, **1**:762–63, 1913.

6. Fothergill, W. E.: Anterior colporrhaphy and amputation of the cervix combined as a single operation for use in the treatment of genital prolapse. *Am. J. Surg.*, **29**:161, 1915.

7. Fothergill, W. E.: The end results of vaginal operations for genital prolapse. *J. Obst. & Gynaec. Brit. Emp.*, **28**:251–55, 1921.

8. Mackenrodt, A.: Ueber die Ursachen der normalen und pathologischen Lagen des Uterus. *Arch. f. Gynäk.*, **48**:394–421, 1895.

9. Mackenrodt, H.: Alwin Mackenrodt. *Zentralbl. f. Gynäk.*, **50**:1041–50, 1926.

10. Obituary: William Edward Fothergill, M.D., B.Sc.Edin. *Lancet*, **211** (2): 1034–35, 1926.

11. Obituary: Archibald Donald, M.D.Edin., F.R.C.P.Lond., F.C.O.G. *Lancet*, **1**:1078–80, 1937.

12. Obituary: Archibald Donald, LL.D., M.D., F.R.C.P., F.C.O.G. *Brit. M. J.*, **1**:891–93, 1937.

13. Ricci, J. V.: *One Hundred Years of Gynaecology: 1800–1900.* Blakiston Co., Philadelphia, 1945, pp. 269–97.

14. Schultze, B. S.: Ueber Versionen und Flexionen, special über die mechanische Behandlung der Rückwärtslagerungen der Gebärmutter. *Arch. f. Gynäk.*, **4**:373–417, 1872.

15. Shaw, W. F.: Archibald Donald. *J. Obst. & Gynaec. Brit. Emp.*, **44**:527–35, 1937.

16. Shaw, W. F.: The Manchester operation for genital prolapse. *J. Obst. & Gynaec. Brit. Emp.*, **54**:632–35, 1947.

Anders Adolf Retzius
and the Prevesical Space

The constantly changing volumetric relations of the bladder require a distensible and elastic environment that can accommodate to the filling and emptying of this viscus. Nature has met this need in admirable fashion, partly encompassing the bladder, like the rectum, with a cushion of areolar connective tissue, encased in the resilient prevesical space, or space of Retzius. Part of the potential extraperitoneal space that extends from the pelvic floor to the umbilicus, and bounded anteriorly by the posterior surface of the pubes and the posterior sheath of the rectus muscles, the space of Retzius limits the spread of infection, hemorrhage, and urinary extravasation from extraperitoneal injury to the bladder.

Primarily the province of the urologist, the space of Retzius also recognizes the rights of the obstetrician-gynecologist to its recesses. The latter's long familiarity with this space, acquired over the years in the performance of pubiotomy, extraperitoneal cesarean section, and anterior colporrhaphy for cystourethrocele, has been greatly augmented by a host of newer gynecologic procedures, such as the sling operations for urinary incontinence, suprapubic suspension of the urethra, and the radical operations for uterine cancer.

RETZIUS' DESCRIPTION OF THE PREVESICAL SPACE

The prevesical space and its contents were first mentioned by Retzius, but only in an incidental manner, in his 1849 description of the pubo-prostatic ligament.[5] Wrote Retzius:

116

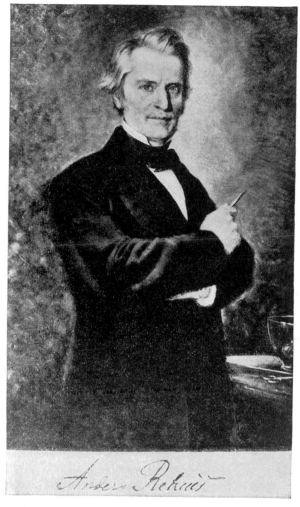

Fig. 15-1. Anders Adolf Retzius (1796–1860).

The thin capsule of the urinary bladder, which membrane is usually described as a part of the pelvic fascia and continues laterally into the arcus tendineus, proceeds from the inferior part of the bladder over the prostate. After reaching this organ it becomes firmly attached to the gland. The anterior part of the levator ani lies adjacent to the side of this capsule, without the support of a fascia of its own. Thinnest at the posterior surface of the gland, the fascia descends between it and the rectum, proceeds under the prostate, covers the posterior part of the muscular apparatus of the urethra near the site where Cowper's glands are embedded in the latter, and stretches laterally to the ascending rami of the ischium, to which it attaches. Between these places of insertion it descends loosely behind the urethral bulb and ends in a sharp angle at the so-called triangular ligament. It proceeds laterally to the sides of the prostate, where the capsular ligament is strongest, to attach to the rami of the respective ischium and pubis. The sides of the capsule are thus stretched like a tent, and after leaving the prostate, cover the rich venous pudendal plexus lying alongside it, together with the accompanying arteries and nerves. The attachment at the lateral margins of the pelvic opening extends from the horizontal ramus of the pubis to the vicinity of the ischial tuberosity. The anterior margins of these lateral parts comprise the aponeurotic part of the puboprostatic (pubovesical) ligament; the posterior, which extend over the bundles of the urethral muscle arising from the ischii, stretch out into two strands, like the corners of a four-cornered tent. . . . Superiorly the capsule wall touches only a small part of the prostate; and after leaving the prostate and bladder, is stretched out by muscle strands from the latter, to reach the adjacent surface of the pubes. . . . The pubovesical ligaments are the stretched, strandlike bands thus formed. Between them, above the urethra and prostate, and behind the symphysis . . . the capsule forms a deep fossa.

The surgical-anatomic significance of the properitoneal space was later elucidated by the distinguished Viennese anatomist Hyrtl, in his *Handbuch der Topographischen Anatomie.*[1] He wrote:

Most important is the cellular layer between the inner surface of the transverse abdominal muscle (or actually the transversalis fascia) and the peritoneum. It is particularly well developed, adipose, and multilayered in the lower abdominal region. . . . The extensibility, the laminated structure of this connective tissue layer, and the ease with which it can be dissected, make it possible to separate the peritoneum from the abdominal muscles with the palm of the hand and to perform certain abdominal operations, such as extraperitoneal cesarean section and ligation of the aorta or the external iliac artery within the pelvis, without opening the abdominal cavity. It becomes even more important in the case that rather large masses of fat developing in it dilate the small openings in the abdominal aponeuroses for the blood vessels, as a result of abdominal pressure, or project through normal openings in the abdominal wall and present outwardly as fatty hernias (which are probably often taken for incarcerated omental hernias). . . . It is noteworthy that abscesses forming in this deep layer of connective tissue are more likely to rupture toward the outside, through all the layers of the abdominal wall, than inwardly into the peritoneal cavity.

The relations of the anterior abdominal extraperitoneal space were further elaborated by Retzius at the November 4, 1856, meeting of the Swedish Medical Society in Stockholm,[6] in which presentation the prevesical space was described accurately and in detail for the first time. Retzius also communicated his observations privately to his Viennese friend and colleague, Hyrtl, together with three colored plates; and at the March 26, 1858, meeting of the Royal Scientific Academy in Vienna, Hyrtl publicized Retzius' discovery and referred to the prevesical space as the *Cavum praeperitoneale Retzii*. In the published account of Hyrtl's report,[2] the observations of Retzius were summarized in nine statements:

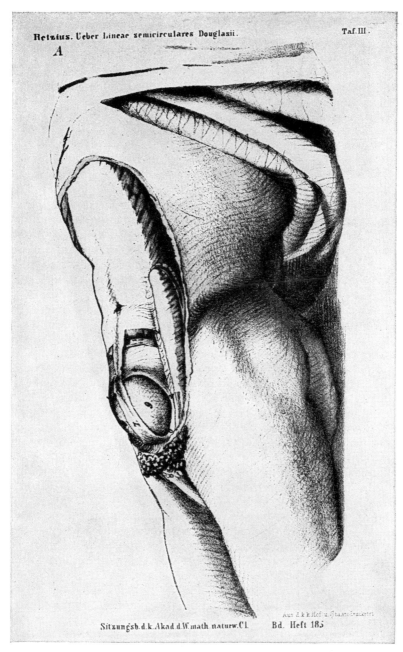

Fig. 15-2. One of Retzius' illustrations of the prevesical space, occupied by the full bladder (9). (Published by Hyrtl.[2])

1. The transversalis fascia, which forms a fibrocellular layer lying on the inner surface of the transverse abdominal muscles, fuses with the lower border of the posterior, incomplete sheath of the rectus muscles, which is formed by the aponeurosis of the transverse abdominal muscles. This fusion corresponds to the semicircular line of Douglas.

2. The transversalis fascia and the aponeurosis of the transverse abdominal muscle do not end at the semicircular line of Douglas, however, as they appear to, but they both fuse into a simple fibrous sheet that continues in the same direction and also laterally and posteriorly, and covers the part of the peritoneum that forms the posterior sheath of the rectus, from the line of Douglas down to the pubic symphysis. . . .

3. There thus results a space or a cavity in the lower part of the anterior abdominal wall, which Professor Retzius calls *Cavum praeperitoneale* and in which the distended bladder rises up from below.

4. The part of the fibrous leaf that joins with the peritoneum, arrives in its descent neither at the pubic symphysis nor at Poupart's ligament, but instead goes behind the bladder and down into the pelvic cavity, where it joins with the pelvic fascia.

5. The semicircular lines of Douglas, projected laterally and inferiorly in an arch, fuse with the transversalis fascia, which follows the body of its muscle almost to the external edge of the rectus tendons.

6. A ring or opening thus results, bounded by fibrous edges that form a sort of entrance to the aforementioned *Cavum praeperitoneale*. If the full bladder invades this space, its anterior and posterior walls are separated widely from each other. Its anterior wall is then formed by the lower ends of the rectus muscles and the outer leaf of their sheath; its posterior wall, by the peritoneum, which is covered with the surrounding aponeurosis extending from the lines of Douglas posteriorly; and its lateral walls, by the folds of Douglas and their semilunar processes.

7. Filling this space is a type of connective tissue which, because of its extensibility and pliability, offers no resistance to the rise and fall of the fundus of the bladder in the filling and emptying of this organ.

8. In order to see these relations simultaneously and to appreciate their actual existence, it is necessary to remove the external and internal oblique abdominal muscles in such a way that only a narrow rim of aponeurosis remains attached to the rectus sheath. The rectus sheaths are opened from umbilicus to pubis by means of two longitudinal incisions, one on either side of the linea alba, the muscles are removed, the semicircular lines of Douglas and their curved continuations put on a stretch with a hook . . . the peritoneum with its fibrocellular layer depressed, and the bladder made to rise into the *Cavum praeperitoneale* by filling with air or water.

9. Concerning the linea alba, Retzius observes that below the umbilicus this shows no fibrous septum that could separate the two rectus muscles from each other completely (as is the case above the umbilicus), but presents instead only a thin strip of connective tissue, which separates the recti from each other only incompletely and continues into the connective tissue that occupies the *Cavum praeperitoneale*.

In a gracious tribute to Retzius, Hyrtl concluded:

Any further discussion of this condition I consider as *Ilias post Homerum*. All the discoveries of my learned friend have assumed an incontestable place in science, and through the proposed publication of this report by the Royal Academy a similar place will also be accorded the *Cavum praeperitoneale* and the *Porta vesicae Retzii*.

RETZIUS' LIFE

Anders Adolf Retzius was born October 13, 1796, in the university town of Lund, Sweden, where his father, the author of an important work on the fauna of Sweden, occupied the chairs of natural history and chemistry.[3,4,7,8] Influenced toward the natural sciences by Arvid Florman, professor of anatomy in the university, young Retzius studied there until the age of 19, when he transferred to the University of Copenhagen, attracted by the Danish anatomist Ludwig Jacobsson. Returning to his native city, he received his medical degree in 1819 after publication of his graduation thesis on the structure of sharks and rays. In his investigation of elasmobranchs, Retzius discovered the interrenal organ, later shown to be homologous with the adrenal cortex of higher forms. After completing a subsequent course of study for master of surgery at the Carolinian Institute in Stockholm, he spent four years in the military service as surgeon to a regiment of hussars, following which he was chosen professor of comparative anatomy in the Veterinary School of Stockholm.

In a debate in 1824 on the anatomy of the eye Retzius showed such wide knowledge that Jacob Berzelius, the head of the Carolinian Institute, arranged for his appointment to the chair of human anatomy and physiology in the institute. For several years Retzius was permitted to retain his position in the veterinary school as well, because of the larger stipend it provided, but he relinquished this post in 1830, and soon thereafter was made rector of the institute. In the ensuing years he made several trips to England and the Continent, cultivating close personal friendship and scientific collaboration with Purkinje, Johannes Müller, and many other outstanding medical scientists of Europe, with whom he maintained an extensive correspondence. In 1839 he was appointed professor of anatomy in connection with painting at the Royal Academy of Arts. Retzius never engaged in private practice but achieved wide renown as a teacher. Despite the fact that the Carolinian Institute lacked the authority for conferring a medical degree at that time, many students from Upsala and Lund were attracted to his courses in anatomy, returning to their own universities for their examinations. In 1858 Retzius was elected president of the Royal Academy of Sciences of Stockholm, and was honored by the King with the Order of the Lion of the Netherlands. He died of a volvulus on April 18, 1860. Gustav, his son, later wrote of him in a letter:

And each Spring when the ice broke up, he took me with him to Kungsholm-brunn, where we clattered down on the stone piers to the water's edge and gathered small water animals, infusoria, bryozoans, and worms, which we took home to the aquaria. I shall never forget my father's enthusiasm when he observed under the microscope the wonderful life which was unfolded in the waters of these aquaria, and of which he with his spirited descriptive art tried to give me an inkling.*

Although he produced no single work of outstanding magnitude, Retzius, like Johannes Müller, contributed an impressive list of monographs in a wide variety of scientific fields. The titles of his publications fill three closely printed pages in the *Swedish Biographical Lexicon*. His interest in marine fauna persisted throughout his life. Other contributions included his demonstration of the connections between the anterior as well as the posterior spinal nerve roots and the sympathetic chain; studies on the finer structure of the avian lung, the atrial septum and semilunar valve of the heart, the transverse processes of the thoracic and lumbar vertebrae in human beings and various other species, the histology of the liver, and the pyloric antrum and abnormalities of its orifice. He conducted experiments on the ligation of arteries and the effect of vagotomy on the digestive process; described the ciliary and sphenopalatine ganglia in the horse; discovered the peripheral canal of the cornea, later called the canal of Schlemm; undertook a microscopic dental investigation that led to his description of the brown striae of the teeth, or contour lines of Retzius; discovered the small convolutions between the hippocampus and dentate nucleus of the brain, later named the gyri of Retzius by his son; and described a ligament of the ankle, known as the ligament of Retzius. Named for him also are the veins of Retzius, which unite the radicles of the splenic and mesenteric trunks of the portal vein with the branches of the inferior vena cava. Together with Müller, who accompanied him on a trip to the coast of Sweden in 1841, Retzius described the morphology of amphioxus and clarified some problems of its physiology. He also carried out horticultural experiments, introducing many new plants into Sweden; published an essay on the castration of cattle; and wrote on sanitation and the water supply of Stockholm.

Retzius is perhaps best remembered as an anthropologist. The races of mankind had been classified on the basis of skin color and geographic habitat until 1842, when Retzius introduced the new science of craniometry and proposed a classification based on the cephalic index, distinguishing between the dolichocephalic and the brachycephalic races. His ethnographic inquiries led to the study of exhumed skulls of the early inhabitants of Sweden and culminated in his description of the skull form later designated as typically

---

* Reprinted by permission of the publishers, Abelard-Schuman Limited. From *Annals of Medical History*. Copyright 1924.

Nordic. In recognition of his pioneering efforts in physical anthropology the Association of Scandinavian Naturalists elected him chairman of its section for ethnology.

The faculty with which Retzius was identified during most of his professional life now has the honored responsibility for awarding the Nobel prize in medicine. The institution's present distinction is traceable in large measure to the energy, administrative ability, and personality of Anders Retzius and the scientific tradition he helped establish.

REFERENCES

1. Hyrtl, J.: *Handbuch der Topographischen Anatomie, und ihre Praktisch Medicinisch-Chirurgischen Anwendungen*, 3rd ed. Braumüller, Vienna, 1857, Vol. 1, p. 513.

2. Hyrtl, J.: Notiz über das Cavum praeperitoneale Retzii in den vorderen Bauchwand des Menschen. *Sitzungsb. d. k. Akad. d. Wissensch. Math.-naturw. Cl.,* **29**:259–64, 1858.

3. Larsell, O.: Anders Adolf Retzius (1796–1860). *Ann. M. Hist.,* **6**:16–24, 1924.

4. Obituary: Andreas Retzius. *Lancet,* **1**:483, 1860.

5. Retzius, A.: Om Ligamentum pelvioprostaticum eller den apparat med Lvilken bläsan, prostata och urinröret äro fästade vid nedre bäckenöppningen. *Hygiea,* **11**:321–26, 1849. Translated from the Swedish by F. Creplin: Ueber das Ligamentum pelvioprostaticum oder den Apparat, durch welcher die Harnblase, die Prostata und die Harnröhre an der untern Beckenöffnung befestigt sind. *Arch. f. Anat., Physiol. u. wissensch. Med.,* 182–90, 1849.

6. Retzius, A.: Den stora öppningen, som förefinnes på den främre bukväggens bakre sida, emellan nafveln och blygdknölarna, och som uppkommer genom den egna gången af fascia transversa, för hvilken öppning Hr. R. föreslår benämringen af blåsporten. *Hygiea,* **18**:792–94, 1856.

7. Retzius, G.: *Skrifter I Skilda Ämnen Jämte Några Bref af Anders Retzius.* A. B. Nordiska Bokhandeln, Stockholm, 1902.

8. Wilson, C.: Obituary notice of Professor Anders A. Retzius, foreign corresponding member of the Medico-Chirurgical Society of Edinburgh. *Edinburgh M. J.,* **6**:777–83, 1861.

William Hunter, in his *Medical Commentaries,*[6] stated: "It is remarkable, that there is scarce a considerable character in anatomy, that is not connected with some warm controversy. Anatomists have ever been engaged in contention. And indeed, if a man has not such a degree of enthusiasm, and love of art, as will make him impatient of unreasonable opposition, and of encroachments upon his discoveries and his reputation, he will hardly become considerable in anatomy, or in any other branch of natural knowledge." This philosophic comment, which accompanied Hunter's reply to Monro's attack on him, scarcely anticipated the intrigue, calumny, and vituperation associated with the search for the neural apparatus of the human uterus. In their zealous efforts to trace the pathways by which pain of uterine origin is mediated and through which uterine contractility is effected, anatomists have long sought to demonstrate the complex nervous connections in the pelvis. Modern gynecologists have shown renewed interest in these structures, because of their possible importance in vascular disturbances in the pelvic viscera and because of the impaired function of adjacent organs, especially the bladder, resulting from radical hysterectomy for cervical cancer.

From the early-eighteenth century de Graaf, Eustachius, John Hunter, and others had claimed to follow the pelvic nerves into the uterus, but their illustrations were schematic and their descriptions inadequate. As recently as 1829 Osiander, in the second edition of his textbook of obstetrics,[18] recanted his previous statements concerning the presence of nerves within

124

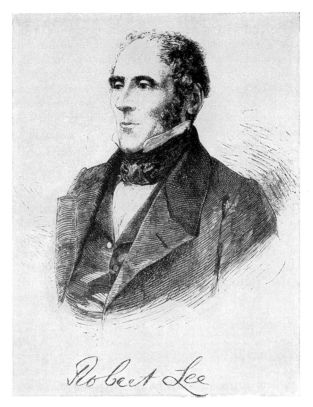

Fig. 16-1. Robert Lee (1793–1877).

the uterus, stating that he had been deceived by the authority of more learned anatomists, but that he now felt quite certain that the nerves of the human uterus had never been seen, by him or any other anatomist. Yet every obstetrician of experience had felt against his arm the great contractile force of which the uterus is capable in response to the stimulation of internal version. Of the existence of nerves in such an irritable organ there could be no doubt.

LEE'S ACCOUNT OF UTERINE INNERVATION

The first good description of the nervous structures of the uterus was by Robert Lee, who presented his findings to the Royal Society of London on June 17, 1841. In his account, published in the *Philosophical Transactions,*[7] Lee wrote:

The uterus and its appendages are wholly supplied with nerves from the great sympathetic and sacral nerves. At the bifurcation of the aorta, the right and left cords of the great sympathetic nerve unite upon the anterior part of the aorta, and form the aortic plexus. This plexus divides into the right and left hypogastric nerves, which soon subdivide into a number of branches to form the right and left hypogastric plexus. Each of these plexuses, having the trunk of the hypogastric nerve continued through its centre, after giving off branches to the ureter, peritoneum, rectum, and trunks of the uterine blood-vessels, descends to the side of the cervix, and there terminates in a great ganglion, which, from its situation and relations, may be called the hypogastric ganglion, or utero-cervical ganglion.

This ganglion is situated by the side of the neck of the uterus, behind the ureter, where it is passing to the bladder. In the unimpregnated state it is usually of an irregular, triangular or oblong shape, with several lobes or processes projecting from it where the nerves enter, or are given off from it. In the long diameter it usually measures from half an inch to three-quarters of an inch, varying in dimensions with the size of the nerves with which it is connected. The hypogastric ganglion always consists of cineritious and white matter like other ganglia, and gray and white nerves issue from it, which proceed to the rectum, bladder, uterus, and vagina. It is covered with the trunks of the vaginal and vesical arteries and veins, and the ganglion has an artery of considerable size, which enters it near the centre, and divides into branches which accompany the nerves given off from its inner surface, and from its anterior and inferior borders. The hypogastric nerve, after separating into a plexus, enters its upper edge, and branches from the third and other sacral nerves its posterior border, and the whole of its outer surface. . . .

From the inner surface of each hypogastric ganglion numerous small, white, soft nerves pass to the uterus, some of which ramify upon the muscular coat about the cervix, and others spread out under the peritoneum, to coalesce with the great ganglia and plexuses situated on the posterior and anterior surfaces of the organ. Large branches also go off from the inner surface of the hypogastric ganglion to the nerves surrounding the blood-vessels of the uterus, which they accompany in all their ramifications throughout its muscular coat. Other branches of nerves pass down from the ganglion between the vagina and bladder. Soon after conception the blood-vessels of the nervous ganglia and plexuses now described enlarge, and the ganglia and plexuses themselves expand with the uterus. The long diameter of the hypogastric ganglion at the end of the ninth month measures about an inch and a half.

Thus was the demand for an explanation of uterine function temporarily satisfied. Lee concluded:

These dissections prove that the human uterus possesses a great system of nerves, which enlarges with the coats, blood-vessels and absorbents during pregnancy, and which returns after parturition to its original condition before conception takes place. It is chiefly by the influence of these nerves, that the uterus performs the varied functions of menstruation, conception, and parturition, and it is solely by their means, that the whole fabric of the nervous system sympathises with the different morbid affections of the uterus. If these nerves of the uterus could not be demonstrated, its physiology and pathology would be completely inexplicable.

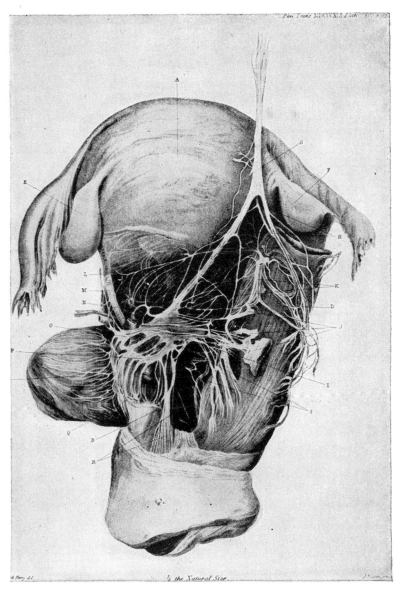

Fig. 16-2. Illustration from Lee's paper,[7] showing a posterolateral view of the uterus in the fourth month of pregnancy, with the great uterocervical ganglion and its nervous connections to the uterus, vagina, rectum, and bladder.

LEE'S LIFE

Robert Lee was born in 1793 in Melrose, Roxburgh, Scotland.[3,17] He received his medical degree at Edinburgh in 1814, and three years thereafter set out on the well-traveled road to London. After a period of anatomic study in Paris he returned in 1823 to England, where he was licensed by the Royal College of Physicians, and began the practice of obstetrics. He soon abandoned this, however, because of illness and the offer of an appointment as domestic physician to the family of the Prince of Woronzow, governor-general of the Crimea and Russian provinces on the Black Sea. In 1826 Lee returned to his obstetric practice in London and was elected physician to the British Lying-In Hospital. In 1834 he was appointed professor of midwifery in the University of Glasgow, but again he soon returned to England, this time to the chair of midwifery at St. George's Hospital, where he remained for 30 years, until his resignation in 1866. He died February 6, 1877, at the age of 84.

The uterocervical ganglion is sometimes spoken of today as Lee's ganglion, but proper recognition of Lee's discovery was retarded by the collusion of his antagonists and the shameful devices of T. Snow Beck, who vied with Lee for the Royal Medal in Physiology. Beck, a former student of Lee's, in an effort to further his own aims, surreptitiously mutilated Lee's preparations in the museum of the Royal College of Surgeons, and Beck's friends on the committee of physiology of the Royal Society's Council collaborated in the fraud by holding an unauthorized meeting to discuss the award, concealing their illegal transactions, and even resorting to an erasure of a confirmed minute from the council's journal book. The complex details of the ensuing controversy are related in a series of letters to the editor of the *Lancet,*[1,2,8,9,10,11,12,13,14] who, finally convinced of Beck's duplicity, roundly reprimanded him and closed the journal's columns to further discussion of the matter.

FRANKENHÄUSER'S ACCOUNT OF UTERINE INNERVATION

A quarter century after Lee's publication a monograph [4] appeared, redescribing in greater detail the innervation of the uterus, its plexuses, and its ganglia. Since then these structures have been associated with the name of the author, Ferdinand Frankenhäuser, who wrote:

One can convince himself most easily of the existence of the uterine ganglionic mass in the human by examining the cadaver of a newborn. After removing half of the pelvis, without having to perform much dissection, one sees here, lying against the upper part of the vagina, a sickle-shaped ganglion several lines thick. . . . It is a solid mass, quite discrete but not very thick, composed of ganglia and nerves. Since no dissection is necessary in this case no artefact can be produced, and the existence of a definitely circumscribed ganglion at the cervix is proved with certainty. Its demonstration in adults is more difficult. . . . At the internal aspect of the vertical part of the pelvic fascia, that is, in the lateral wall of the cul-de-sac, the hypogastric plexus extends to the lateral part of the vaginal vault. A part of this nerve trunk, the inner and upper, goes directly to the cervix,

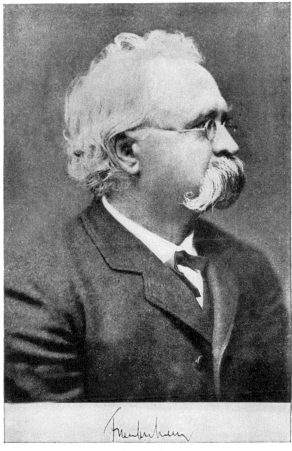

Fig. 16-3. Ferdinand Frankenhäuser (1832–1894).

while another part of it penetrates the fascia somewhat remote from the cervix and enters the cervical ganglion located at the outer aspect of the fascia. The fascia itself, attached to the cervix and upper part of the vagina, sends considerable masses of elastic fibers into these organs, and a considerable number of these fibers accompany the nerves going from the cervical ganglion into the uterus. . . . The cervical ganglion is located at the outer aspect of the horizontal part of the fascia; and since the middle and lower part of the hypogastric plexus enters it, one must follow its course through the fascia in dissecting it. . . . The sacral nerves as well as the branches from the sympathetic chain naturally lie outside the fascia, approaching it only at its junction with the cervical ganglion. It is thus clear that only the anterior part of the ganglion, which is located on the vaginal vault, lies entirely outside the pelvic fascia; the posterior and upper part, into which the sacral, sympathetic, and hypogastric nerves enter, being located in the fascia itself. . . . For a clear picture of this relationship it is absolutely necessary to remove the fascia. . . .

In viewing it from the exterior, one first sees a white tissue mass, about one line thick in the nonpregnant, lying against the posterior part of the vaginal vault and the side wall of the cul-de-sac, and in contact with the anterior part of the rectum, where nerves from the second, third, and fourth sacral foramina come

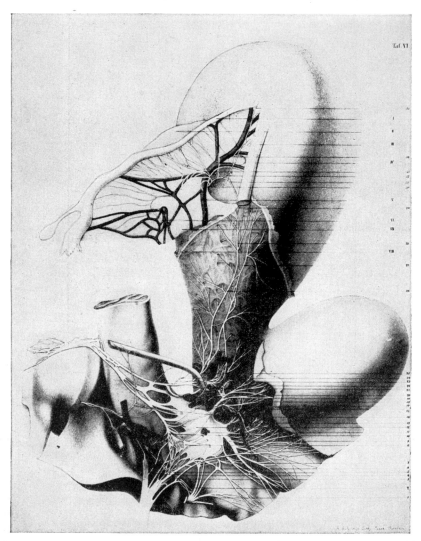

Fig. 16-4. Illustration from Frankenhäuser's monograph,[4] showing the cervical ganglion and sacral and uterine nerves of the right side of a pregnant uterus.

together . . . the main part proceeding to the bladder, vagina, and rectum. . . . In Plate 6 [Fig. 16-4] I have dissected away the nerve trunks covering the cervical ganglion, and its compact tissue layer is seen there. . . . This consists, as shown by microscopic examination, of ganglion cells compactly arranged in a flat surface and permeated by nerves. The size of this ganglionic mass differs quite considerably in the nonpregnant and pregnant. In the former it measures about ¾ inch in length and somewhat more than ½ inch in breadth. . . . In the pregnant or recently parturient uterus the length of the ganglion measures almost 2 inches, its width 1¼–1½ inches. Its long axis lies in the same direction as that of the vagina and rectum. Its thickness is not uniform. The part lying on the vaginal vault is the thickest, measuring up to 1½ lines. Posteriorly and above, on the other hand, it flattens out, becoming membranous where the nerves enter. Its form is roughly triangular, with pointed projections where the nerves enter and leave. . . .

Most of the uterine nerves arise from this ganglion. A smaller part arises from the hypogastric plexus . . . before it joins with the ganglion and branches along the lateral and posterior aspects of the uterus. . . . In addition to the uterus, the ganglion also sends nerves to other organs. . . .

The neural plexuses associated with Frankenhäuser's ganglion he described as follows:

About 1½ inches below the bifurcation of the aorta, directly over the promontory, this nerve plexus divides into two trunks (*plexus uterinus magnus*), which encircle the rectum from either side and continue toward the upper part of the vagina. . . . They are not simple nerves by any means, but should rather be called a nerve plexus, since they have a bandlike form and contain many interstices. These spaces are only small at the beginning of the course of these nerve trunks, but get progressively larger as the plexus becomes broader. The plexus finally disappears into its small end branches. In their course in the pelvis they travel at first along the inner aspect of the pelvic vessels and directly against the posterior wall of the rectum, with which they are intimately bound by connective tissue. They then proceed under the vessels and finally lie along their outer aspect near the uterus. . . . These nerve trunks lie on the upper pelvic fascia; they fuse in part with its fibers, however, in the vicinity of the vaginal vault. The hypogastric nerves are 3½–4 inches long, from the bifurcation of the aorta to their junction with the uterine ganglia. On their external or inferior aspect they are joined by extraordinarily numerous nerve branches of the fifth lumbar and first, second, and third ganglia of the sympathetic chain. On the other hand, they give off very numerous nerves again from their inner aspect. . . . Quite a number of nerves also proceed from the hypogastric plexus into the mesentery of the sigmoid, several very large branches coursing along the hemorrhoidal artery on either side and into the mesorectum directly adherent to the bowel. The hypogastric plexuses are thus bound extraordinarily intimately with the rectum; they must therefore follow all its motions and are even compressed by fecal masses. But they are also most easily accessible there for therapeutic intervention. Having arrived at the side of the rectum, the hypogastric nerves split into two branches. The smaller one remains on the inner aspect of the pelvic vessels and branches directly at the posterior and lateral part of the uterus; the other proceeds under the vessels and in part joins the great cervical ganglion, in part the sacral nerves. . . .

Frankenhäuser's dissections were carried out with the critique of the physiologist seeking an explanation for the clinical phenomena of practical significance to the obstetrician and gynecologist. He wrote:

Compression of the aorta is a well-known means of arresting severe postpartum hemorrhage, and it is believed that closure of the aorta is important in accomplishing this. But this is highly improbable, for the ovarian vessels, extraordinarily dilated during pregnancy, still continue to carry enough blood to maintain the bleeding. Aortic compression is nevertheless effective . . . the bleeding stops simply because of the strong uterine contractions that occur as a result of stimulation of the nerves coursing along the aorta in the process of compressing it. Continuous compression of the aorta is quite superfluous for this purpose, of course; gentle back-and-forth stroking with the finger tips over the pulsating vessel is sufficient to induce contractions and thus stop the bleeding.

As long as they course along the aorta the nerves are protected from pressure by means of their supports. Directly in front of the promontory, however, where the bifurcation into the two hypogastric plexuses occurs, they can easily be compressed in cases of contracted pelvis with prolonged engagement of the head in the pelvic inlet; and this possibly explains the sudden occurrence of uterine inertia in such cases.

The nerves of the rectum are readily accessible for therapeutic electrical stimulation: one can easily pass electrodes up as high as the promontory and immediately stimulate uterine contractions. . . . Medication for the purpose of stimulating or stopping labor pains works infinitely more surely, quickly, and in smaller dosage, if administered as an enema in the direct vicinity of these nerves than when given in the usual manner. . . . The effect of opium is then often surprisingly rapid; similarly in cases of uterine cramps or menstrual colic resulting from uterine fibroids. . . .

Several other phenomena, e.g., unusually strong borborygmi, which often appear immediately before a labor pain and which are observed in many uterine disturbances and during menstruation, are explained by this intimate neural relation. In animals, certainly, with each stimulation of the uterine nerve, one sees a very vigorous movement of the intestines, beginning at the same time as contraction of the uterus.

FRANKENHÄUSER'S LIFE

Ferdinand Frankenhäuser was born in 1832, but neither the birthplace nor the exact date is now known.[5,15,16] The details of his youth and early education likewise remain obscure. He first became the object of recorded notice as an assistant to Edward Martin in Jena, and in 1858 drew considerable attention as the author of a paper entitled "Über einige Verhältnisse, die Einfluss auf die stärkere oder schwächere Entwicklung der Frucht während der Schwangerschaft haben," statistically correlating the sex and development of the infant and the weight and parity of the mother. The following year he published "Über die Herztöne der Frucht und ihre Benutzung zur Diagnose des Lebens, der Stellung, der Lage und des Geschlechtes derselben," which purported to predict the infant's sex from the fetal heart rate. This idea, although not original with Frankenhäuser, created violent controversy at the time, and has been the subject of repeated investigation since then. He next turned his attention to the innervation of the uterus, both in the rabbit and the human, and it was in this field that he achieved his greatest laurels. In 1872 Frankenhäuser was called to Zürich as professor of obstetrics and gynecology, where he remained until 1888. Here he was instrumental in the creation of a new lying-in hospital; and under his direction the maternal mortality rapidly decreased, reaching a new low of one per thousand. The operative era of gynecology was just getting into swing, but Frankenhäuser remained loath to undertake major abdominal surgery because of his dissatisfaction with the available methods of antisepsis. He confined himself instead to vaginal operations, for which he soon achieved great fame. He became especially well known for his vaginal myomectomies, removing tumors of any size, as long as they could be approached through the uterine cavity. With the aid of laminary tents he would dilate the cervix for several days in preparation for the operation which, in the case of the larger tumors, consisted in incising the capsule from below, applying traction with a tenaculum, and removing the mass in stages, depending upon the assistance of uterine contractions for delivery of the tumor.

Frankenhäuser was an ardent student of the obstetric pelvis and possessed an excellent collection of specimens. He taught that the aftercoming head could come through a flat pelvis more easily than the foregoing head, but not so in a generally and equally contracted pelvis. He is said to have employed the method of pelvic mensuration later named for P. Müller, of impressing the head over the pelvis to test its adequacy. Suffering from a severe depression, and with his faculties failing, he returned in 1888 to Jena, where he died February 3, 1894.

REFERENCES

1. Beck, T. S.: Nerves and ganglia of the uterus. *Lancet*, **2**:173–74, 1856.

2. Beck, T. S.: The nerves and ganglia of the uterus and heart. *Lancet*, **2**:393–94, 1856.

3. Biographical sketch of Robert Lee, M.D., F.R.S. *Lancet*, **1**:332–37, 1851.

4. Frankenhaeuser, F.: *Die Nerven der Gebaermutter und ihre Endigung in den Glatten Muskelfasern*. Mauke, Jena, 1867.

5. Frankenhäuser, Ferdinand (1832–1894). *Zürcher Spitalgeschichte*, **2**:289–93, 1951.

6. Hunter, W.: *Medical Commentaries. Part I. Containing a Plain and Direct Answer to Professor Monro jun. Interspersed with Remarks on the Struc-*

ture, Functions, and Diseases of Several Parts of the Human Body, 2nd ed., Suppl. [iii]. S. Baker & G. Leigh, London, 1777.

7. Lee, R.: *On the Ganglia and the Other Nervous Structures of the Uterus.* Richard & John E. Taylor, London, 1842.

8. Lee, R.: Proceedings of the Royal Society relative to the discovery of the nervous system of the uterus. *Lancet,* **1**:3–4, 119–21, 207–8, 1855.

9. Lee, R.: The nerves of the uterus. *Lancet,* **2**:56, 1856.

10. Lee, R.: Nerves and ganglia of the uterus. *Lancet,* **2**:146–47, 1856.

11. Lee, R.: The nervous structures of the uterus and heart. *Lancet,* **2**:290–91, 1856.

12. Lee, R.: Ganglia and nerves of the uterus. *Lancet,* **2**:316–17, 1856.

13. Lee, R.: History of the discovery of the ganglia and other nervous structures of the uterus and heart. *Lancet,* **2**:377–78, 1856.

14. Lee, R.: The controversy between Dr. Lee and Dr. Snow Beck. *Lancet,* **2**:473–74, 1856.

15. Medicinisch-naturwissenschaftlicher Nekrolog des Jahres 1894. *Arch. f. path. Anat. u. Physiol.,* **139**:554, 1895.

16. Meyer-Ruegg, H.: Prof. Dr. F. Frankenhäuser. Biographische Skizze. *Gynaec. helvet.,* **9**:278–86, 1909.

17. Munk, W.: *The Roll of the Royal College of Physicians of London.* Vol. 3 (1801 to 1825). London, 1878, pp. 260–69.

18. Osiander, F. B.: *Handbuch der Entbindungskunst,* 2nd ed. Christian Friedrich Osiander, Tübingen, 1829, Vol. 1, pp. 145–47.

Cloquet's Node, Basset's Operation, and Cancer of the Vulva*

Surgical operations for the cure of cancer are based in large measure on the lymphatic drainage of the affected organ or region. It is not surprising, therefore, that of the two eponymics associated with the development of radical vulvectomy for cancer, namely, the node of Cloquet and the Basset operation, one designates a lymph node and the other a technique for en masse lymphatic extirpation.

CLOQUET'S NODE

The node of Cloquet was first described not in relation to the cancer operation, however, but in a detailed exposition of the surgical anatomy of the parts concerned in inguinal and femoral hernias.[4] In this monograph, published by Jules Cloquet in 1817, there is not even a suggestion that the lymph node in the femoral canal, later to be named for him, should be an object of attention in the treatment of vulval cancer, the modern operation for which was still far from development. In 1835 Andrew Melville McWhinnie published an English translation from the French of Cloquet's lengthy treatise, from which the following two paragraphs, describing the eponymic node and its relations, are taken:

The upper surface of the Septum Crurale is towards the abdominal cavity; it is concave: the inferior, directed towards the crural canal, is convex: each surface

---

* This chapter originally published in *Cancer,* **8**:1083–86, 1955; reprinted by permission. Copyright, 1955, by the American Cancer Society, Inc.

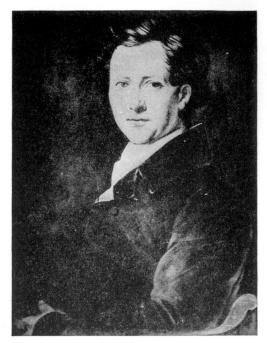

Fig. 17-1.   Jules Germain Cloquet (1790–1883).

is, however, sometimes level. This septum is always perforated by small apertures for the passage of lymphatics, and which are sometimes so numerous, that the superior part of the canal appears to be closed simply by a fibro-cellular net-work. One of these apertures, more considerable than the others, is central, and is sometimes occupied by an elongated absorbent gland; it is sufficiently large to admit the point of the little finger, which, when introduced, will be girt by it as by an elastic fibrous ring. Internally, another tolerably large foramen is also sometimes found, near to Gimbernat's ligament.

The absorbent vessels and glands of the groin vary as to their number and situation, as well as in their mode of communication. In front of the anterior wall of the crural canal there are absorbent glands, which communicate with others which are placed behind it; they cover the opening for the vena saphena, and are continued into the crural canal to accompany the femoral vessels: there are usually one or two, of an elongated form, situated in the groove, which separates the external iliac artery from the vein, where they enter the crural canal. The lymphatic trunks form in this canal a net-work more or less considerable, which, being interwoven with small veins and the septum crurale, afford an obstacle to any protrusion of the abdominal viscera.

CLOQUET'S LIFE

Jules Germain Cloquet was born in Paris, December 28, 1790, the son of an art teacher.[3] He was educated in the natural sciences together with

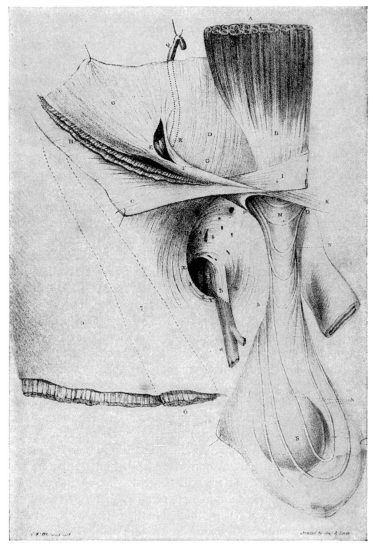

Fig. 17-2. An illustration from Cloquet's thesis,[4] showing the right inguinal and crural canals. (Reproduced from a lithograph in McWhinnie's translation.)

his elder brother, Hippolyte, to whom he was deeply devoted, but whose later brilliant career as a surgeon was prematurely terminated by an apoplectic stroke. Early in his medical studies in Paris, Jules showed great aptitude for anatomic investigation, and his drawings and *moulages* attracted wide attention from the faculty. Because of his exceptional ability the assembly of professors of the university requested his exemption from military service, which was granted by a special decree of Napoleon dated December 27, 1812. The following year Cloquet received first prize in anatomy and physiology. In 1815, at the age of 25, he was appointed prosector on the medical faculty. Receipt of his doctorate in medicine, two years later, was the occasion of his famous *Recherches anatomiques sur les hernies de l'abdomen,* a purely anatomic study based on the dissection of 340 hernia cases. This was later followed by a companion work, *Recherches sur les causes et l'anatomie des hernies abdominales,* encompassing observations on 500 cadavers and describing the mechanisms of hernia formation, the development and anatomy of hernia sacs, and methods for their reduction. Between these two investigations, however, he actively pursued other interests. In 1818 he demonstrated for the first time the sexual differences in the intestinal parasite *Ascaris lumbricoides;* and in the same year he published an important paper showing the structure of the human fetal pupillary membrane, the existence of which had been in question. His subsequent studies on the crystalline lens and its development led to the eponymic association of his name with the hyaloid canal of the vitreous. Cloquet was not unmindful of his accomplishments, his broad knowledge of human anatomy, and his proficiency as a teacher, nor did he make any effort to conceal his academic aspirations. In 1819, therefore, when the position of chief of anatomy, previously occupied by the distinguished Béclard, was vacant, no one was surprised to witness Cloquet, although only 29 years of age at the time, enter into open dispute over the position with Breschet, a man of much greater age and long-established reputation.

Cloquet had also trained himself in clinical surgery, and in 1819 was named surgeon and chief adjunct to the St. Louis Hospital, the first of a succession of clinical posts of increasing importance that culminated in his appointment in 1852 as consultant surgeon to Emperor Napoleon III. In 1829, before the advent of chloroform anesthesia, he succeeded in painlessly removing a cancerous breast from a Madame Plantin, whom he had previously hypnotized. Although the patient conversed with him during the operation, she had no recollection of it afterward. Cloquet was also greatly impressed with the value of the Oriental practice of acupuncture for neuralgia and rheumatism, and his observations on this method of therapy were incorporated into a treatise on the subject by Dantu in 1824.

Cloquet's bibliography, which appears in a biography of him written by a grandnephew,[3] contains an impressive list of titles in anatomy, surgery, surgical pathology, and therapeutics. Of interest to the obstetrician is his paper, *Modifications des ligaments ronds de l'utérus pendant la grossesse,* based on the postmortem study of women who died soon after delivery. His analysis of the active and passive phases of respiration, his study of the pathogenesis and treatment of urinary stones, and his description of the lacrimal apparatus of snakes illustrate the continuing range of his interests throughout his highly productive life. In 1821 Cloquet began the publication of what many believe to have been his most important work, his *Anatomie de l'homme,* an effort comprising five volumes and including 300 plates and 1300 figures, most of which he personally designed with the help of his sister. This treatise went into many editions, including an English translation by John Godman, published in Boston.

Cloquet's greatest ambition, admission to the Académie des Sciences, was realized in 1854, after which he stopped operating, stopped writing, and gradually withdrew into retirement, surrounded by honors, riches, and a wide circle of friends. He died suddenly on February 24, 1883, at the age of 92.

BASSET'S OPERATION

Radical vulvectomy for carcinoma was beautifully described and illustrated in the thesis of Antoine Basset, published in Paris in 1912.[2] This procedure, subsequently popularized in the United States by Taussig, has since been known as the Basset operation. Widely adopted as the treatment of choice for malignant tumors of the vulva, it has been extended in scope only very recently in an effort to improve the rather disheartening cure rate usually associated with this disease.

Basset's important paper reported his study of 147 cases of primary carcinoma of the clitoris. Careful study of the lymph nodes in each case led him to the conclusion that early and bilateral nodal involvement was the rule, and this is the premise upon which the routine application of his operation to all suitable patients with carcinoma of the clitoris was based. Wrote Basset:

Among the cancers of the clitoris and the prepuce the cancerous adenopathy should be regarded as ever present, at least after a relatively short time (six months or less, on the average) after the apparent onset of the disease as indicated by the recognition of the tumor. It is thus a *precocious* adenopathy. It is furthermore usually, if not always, *bilateral.* Finally this adenopathy strikes the superficial and deep inguinal-crural nodes and the external and internal retrocrural nodes, at the same time or sequentially according to the initial location of the neoplasm in the prepuce or body of the clitoris.

The principles of treatment recommended by Basset logically followed from these surgical-pathologic findings:

In the presence of a duly diagnosed epithelioma of the clitoris and in the present state of surgery, we have seen which treatment is indicated: extirpation of the tumor, the lymphatics, and the nodes. The only surgical contraindications would be those resulting from too great a local extension, or nodal invasion so remote as to render impossible complete ablation of the tumor and of the involved lymphatic region, or necessitate enormous mutilation, and a fortiori a state of cachexia of the patient indicating widespread dissemination.

Basset's description of the operation itself similarly stresses the groin lymphatics and their surgical-anatomic relations:

We thus see that there exist two lymphatic pedicles extending from the clitoris.
One, the superior pedicle, which one might call the pedicle of the round ligament, accompanying the latter in its inguinal course, extends to the most anterior and most external of the neighboring nodes of the external iliac artery, the external retrocrural node.

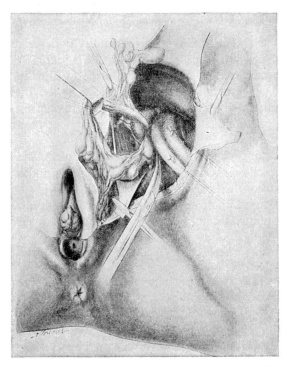

Fig. 17-3. An illustration from Basset's thesis,[2] showing extent of his operation, complete freeing of the lymphatic pedicle.

The other, the inferior pedicle, extends first to the superficial and deep inguinal nodes, located in front of the vein, then alongside it to Cloquet's node and the internal retrocrural node.
The crural and retrocrural nodes would thus represent the true regional nodes of the clitoris.
The crural nodes are very small and therefore very hard to see and to distinguish from the superficial inguinal nodes in the young subjects on whom we have operated. The largest of these nodes, the node of Cloquet, appeared rather incon-

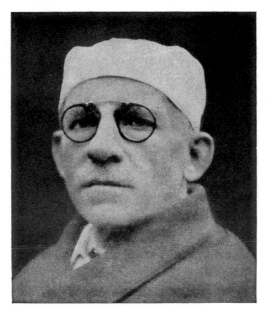

Fig. 17-4. Antoine Basset (1882–1951).

stant to us. Only 10 times out of 20 were we able to inject it and it seemed to us that it was chiefly in the cases in which the internal retrocrural node was very well developed that it [Cloquet's node] was absent. . . .

Our investigations and various attempts on the cadaver to find an operative procedure which met the requirements that we have just described have led us to propose the following operative technique:

First step.—Outline of the incision.

Second step.—Dissection of the round ligament and fatty tissue of the inguinal canal up to the iliac vessels.

Third step.—Isolation of the inferior pedicle by the crural route.

Fourth step.—Section of the crural arcade. Isolation of the internal retrocrural group of nodes.

Fifth step.—Extirpation of the tumor.

Sixth step.—Repair and suture.

The following excerpts from Basset's summary embody the philosophy of the modern cancer surgeon—frank acknowledgment of the prognosis, recognition of the importance of early diagnosis and treatment, and determination to perform the most complete and anatomically sound operation possible in an effort to eradicate the tumor:

The evolution of the disease appears to be rather rapid without surgical treatment, at least after the tumor is ulcerated, and the prognosis is then always fatal. It is still very somber after the mutilating operation, because of the great frequency of local, and above all nodal, recurrence. But this seems amenable to improvement by early and systematic extirpation including all the lymphatics and nodes [that drain] the clitoris.

. . . One should in every case strive to remove in a single mass all the tissues to be extirpated. It will always be preferable to start with the nodes and lymphatic pedicles on each side, carrying out removal of the tumor only as the last step.

BASSET'S LIFE

Antoine Basset was born in Paris, June 3, 1882.[1,5] He received his medical training under a distinguished group of clinicians, including Renault, Pozzi, and Delbet; and, after his initial academic appointment in 1908 as aide in anatomy, became Delbet's chief of clinic in 1911, and assistant to Pierre Duval in 1922. He served in the French Army during World War I and received a number of military decorations. In 1943 he was appointed to the rank of honorary professor in the faculty at Paris. He served at various times as president of the Académie de Chirurgie, the Société de Gastro-entérologie de Paris, and the Société de Gynécologie et d'Obstétrique de Paris. Basset is best known, of course, for his thesis and the operation named for him; but he was also greatly interested in gastrointestinal and orthopedic surgery. His published works on the anatomy, radiology, and surgery of the knee and shoulder were regarded as significant contributions. Basset died on May 7, 1951.

REFERENCES

1. Ameline, A.: Antoine Basset (1882–1951). *Gynéc. et obst.,* **51**:91–92, 1952.

2. Basset, A.: *L'épithélioma primitif du clitoris; son retentissement ganglionnaire et son traitement opératoire.* (Thesis.) G. Steinheil, Paris, 1912.

3. Cloquet, G.: *Jules Cloquet; sa vie—ses oeuvres; 1790–1883.* (Thesis.) J. Rousset, Paris, 1910.

4. Cloquet, J.: *Recherches Anatomiques sur les Hernies de l'Abdomen.* Paris, 1817; also transl. by A. M. McWhinnie: *Anatomical Description of the Parts Concerned in Inguinal and Femoral Hernia.* S. Highley, London, 1835.

5. Lantuéjoul, P.: Notice nécrologique sur M. Antoine Basset. *Bull. Acad. nat. méd.,* **135**:370–72, 1951.

Jean-Louis Baudelocque and the External Conjugate of the Pelvis

CHAPTER

18

Obstetric interest in pelvic mensuration dates back over 200 years, to the realization that the bony pelvis is a rigid, unyielding structure, indistensible at its joints, and that deformity of its contours or contraction of its diameters may result in dystocia, previously ascribed to other causes. The principles of clinical pelvimetry must be credited to William Smellie, but its widespread acceptance and popularization as an essential part of the obstetric examination are due in large measure to those who followed him. One of the foremost teachers of pelvic mensuration was Jean-Louis Baudelocque, who, with André Levret, was one of the two outstanding figures in French obstetrics of the eighteenth century.

BAUDELOCQUE'S TECHNIQUE OF PELVIC MENSURATION

Baudelocque's instructions for measuring the pelvis were set forth in his famous textbook, *L'Art des Accouchemens,*[1] published in 1781, in a chapter (Section XII) bearing the title, "Concerning the Examination Necessary to Determine If the Pelvis Is Adequate or Malformed." The importance of this examination he described in the first two paragraphs, as follows:

One cannot be indoctrinated with certain fundamental truths of the art of obstetrics without knowing the full importance of this examination; but its difficulties are only appreciated by those who are obliged to carry out these researches; and

143

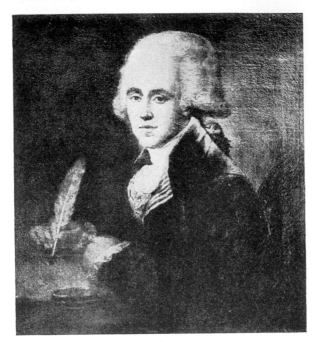

Fig. 18-1. Jean-Louis Baudelocque (1746–1810).

experience acquired through frequent practice on the cadaver can only remove part of the obstacles that one encounters.

If the accoucheurs had applied themselves more diligently to this examination, and if all women in any way malformed had submitted themselves for examination and study, we might now not be witnessing the unhappy practices of our art * that have taken so many victims, for the few mothers or few children that they have definitely saved from danger.

* Cesarean section, symphysiotomy, and destructive operations on the fetus.

With his marginal note warning that "inspection of the vertebral column and the lower extremities is just as significant in leading us astray as in instructing us," Baudelocque continued:

Inspection of the dorsal spine and of the lower extremities of women can only shed very little light on the interior of the pelvis, for the deformities of those parts do not always affect the latter adversely for delivery; and we often see the same childhood deformities disappear during adolescence while the pelvis alone retains the ineradicable imprint of the rickets that produced them.

The external characteristics of the pelvic region nevertheless received much of Baudelocque's attention. He wrote:

The external shape of the pelvis can help us a great deal in the examination of this part. The roundness of the hips, their symmetry, in height as well as width, the convexity of the pubis; the superior part of the sacrum slightly concave; a distance of 4 to 5 inches from this point to the tip of the coccyx; a diameter of 7 to 8 inches, in women of average girth, from the point of the spinous process of the last lumbar vertebra to the middle of the mons veneris; 7 to 8 inches distance between the anterior superior spines of the ilia, characterize the well-formed pelvis.

Baudelocque recognized narrowing of the anteroposterior diameter as the commonest type of inlet contraction, but he erred in teaching that this diameter could be estimated reliably from external measurements:

Whenever the superior strait is contracted from front to back, the pubis is more flattened and the small of the back more curved, because the base of the sacrum is carried forward and its lower end more outward.

The thickness of the pelvic bones being almost the same in all women, abnormally built or not, one can determine, within one or two lines, to what degree the superior strait is abnormal in this regard, by measuring the thickness of the woman from the middle of the pubis to the tip of the spine of the last lumbar vertebra . . . and by subtracting 3 inches from this measurement in women who are thin and a little more in others; the thickness of the base of the sacrum and of the os pubis in front being only 3 inches.

This external measurement, the external conjugate of the pelvis, has been identified so closely with the name of Baudelocque by subsequent generations of obstetricians that it is usually referred to as Baudelocque's diameter or abbreviated simply as B. D. For a century and a half great reliance was placed on it as an index of the capacity of the superior strait. Only with the recent application of roentgenography to pelvic mensuration has the inadequacy of external pelvimetry for the estimation of the internal pelvic measurements been brought to light.

Considering the external manifestations of the transversely contracted inlet, Baudelocque wrote:

When this same strait is contracted transversely, the pubic region is protuberant rather than flattened, as in the preceding case; the anterior part of the pelvis forms an obtuse angle, and not the rounded girdle that characterizes the well-formed pelvis. Although it is more difficult to evaluate narrowing that affects only one side of this strait, this impedes delivery less than the type of contraction we have just discussed.

Baudelocque's examination proceeded then to an evaluation of the inferior strait:

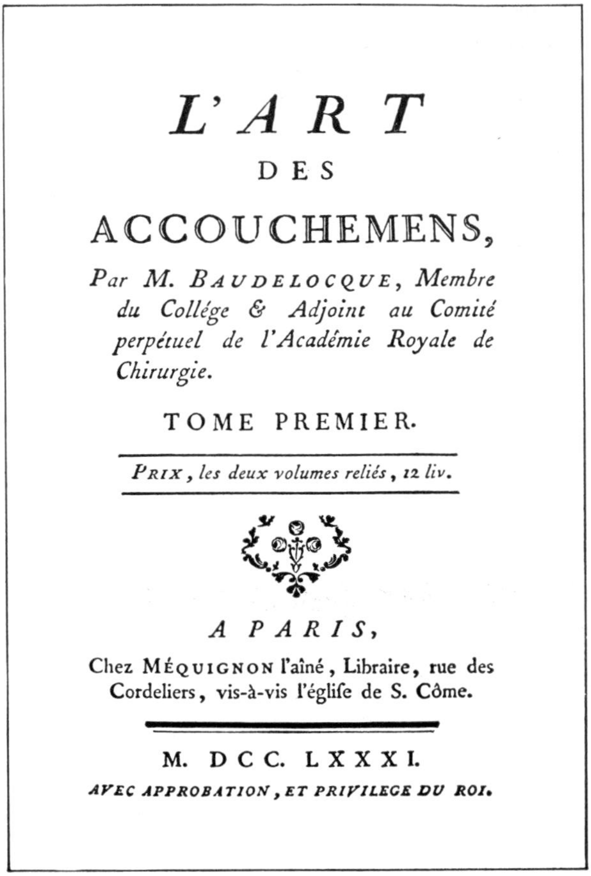

L'ART

DES

ACCOUCHEMENS,

*Par M. B A U D E L O C Q U E , Membre
du Collége & Adjoint au Comité
perpétuel de l'Académie Royale de
Chirurgie.*

TOME PREMIER.

Prix , les deux volumes reliés , 12 liv.

A P A R I S ,

Chez Méquignon l'aîné , Libraire, rue des
Cordeliers, vis-à-vis l'églife de S. Côme.

M. D C C. L X X X I.

Avec approbation , et privilege du roi.

Fig. 18-2. Title page of Baudelocque's textbook.

When the thighs and legs are flexed, or with the patient squatting, as one vulgarly says, one easily distinguishes by touch the ischial tuberosities, the tip of the coccyx, and the lower margin of the pubic symphysis, to evaluate their distance and to determine the size of the inferior strait with the precision necessary to avoid committing gross errors in practice.

Despite Smellie's introduction of the internal, or diagonal, conjugate a quarter century earlier, internal pelvimetry was just beginning to take root in French obstetrics, as evidenced by Baudelocque's meager paragraph on "Another Method of Estimating the Width of the Pelvis":

Whenever the condition of the patient under examination permits the insertion of the finger into the vagina, one should not fail to do so. One could even insert his whole hand if necessary and if conditions were favorable enough to permit it, as, for example, at the time of delivery. These procedures lead us still more surely to an understanding of the pelvis, as they enable us to learn things that cannot be recognized by simple external examination, such as the exostoses that are sometimes present.

The chapter on pelvimetry concludes with the following description of the methods for measuring pelvic depth and the height of the pubic arch:

The depth of pelvis posteriorly is measured by the length of the sacrum; laterally, by half the height of the ilium, from its anterior superior spine to the ischial tuberosity; finally, one establishes the depth anteriorly by the extent of the pubic symphysis.

It is easy to find the elevation or the height of the pubic arch by subtracting the length of the symphysis from the length of the sides of the pelvis. For example, if the first is 15 to 18 lines and the lateral depth of the pelvis is 3¼ or 3½ inches, the height of the arch will be 2 inches.

In an earlier chapter (Section X), "Concerning the Structural Abnormalities of the Pelvis in Relation to Childbirth," Baudelocque considered the effects of pelvic contraction. This chapter so well illustrates his clinical acumen and experience against a background of eighteenth-century obstetrics, that it is reproduced here in its entirety, with only minor elisions, unimportant to the content:

The different conditions of the pelvis that may interfere with the normal mechanism of birth and render it moie or less difficult, ought to be considered just as much as the functional abnormalities in this regard. They all consist in excessive or insufficient width of this cavity.

These main defects may affect all parts of the pelvis or only one, and often one is the result of the other, or results from the same cause. Their slight variations are so numerous that one would be wrong in attempting to distinguish among them by touch. We will speak here only of the most important.

It seems at first that the wider the pelvis the easier the delivery ought to be, but the opposite has often been observed; for women who are blessed with such a conformation, at first thought advantageous, are subject more often than others to obliquity [retroversion] of the uterus and its descensus, above all at the time of delivery, when this organ, already laden with the weight of the infant, is subjected to the expulsive force of the abdominal muscles.

It is easy indeed to prevent this latter accident and to remedy the others. In order to prevent the uterus from partly projecting at the time of delivery, one keeps the patient in a horizontal position; one advises her not to assist her pains, that is, to make no voluntary effort; one supports the edge of the cervix until the head is already out; and one takes care that this organ is not pulled out by the infant's shoulders.

When the uterine cervix, filled by the infant's head, is pushed all the way down to the introitus, so that the head appears to be completely out of the pelvis, one must begin by extracting the infant with proper precautions, in order not to aggravate the bad situation already existing; and then the uterus, its volume diminishing, will go back into the pelvis easily. . . .

Contraction of the pelvis, in relation to delivery, may be relative or absolute. The former results from an extraordinarily large size of the infant's head, and the latter from the actual shape of the pelvis. To determine accurately the various degrees of each, and to establish the possible consequences, one would have to know the precise size of the specific pelvis and the volume of the head that must pass through it, which is impossible as far as the latter is concerned, but which we ordinarily assume to be 3 inches 6 lines from one parietal boss to the other.

Absolute contraction, to which we will confine ourselves here, is rarely found in all parts of the pelvis at the same time. Most often this abnormality affects only one strait, and rather often in this case the other is a little larger than usual. It is present more often in the superior strait than in the inferior. One notices that it almost always exists from front to back, sometimes only on one side, and very rarely in the transverse diameter. The opposite is seen with respect to the inferior strait, for here the ischial tuberosities are usually too close together.

With respect to the relationship of the width of the infant's head to the smallest diameter of the average-sized pelvis, one sees that the latter could be a little narrower, still without being inadequate for delivery; so that one need only ascribe the first degree of contraction to a width of 3½ inches in the diameter concerned; and the other [degrees of contraction] from this width down to the smallest.

The difficulty of delivery, everything else being favorable, is proportional to the narrowness of the pelvis. When this abnormality allows only a 3¼-inch space, labor becomes long, in proportion to the increased pressure the head must endure in passing through this part.

The difficulties of delivery are much greater when the pelvis is only 3 inches in its smallest diameter. It is possible, however, despite this obstacle, for it to occur naturally, even in cases where this diameter is only 2¾ inches, as we have observed several times; still these deliveries should only be considered exceptions to the rule. In these cases the cranial bones of the infant have an unusual degree of pliability, which favors molding of the head and the changes necessary for its delivery.

When the pelvis is so contracted that it is only 2½ inches in its smallest diameter, birth of a term infant cannot occur by this route. Cesarean section, pubiotomy, and premature delivery have been recommended in these cases. The first is the only one that surgery has sanctioned to date. One will be able to form his own opinion of the second later. As for premature delivery, the law absolutely prohibits it.

If the woman can deliver by herself when the contracted pelvis is more than 2½ inches in its smallest diameter, it is not always without danger to her and the infant. . . . The soft parts that line the pelvis, being subjected to strong compression, become irritated, painful, and are sometimes threatened by gangrene.

. . . The cranial bones of the infant, overriding each other, compress the brain, causing its congestion and hemorrhage within it, often fatal.

These effects appear sooner or later, according as the superior or inferior strait is abnormal. When both are, the expulsive forces often become so exhausted in the face of the difficulties presented by the superior strait, that the head is arrested there or, having been pushed into the pelvic cavity, it cannot advance further, so that it remains stuck there until the weakened forces are sufficiently recovered to expel it, or skilled aid comes to the rescue.

In the last case the head, being in a space larger than the strait that it has already negotiated, and not being subjected to the same pressure, restitutes itself more or less to its original state and changes back from the shape it has acquired earlier, which is still necessary for its passage through the inferior strait. . . .

When the superior strait alone is contracted, the infant's head advances with great difficulty at first; but once the parietal bosses have passed this strait, the other parts of the pelvis being relatively or absolutely larger, the head negotiates them with such ease that a few pains often suffice to bring about delivery.

The opposite is seen when the inferior strait is abnormal, the first [superior strait] being of average width. The head engages easily into the pelvis, from which it cannot emerge without overcoming obstacles that impede its progress, making it difficult and laborious. . . . The effects . . . become apparent later than in the former case.

The accoucheur, who even through long experience has not come to appreciate the forces of nature, can easily make a mistake in such cases; in the first case, by judging delivery to be impossible; and in the second case, by announcing it as very easy, when difficulties exist that either prevent delivery or render it so difficult that it can be accomplished only by the exercise of great skill.

Very rarely the midpelvis is found to be narrower than the straits, but this abnormality, which can result only from some exostosis or from a defect in curvature of the sacrum, could produce no other effects than those we have just described.

It is not the same in the case of abnormal depth, the commonest cause of which is excessive curvature of the sacrum. Besides being more frequent than the preceding, this interferes with delivery much more; not only because the straits of the pelvis are usually contracted, but because of this the progress of the head is arrested by the lower part of the sacrum before the occiput has descended enough to engage under the pubic arch.

Excessive width of the pubic symphysis, deficient height and smallness of its arch, abnormal length and direction of the ischial spines, as well as the firm fusion of the coccyx with the lower end of the sacrum, can also make delivery difficult, in the same way.

. . . One cannot praise the teaching of some with respect to the last of these abnormalities * without accusing the majority who practice obstetrics of abusing it; for most often one attributes to fusion of the coccyx that which is, in reality, only the effect of resistance of the external parts.

* The teaching consists of pushing the coccyx backward when the engaged head cannot be delivered easily.

BAUDELOCQUE'S LIFE

Jean-Louis Baudelocque was born in Heilly, a village in Picardie, France, in 1746,[2,3] the precise date being unknown. Following the career of his father, a surgeon, he went to Paris for his education, there devoting himself chiefly to the study of anatomy, surgery, and obstetrics. He became the outstanding disciple of the distinguished obstetrician, Solayrès de Renhac, at the Charité Hôpital; and when the master on one occasion took sick, Baudelocque, still a student, brought great credit upon himself by taking over the lectures and delivering them with clarity and authority. Only a year later he took his own rightful place among the professors, and from this time his reputation mounted rapidly. In 1776 he was made a member of the Collége de Chirurgie, his thesis on this occasion speaking out strongly against the practice of symphysiotomy in the management of dystocia.

After the French Revolution the scientific institutions were reorganized; and in 1798, with the replacement of the Faculté de Médecine and the Collége de Chirurgie by the newly established École de Santé, Baudelocque was made professor of obstetrics in the last and director of the Maternité, where he supervised the training of midwives and the 1700 to 2000 deliveries that occurred there annually. His private practice thrived and he soon became the acknowledged master accoucheur in France, being referred to as *le grand Baudelocque*. Engaged by Napoleon to attend the Empress Marie-Louise in her first confinement, he was also called upon by the Queen of Holland and the Grand Duchess of Berg. Together with Baudelocque's rapidly acquired fame came a full measure of envy and villification by a few articulate contemporaries, the foremost of whom, Sacombe, drew him into trial in open court because of the death of a patient. Baudelocque's advocacy of cesarean section for certain cases of pelvic contraction drew from Sacombe the epithet of assassin and even led to the formation of an anti-cesarean society.

Baudelocque's renown was based largely on his teaching ability and the clarity with which he expressed the principles of his art. The Maternité, with its excellent clinical facilities for instruction, unique in Europe in Baudelocque's day, became the French center for the training of midwives. Here he taught about 150 students a year in the principles and techniques of obstetrics, including version and the use of forceps, and these women in turn spread Baudelocque's name and precepts throughout France. In addition to his *L'Art des Accouchemens,* Baudelocque in 1775 published a manual for midwives, *Principes sur l'Art des Accouchemens,* which went through five editions. The other obstetric contributions for which he is best known include his pelvimeter and his forceps, the latter based on the earlier model of Levret. Baudelocque died on May 1, 1810, but the name was kept alive in French obstetrics by two nephews: Caesar-Auguste Baudelocque (1795–1851), *agrégé* in the medical faculty; and Louis-Auguste Baudelocque (1800–1864), professor in the medical faculty and inventor of a cephalotribe.

REFERENCES

1. Baudelocque, J. L.: *L'Art des Accouchemens.* Méquignon, Paris, 1781, Vol. 1, pp. 38–45, 54–58.
2. Bayle and Thillaye: *Biographie Médicale.* Delahays, Paris, 1855, pp. 700–702.
3. *Biographisches Lexikon der hervorragenden Ärzte aller Zeiten und Völker,* 2nd ed. Ed. by W. Haberling, F. Hübotter, and H. Vierordt. Urban & Schwarzenberg, Berlin & Vienna, 1929, Vol. 1, pp. 379–80.

Gustav Adolf Michaelis

and Michaelis' Rhomboid

CHAPTER

19

External pelvimetry still draws an occasional gasp but its days are numbered, its uselessness in clinical obstetrics fully recognized within the past few years. As roentgen pelvimetry has demonstrated in convincing manner the futility of external pelvic measurements, these have been virtually abandoned by obstetricians and consigned at last to the limbo of outmoded procedures. External pelvic mensuration will ever remain an inglorious tribute to the conservatism of the medical profession and its reluctance to reject what it has once embraced, for a full century elapsed between Michaelis' demonstration of the inadequacy of external pelvimetry and the full acknowledgment of its deficiencies by obstetric textbooks. It is but one of a succession of ironies in the career of this obstetric pioneer, who first spoke out in a clear voice against the reliance on external measurements, that his name should have been perpetuated among the eponyms of obstetrics in association with an external pelvic landmark, "the rhomboid of Michaelis."

MICHAELIS' DESCRIPTION OF SACRAL QUADRANGLE

Michaelis' comparison of normal with contracted pelves had shown that although the maximum measurement between the posterior superior iliac spines in the former group exceeded that of the latter, the minimum measurements were practically identical in both groups. Similarly, he encountered

152

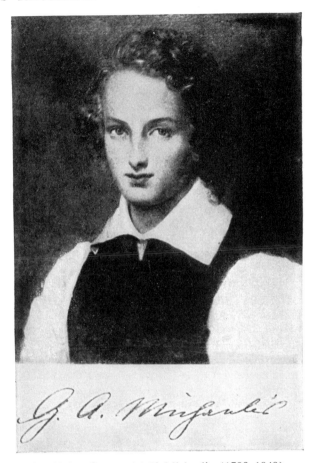

Fig. 19-1. Gustav Adolf Michaelis (1798–1848).

great variations in sacral length in both the normal pelves and the contracted rachitic. He was struck, however, by the variations in size and form of the diamond-shaped area demarcated by the medial borders of the gluteal muscles, the dimples overlying the posterior superior iliac spines, and the depression over the sacrum, and by the possibility of correlating variants of this outline with specific pelvic forms. Wrote Michaelis:

The surface of the sacrum . . . presents markedly different appearances in different pelves. In the normal pelvis of a strong, healthy, and well-developed patient, it is usually flat and lies rather embedded among the surrounding muscles. When feminine fullness is lacking, as well as in cases of contracted pelvis, it is often arched, projecting above the surrounding tissues; but the pelvis may also be large in cases of this type. Especially characteristic, however, is the different border of the surface. In normal pelves the sacral surface forms an elongated quadrangle, bounded by the borders of the glutei maximi and by two lines, which connect the region of the posterior spines of the ilium with the depression over the sacrum; and in the better body conformation this quadrangle approaches a rhomboid. In cases of abnormal body configuration, especially those with rachitic distortion, the upper angle becomes more obtuse at the depression over the sacrum and may even disappear completely, the sacral surface then presenting the appearance of a triangle. This latter form, also characteristic of the male, lacks the fullness that normally typifies this region in women. Some pathologic pelvic forms, especially Naegele's obliquely contracted pelvis and Robert's transversely contracted pelvis, can only be recognized through changes in the sacral area to the extent that this is lacking on one or both sides.

If one visualizes a straight line connecting the two posterior superior spines of the ilium and measures the height of the sacral depression above this line, this measurement provides the principal feature of this surface.

The following table summarizes Michaelis' measurements in 61 cases (the units of measurement presumably being inches and lines).

**HEIGHT OF THE UPPER BORDER OF THE SACRUM
ABOVE THE POSTERIOR SUPERIOR SPINES OF THE ILIUM**

	Maximum	*Minimum*	*Average*
Normal pelvis, normal body habitus	2″3″ ′	1″3″ ′	1″9″ ′
Normal pelvis, abnormal body habitus	0″8″ ′	0″0″ ′	0″4″ ′
Contracted nonrachitic pelvis	1″6″ ′	0″6″ ′	1″1″ ′
Contracted rachitic pelvis	1″4″ ′	0″0″ ′	0″9″ ′

Referring later to the distortion of his "rhomboid" in the rare case of a Robert pelvis, Michaelis wrote:

The sacral surface must have a most characteristic shape; for the posterior superior spines of the ilium almost touch each other, even covering the spinous process of the fifth lumbar vertebra. Thus in such a case no true sacral surface is present at all, the buttocks being in contact with each other well up to the vertebral column. As a result, the gluteal cleft has to be unusually long, extending high up and merging directly with the furrow-like depression over the vertebrae.

In the Naegele pelvis, Michaelis explained:

. . . the surface of the sacrum is quite asymmetrical in its lateral parts. Specifically, on the side of the ankylosis the posterior superior spine of the ilium is located very close to the midline, or actually in the midline, while the spine maintains its normal position.

This description of Michaelis' rhomboid, actually one of his lesser contributions, is taken from his monumental work, *Das Enge Becken,*[3] which was completed and published in 1851, three years after Michaelis' death, by his

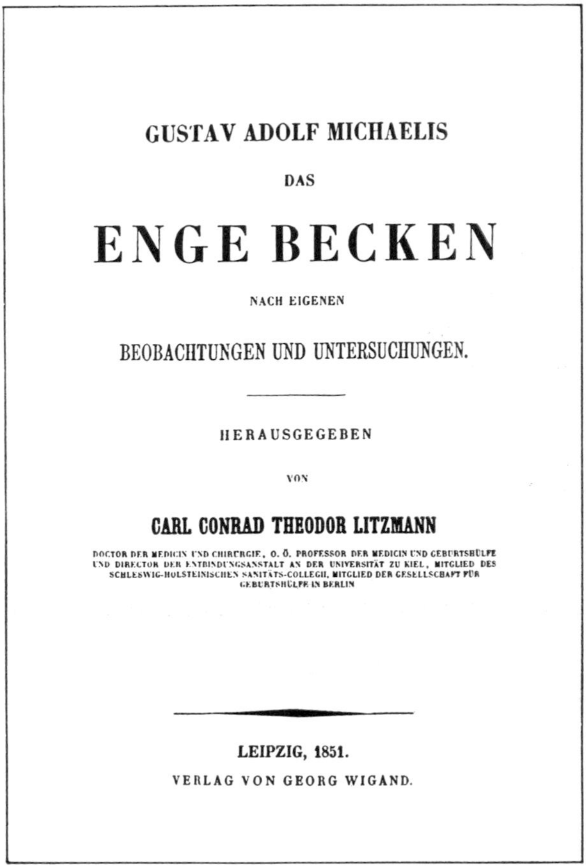

GUSTAV ADOLF MICHAELIS

DAS

ENGE BECKEN

NACH EIGENEN

BEOBACHTUNGEN UND UNTERSUCHUNGEN.

HERAUSGEGEBEN

VON

CARL CONRAD THEODOR LITZMANN

DOCTOR DER MEDICIN UND CHIRURGIE, O. Ö. PROFESSOR DER MEDICIN UND GEBURTSHÜLFE
UND DIRECTOR DER ENTBINDUNGSANSTALT AN DER UNIVERSITÄT ZU KIEL, MITGLIED DES
SCHLESWIG-HOLSTEINISCHEN SANITÄTS-COLLEGII, MITGLIED DER GESELLSCHAFT FÜR
GEBURTSHÜLFE IN BERLIN

LEIPZIG, 1851.
VERLAG VON GEORG WIGAND.

Fig. 19-2. Title page of Michaelis' book on contracted pelves.

friend and associate, Carl Litzmann, who achieved eponymic distinction on his own through his description of posterior asynclitism. *Das Enge Becken* is now recognized universally as one of the great contributions to obstetric literature. John Whitridge Williams was fond of saying that no obstetrician could pretend to understand contracted pelves until he had read it. Ironically, however, the value of this book was overlooked for several years. Indeed, only a small part of the first edition was ever sold, the publisher marking the remainder as unsalable. Not until 1865 had the importance of the book attained sufficient recognition to warrant its reprinting.

The material for *Das Enge Becken* was derived from Michaelis' measurement and study of a thousand obstetric pelves, in 72 of which the true conjugate was 8.75 cm or less. A third of these contractions he attributed to rickets, the remainder chiefly to hereditary factors. Pelvic contraction, Michaelis insisted, was more prevalent than had been recognized previously; but pelvimetry rather than body build was the only reliable criterion for diagnosis. The intertrochanteric, iliac interspinous, and intercristal measurements he dismissed as worthless for estimating the internal pelvic diameters, and Baudelocque's diameter as unreliable as an index of the true conjugate. He demonstrated the relation of the contracted pelvis to abnormalities of fetal position and to the mechanism of labor more clearly than had ever been done before.

In his management of cases of contracted pelvis Michaelis resorted to dietetic restriction during pregnancy for the majority, coupled with abdominal binders near term for patients with a pendulous abdomen, to promote a favorable fetal lie. For high degrees of pelvic contraction, he favored the induction of premature labor, unless cesarean section appeared absolutely indicated. Craniotomy was reserved for cases in which the fetus was already dead. He acknowledged symphysiotomy as justifiable in certain cases but did not use it himself.

Michaelis' conclusions added fresh emphasis to the need for actual pelvic measurement in clinical diagnosis. He wrote:

Only pelvic mensuration can be relied upon as a sure means of recognizing pelvic contraction. Nevertheless, certain bodily deformities, when present in marked degree, can probably be correlated with certainty with a contracted pelvis. These cases are very rare, however, and in the final analysis even they demand measurement for an estimation of the degree of pelvic contraction, to determine which ones require the most formidable therapeutic measures, such as cesarean section.

In the large majority of cases of pelvic contraction, no definite signs exist other than measurement; although contraction may be suspected from a history of illnesses that commonly deform the pelvis [Michaelis included in this category rickets, osteomalacia, tuberculosis, osteotomas, and pelvic fractures], from body form [including scoliosis and abnormally short stature], or from the course of labor. The last certainly provides a definite disclosure in some cases . . . but it gives us this information too late to permit the institution of rational therapy in time to safeguard the mother and infant. How many infants, how many mothers fall victim to premature intervention, to lethal interference, in this condition, merely because the obstetrician did not anticipate the pelvic contraction he had to deal with? . . . Only short stature of extreme degree, whether the result of rickets or truly symmetrical dwarfism, indicates a contracted pelvis; whereas unusually large body size, even if associated with large extremities, is not always accompanied by a correspondingly large pelvis.

With complete candor Michaelis related his difficulties in measuring the pelvic outlet:

I will frankly confess that until now I have never recognized a contraction of the outlet with certainty by measurement. It may indeed be mere chance that I have never encountered this in marked degree; but that it is surely recognizable I do not doubt at all. I have repeatedly sought to extend the general measurements to the outlet but always failed in this, never obtaining consistent results. The ischial tuberosities could not be measured externally, nor the distance between them in the living subject. I have been just as unsuccessful in measuring them internally, however, partly because the great sensitivity of these parts does not permit the pressure necessary for this purpose, and partly because I could discover no satisfactory place to put my finger for this measurement. I have learned that equally little satisfaction could be obtained with instruments. The distance between the lower border of the pubic symphysis and the coccyx appears to be more easily measurable, but I found it also just as difficult to measure, never yielding results that agreed with one another to a half-inch. Particularly vexing is the fact that the tip of the coccyx is not sharply defined; also the fact that the inclination of the pubic symphysis intersects the measuring line in a sharp angle, as a result of which the proper point on the symphysis can be marked only inaccurately on the measuring finger. External measurement with calipers works best. This measurement is of little significance, however, because of variations of about 1 to 2 inches in the length of the coccyx. But to find the end of the sacrum with certainty and to measure the distance to it are beset with such difficulties, that only in the rarest case does the importance of this measurement justify the trouble and pain it entails.

A century later, obstetricians continue to share Michaelis' frustration over clinical mensuration of the pelvic outlet.

MICHAELIS' LIFE

Gustav Adolf Michaelis was born July 9, 1798, in Harburg, Germany, where his father practiced medicine.[1,2,4] Upon the latter's early death, young Michaelis went to Kiel to live with his uncle, C. R. W. Wiedemann, who was professor of medicine and director of the school for midwives in that city. Here the young boy's interest in natural science was carefully nurtured, and he was encouraged to follow the profession of his father and uncle. After attending gymnasiums in Kiel and Göttingen, he entered the former city's medical school, from which he graduated in 1820. While pursuing his medical studies he managed to maintain an active interest in mathematics and archaeology as well. Similarly, while continuing his postgraduate studies in the hospitals of Paris, he found ample time for artistic and literary pursuits. In 1823 Michaelis returned to Kiel, where he entered practice and served as assistant to Wiedemann in the lying-in hospital. His dissertation on sclerema neonatorum was published in 1825, under the title *De induratione telae cellulosae recens natorum*. Even while developing an extensive practice and devoting himself assiduously to his academic duties, he still maintained an interest in natural history; and in 1846 he served as first president of the biologic congress in Kiel. He carried out original observations on the phenomenon of phosphorescence in marine forms, one species of which has been named for him, the flagellate *Peridinium michaelis.* In 1836 he was named official physician (Physikus) to the city of Kiel; he also replaced his ailing uncle at the lying-in hospital, of which he was made director after Wiedemann's death in 1841. In 1839 he was elevated to the rank of extraordinary professor of obstetrics at the university, but he was never given the full recognition of ordinarius. As a result, he did not participate in the examinations by the medical faculty and never attracted more than a small number of students. In 1842 Michaelis published his textbook for midwives, *Unterricht für Hebammen.*

In his later years Michaelis, taking an active part in communal affairs, became increasingly preoccupied with the social and personal problems of his fellow citizens. His long-standing tendency toward depression worsened, and in 1846 the political turmoil within the state provided an additional stimulus to his agitation. To add to his troubles, an epidemic of puerperal infection broke out in the wards of the lying-in hospital, taking the lives of many patients. In time, the scourge of sepsis began to invade his private practice. Michaelis had been one of the very first to recognize the importance of Semmelweis' contribution to the understanding and prevention of childbed fever, and had stood almost alone in the latter's defense. Despite his efforts at asepsis, however, a beloved cousin succumbed to infection after he had attended her at delivery. This was the last straw! Overcome by an intense feeling of personal guilt, he was plunged into a profound depression, from which he never recovered. A vacation failed to help, and on August 8, 1848, at the age of 50, the final irony in the life of this great man was enacted when he hurled himself under the wheels of a moving train.

REFERENCES

1. Dohrn, R.: *Geschichte der Geburtshülfe der Neuzeit.* Part 1 (1840–1860). Pietzcker, Tübingen, 1903, pp. 56–60.
2. Findley, P.: *Priests of Lucina: The Story of Obstetrics.* Little, Brown & Co., Boston, 1939, pp. 254–57.
3. Michaelis, G. A.: *Das Enge Becken nach eigenen Beobachtungen und Untersuchungen.* Ed. by C. C. T. Litzmann. Wigand, Leipzig, 1851.
4. Michaelis, Gustav Adolph. *Allegemeine Deutsche Biographie.* Duncker & Humblot, Leipzig, 1885, Vol. 21, pp. 679–81.

Carl Gustav Carus and the Parturient Axis

Recognition of the purely passive role of the fetus in the birth process, over two centuries ago, stimulated obstetricians to increased concern with the mechanics of labor and with efforts to determine the shapes, planes, and axes of the pelvis, as well as the expulsive forces of the parturient uterus. In the words of James Matthews Duncan: [1]

> The ovum or foetus, in its passage through the developed genital canal, is subjected, in various circumstances, to various rotations on some more or less longitudinally directed axis. It is also subject, in various circumstances, to various revolutions or sinuous deflections, in which its long axis moves through portions of curves which are measured by corresponding angles.

This path of egress of the fetus, known as the axis of parturition, is determined largely by the axis of the pelvic canal, a curve resulting from perpendiculars erected at the midpoints of an infinite number of imaginary pelvic planes, from the superior to the inferior strait.

The first attempt at an accurate description of the axis of the birth canal was a terse, one-sentence statement in 1701 by the famous Dutch obstetrician Hendrik van Deventer: [5]

> Cavitas Pelvis longitudine sua non secundum longitudinem spinae dorsi tendit, sed *ab imo oblique anticam versus ascendendo* progreditur, quasi per eam umbilicum ventris attingere velis; quare quaerentes os uteri non recta versus curvatum Os sacrum digitos intrudere debent, sed ab imo sursum tendere, quasi per

159

muliebria umbilicum ventris manu attingere vellent. [The Cavity of the *Pelvis* does not tend in its Length according to the Length of the Back-Bone, but rising from the Bottom obliquely, it ascends forwards, and so proceeds, as if through it you would touch the Navle, wherefore those that seek the Mouth of the Womb must not thrust their Fingers strait towards the bending of the *Os Sacrum,* but moving them upwards from the Bottom, as if through the Private Parts they would touch the Navel with their Hands.]

LEVRET'S DESCRIPTION OF THE PARTURIENT AXIS

During the ensuing century the problem received the attention of Johann Jacob Müller (1745), Röderer (1751), Smellie (1751), Levret (1753 and 1761), Peter Camper (1759), Saxtorph (1764), Georg Wilhelm Stein, the elder (1770), Baudelocque (1781), J. C. Sommer (1791), C. C. Creve (1794), G. W. Stein, the younger (1797), Osiander (1802–1818), and others, whose contributions were reviewed in a critical and scholarly fashion in 1825 by Naegele.[13] Outstanding among these were the geometric formulations of Levret,[9] which delineated for the first time the three pelvic planes of chief obstetric significance. Levret's description assumed the woman in the standing posture and the planes determined by the following (Fig. 20-1):

1. A line from the top of the pubic symphysis to the junction of the last two sacral vertebrae, corresponding to the horizon. [Levret erred here, for this line, corresponding to the plane of the midpelvis, is inclined rather than horizontal in the standing woman.]
2. A line from the same point on the pubic symphysis to the middle of the lower edge of the last lumbar vertebra, forming an angle of about 35° with the former. [Here again Levret was in error, for the plane of the superior strait is normally inclined at an angle of about 55° to the horizontal.]
3. A line parallel to 2, from the tip of the coccyx and extending to the lower part of the vulva [corresponding to the plane of the inferior strait].

"In order to understand perfectly the inclination of the pelvic cavity," Levret continued, "it is necessary to consider three different axes, all of which intersect the parabolic line." Levret's parabola represented the first attempt to illustrate the path of the fetal head in labor by means of a curve. He proceeded to define the axes as follows: The first is perpendicular to line no. 2, described above, and intersects it at its midpoint; the second is perpendicular to line no. 1 and intersects it at its midpoint; and the third axis forms a right angle with line no. 3 at its midpoint. If these axes are projected inferiorly, the first meets the lower end of the sacrum, the second the tip of the coccyx, and the third the anus. If a diagonal is now drawn from behind forward and from above downward, between the parallel lines nos. 2 and 3, then this diagonal, where it intersects the axes, together with the parabolic curve, shows the principal changes in the direction of the head as it moves through the pelvis in normal labor.

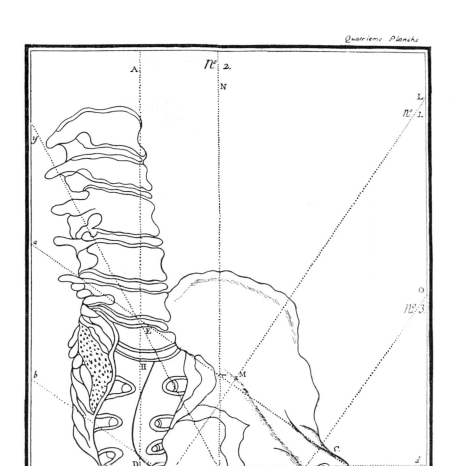

Levret Sculp.
PRINCIPES FONDAMENTAUX DU MECHANISME DE L'ACCOUCHEMENT RELATIVEMENT
AU VUIDE DU BASSIN SEULEMENT.
Découvert et démontré par M. André Levret Accoucheur de Madame La Dauphine &c.

Fig. 20-1. Levret's concept of the pelvic planes and axes, published in 1761,[9] showing the first curvilinear representation of the axis of parturition.

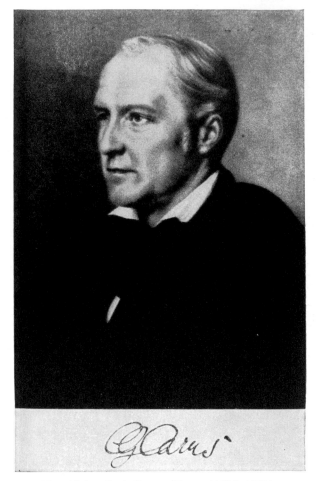

Fig. 20-2. Carl Gustav Carus (1789–1869).

The complexity of Levret's diagram, coupled with the welter of errors it contains, including a lack of agreement between its labeling and the textual description, soon leaves the reader in a state of hopeless confusion. Despite Levret's reminder, conspicuously affixed to the foot of his illustration, that he was "Accoucheur de Madame La Dauphine," it is little to be wondered that his "discovery and demonstration" of the axis of parturition failed to achieve sustained acceptance.

CARUS' DESCRIPTION OF THE PARTURIENT AXIS

In contrast to the absurd and meaningless intricacy of Levret's system of planes, axes, and curves, there appeared in 1820 another formulation of the parturient axis, so simple in principle and clear in presentation that it found wide and immediate appeal among obstetricians of all lands. The curve of Carus, as it soon came to be known, suffered from imperfections also, as pointed out by subsequent students of the problem; but the charm of its simplicity soon entrenched this arc so deeply in obstetric teaching that the term "curve of Carus" came to be used by some as synonymous with "axis of parturition."

Carus' consideration of the path of the fetal head appears in paragraphs 43 and 44 (Fig. 20-3) of Part 1 of his *Lehrbuch der Gynäkologie*.[2] He wrote:

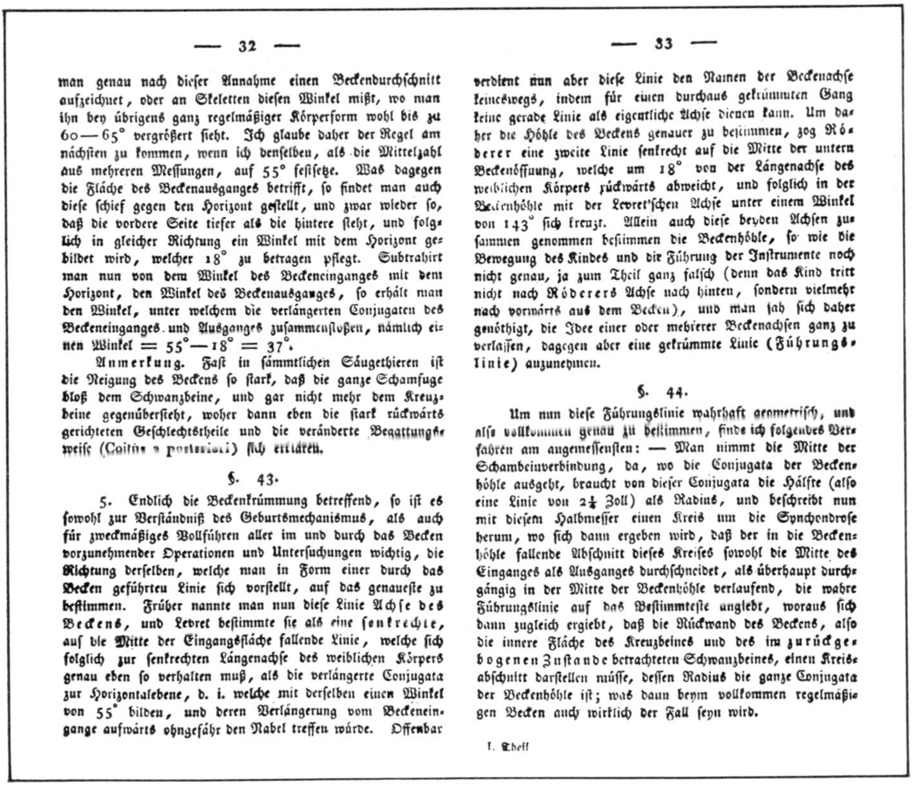

— 32 —

man genau nach dieser Annahme einen Beckendurchschnitt aufzeichnet, oder an Skeletten diesen Winkel mißt, wo man ihn bey übrigens ganz regelmäßiger Körperform wohl bis zu 60—65° vergrößert sieht. Ich glaube daher der Regel am nächsten zu kommen, wenn ich denselben, als die Mittelzahl aus mehreren Messungen, auf 55° festsetze. Was dagegen die Fläche des Beckenausganges betrifft, so findet man auch diese schief gegen den Horizont gestellt, und zwar wieder so, daß die vordere Seite tiefer als die hintere steht, und folglich in gleicher Richtung ein Winkel mit dem Horizont gebildet wird, welcher 18° zu betragen pflegt. Subtrahirt man nun von dem Winkel des Beckeneinganges mit dem Horizont, den Winkel des Beckenausganges, so erhält man den Winkel, unter welchem die verlängerten Conjugaten des Beckeneinganges und Ausganges zusammenstoßen, nämlich einen Winkel = 55°—18° = 37°.

Anmerkung. Fast in sämmtlichen Säugethieren ist die Neigung des Beckens so stark, daß die ganze Schamfuge bloß dem Schwanzbeine, und gar nicht mehr dem Kreuzbeine gegenübersieht, woher dann eben die stark rückwärts gerichteten Geschlechtstheile und die veränderte Begattungsweise (Coitus a posteriori) sich erklären.

§. 43.

5. Endlich die Beckenkrümmung betreffend, so ist es sowohl zur Verständniß des Geburtsmechanismus, als auch für zweckmäßiges Vollführen aller im und durch das Becken vorzunehmenden Operationen und Untersuchungen wichtig, die Richtung derselben, welche man in Form einer durch das Becken geführten Linie sich vorstellt, auf das genaueste zu bestimmen. Früher nannte man nun diese Linie Achse des Beckens, und Levret bestimmte sie als eine senkrechte, auf die Mitte der Eingangsfläche fallende Linie, welche sich folglich zur senkrechten Längenachse des Körpers genau eben so verhalten muß, als die verlängerte Conjugata zur Horizontalebene, d. i. welche mit derselben einen Winkel von 55° bilden, und deren Verlängerung vom Beckeneingange aufwärts ohngefähr den Nabel treffen würde. Offenbar

— 33 —

verdient nun aber diese Linie den Namen der Beckenachse keinesweges, indem für einen durchaus gekrümmten Gang keine gerade Linie als eigentliche Achse dienen kann. Um daher die Höhle des Beckens genauer zu bestimmen, zog Röderer eine zweite Linie senkrecht auf die Mitte der untern Beckenöffnung, welche um 18° von der Längenachse des weiblichen Körpers rückwärts abweicht, und folglich in der Beckenhöhle mit der Levret'schen Achse unter einem Winkel von 143° sich kreuzt. Allein auch diese beyden Achsen zusammen genommen bestimmen die Beckenhöhle, so wie die Bewegung des Kindes und die Führung der Instrumente noch nicht genau, ja zum Theil ganz falsch (denn das Kind tritt nicht nach Röderers Achse nach hinten, sondern vielmehr nach vorwärts aus dem Becken), und man sah sich daher genöthigt, die Idee einer oder mehrerer Beckenachsen ganz zu verlassen, dagegen aber eine gekrümmte Linie (Führungslinie) anzunehmen.

§. 44.

Um nun diese Führungslinie wahrhaft geometrisch, und also vollkommen genau zu bestimmen, finde ich folgendes Verfahren am angemessensten: — Man nimmt die Mitte der Schambeinverbindung, da, wo die Conjugata der Beckenhöhle ausgeht, braucht von dieser Conjugata die Hälfte (also eine Linie von 2¼ Zoll) als Radius, und beschreibt nun mit diesem Halbmesser einen Kreis in die Synchondrose herum, wo sich dann ergeben wird, daß der in die Beckenhöhle fallende Abschnitt dieses Kreises sowohl die Mitte des Einganges als Ausganges durchschneidet, als überhaupt durchgängig in der Mitte der Beckenhöhle verlaufen, die wahre Führungslinie auf das Bestimmteste angiebt, woraus sich dann zugleich ergiebt, daß die Rückwand des Beckens, also die innere Fläche des Kreuzbeines und des im zurückgebogenen Zustande betrachteten Schwanzbeines, einen Kreisabschnitt darstellen müsse, dessen Radius die ganze Conjugata der Beckenhöhle ist; was dann beym vollkommen regelmäßigen Becken auch wirklich der Fall seyn wird.

I. Theil

Fig. 20-3. Carus' description of the parturient axis, pages from his textbook.[2]

With respect to the pelvic curvature, it is important to determine its direction, as much for an understanding of the mechanism of birth as for the proper performance of all pelvic examinations and operations. This direction, pictured as a line drawn through the pelvis so that it can be defined more precisely, was formerly called the pelvic axis. Levret defined it as a line perpendicular to the middle of the plane of the inlet, which line must therefore maintain precisely the same relation to the vertical longitudinal axis of the female body as the extended conjugate does to the horizontal; that is, forming an angle of 55°. . . .

Now obviously this line does not merit at all the designation of pelvic axis, for no straight line can serve as an exact axis for a passage curved in its entirety. In order to define the pelvic cavity more precisely, therefore, Röderer drew a second line, perpendicular to the middle of the pelvic outlet, which deviates posteriorly about 18° from the longitudinal axis of the female body and then intersects the axis of Levret at an angle of 143°. But these two axes taken together still do not precisely determine the pelvic cavity nor the movement of the fetus and the introduction of instruments. Indeed they denote the pelvic axis quite inaccurately in part, for the fetus does not make its exit from the pelvis in a posterior direction, as indicated by Röderer's axis, but much more anteriorly. It was therefore found necessary to abandon entirely the idea of one or several pelvic axes and to adopt a curved line (Führungslinie) instead.

Carus, it will be noted, has mistakenly referred to Levret's axis of the superior strait as Levret's axis of the pelvis, a totally unwarranted over-simplification and a further distortion of Levret's already faulty scheme. Carus' historic perspective was also somewhat distorted in the statement that Röderer *added* a second line to Levret's, for the first edition of the latter's book post-dated Röderer's publication by two years. Carus continued in his description of the curve that now bears his name:

Now in order to define this pelvic axis truly geometrically and thus completely precisely I find the following procedure to be the most suitable:—One takes the middle of the pubic symphysis, where the conjugate of the pelvic cavity begins, and using a radius of 2¼ inches, describes a circle around the synchondrosis,

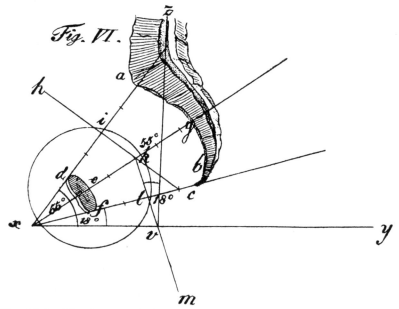

Fig. 20-4. The "curve of Carus" as originally illustrated by the author.[2]

whereupon it will then be seen that the arc of this circle falling inside the pelvic cavity transects the middle of the inlet as well as the outlet [Fig. 20-4]. Coursing in general through the middle of the pelvic cavity, it indicates the true axis of the pelvis in the most precise way. It thus follows that the posterior wall of the pelvis, that is, the inner surface of the sacrum and the posteriorly retracted coccyx, must represent an arc of a circle whose radius is the whole conjugate of the pelvic cavity; and this will actually be the case in the completely regular pelvis.

Cognizant of pelvic variability, Carus added the comment:

The female pelvis shows itself as normal in all respects much less often than seems to be generally believed; and I have found this to be the case particularly with the curvature of the pelvic cavity, in which respect scarcely one pelvis whose curvature measures up completely to the true norm is likely to be found among a considerable series of otherwise rather well-formed pelves.

Soon after the publication of Carus' book, Naegele [13] pointed out the short-comings of the circle of Carus as the track of the fetal head, at the same time presenting his own version of this axis. Naegele correctly pictured the path of parturition for the first time, as a straight line in its upper half, to the level of the midpelvis, and curved in its lower, to the outlet. Two centuries later, this concept has finally achieved universal acceptance as best portraying the true axis of the pelvis.

Until the end of the nineteenth century, however, a few authors of obstetric textbooks remained captivated by the greater simplicity of Carus' circle, which they continued to teach as the birth axis. The illustrious and bombastic Meigs of Philadelphia, for example, wrote in his *Obstetrics*,[12] published in 1849:

Such is Carus's curve, or Carus's circle; which is the bent axis of the pelvic canal, an important item of midwifery knowledge; one without which a practitioner is incompetent scientifically to deliver a placenta, and far less to extract a child by turning, or to apply, and deliver with, the forceps, or the crotchet. I caution the student not to fail in understanding this point very perfectly. If he should make himself perfectly familiar with the curve of Carus, I see not how he could make any mistake as to the appropriate direction of his efforts in any act of delivery, whether with the hand alone, or with instruments.

As late as the latter part of the nineteenth century Barnes wrote, in his *Manual of Midwifery:* [1] "The general axis of the pelvis is called the curve of Carus." Dorland, in his *Manual of Obstetrics*,[6] taught that "the axis of the pelvic cavity, or canal, also termed the *curve* or *circle of Carus* . . .* represents the path followed by the fetus during parturition." Meadows also, in the early editions [10] of his *Manual of Midwifery,* stated that "the circle of Carus . . . corresponds with the course followed by the foetus in its passage through the pelvis," but recanted in later editions [11] of his popular text with the revised statement: "The circle or curve of Carus . . . was formerly supposed to indicate the complete axis of the entire pelvic canal, and to represent the course which the child took in its passage through the pelvis. . . . This, however, is now known to be an error, for the pelvic canal is not a simple cylinder, and no such circle or curve can represent its axes at different points from brim to outlet." Hodge had already registered an American note of dissent much earlier, in his famous *Principles and Practice of Obstetrics,*[8] with the statement: "The 'curve of Carus,' the distinguished Professor of Dresden, although by many in this country regarded as true, seems to us very erroneous. . . . This gives a curved line as the axis of the superior strait, instead of acknowledging its straight character until it reaches the level of the sub-pubic ligament."

Most twentieth-century textbooks of obstetrics continue to describe the curve of Carus, but only for its historic interest.

CARUS' LIFE

Carl Gustav Carus was born January 3, 1789, in Leipzig, Germany.[4] The details of his youth are retold with sensitivity and charm in his philosophic autobiography,[3] published in 1866. As a boy he became interested in natural science, and in 1811 received both his doctorate of philosophy and medical degree from the University of Leipzig, his dissertation for the latter degree being titled *De uteri rheumatismo.* Following graduation he taught comparative anatomy at the university while carrying out investigations on the comparative anatomy of the nervous system, and then served for a period as medical officer in the lying-in hospital of Trèves. When the medical-surgical academy opened in Dresden in 1814 Carus was made professor of obstetrics and director of the lying-in hospital. Here he remained for 13 years, so happy in his work and surroundings that he declined invitations to the universities of Erlangen, Göttingen, Breslau, and Berlin. In 1827 he was appointed royal physician and given a position of high authority in the state regulation of medical practice.

Despite his large practice, which included many of the nobility, Carus found time for a prodigious literary production of about 100 works, which included 40 books, five volumes of his memoirs, and an extensive correspondence. He drew many of his illustrations himself. The multiplicity of Carus' interests is revealed by the titles in his bibliography, listed in his autobiography. His works included books on zoology, comparative anatomy, physiology, art, psychology, philosophy, obstetrics, archaeology, and anthropology. Carus has been referred to as the Harvey of entomologists. For his discovery of a blood circulation mediated by the heart of larval insects he was awarded the gold medal of the French Institute.

A disciple of Goethe, Carus has likewise been regarded as one of the outstanding romanticists of the nineteenth century. He also lived in the spirit of Goethe, his home in Dresden being graced almost constantly by some of the best-known artists, singers, musicians, actors, and philosophers of the day. Jenny Lind sang there, Purkinje and Remak, the neurophysiologists, lectured there, and Henrik Ibsen sought his frequent companionship. Carus died on July 28, 1869.

REFERENCES

1. Barnes, F A.: *A Manual of Midwifery, for Midwives and Medical Students.* Henry C. Lea, Philadelphia, 1879, p. 17.

2. Carus, C. G.: *Lehrbuch der Gynäkologie, oder Systematische Darstellung der Lehren von Erkenntniss und Behandlung Eigenthümlicher Gesunder und Krankhafter Zustände, sowohl der nicht Schwangern, Schwangern und Gebärenden Frauen, als der Wöchnerinnen und Neugeborenen Kinder.* G. Fleischer, Leipzig, 1820, Part 1, pp. 32–33, Fig. 6.

3. Carus, C. G.: *Lebenserinnerungen und Denkwürdigkeiten.* F. A. Brockhaus, Leipzig, 1866. In Knoll, A. G.: *Vom Wirken Berühmter Ärzte aus Vier Jahrhunderten.* Chemische Fabriken, Ludwigshafen a. Rh., 1936.

4. Clemens, P.: Zum Gedächtnis von Carl Gustav Carus, dem grossen Arzt und Naturforscher, Künstler und Philosophen. *München. med. Wchnschr.,* **86**: 700–702, 1939.

5. Deventer, H. van: *Operationes Chirurgicae Novum Lumen Exhibentes Obstetricantibus, quo fideliter manifestatur ars obstetricandi, et quidquid ad eam requiritur: Instructum pluribus figuris aeri incisis. . . . .* Dyckuisen, Leyden, 1701, Cap. 3, pp. 21–22. English translation from *The Art of Midwifery Improv'd. Fully and Plainly laying Down Whatever Instructions Are Requisite to Make a Compleat Midwife. And the Many Errors in All the Books hitherto Written upon this Subject Clearly Refuted. Written in Latin by Henry à Deventer. Made English by an Eminent Physican.* E. Curll, F. Pemberton, & W. Taylor, London, 1716, p. 26.

6. Dorland, W. A. N.: *A Manual of Obstetrics.* W. B. Saunders Co., Philadelphia, 1896, pp. 26–27.

7. Duncan, J. M.: The curves of the developed genital passage. In *Contributions to the Mechanism of Natural and Morbid Parturition Including that of Placenta Praevia.* Adam & Charles Black, Edinburgh, 1875, pp. 37–62.

8. Hodge, H. L.: *The Principles and Practice of Obstetrics.* Henry C. Lea, Philadelphia, 1864 (1866), p. 47.

9. Levret, A.: *L'Art des Accouchemens, Demontré par des Principes de Physique et de Méchanique,* 2nd ed. Le Prieur, Paris, 1761, pp. 7–8, 299–303, and Fig. 4. (First edition, published in 1753, lacked Fig. 4.)

10. Meadows, A: *A Manual of Midwifery, Including the Signs and Symptoms of Pregnancy, Obstetric Operations, Diseases of the Puerperal State, etc., etc.,* 1st American ed. from 2nd London ed. Lindsay & Blakiston, Philadelphia, 1871, p. 36.

11. Meadows, A., and Venn, A. J.: *A Manual of Midwifery,* 4th ed. G. P. Putnam's Sons, New York, 1882, pp. 14–15.

12. Meigs, C. D.: *Obstetrics: The Science and the Art.* Lea & Blanchard, Philadelphia, 1849, pp. 47–48.

13. Naegele, F. C.: *Das Weibliche Becken Betrachtet in Beziehung auf seine Stellung und die Richtung seiner Höhle nebst Beyträgen zur Geschichte der Lehre von den Beckenaxen.* Müller, Carlsruhe, 1825.

Franz Carl Naegele, Naegele's Rule, Naegele's Asynclitism, and the Naegele Pelvis; Ferdinand Robert and the Robert Pelvis

NAEGELE'S RULE

Estimation of the onset of pregnancy and prediction of its date of termination must be based on retrospective evaluation of circumstantial evidence, often of uncertain credibility. This difficulty in determining the precise time of conception was discussed by Montgomery,[6] who stated a century ago:

[It] can hardly be otherwise until we meet in society more numerous imitators of Zenobia, the beautiful Queen of Palmyra, who, if we are to credit Trebellius Pollio, "never admitted her husband's embraces but for the sake of issue; if her hopes were baffled in the ensuing month, she reiterated her experiment": but in the existing rarity of such instances of self-command, we are obliged to acknowledge, with regret, that "as it is difficult to conceal the termination of pregnancy, so it is equally difficult to ascertain its commencement."

Thus, although conception can sometimes be dated accurately from isolated coitus or artificial insemination, in the majority of cases the duration of pregnancy must be reckoned from the last menstrual period. Invoking Christian dogma, William Harvey[5] wrote in the early-seventeenth century:

Unquestionably the ordinary term of utero-gestation is that which we believe was kept in the womb of his mother by our Saviour Christ, of men the most perfect; counting, viz. from the festival of the Annunciation, in the month of March, to the day of the blessed Nativity, which we celebrate in December

169

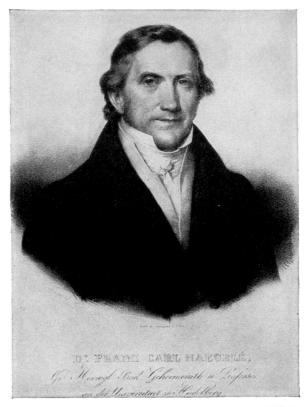

Fig. 21-1. Franz Carl Naegele (1778–1851). (Courtesy of National Library of Medicine, Washington, D. C.)

[275 days]. Prudent matrons, calculating after this rule, as long as they note the day of the month in which the catamenia usually appear, are rarely out of their reckoning; but after ten lunar months have elapsed, fall in labour, and reap the fruit of their womb the very day on which the catamenia would have appeared, had impregnation not taken place.

In actual practice the date of labor has long been estimated by the simple calculation: adding seven days to the first day of the last menstruation and counting back three months. This formula, found in all obstetric texts, is designated as Naegele's rule. Nineteenth-century teaching, although hazy concerning the fertile days of the menstrual cycle, was quite explicit for calculating the expected date of confinement. The following excerpt from Bedford's *Principles and Practice of Obstetrics* [1] is representative of the texts of that era:

A very common mode of calculation, both among the profession and women themselves, is to take the last catamenial turn as the starting point. . . . I think the fact is very generally conceded, that the most likely time for a female to become fecundated is immediately after a menstrual crisis; but, it is equally well established, that impregnation will occasionally occur just before the catamenial period, and sometimes during the menstrual flow, while, on the other hand, it must not be forgotten that conception is possible at any time between the two menstrual turns. . . . I have, for several years, adopted a rule which, I believe, was originally suggested by the celebrated Naegele; with some exceptions, I have found it generally quite reliable, and far more satisfactory in its results than any plan which has yet been proposed. Imagine, for example, the termination of the last menstrual period to be on the 10th day of January; then count back three months, which will correspond with the 10th day of October; now from the 10th of October, add seven days—this will bring you to the 17th day of October—the day on which the labor will commence.

The reader will be quick to note Bedford's apparent inaccuracy in taking the last day of the menstrual period, rather than the first, as the point of reference. More likely to be overlooked, however, is the author's mistake in crediting this formula to Naegele, an error that has been kept alive for over a century and is still being perpetuated by the most recent obstetric texts. Naegele neither formulated nor made any claim to the "rule" that bears his name. He clearly presented it, rather, in the form of a direct quotation from Boerhaave, properly annotated bibliographically, and indeed in Boerhaave's original Latin,[2] which sets the passage off quite sharply from the German of Naegele's text: [7]

Feminae plerumque post finem mensium impraegnantur: id confirmant numerosa experimenta in Galliis capta: ex centum enim partubus omnino nonaginta & novem fiunt nono mense post menstrua ultima, numerando unam septimanam post menses ultimos, & ab ea epocha repetendo novem gestationis menses. Tunc enim uterus repurgatus & vacuus est, & exhausta plethora, neque metus adest, conceptum adeo cito expulsum iri. . . . [Women are usually impregnated after the end of their menstrual flow. This is proved by numerous observations in France; for 99 out of 100 births occur in the ninth month after the last menstruation, adding a week after the last menses and counting nine months of gestation. For at this time the fetus will soon be expelled, the uterus is emptied and cleaned, and the plethora removed.]

"Naegele's rule" as originally stated by Boerhaave, is ambiguous in respect to the date of reference. Bedford was therefore equally justified in counting from the end of the last menstrual period as is the more modern practice of calculating the date of confinement from the day of the last menses' onset. Some recent studies have even suggested that the former method agrees more closely with actual experience. In any case the designation "Naegele's rule" is one of the outstanding examples of misplaced credit in obstetric terminology.

Hermann Boerhaave, the probable author of Naegele's rule and one of the most famous physicians of the eighteenth century, was born in Voorhout,

Holland, December 31, 1668. In 1709 he was made professor of medicine and botany at the University of Leyden, and five years later was elevated to the position of rector of the university and president of the Chirurgical College. He achieved the reputation as the outstanding medical consultant of his time, one measure of his success being a fortune of 2 million florins he left at his death on September 23, 1738. Among his many pupils was Albrecht von Haller, who later published Boerhaave's academic lectures. Boerhaave is said to have left an elaborately bound volume, which was to contain all the secrets of medicine. When it was opened, after his death, all the pages were found blank save one; and on it was inscribed but one sentence: "Keep the head cool, the feet warm, and the bowels open."

NAEGELE'S ASYNCLITISM

Understanding of the precise positions of the fetal head during its engagement and descent through the pelvis was long hampered, until the advent of radiography, by a number of factors: the lack of precise methods of observation; the failure to appreciate the transcendent importance of pelvic type in determining the mechanism of labor; and the inadequate recognition of asynclitism, a lateral flexion of the neck, as an accessory mechanism in the birth process. For many years the fetal head was believed to enter the superior strait in all normal cases with its sagittal suture in the direct anteroposterior diameter. We now know that this rarely occurs, and that in the majority of cephalic presentations engagement occurs in the transverse, with the sagittal suture parallel to the transverse diameter of the inlet. When the sagittal suture lies equidistant from the sacral promontory and pubic symphysis, the head is said to be synclitic. More often, however, the sagittal suture deviates, to a greater or lesser degree, toward the promontory or symphysis, anterior or posterior asynclitism resulting according as the anterior or posterior parietal bone becomes the presenting part.

Anterior asynclitism, or anterior parietal presentation, is often referred to as Naegele's obliquity, for it was Naegele who stressed its normalcy in the mechanism of labor. Naegele's description of anterior asynclitism appeared in 1819, in his monograph, *Ueber den Mechanismus der Geburt.*[8] He wrote:

In the most frequent cephalic presentation [L O A], the head presents not with the occiput, but rather with the right parietal bone, the posterior fontanelle being directed toward the left acetabulum during labor.

On examination at the beginning of cervical dilatation, and even earlier in multiparas, at the very onset of labor, the examining finger, introduced toward the center of the pelvic cavity, will encounter the head in the region of the right parietal boss. The two fontanelles are usually at the same level; occasionally the anterior, but more often the posterior, is a little lower. The head assumes an oblique rather than a vertical position at the pelvic inlet, so that neither the vertex nor the sagittal suture, but rather the right parietal bone, is the presenting part. The sagittal suture is much closer to the sacral promontory than to the pubis, and divides the cervical os, which faces posteriorly and usually somewhat to the left, into two unequal segments. In some circumstances . . . swelling of the scalp [caput succedaneum] occurs soon after the cervix has begun to dilate, this swelling gradually disappearing as the cervix changes in condition and position and as the head also changes its relation to it. Still, as the cervix dilates, the caput remains palpable for some time, although it becomes much softer. In the cephalic position here under consideration [L O A] the caput is situated over the *right* parietal bone, near its upper edge, and equidistant from both ends.

Naegele's concept of asynclitism as an auxiliary factor in the birth mechanism has been amply corroborated, but he erred in regarding the obliquity as constant throughout the greater part of labor:

Because of the oblique position of the head, the greatest diameter of the skull, from one parietal boss to the other as well as at the base, can never coincide with the diameters of the pelvic inlet as the head passes through it. . . . When the head is completely engaged and nearing the outlet, the posterior fontanelle is still found directed toward the left obturator foramen. If the finger now be introduced under the center of the pubic arch and continued along the course of an imaginary median line projected outward from the pelvic cavity, the finger tip will impinge upon the right parietal bone, rather precisely at the middle of its superior and posterior quadrant, occasionally at the middle of its posterior half.

It is not the center of the occiput that advances under the pubic arch; instead the head approaches the external os with the posterior and superior part of the right parietal bone presenting, and it maintains this position until its greatest circumference has passed through the pelvic outlet. . . . In this position the right parietal boss will be distinctly felt clearing the labia some time before the left.

Considering the cephalic relations when the occiput lies on the right side of the pelvis, Naegele wrote:

Just as the *right* parietal protuberance is the most dependent part in the first position of the head [L O A], in this case it is the *left*. If the finger tip is brought into contact with the head in the midline of the pelvic cavity, it encounters this parietal boss . . . and as the head advances progressively nearer to the outlet, the posterior and superior quadrant of the left parietal bone becomes palpable under the pubic arch . . . and it is precisely this part that first distends the labia as the head advances further . . . and upon which the caput succedaneum forms.

. . . Just as the caput is usually limited to the superior and posterior quadrant of the *right* parietal bone in cases where the vertex is in the first position [L O A], so in this case it is found on the *left* parietal bone. Similarly, just as the right half of the cranium is higher, and the right parietal bone elevated above the left, immediately after delivery from the first position [L O A], so in this case the opposite relations prevail. This difference in the contour of the head cannot be mistaken, even at a glance, and these two manifestations (*the shape of the head* and *the location of the caput succedaneum*) are so *remarkable* and *striking,* that even if one had not examined the patient during labor, they would usually enable him to determine whether the head had taken the first [L O A] or third [R O P] position during labor. . . .

THE NAEGELE PELVIS

Soon after the bony pelvis became recognized as a rigid, unyielding structure, obstetricians began to concern themselves with its deviations from the normal. Few, however, have developed personal acquaintance with the bizarre pelvic abnormality associated with the name of Naegele, because of its rarity as well as the difficulty of recognizing it by clinical examination of the living subject.

Following his initial discovery of this interesting pelvic form, Naegele embarked on a thoroughgoing search, extending over a period of years, for other examples of the malformation. By 1834 he had collected nine cases, which he published in the *Heidelberger Klinische Annalen.* Continuing inquiry and study culminated in his monumental monograph, *Das Schräg Verengte Becken,*[9] published in 1839, which reported 35 female and 2 male pelves of this type, including one in an Egyptian mummy. The peculiar characteristics of these malformed pelves were summarized by Naegele in these words:

1. Complete ankylosis of one sacroiliac synchondrosis or complete fusion of the sacrum with one innominate bone.
2. Atrophy or faulty development of the lateral half of the sacrum and a diminished width or narrowed lumen of the anterior sacral foramina on the side of the ankylosis.
3. Reduced width of the innominate bone and its sacrosciatic notch on the affected side. The distance between the anterior superior spine of the ilium and its posterior superior spine is thus shorter than between the corresponding bones of the other side, as is a line drawn at the pelvic inlet, beginning at about the place where the (missing) sacroiliac joint should be and extending along the innominate line and the crest of the pubic bone to the symphysis. In addition, the region of the posterior part of the inner surface of the innominate bone, where it joins with the sacrum, is not as long, nor does it extend so far down, on the ankylosed side as on the other side and as in the normally formed ilium. . . .
4. The sacrum appears deviated toward the side of the ankylosis, and its anterior surface is also turned more or less toward this side, while the pubic symphysis is forced over toward the opposite side. The symphysis is therefore not directly in front of the promontory but rather oblique to it.
5. The inner surface of the pelvic side wall and of the lateral half of the anterior pelvic wall is less concave, or flatter, on the side of the ankylosis than in the normal pelvis. We have never observed, in the pelves under consideration, the inward pro-

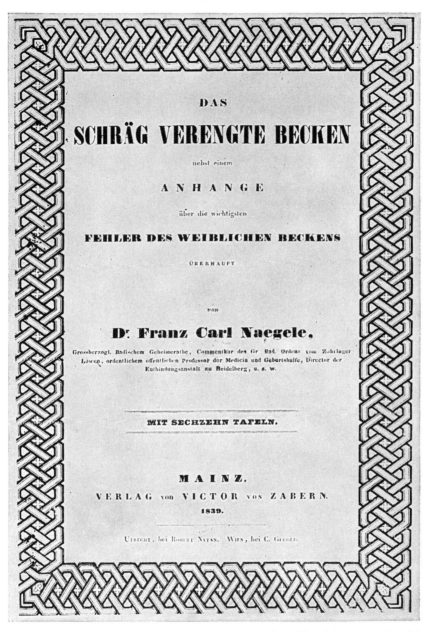

Fig. 21-2. Title page of Naegele's monograph on the obliquely contracted pelvis.

trusion of the superior ramus of the pubis that occurs as a result of . . . adult osteomalacia.

6. The other lateral half of the pelvis, in which the sacroiliac synchondrosis is present, likewise varies from the normal. At first glance . . . one can easily be deceived into believing that the other half is normal. This is not so, however; for if one visualizes such a pelvis, with the sacroiliac ankylosis on the left side, divided anteroposteriorly so that the cut divides the sacrum and pubic symphysis vertically in the midline; and if one were to put the right side of this pelvis together with the left side of a pelvis that was identical except that its ankylosis was on the left side, so that the cut surfaces of both divided sacrums were brought together in contact with each other; then the pubes would be 3 to 4 inches apart. The side of the pelvis uninvolved by ankylosis thus shares with the ankylosed side not merely an abnormal position or direction of the bones, but also an abnormal shape. . . . As a result of the above:

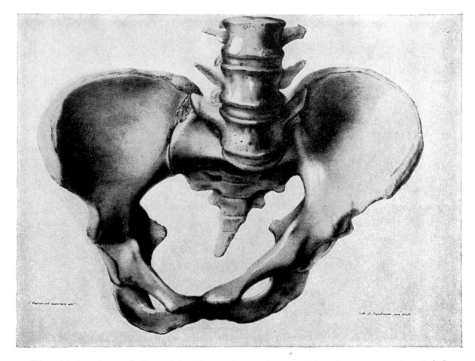

Fig. 21-3. One of Naegele's illustrations of the obliquely contracted pelvis.[9]

7(a). The pelvis is oblique, being contracted in the axis that crosses the line connecting the ankylosis and the acetabulum of the opposite side; while the latter axis is not contracted or is even wider than usual, especially in cases of pronounced deviation. Therefore, the plane of the pelvic inlet . . . and the plane of the midpelvis . . . simulate an oblique oval . . . whose transverse or small diameter corresponds to the contracted oblique diameter of the inlet and pelvic cavity, and whose longitudinal or large diameter corresponds to the other oblique of the pelvis. Thus the term *obliquely oval pelvis* (schrägovales Becken, Pelv. oblique-ovata, Bassin obliq' ovalaire) would probably be an appropriate designation. . . .

(b). The distance between the promontory and the area over one or the other acetabulum (sacrocotyloid distance), and the distance from the tip of the sacrum laterally to one or the other ischial spine, are shorter on the side of the ankylosis than on the other.

(c). The distance between the ischial tuberosity on the side of the ankylosis and the posterior superior spine of the ilium on the other side, and the distance between the spinous process of the last lumbar vertebra and the anterior superior spine of the ilium on the ankylosed side, are shorter than the corresponding measurements on the opposite side.

(d). The distance between the lower edge of the pubic symphysis and the posterior superior spine of the ilium is greater on the ankylosed side. . . .

(e). The pelvic side walls converge obliquely downward to some extent, and the pubic arch is more or less narrowed, because of the abnormal direction in which the joint faces the flattened pelvic wall. As a result, the pelvic shape approaches the male type. . . .

(f). The acetabulum on the flattened side faces forward to a greater degree than in the normal pelvis; on the other side, however, it faces almost completely outward. When one looks at the pelvis from in front, therefore, one looks into the former acetabulum but past the latter, or sees only a small part of its cavity.

His over-all impression of this pelvic type Naegele passed on to the reader "in order to provide, as far as possible, the correct picture for those who have not yet seen such pelves":

. . . At first glance these pelves give the impression of having been compressed from without by a force applied in an obliquely upward direction at one lateral half of the anterior pelvic wall and the region of the acetabulum; while at the same time the other half appears compressed inwardly at its posterior wall.

A further peculiarity of these pelves is that they all differ from one another only in degree of deviation and in the side on which the sacrum is fused with the innominate bone. In all other respects, however . . . they are as similar as one egg is to the next. This similarity is so pronounced that even an experienced person who is unaware of it, if he has once seen such a pelvis and then happened upon another example of it subsequently, would be inclined to take it for the same one he had seen previously.

Naegele ascribed this deformity to a developmental fault, for the bones were of normal size and strength and showed no evidence of rickets, infection, or injury. His view of its etiology still prevails.

All of Naegele's patients with a recorded obstetric history were young, healthy, and otherwise well-formed primigravidas; in each case both mother and child perished in labor. Subsequent experience has confirmed the impossibility of vaginal delivery of a term-sized infant in all but mildest forms of the Naegele pelvis. Williams,[12] however, has reported the case of a patient who spontaneously delivered six viable infants through such a pelvis before suffering rupture of the uterus in her seventh labor, following a failed forceps operation and a version and extraction.

In Naegele's day the deformity had never been recognized in a living person, for it caused little, if any, limp and resulted in no obvious external manifestations. Acknowledging the greater difficulties in recognizing this condition than the more common types of pelvic contraction, Naegele suggested the following external measurements as diagnostic aids, significant differences between the measurements of the two sides pointing to the obliquely oval pelvis:

1. From the ischial tuberosity on one side to the posterior superior spine of the ilium on the other.
2. From the anterior superior spine of one innominate bone to the posterior superior spine of the other.
3. From the spinous process of the last lumbar vertebra to the anterior superior spine of each innominate bone.
4. From the greater trochanter on one side to the posterior superior spine of the ilium on the other.
5. From the middle of the lower border of the pubic symphysis to the posterior superior spine of each innominate bone.

NAEGELE'S LIFE

Franz Carl Naegele was born July 12, 1778, in Düsseldorf, Germany, where his father was a professor in the medical school.[3,4,11] After study in Strassburg, Freiburg, and Bamberg, where he received his doctorate in medicine, followed by a period of travel, young Naegele accepted a position as official physician to the towns of Barmen and Beyerburg in the grand duchy of Berg. He began at once to interest himself in the problems of obstetrics. In 1807 he was called to Heidelberg as extraordinary professor of physiology and pathology, a move arranged by Professor Mai, his prospective father-in-law. Three years later, when Mai retired, Naegele succeeded him as ordinary professor and director of the lying-in hospital, where he spent the next 40 years, until his death on January 21, 1851. In 1813 he assumed the additional position of chief obstetrician for the Neckar, Main, and Tauber regions, a function he passed on to his son, Franz Josef, in 1838.

Naegele became the outstanding personality among the professors of Heidelberg's medical faculty in the first half of the nineteenth century. His renown was based on his obstetric work exclusively, for Naegele scarcely interested himself in gynecology, which was practiced at that time largely by the surgeons and internists. His first studies on the obstetric pelvis resulted in a richly documented monograph, *Das Weibliche Becken,* published in 1825. In this work he took issue with the previously held view that the axis of the pelvis is affected by changes in the position of the body. His study of the mechanism of labor, in addition to pointing out the important phenomenon of asynclitism, called attention to the frequency of spontaneous rotation of the occiput from R O P to L O A, attributing this to the resistance of the pelvic floor. Naegele's *Lehrbuch der Geburtshülfe,* published in 1830 for midwives, found favor among physicians also, and enjoyed the success of 14 editions.

THE ROBERT PELVIS

Shortly after Naegele's description of the pelvic malformation that bears his name, Ferdinand Robert encountered a related but even rarer anomaly, which has since been known as the Robert, or double Naegele, pelvis. In this form the sacral alae are lacking bilaterally, extreme transverse narrowing of the pelvis resulting. The rarity of the Robert pelvis finds its counterpart in the scarcity of Robert's monograph [10] describing it. I am indebted to the University of Chicago Library for the loan of one of the few known copies.

The patient was Elizabeth Reuter, a 31-year-old, illegitimately pregnant primigravida. Robert described her as:

. . . of small stature and gracile habitus. From her youth she had always been well and never suffered from scrofula nor any other diseases that affect the osseous system. Her pregnancy also progressed uneventfully to its calculated date of termination. Labor began on March 9, 1837; on the 11th the water began to leak out. Up until the morning of the 13th the midwife could make out no presenting part of the fetus by internal examination. She therefore summoned Dr. Dittmayer. . . . At 10 A.M. he found the patient in very irregular labor. The abdomen was distended transversely; the cervix was so high that the anterior lip could scarcely be reached; no fetal part could be felt through the vaginal vault. Internal examination revealed such transverse narrowing of the pelvis that there was not enough room for two fingers alongside each other. The patient had felt no fetal movements for several hours. . . . Under the circumstances Dr. Dittmayer considered cesarean section indicated, since he regarded it as the only means of saving the mother's life in such a case of absolute pelvic contraction. . . . The operation was carried out the same day, through a midline incision. . . . The fetus lay in the transverse, and as suspected, was dead. . . . The wound suppurated and there was hope of a favorable outcome. At the same time neither pus nor lochia drained from the vagina. But on the fifth day the patient committed an error of diet, as a result of which she died the following night.

After autopsy, Robert carefully preserved and measured this bizarre pelvis. He reported:

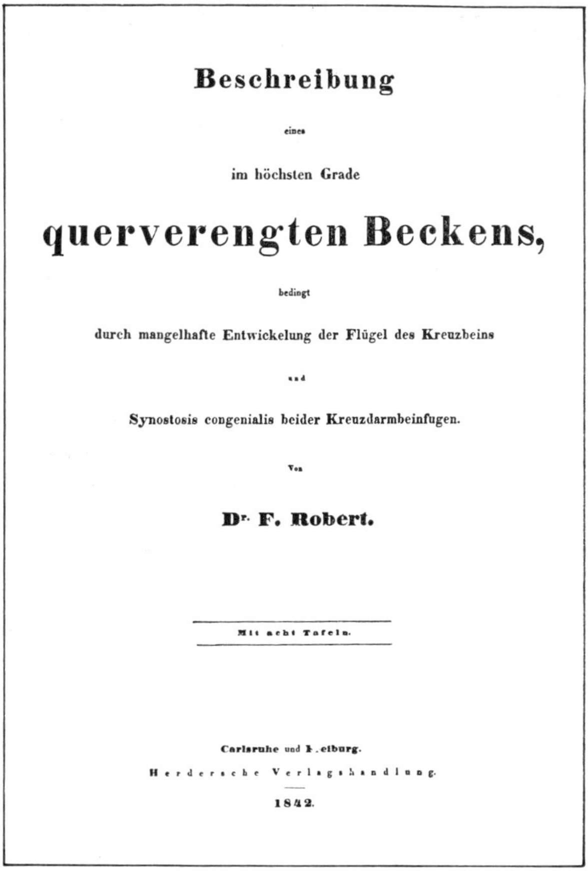

Beschreibung

eines

im höchsten Grade

querverengten Beckens,

bedingt

durch mangelhafte Entwickelung der Flügel des Kreuzbeins

und

Synostosis congenialis beider Kreuzdarmbeinfugen.

Von

Dr. F. Robert.

Mit acht Tafeln.

Carlsruhe und Freiburg.
Herdersche Verlagshandlung.
1842.

Fig. 21-4. Title page of Robert's monograph describing the pelvic malformation associated with his name.

Its bony structure, strength, texture, and color are entirely normal. Its tissue shows no trace of any change that could be the result of previous or present bone disease. Nor are any curvatures or similar malformations apparent that could have resulted from mechanical influences, such as a thrust, fall, blow, or pressure. The pelvis presents to the observer a completely symmetrical picture; every experienced osteologist will be convinced of its normal bony structure. . . . It differs from the normally formed pelvis, however, in two essential respects:

1. *All the anteroposterior measurements* (with the exception of the pelvic inlet) *are increased in relation to the normal; all the transverse measurements are shortened correspondingly; the pelvis belongs to the group of absolutely contracted pelves; and it is comparable in form to those of the human fetus and of the mammals.*

2. *The sacrum is fused with both innominate bones into one single bone as a result of complete ankylosis of both sacroiliac synchondroses, forming an integrated bony ring, which is interrupted only anteriorly by the pubic symphysis.*

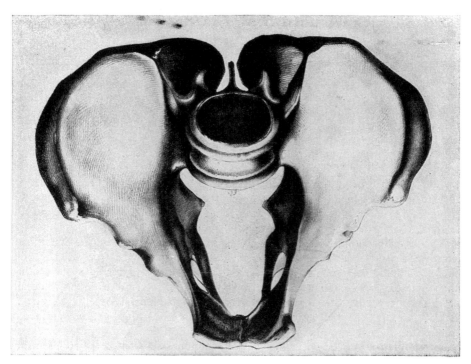

Fig. 21-5. Illustration from Robert's monograph,[10] showing inlet view of pelvis.

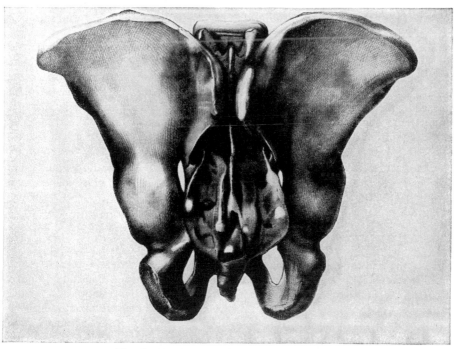

Fig. 21-6. Robert pelvis, posterior view.[10]

After presenting a detailed description of the pelvis and meticulous measurements of its parts, Robert considered the bony structure from the obstetric standpoint. He wrote:

Viewing the entire pelvis in outline, we must classify it with the wedge-shaped pelves, whether regarded from above or below. The apex of its very sharp wedge lies at the symphysis; the posterior surface of the iliac bones forms the blunt end. The profile view presents a pentagon elongated on one side. Regarded from the front and back it has the outline of a narrow wedge with a gentle outward curve. . . . The upper pelvis is not oval, as is the normal pelvis, but funnel-shaped instead, or rather pointedly heart-shaped, the symphysis forming the apex, the promontory the deep impression, and the iliac fossae the two halves of the heart. . . .

The lateral compression of the pelvis and the elongation of the innominate bones and sacrum have markedly affected the cavity of the true pelvis. While the acetabula have retained their direction and have approached each other, the obturator and ischiatic foramina have been displaced more directly laterally from their respective anterior and posterior lateral positions. The pelvic canal . . . has acquired the shape of an elongated rectangle, of which the anterior surface of the sacrum forms the posterior side; the ischiatic notches, the obturator foramina, the posterior wall of the acetabular socket, the inner surface of the ischium, and the ascending and horizontal rami of the pubis, the lateral sides; and the posterior surface of the pubic symphysis and the bodies of the pubic bones, the anterior side. . . . The canal also deviates from the normal in its course from above downward, in that it is much more elongated and curves anteriorly more rapidly at the pelvic outlet. . . .

Because of the fusion of the sacrum with both ilia, the pelvis under discussion resembles the pelves of those animals such as the birds, Bradypus, Manis, Echidna, Talpa, and the bats, in which these three bones are normally combined into one. . . . Moreover, the present pelvis closely resembles that of the orangutan, approaching the latter, as it does the pelves of most quadripeds, in the relations of its diameters to one another. Most animal pelves differ essentially, however, in having a lower position of the symphysis and a greater inclination of the pelvic inlet.

Comparing his specimen with the Naegele pelvis, Robert recognized the former as apparently comprised of two abnormal halves of the Naegele type. From this similarity he concluded that the same cause factors produce both malformations. Emphasizing the absence of any evidence or history of illness or injury, he concurred with Naegele:

. . . the malformation results primarily from faulty development . . . and . . . the anomalies of the sacrum are primary, the abnormal shapes and connections of the other bones resulting secondarily from the sacral defect. . . . The structure of the sacroiliac synostoses, their completeness, neatness, the total absence of intermediate substance, and the secondary deformity of the innominate bones, provide evidence that the genesis of the abnormalities coincides with the ossification process of the whole pelvis. *Congenital synostosis of both sacroiliac joints* would be an appropriate name for the condition.

The Robert pelvis produces very pronounced narrowing of the patient's hips. On pelvic examination, Robert pointed out:

The examiner, placing his hand at the pelvic outlet, will detect the convergence of the pubic bones and the angularity of the arch. From this alone he will be able to recognize at once the transverse narrowing of the entire pelvic cavity. . . . On internal examination he will determine the distance between the ischial spines with one or two fingers. Since the greatest narrowing occurs here, and since the indication for obstetric intervention in a case of contracted pelvis is determined by the site of greatest contraction, the examiner can formulate his prognosis and indication from this measurement.

In any event one would reach neither the sacrum nor its promontory in such a pelvis. . . . This is quite unnecessary, however, for since the contraction is greater in the transverse diameters of the pelvic cavity and outlet than in the anteroposterior, the readily detectable former determines the prognosis and indication.

Considering finally the problem of labor, Robert recognized the impossibility of vaginal delivery of a viable child. Intervention, he concluded, is essential. He stated:

Forceps extraction of the infant from such a pelvis is impossible, for even with a favorable lie and position, the head could be brought into the pelvis neither by the force of the uterus nor by means of the forceps. Version and extraction would also be impossible, for one could not get his hand through the true pelvis into the upper pelvis; and even if this were possible, he would still be unable to extract the infant.

The question whether any help might be expected from the cephalotribe must also be answered in the negative, for the distance between the two blades surrounding the compressed head is greater than the interspinous diameter. The question still remains whether recourse might be had to forced premature delivery. If this procedure were considered in the interests of the infant, then it would not be indicated, because no viable fetus could be pushed or pulled through so narrow a pelvis . . . [and because of the mechanical difficulties, this approach would likewise be contraindicated for purely maternal reasons]. Whether the infant be alive or dead, only cesarean section remains.

ROBERT'S LIFE

Heinrich Ludwig Ferdinand Robert was born May 29, 1814, in Marburg, Germany, where his father was vice-chancellor of the university. He studied in Göttingen, Berlin, and Würzburg, and later married the daughter of Professor d'Outrepont of the last university. After receiving his medical degree in Marburg in 1838, he entered general practice in that city. He held the title of extraordinary professor in the University of Marburg, lecturing on surgery, ophthalmology, and materia medica from 1843 to 1850, when he left on an extended sabbatical to England and France. He then relinquished his position in Marburg and moved to Coblenz, and in 1863 moved again to Wiesbaden, where he continued in general practice until his death on November 22, 1878. There is no known portrait of him. In addition to his famous monograph on the Robert pelvis, he published in 1853 the description of a pelvic distortion resulting from mechanical injury, and in 1855 two contributions to the anatomy, physiology, and pathology of the knee joint.

REFERENCES

1. Bedford, G. S.: *The Principles and Practice of Obstetrics,* 5th ed. William Wood & Co., New York, 1871, p. 306.

2. Boerhaave, H.: *Praelectiones Academicae in Proprias Institutiones Rei Medicae.* Ed. by A. von Haller. Vandehoeck, Göttingen, 1744, Vol. 5, Part 2, p. 437.

3. Findley, P.: *Priests of Lucina: The Story of Obstetrics.* Little, Brown & Co., Boston, 1939, pp. 252–54.

4. Haberling, W.: Die Geschichte der Düsseldorfer Aerzte und Krankenhäuser bis zum Jahre 1907. *Düsseldorfer Jahrbuch.* Lintz, Düsseldorf, 1936, Vol. 38, p. 48.

5. Harvey, W.: *The Works of William Harvey, M.D.* Translated from the Latin by R. Willis. Sydenham Society, London, 1847, p. 529.

6. Montgomery, W. F.: *An Exposition of the Signs and Symptoms of Pregnancy,* 2nd ed. Longman, Green, Longman, Roberts, & Green, London, 1863, p. 495.

7. Nägele, F. C.: *Erfahrungen und Abhandlungen aus dem Gebiethe der Krankheiten des Weiblichen Geschlechtes. Nebst Grundzügen einer Methodenlehre der Geburtshülfe.* Loeffler, Mannheim, 1812, p. 281.

8. Naegele, F. C.: Ueber den Mechanismus der Geburt. *Deutsche Arch. f. d. Physiol.,* **5**:483–531, 1819.

9. Naegele, F. C.: *Das Schräg Verengte Becken nebst einem Anhange über die Wichtigsten Fehler des Weiblichen Beckens überhaupt.* Von Zabern, Mainz, 1839.

10. Robert, F.: *Beschreibung eines im höchsten Grade Querverengten Beckens, bedingt durch Mangelhafte Entwickelung der Flügel des Kreuzbeins und Synostosis Congenialis beider Kreuzdarmbeinfügen.* Herder, Carlsruhe & Freiburg, 1842.

11. Stübler, E.: *Geschichte der Medizinischen Fakultät der Universität Heidelberg, 1386–1925.* Winters, Heidelberg, 1926, pp. 242–47.

12. Williams, J. W.: A clinical and anatomic description of a Naegele pelvis. *Am. J. Obst. & Gynec.,* **18**:504–14, 1929.

Thomas Wharton
and the Jelly of the
Umbilical Cord*

CHAPTER

22

The lifeline of the fetus, the umbilical cord, contains a unique type of mucoid matrix, Wharton's jelly, in which are embedded the umbilical vessels and which imparts to the cord its soft, ropelike character. Because of its gelatinous consistency Wharton's jelly is admirably adapted as a medium and casing, as well as a cushion, for the fetal vessels, easily accommodating to the pulsatile changes in the arteries during the intrauterine life of the fetus and permitting the rapid constriction of the vessels that occurs immediately after its birth. Bathed in its normal environment of amniotic fluid, the cord remains soft and pliable; exposed to the desiccating effect of the atmosphere, Wharton's jelly rapidly shrivels, allowing the umbilical stump to wither and drop off.

WHARTON'S DESCRIPTION OF UMBILICAL-CORD JELLY

Three centuries have elapsed since Thomas Wharton's description of the umbilical-cord jelly and the expression of his views concerning its origin. In his famous *Adenographia* (Fig. 22-2), published in 1656,[3] Wharton wrote (Fig. 22-3):

* This chapter originally published in *Obst. & Gynec.*, **8**:380–82, 1956; reprinted by permission. Copyright © 1956, by the American College of Obstetricians and Gynecologists.

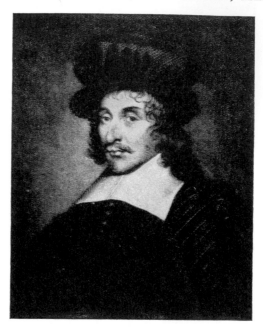

Fig. 22-1.   Thomas Wharton (1614–1673).

Although we are not able, in truth, to follow their rivulets all the way to the placenta, we can, nevertheless, discern a certain copious jelly in the umbilical cord itself that covers all the other vessels. In the cow's fetus this jelly clearly has the same odor as the tense amniotic fluid and it is very likely that this fluid emanates from the same copious source. On the other hand, something else is also true: that this jelly is in a space in the vessels or in the trunk of the vessels, through which the amniotic fluid is supplied. And further, this jelly ends unevenly in innumerable tiny papillae encircling and extending along the whole length of the cord. But notice, the fetus does not supply the umbilical cord. It is certain, there-fore, that this jelly takes its origin from the placenta and turns around to flow into the umbilical cord. Indeed, it cannot come from the fetus, not only because the jelly is separated from the vessel in the umbilical cord itself, but also be-cause none of this kind of material is found next to the umbilicus, and also because very similar material is found in the chorion of the placenta. On the other hand, the arteries and veins (which are companions in the placenta), returning from the same source, are enveloped and obscured by a covering of the same material. Thus when several of these veins, with the accompanying arteries, come together into great trunks, the jelly enveloping them may be seen more easily. For the arteries and veins lead away from the chorion by a separate path and pass out of view into the funis, constituting two prominent branches of one sort or another; it being no less evident that they are encased in a covering of this material than are the vessels in the cord themselves. I am positive that this particular jelly of the vessels is secreted as a function of the lymph ducts. Even though some may doubt

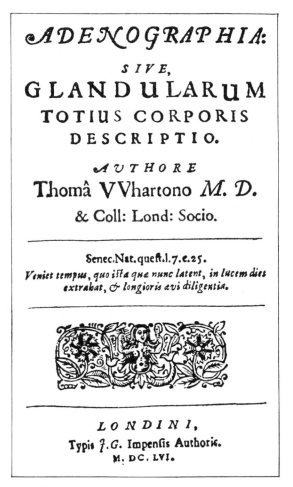

Fig. 22-2. Title page of Wharton's *Adenographia*.

what I say here, they need only follow my reasoning in the same logical fashion to be convinced.

WHARTON'S LIFE

Thomas Wharton was born August 31, 1614, in Winston-on-Tees, England.[1] He was admitted to Pembroke College, Cambridge, in 1638 but later continued his studies at Trinity College, Oxford, where he also served as a tutor. In 1642 he went to Bolton for three additional years of preparation before embarking on the study of medicine under John Bathurst in London. Returning to Oxford in 1646, Wharton received his medical degree there on May 7, 1647. Three years later he was made a fellow of the Royal College

Cap. XXXV.   *uterina.*   243

famq;aquam, in qua embryo natat, quaq; ex parte nutritur, fuppeditare. Ideóque, vi-vo animali, ad ea indaganda, acceffus non datur; & poft mortem, ceffante lymphæ profufione, compreffisque nonnihil ex ipfo frigore membranis, ita concidunt, ut eorû minores ramuli cerni vix poffint, neq; obvium eft, ligatura injectâ præcavere, ne in hunc modum fe exonerent & fubfidant.

Quanquam verò apertè rivulos eorum ad placentam ufque profequi non poffu-mus; in ipfo tamen funiculo umbilicali gelatinam quandam adeò copiofam cerni-mus, ut vafa alia omnia inveftiat. Hæc *Eos gela-* *tina fpe-* *ciem re-* *ferc.* gelatina in fœtu vaccino ejufdem planè fa-poris eft cum liquore in amnio contento; & verifimile eft, liquorem hunc ab ea-dem fcaturigine promanafie: immo hanc ipfam quoq; gelatinam loco vafis effe aut trunci vaforum, per quem liquor in am-nio contentus fuppeditetur. Gelatina e-nim hæc in innumeras papillulas minutulas totam funiculi longitudinem ambientes, afperamque reddentes terminatur; fœ-tús autem umbilicum non penetrat. Cer-tum igitur eft, hanc gelatinam à placenta originem ducere; & verfùs inteftinulum umbilicale fluere. Non enim á fœtu pro-venire poteft, quia non tantùm vafe ca-ret *Et exonerat varia in papillas: Hc um vaforum exortur:*

R 2   ret

244   *Placenta*   Cap.XXXV.

ret in ipfo umbilico, fed & nihil iftiufmo-di materiæ juxta umbilicum reperitur; è contrà in placenta chorii, materia confi-milis deprehenditur: immo arteriæ & ve-næ (quæ comites in placenta funt) ab ea-dem redeuntes, capfula ejufdem materiæ fubobfcurè involvuntur: quando verò plures harum venarum, comitantibus ar-teriis, in truncos majufculos coeunt, gela-tina eas involvens magis confpicuè cer-nitur. Nam arteriæ & venæ per aliquod fpa-cium antequam chorion deferunt & funi-culum fubintrant, duos infignes utriufque generis ramos conftituunt: quæ non mi-nus evidenter materiæ hujus theca amici-untur, quàm vafa illa in ipfo funiculo; certum ergo mihi eft, gelatinam hanc vaforum quorundam, nempè *lymphæ-ductuum*, munere defungi. Quia vero alii de hac re adhuc dubitaverint, rationes fequé-tes ad ejufdem confirmationé adnectam. *Gelati-nom lym-phæ-ctuum mu-nere fun-gi.*

1. Video in illis perfectorum animali-um partibus, quæ placent maximè re-fpondent, *lymphæductus* confpicuos repe-riri; ut in mammis, tefticulis, utero, me-fenterio, aliifque plurimis membranis; curque hifce partibus iidé, aut vafa eorum vicaria denegentur, haud facile ex-plicatu arbitror. *Probatur*

2. Vi:

the body, more accurate and detailed than any previous, were based on his own dissections and experiments. Particularly noteworthy was his study of the minute anatomy of the pancreas. In addition to the jelly of the umbilical cord, his name is eponymically associated with the duct of the submaxillary salivary gland.

Little is known of Wharton's nonprofessional interests. He composed a few English verses, as a prefix to a book by one of his friends. His enthusiasm for fishing is suggested by the following note in Izaak Walton's *Compleat Angler:* [2]

. . . and yet I will venture to tell you a real truth concerning one [fish] lately dissected by Dr. Wharton, a man of great learning and experience, and of equal freedom to communicate it; one that loves me and my art; one to whom I have been beholden for many of the choicest observations that I have imparted to you. This good man, that dares do any thing rather than tell an untruth, did, I say, tell me he lately dissected one strange fish and he thus described it to me.

"The fish was almost a yard broad, and twice that length; his mouth wide enough to receive or take into it the head of a man; his stomach seven or eight inches broad. He is of a slow motion, and usually lies or lurks close in the mud, and has a movable string on his head about a span, or near unto a quarter of a yard long, by the moving of which, which is his natural bait; when he lies close and unseen in the mud, he draws other smaller fish so close to him, that he can suck them into his mouth, and so devours and digests them."

REFERENCES

1. Lee, S. (ed.): *Dictionary of National Biography.* The Macmillan Co., New York, 1909, Vol. 20, pp. 1327–28.
2. Walton, I.: *The Compleat Angler, or the Contemplative Man's Recreation.* London, 1653, Part 1, Chap. 19.
3. Wharton, T.: *Adenographia: sive, Glandularum Totius Corporis Descriptio.* R. Marriot, London, 1656, pp. 243–44.

Nicolaas Hoboken and the Valves and Nodes of the Umbilical Vessels

Until the rather recent application of contrast radiography to the study of blood flow, knowledge of the hemodynamics in the fetus had been largely a matter of surmise, based on anatomic observations. S. R. M. Reynolds and his group are currently providing, for the first time, data on the umbilical circulation by means of radiokinescopic studies in the fetal sheep. Previous physiologic investigation of the umbilical vessels had been limited to a few blood pressure measurements.

Functional differences between these vessels and the others of the body were long suspected, however, because of the morphologic differences between them. The umbilical artery possesses a remarkably thick muscular layer. In contrast to other arteries of comparable size the internal elastic lamina is absent, elastic tissue fibrils being dispersed instead within the media. The umbilical vessels contain neither an adventitia, vasa vasorum, nor a clearly demonstrable nerve supply. True valves are lacking in the veins, but within them, and more noticeably within the arteries, are intraluminal folds or projections, for which a valvelike function has been affirmed by some students and denied by others. These structures are known as the valves or folds of Hoboken. When an umbilical artery is examined in the fresh state, constrictions are seen in its outer surface partially encircling the vessel and dividing it into segments of varying length like uneven links in a chain of sausages. The dilatations in the vessel lying between consecutive constrictions have

190

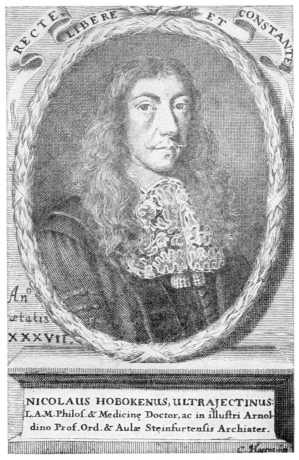

RECTE LIBERE ET CONSTANTE

Anⁿ ætatis XXXVII.

NICOLAUS HOBOKENUS, ULTRAJECTINUS: L.A.M.Philoſ.& Medicinę Doctor,ac in illuſtri Arnol- dino Prof.Ord.& Aulæ Steinfurtenſis Archiater.

Fig. 23-1. Nicolaas Hoboken (1632–1678).

been referred to as cellulae of Ruysch, cochleae of Hebenstreit, tubercula of Böhmer, genicula, aneurysmata of Eysson, varices arteriarum, elevationes arcuatae, eminentiae leves of Wrisberg, gemmulae of Hoboken, and the nodules of Hoboken.[5] Longitudinal sections through the folds of Hoboken in the umbilical artery show a moundlike thickening of the vessel media, with a thinning out of this layer in the adjacent, saccular "nodule."[7] The folds within the veins, on the other hand, although comprised also of a layer of muscle, follow a spiral or "semilunar" course within the lumen and fail to cause any distortion of the vessel's exterior. Modern students of these structures, having found them functionally incompetent as valves, have suggested their possible function to be in aiding closure of the vessels after birth. The possibility of their being postnatal artefacts, present only in the contracted vessels, has not been completely excluded.

HOBOKEN'S DESCRIPTION OF VALVES AND NODES

"Valvulae" and "plicae" in the umbilical arteries were described by Jean Riolan (1580–1657) and Werner Rolfinck (1599–1673),[3] contemporaries of Hoboken. But Hoboken's *Anatomia Secundinae Humanae*,[4] published in 1669, gave the first full account of these folds, and it is his name, therefore, that has since been eponymically associated with them and the arterial irregularities. Hoboken's description, as follows, appears as Article 6 of his book, under the title, "Interior Funis, Constitutio Explicate Tradititur, Praesertim Vasorum Umbilicalium Exteriora Narrantur," or "The Internal Structure of the Cord Described in Detail, with Special Reference to the Exterior of the Umbilical Vessels."

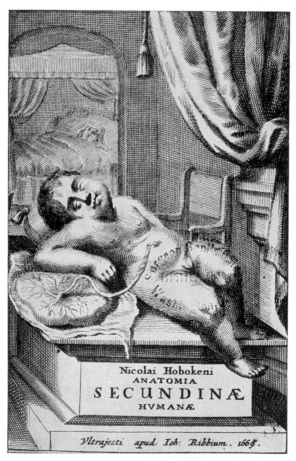

Fig. 23-2.   Frontispiece from Hoboken's *Anatomia Secundinae Humanae.*

1. Et funis interiora tunc perlustrans, inveni substantiam ejus totam fibrosam, membranosam, et humidam; cui affabre inserta quasi, delitescebant vasa teretia, numero tantum tria.

2. Duo quidem tenuiora, & albicantia, quae arteriae erant: & tertium crassius, ac rubicundius aequaliter visum, quod manu & unicam referebat venam: juxta delineationes Figurae iv, xiii, & xv.

3. In quibus perquirendis & examinandis, quam licuit, operam impendi. Et primo (preter dictum differentem colorem, & magnitudinem ac crassitiem) eam observabam inter venam atque arterias diversitatem: qua venam medio fere tramite, & aequali ductu transeuntem comperiebam.

4. Arterias vero instar tubulorum flexibilium, varie intorqueri, & inaequales illas efformare convolutiones.

5. Insuper venam adeo firmiter innexam deprehendi, ut difficillime eam, vel ad aliquantillam partem, a funis substantia memorata separarem. Juxta Figuram xv.

6. Arterias autem facile integras separabam: juxta nutum Figurae xiii. Et has ni sanguinis, contenti hic atque illic ulteriore examine observassem vestigia, jurassem fere nervos esse.

7. Deinceps in vena nullum invenire potui nodum: uti quousque in ipso fune delitescit valvulam notabilem nullam.

8. Sed extra funis ejusdem tractum, circa venae ramificationes, & harum per placentam facta divortia, esse valvulas varias conjicere licuit. I. Quia sanguinem contentum, vel digito extrinsecus admoto, ultro citroque promovere quidem potui, in ipso dum delitescit fune. In placentae vero insertis venae ejusdem ramificationibus ea observata fuit differentia; qua sanguinem facile quidem versus funem moverem, retrorsum autem versus placentam minus.

9. Et 2. stylum convenientem ab una alteram venae dictae extremitatem inturbate inferui, hinc atque illinc, quousque func involveretur. Sed per superficiem placentae discurrentes ramos aliter se habere comperi: quippe qui versus placentam factam insertionem minus admitterent, libere concessa ea versus funem, & foetus umbilicum.

10. Et in arteriis quousque fune comprehenderentur, I. nodulos varios, ad gemmularum speciem se habentes, observavi.

11. Quos dum perquirerem, eos deprehendi ratione sanguinis, referre maculas praenominatas. Juxta Figuras v. x. & xiii.

12. Et eos aperiens (2.), valvulas, ex tunicae laxioris plicatura orbiculari efformatas, reperi, recursum sanguinis arteriosi a placenta versus umbilicum foetus inhibentes: media gemmulae tunica a copiosiore sanguine distensa. Quemadmodum Figurae demonstrant vi & vii.

13. Et quomodonam vasa haec (vena et arteriae) terminarentur circa foetus umbilicum demonstrat Figura i. Circa placentam vero quomodo concurrerent demonstrat Figura viii.

[1. And the interior of the cord being examined then, its substance is found to be all fibrous material, membrane, and fluid, and the smooth vessels contained within are arranged in artistic fashion.

2. Of the last, the two that proceed as arteries are thin and whitish; the third,

more reddish to the view and thicker, returns alongside as a vein, these being shown in Figures 4, 13, and 15.

3. With respect to these structures, I intensified my efforts in examining and studying them, and was rewarded. Immediately I noticed (in addition to what I have already said concerning the differences in color, size, and thickness) a difference between the vein and the arteries: as I clearly discerned the vein almost in the middle of the section, maintaining a constant size.

4. The arteries in truth had the appearance of flexible tubes, greatly twisted into uneven shapes.

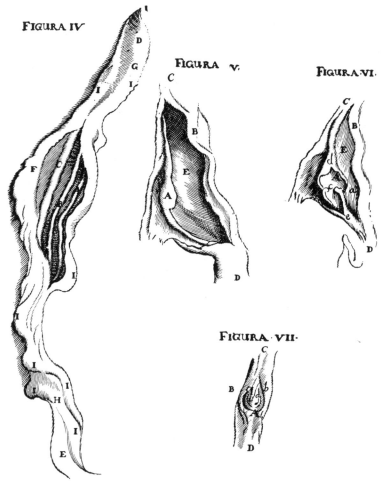

Fig. 23-3. Illustrations from the *Anatomia Secundinae Humanae,*[4] showing the umbilical vessels, their "folds," "valves," and "nodes." See also Figure 23-4.

5. I approached the twisted vein to grasp it, but was able to separate even this small part from the above-noted substance of the cord only with the greatest difficulty. See Figure 15.

6. Moreover I separated the arteries easily in their entirety, as shown in Figure 13. And in the subsequent examination of them I noticed here and there traces, not of blood, but of what I would almost swear were nerves.

7. Next I was able to find a tiny nodule inside the vein: a tiny valve is also visible inside the same vessel.

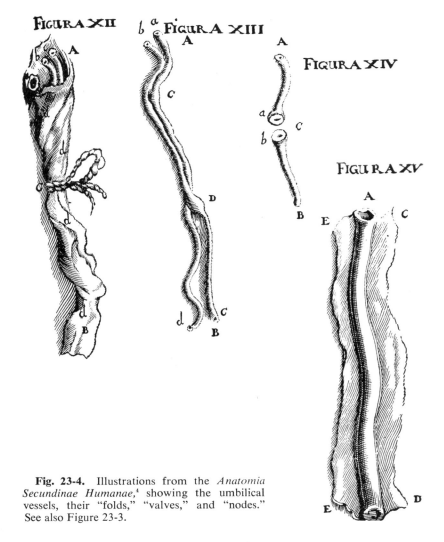

Fig. 23-4. Illustrations from the *Anatomia Secundinae Humanae,*[4] showing the umbilical vessels, their "folds," "valves," and "nodes." See also Figure 23-3.

8. But beyond the extent of this vessel, around the ramifications of the vein, and at their site of divergence in the placenta, one may be permitted to conjecture that there are various little valves. First, because the blood is held back by external pressure with the finger, and I was even able to move the blood contained within the cord back and forth. Even in the branches of this vein in the placenta this

difference was observed: that I could move the blood toward the cord easily indeed, but less so in a reverse direction toward the placenta.

9. Second, I concluded that the pattern was consistent from one end of the vein to the other, the vein being embedded in the cord throughout its entire length. But I learned that the branches coursing over the surface of the placenta are arranged differently; indeed there are only a few who would assert that the direction of flow is toward the placenta, it being generally conceded to be toward the cord and the umbilicus of the fetus.

10. And I observed (1) that the various nodules, having the appearance of little buds, are joined together in the arteries and also in the cord.

11. While seeking these out, I discovered that these previously mentioned nodes are the result of collections of blood. See Figures 5, 10, and 13.

12. And opening these, I found (2) circular valves, formed by the plication of a rather loose tunic, inhibiting the back flow of the arterial blood from the placenta toward the umbilicus of the fetus; the tunic of the little bud being distended in the middle by a copious collection of blood. See Figures 6 and 7.

13. And Figure 1 shows how these vessels (the vein and arteries) are terminated around the umbilicus of the fetus. Figure 8 shows how they course around the placenta.]

HOBOKEN'S LIFE

Nicolaas Hoboken was born in Utrecht, Holland, in 1632.[1,2,6] After receiving his doctorate of philosophy in 1658, he studied medicine there under Diemerbroeck, graduating in 1662. The following year he was named to the chair of medicine and mathematics at Steinfurt in Westphalia, and while at this post was chosen as personal physician to Count Bentheim. In 1669 Hoboken was called to Harderwyck as ordinary professor of medicine and extraordinary professor of mathematics, and here he achieved a considerable reputation for his clinical prowess. Because of the approach of the French Army, he suddenly left Harderwyck in 1672, never to return, and died in Utrecht in 1678. Hoboken's writings encompass a variety of topics, including anatomy, physiology, pathology, mathematics, politics, and philosophy. His inaugural thesis, published in 1661, was on the salivary gland. Hoboken is best known today for his personally illustrated *Anatomia Secundinae Humanae,* describing the human placenta, cord, and fetal membranes.

REFERENCES

1. Banga, J.: *Geschiednis van de Geneeskunde en van hare beoefenaren in Neder-land.* Eekhoff, 1868, Vol. 1, pp. 396–99.

2. Bayle and Thillaye: *Biographie Médicale.* Delahays, Paris, 1855, Vol. 1, p. 498.

3. Boehmer, P. A.: *De Necessaria Funiculi Umbilicalis vi Vasorum Structurae in Nuper Natis Deligatione.* Halle, 1745. Republished in Haller, A. von:

Disputationum Anatomicarum Selectarum. Göttingen, 1750, Vol 5, p. 639 (footnote to par. 11).

4. Hoboken, N.: *Anatomia Secundinae Humanae, Quindecim Figuris ad Vivum Propria Autoris Manu Delineatis, Illustrata.* Joannes Ribbius, Utrecht, 1669, pp. 28–34.

5. Hyrtl, J.: *Die Blutgefässe der Menschlichen Nachgeburt.* Wilhelm Braumüller, Vienna, 1870, pp. 28–29.

6. Siebold, E. C. J. von: *Versuch einer Geschichte der Geburtshülfe,* 2nd ed. Tübingen, 1902, Vol. 2, p. 255.

7. Spivack, M.: On the anatomy of the so-called "valves" of umbilical vessels, with especial reference to the "valvulae Hobokenii." *Anat. Rec.,* **66**:127–48, 1936.

Theodor Langhans, J. Hofbauer, and the Histology of the Placenta

The manifold functions of the placenta and its progressive changes in metabolism, permeability, active transfer, and synthesis of hormones, vitamins, and other metabolites, are governed in large part by the epithelial investment of the chorionic villi and, probably to a lesser degree, by the villous stroma. The morphologic nomenclature of each of these tissue elements is embellished by an eponymic term: the epithelium by the Langhans layer and the stroma by the Hofbauer cells.

THE LANGHANS LAYER

The placental villi are covered by a membranous blanket whose area has been estimated up to 14 square meters. Its epithelial character was pointed out in 1842 by Dalrymple,[1] with the brief statement that "the membrane enclosing the vessels and capillaries is studded on the exterior by nucleated cells, resembling an irregular epithelium."

Subsequent investigators have learned to distinguish two types of epithelium in the formative stages of the primate placenta: the syncytiotrophoblast, or syncytium; and the cytotrophoblast, or Langhans layer. The latter, consisting of large, discrete, pale-staining cells with relatively large nuclei and glycogen-containing vacuoles, sends streamers or columns into the maternal decidua, producing coagulation necrosis of the host cells and securing a firm attachment for the developing ovum to the uterine wall. The proliferating cytotro-

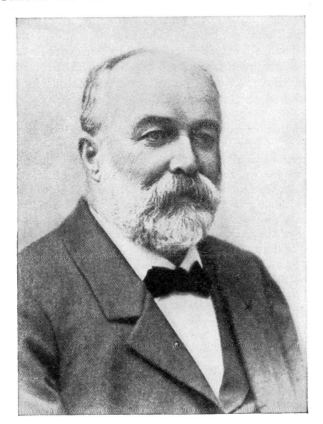

Fig. 24-1. Theodor Langhans (1839–1915). (Reproduced from *Schweiz. med. Wchnschr.,* **64,** No. 23, 1934.)

phoblast probably serves as the germinal zone for the syncytial layer and the chorionic angioblasts as well. In the definitive villi the Langhans layer lies subjacent to the outermost covering of syncytium; as the villi mature the Langhans cells become reduced sharply in number, and are demonstrable only with difficulty in the term placenta. Their period of maximal proliferation corresponds nicely with the stages of greatest concentration of chorionic gonadotrophin in the maternal body fluids; and tissue culture experiments have actually identified this cell type as the source of the hormone.

During the half century that followed Dalrymple's brief paper, the covering of the placental villi became the subject of a host of investigations and reports; and by 1890 Waldeyer [17] was able to formulate ten distinct categories for the published theories of the nature and origin of the chorionic epithelium. Foremost among the nineteenth-century students of the human placenta was Theodor Langhans, whose contributions began with a histologic study published in 1870.[7] In it Langhans dealt at length with the structure of the anchoring villi, intervillous anastomoses, and syncytial knots, but failed to note the cell layer with which he later became identified.

The chorionic epithelium was described in greater detail by Langhans seven years later in a lengthy dissertation [8] that distinguished for the first time between the syncytial covering of the villi and the "Zellschicht," or cell layer, that now bears his name. He wrote:

The epithelium that covers the outer surface of the chorion and villi forms . . . a uniform layer of very bright-appearing, rather homogeneous or finely granular cytoplasm containing nuclei but never showing a clear division into individual cells. Only in younger ova, and very rarely even there, are lines that might represent cell boundaries visible among the nuclei. . . .

The nuclei, which are round or somewhat oval and the size of a white blood cell, have a brilliant nucleolus and a finely granular content that is often separated from the outer border of the nucleus by a bright, narrow band. The nuclei . . . lie in the deeper layer of the cytoplasm, covered by a layer of the latter whose thickness varies with the thickness of the epithelium itself; sometimes it forms a quite narrow band, but often has the same or in some places even twice the thickness of the layer in which the nuclei are embedded. . . .

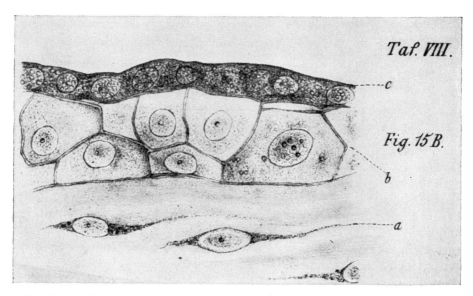

Fig. 24-2. Illustration from Langhans' paper of 1877,[8] which first called attention to the cell layer (Langhans layer) in the placenta. Langhans' Figure 15B is from a specimen of 14 weeks. *a,* chorion; *b,* cell layer; *c,* epithelial layer (syncytium). (Reproduced by permission of Springer-Verlag, Heidelberg.)

The arrangement of the nuclei varies according to location and stage of development. At the placental surface of the chorion the nuclei are always arranged rather irregularly and only moderately concentrated . . . separated from one another on an average by a quarter to a half a nuclear diameter, but up to as much as two or three times this diameter. Here the nuclei are rarely arranged as they usually are in the villi after the fourth month. In the villi during the late months of pregnancy areas of the epithelium that are thin and devoid of nuclei alternate with the nucleus-containing, thicker areas. In addition the nuclei in the villi are arranged into spindles. . . . The nuclei thus lie very close together, almost touching, the cytoplasm being confined to narrow bright bands of varying width. . . .

For a long time epithelial processes have been known that consist only of cytoplasm with nuclei and without a central connective tissue core, representing the forerunners of the villi. They are found at the end of and alongside the villi and at the chorion, are usually numerous in the earlier stages, and of manifold shapes and sizes, cylindrical, club-shaped . . . or with a narrow pedicle; later they become sparser, and in the mature placenta are limited to the fine villi, especially their ends. I have previously [in his 1870 report] found still another form . . . which joins two villous tips together. These appear to belong to the latest stages exclusively. . . . They occur only secondarily, through the fusion of two epithelial processes. . . . The epithelium contains, for the most part, only one layer of nuclei; in the early months, however, numerous thickenings are present containing several layers of nuclei. . . .

The remaining paragraphs of the section on the chorionic and villous epithelium, from which the foregoing is excerpted, are devoted to Langhans' arguments in favor of the fetal rather than maternal origin of the syncytiotrophoblast.

Describing the cytotrophoblast, in his section on the chorion laeve and reflexa, Langhans wrote:

From the sixth week on, at the superficial surface of the chorion, one sees flat, circumscribed areas of a large-celled tissue lying directly on the chorionic stroma and covered with epithelium. . . . Its origin—whether maternal or fetal—is somewhat doubtful. Many considerations point to its being maternal.

Its cells actually differ only slightly from those of the decidua; they are large, of highly variable form, round, polyhedral with pointed processes that project among the neighboring cells, spindle-shaped, or cylindrical; the protoplasm is pale and finely granular; the nucleus large, often multiple . . . its diameter is up to five times, or even more, that of the nuclei in the overlying chorionic epithelium. . . . No intercellular substance is present; nevertheless the cells adhere firmly to one another almost everywhere and follow the chorionic epithelium as its deeper layer. . . . At times they maintain contact with the chorion only by means of narrow, somewhat wedge-shaped processes, among which spaces are present. . . .

These cells form no continuous layer but only individual islands of limited extent, separated from one another by wide spaces. . . . They are present especially at the places free of villi; here and there they enclose villi.

Langhans erred, as he himself later discovered, in his initial labored efforts to determine the origin of the cytotrophoblast. He asked:

Now where do these peculiar islands come from? Seeing this deeper layer under a completely continuous covering of chorionic epithelium, and readily separable from the chorion proper, one is inclined at first to consider it as a part of the epithelium. But very important considerations militate against this conclusion. The completely different form of the cells, the fact that they are sharply separated from the epithelium, as seen in sections, and the later development of intercellular substance, demonstrate the separate identity of each tissue, in my opinion. However, could not the cell layer [cytotrophoblast] be something other than fetal tissue? . . . Could not this subepithelial cell layer be regarded as analogous with the connective tissue of the amnion? I do not believe that this question can be decided definitely at present, but the larger probability does not favor this conjecture. It does not explain the division of the tissue into individual, separate islands; nor is this explained by any peculiarity of the chorionic stroma, for the latter is everywhere the same, at the areas of the subepithelial islands as well as between them.

On the other hand, the similarity between the cell layer and the decidual tissue is so great, that the possibility of deriving the former from the latter will be examined very closely. I suggest at the outset the idea that decidual tissue can separate completely from the parent tissue and cover itself with a layer of proliferating chorionic epithelium, and furthermore that such detached particles might actually produce active penetration into the fetal placenta up to the surface of the chorion. I am most inclined to account for the tissue in question in this manner. . . . One would have to assume that at the chorion laeve these isolated masses of decidual tissue penetrate the chorionic epithelium or destroy it at specific areas and then grow under it and proliferate along the chorionic stroma, gradually spreading and flattening out. Previously visible to the naked eye, they now become fainter and fainter and finally demonstrable only on microscopic examination. The chorionic epithelium can then close over them again completely. . . . In section this subepithelial layer is very often thicker in some places than in others, consisting of several layers of very loose, straight cells, and the chorionic epithelium may be lacking. I regard these pictures as transitional stages between the clearly knot-forming collections of decidual tissue at the superficial surface of the chorion frondosum and the islands covered with continuous epithelium.

At the end of the second month this subepithelial cell layer only forms islands widely separated from one another; at the beginning of the fourth it is already continuous along the entire extent of the chorion, reaching almost but not quite up to the edge of the placenta, stopping about ½ to ¾ cm from it. No relation of any kind is demonstrable with the vascular layer of the chorion frondosum. . . . The cells often form only one layer and are then rather flat; usually, however, several layers are present. . . . I have thus explained the cell layer as decidual tissue.

Not until five years later, in a paper that is usually quoted as Langhans' definitive report on the subject,[9] did he recant his earlier views on the maternal origin of his eponymic cell layer and ascribe a common source to it and the syncytium. He said:

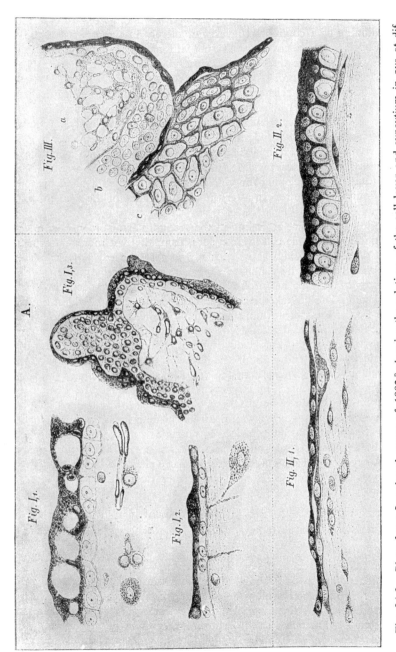

Fig. 24-3. Plate from Langhans' paper of 1882,[9] showing the relations of the cell layer and syncytium in ova at different stages of development. Langhans' Figure I: from an ovum of about three weeks. Figure II: seven or eight weeks. Figure III: fourth month (*a*, villus; *b*, thickened cell layer covered by syncytium; *c*, decidua serotina).

I gladly forego imparting here the basis of these views, for my earlier observations were incomplete and the conclusions drawn from them erroneous.

As a matter of fact, the cell layer of the chorion laeve and frondosum is present from the beginning as a continuous layer, not merely in these parts of the fetal membranes, but . . . also covering all the villi as a continuous subepithelial mantle. Thus we now have three layers in the chorion instead of two: (1) the epithelium, corresponding precisely with the previous descriptions; (2) the cell layer, a layer of large, pale cells containing a single nucleus and clearly separated from one another; and (3) the chorionic connective tissue. Everything that I shall relate concerning the cell layer can be explained most simply on the basis of its development from the ectoderm of the serous membranes. . . .

In the chorion laeve the initially simple cell layer develops into a multilayered one, in individual, isolated areas at first (in the second half of the second month), and then continuously enveloping the villi (in the fourth month) and proceeding in direct continuity with the reflexa after the disappearance of the epithelium [syncytium]. . . .

In the chorion frondosum, beginning in the second half of pregnancy, a similar growth and thickening of the cell layer ensues, from the first more uniform in its entire extent. With the decidua it extends only up to the edge of the placenta. . . . It is replaced in part by canalized fibrin or by connective tissue.

Isolated areas of only partial proliferation of the cell layer occur in the villi; uniform thickening does not take place here. This occurs principally, but not exclusively, at the tips of the villi, forming here small, white, opaque plaques, which I described previously as insular knots of maternal tissue. They arise, after the disappearance of the epithelium [syncytium], in connection with the overlying decidual tissue and thus bring about the firm coalescence of the mass of villi with the serotina. In the other parts of the villi the cell layer becomes thinner and possibly disappears altogether. In any event it can no longer be demonstrated with certainty in the last three months.

The cell layer, where it is preserved in a recognizable form, is thus responsible for creating as firm and lasting a union as possible with the maternal tissue. It appears admirably adapted to this function, for in its very earliest form it bears the greatest similarity to the decidual tissue, and in many places in the mature placenta a boundary between the two tissues can no longer be recognized.

Emphasizing the great reduction in the number of his newly described cells in the placental villi of late pregnancy, Langhans observed:

. . . in the mature placenta the cell layer can no longer be demonstrated with certainty. Much points to its probably still being present, however. Only rarely can sections of a rod-shaped nucleus be seen under the epithelium. . . . Also at the surface, with nuclear stains, one sees in the epithelium large, oval, pale nuclei, up to 0.012 mm long, as much as three times larger than the neighboring nuclei, and the former can be differentiated from the latter as well as from the still smaller stromal nuclei. . . . Whether these nuclei represent rests of the cell layer is a matter of uncertainty. In any event, they are very sparse, much sparser than in the earlier stages. . . . Does the cell layer disappear? Is it compressed and squeezed out by the decidua? Or does it change into a tissue that completely resembles the decidua? [The fate of the Langhans cells still awaits clarification.]

LANGHANS' LIFE

Theodor Langhans was born September 28, 1839, in Usingen, Germany, where his father was a judge.[11,14] He studied medicine in the universities of Heidelberg, Berlin, and Göttingen. In Berlin his teachers included Virchow and Traube, and in Göttingen he came under the influence of Henle, who stimulated Langhans' interest in renal pathology. In 1862 he was made assistant to von Recklinghausen in the pathology institute of Würzburg, and five years later was given a position of greater responsibility in Marburg. Here Langhans began his studies on the structure of the placenta, made two major contributions to the pathology of nephritis, and called attention to the giant cell, also known as the Langhans cell, as an almost invariable component of the tubercle. For a few months in 1872 he occupied the chair of pathologic anatomy in Giessen, but left this post in response to a call to Bern, as successor to Edwin Klebs. As senior member of the illustrious trio that included Kocher and Sahli, Langhans helped bring fame to Bern over the next 40 years, until poor health forced him to relinquish his professorship. His principal investigations here included studies on the pathologic anatomy of goiter and cretinism, renal infections, blood pigments, and the organ with which obstetricians have ever since identified him. He died October 22, 1915, in his seventy-seventh year.

Langhans' reputation has been further enhanced by the placental eponymy of one of his students, Raissa Nitabuch. In her inaugural dissertation,[13] published in 1887, Nitabuch gave a detailed description of the eosinophilic, honeycombed, fibrinoid deposition in the placenta, between the invading trophoblast and the maternal decidua—best known now as Nitabuch's layer of canalized fibrin, but also identified by some as Rohr's stria.

THE HOFBAUER CELLS

The villous stroma of the placenta is made up chiefly of connective tissue and blood vessels, but it contains, in addition, other cellular forms, fewer in number and of less certain function. Toward the close of the nineteenth century Neumann,[12] in a paper on hydatidiform mole, called attention to isolated large cells embedded in the hydropic stroma of the villi. Recent authors [16] have suggested their identity with the stromal elements of the normal placenta later popularized by Hofbauer and since known as Hofbauer cells. These cells, probably histiocytes, are present in the chorionic villi throughout pregnancy, but most abundantly during the early months. In tissue

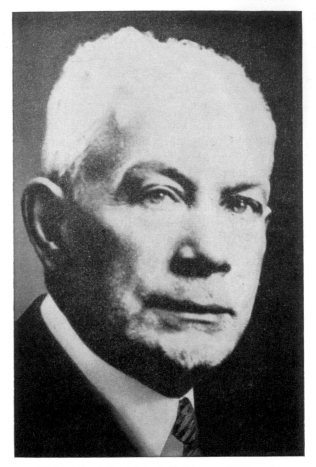

Fig. 24-4. Isford Isfred Hofbauer (1879–   ).

culture experiments Warren Lewis [10] has demonstrated their ability to ingest and destroy bacteria and other foreign particles, and has suggested their possible role in protecting the fetus against bacterial invasion from the mother. Hofbauer called attention to the morphologic characteristics of these cells in his monograph on the human placenta [2] published in 1905. He wrote:

These cellular structures, characteristic of the tissue of the chorionic villi, usually have a spherical shape; their diameter is about 10.5–12.5 microns; their contour is sometimes uniformly circular, but more often stellate or branched, sending out delicate processes, by means of which they are connected with similar structures or with the actual connective tissue elements of the villous stroma. The nucleus of the cells is large, varying between 4.7 and 5.7 microns in diameter; it has a circular or somewhat oval shape and is characterized by an easily stained nuclear membrane, one or two nucleoli, and a dense chromatin network. The cells multiply by mitoses, which are common; . . . occasionally, however, simple fragmentation of the nuclei is seen. The most important characteristic of these cells . . . is the vacuolated, finely granular cytoplasm. In it, grouped in a ring around the nucleus, are small, round, light granules, which enlarge progressively, forming a circumnuclear halo. Adjacent vacuoles, separated from one another at first by slender septa, may coalesce into larger vacuoles. In this manner a honey-combed structure develops in the more peripheral parts of the cytoplasm also. . . . Simultaneously with this complete vacuolization of the cytoplasmic part of the cell, pycnosis of the nucleus occurs, followed by its poor uptake of stain, and finally its complete disappearance. Cytoplasmic granules of variable size must also be mentioned; they stand out sharply with eosin, safranine, and Heidenhain's iron stain. The cell also harbors fat granules.

With regard to their genesis, it should be pointed out that these cells, in their early stages, are connected with the stromal cells of the villi, and must therefore be regarded as derivatives of the connective tissue elements. . . . The cells are not present in extremely young chorionic villi, but appear first toward the end of the fourth week, are abundant in the early placenta, and later decrease progressively as the connective tissue assumes a more fibrous character. The life span of an individual cell is thus limited, as shown by its complete vacuolization and ultimate disappearance. . . . We have established the fact that these cells of the villous connective tissue are surely of histogenic origin. . . . The characteristic chromatin figure . . . the circumnuclear halo, and the usually eccentric position of the nucleus are common to the plasma cells as well as our placental cells, and are reminiscent of von Recklinghausen's conclusion that the plasma cells . . . are to be regarded as embryonal cells of the connective tissue that remain permanently in their primitive state. Finally, these cells of the placenta also show the same forms as plasma cells in their response to vital stains.

Speculating on the physiologic role of the placental histiocytes, Hofbauer added: [4]

We can only say that they probably possess a digestive function,—a view which is supported by the presence of fat in the vacuoles, as well as of neutral red. The phagocytic power is further supported by the fact that at the stage of development when the nucleated red blood cells lose their nuclei, I could demonstrate the disintegration of their nuclei within the fetal capillaries of the chorionic villi, and that the fragments of the nuclei were engulfed by the cytoplasm of a type of cells quite comparable in structure to our vacuolated cells. As this phenomenon could be observed distinctly in various specimens, it became obvious that our cells may be regarded as wandering cells, which had gained access to the fetal blood stream, and thereby constituted a portion of its white cells. . . . A further contribution to the function of the cells in question was afforded by my observation that they possess an elective capacity for the storage of lithioncarmin after vital staining with that dye. . . . The Kupffer cells of the liver, the reticulo-endothelial cells of the spleen, the lymph glands, and the bone marrow, as well as the clasmatocytes of the connective tissue, display an elective affinity for this substance.

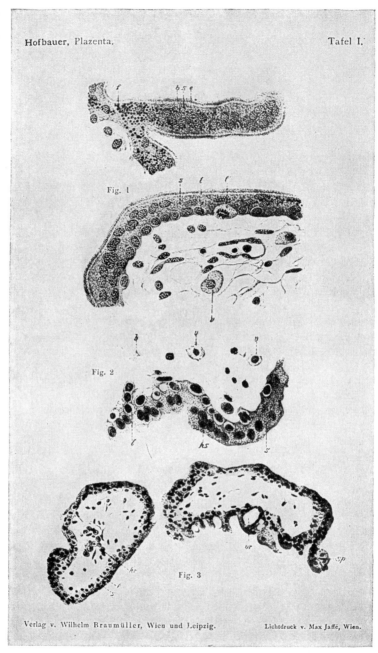

Verlag v. Wilhelm Braumüller, Wien und Leipzig.   Lichtdruck v. Max Jaffé, Wien.

Fig. 24-5. Plate from Hofbauer's monograph of 1905,[2] illustrating the cells now known by his name. Hofbauer's Figures 1 and 2 show these cells (*v*) in the placenta of a 12-mm fetus. (Reproduced by permission of Wilhelm Braumüller, Vienna.)

. . . All these types possess a functional relationship, as they not only store up vital dyes, but also other materials, especially fats and pigments, and are concerned in cellular phagocytosis, as well as in the metabolism of fatty substances. Furthermore, these cells possess a remarkable ability to reproduce themselves after some of them have disintegrated. When inflammation occurs, in the above mentioned organs, all of the cells show a similar reaction and give rise to ameboid phagocytic polyblasts.

The histiocytes of the chorionic villus, as pointed out by Hofbauer, are not peculiar to the placenta, but merely represent a specific localization of the body's wandering cells. The maternal genital tract is richly supplied with them. Cytologic examination [15] has even revealed cyclic variations in their numbers within the vaginal fluid, with marked increases after menstruation, abortion, and parturition, periods associated with additional vaginal debris and augmented vaginal phagocytosis. In 1926 Hofbauer called attention to wandering cells within the parametrium during pregnancy and labor,[5] attributing to them an important function in the maternal defense against infection. These parametrical phagocytes have also come to be known as Hofbauer cells. Wrote Hofbauer:

Whereas in the non-pregnant woman the base of the broad ligament is built up of dense fibrillar connective tissue including but few cell elements and occasional bundles of plain muscle, at term and during labor throngs of well characterized cells make their appearance in this region. These cells are arranged in relation to the course of the lymphatics which accompany the uterine vessels, and can be sharply differentiated into two types. One group consists of cells, to which the name clasmatocyte or histiocyte has been applied; while the other group is represented by cells corresponding to the type of monocytes. When hemorrhage occurs into the parametrium, both groups of cells engulf red blood cells. In such circumstances, either well preserved erythrocytes or their fragments can be seen, which in most instances lie within the cytoplasm adjacent to the nucleus. In other places the cells contain particles of brown pigment. When fresh specimens are subjected to vital staining with neutral red, the majority of these cells exhibit granules which have taken up the dye. By the ready demonstration of this affinity for neutral red and of the ability to ingest red blood cells, clear cut anatomical data as to the phagocytic ability of these strains of cells have been adduced. To these two categories another type of cell must be added, which invariably constitutes a distinct feature of the cell strands mentioned. Close proximity to the smaller blood vessels and the presence of coarse granules in the cytoplasm are quite specific for this type of cell, which may be regarded as the stem-cell of mesenchymal origin from which the clasmatocytes and monocytes are derived. . . .

There is considerable evidence that the monocytes, as well as the clasmatocytes, within the parametrial tissue during pregnancy, develop *in situ*. . . . From the third month of pregnancy on, we can readily trace all stages of their development and maturation, and can see the cytoplasm become more voluminous. . . . A similar metamorphosis likewise occurs in the acquisition of a high phagocytic power; with the result that the essential representatives of the tissue, although derived from cells of diverse morphological type, come to resemble one another closely.

The concentration of these cells in the parametrium was interpreted by Hofbauer as a manifestation of their purposeful role in the pelvic defense mechanism. He wrote: [5]

I wish to emphasize the important point that . . . the occurrence of phagocytic cells is decidedly less abundant in the loose connective tissue, which constitutes the upper part of the broad ligament, than at its base. . . . In the presence of actual infection at the time of labor, it is altogether likely that the bacteria which gain access to the parametrial tissue through smaller or larger cervical tears would give rise to the irritation necessary to stimulate proliferation of the phagocytic tissue, which in all probability would lead to the local limitation of the infectious process, provided the offending bacteria were not of excessive virulence. In other words, the activity of the parametrial tissue in question must be regarded as a most beneficent mechanism in the production of local immunity.

HOFBAUER'S LIFE

Isford Isfred Hofbauer * was born in Vienna, September 11, 1879, of mixed Austrian and Scandinavian parentage. After receiving his medical degree from the University of Vienna he served as assistant to Schauta for three years, followed by a somewhat longer period under Wertheim, in whose clinic Hofbauer carried out his early studies on the placenta. In 1911 he joined the Department of Obstetrics and Gynecology of the University of Königsberg, where he remained until his migration to the United States in 1924 to become a member of Williams' department at Johns Hopkins. Shortly after Williams' death in 1931, Hofbauer moved to Cincinnati, Ohio, where he now resides. Hofbauer was the first to use posterior pituitary extract for the treatment of uterine inertia during labor.[3] In 1929 he called attention to a localization of specialized tissue within the pregnant uterus and suggested its role as a pacemaker, comparable to the conduction apparatus of the heart.[6] He has also written at length on uterine carcinogenesis and the etiology of pregnancy toxemia.

REFERENCES

1. Dalrymple, J.: On the structure and functions of the human placenta. *Med.-Chir. Tr.*, **25**:21–29, 1842.

2. Hofbauer, J.: *Grundzüge einer Biologie der Menschlichen Plazenta mit besonderer Berücksichtigung der Fragen der Fötalen Ernährung.* Braumüller, Vienna & Leipzig, 1905, pp. 28–30.

* Hofbauer's Scandinavian first name has been written more often as Isidro or Jsidro; most of his scientific writings and correspondence are signed simply "J. Hofbauer."

3. Hofbauer, J.: Hypophysenextrakt als Wehenmittel. *Zentralbl. f. Gynäk.,* **35**:137–41, 1911.

4. Hofbauer, J.: The function of the Hofbauer cells of the chorionic villus, particularly in relation to acute infection and syphilis. *Am. J. Obst. & Gynec.,* **10**:1–14, 1925.

5. Hofbauer, J.: The defensive mechanism of the parametrium during pregnancy and labor. *Bull. Johns Hopkins Hosp.,* **38**:255–72, 1926.

6. Hofbauer, J.: A specialized type of muscle in the human pregnant uterus, possibly analogous to conductive system of heart. *J.A.M.A.,* **92**:540–44, 1929.

7. Langhans, T.: Zur Kenntniss der menschlichen Placenta. *Arch. f. Gynäk.,* **1**:317–34, 1870.

8. Langhans, T.: Untersuchungen über die menschliche Placenta. *Arch. f. Anat. u. Physiol., Anat. Abth.,* 188–267, 1877.

9. Langhans, T.: Ueber die Zellschicht der menschlichen Chorion. In *Beiträge zur Anatomie und Embryologie als Festgabe Jacob Henle zum 4. April 1882 dargebracht von seinen Schülern.* Max Cohen & Sohn, Bonn, 1882, pp. 69–79.

10. Lewis, W. H.: Hofbauer cells (clasmatocytes) of the human chorionic villus. *Bull. Johns Hopkins Hosp.,* **35**:183–85, 1924.

11. Lubarsch: Theodor Langhans. *Deutsche med. Wchnschr.,* **42**:392–93, 1916.

12. Neumann, J.: Beitrag zur Kenntnis der Blasenmolen und des "malignen Deciduoms." *Monatschr. f. Geburtsh. u. Gynäk.,* **6**:17–36, 157–77, 1897.

13. Nitabuch, R.: *Beiträge zur Kenntniss der menschlichen Placenta.* Stämpfli'sche Buchdruckerei, Bern, 1887.

14. Obituary: Dr. Theodor Langhans, *Lancet,* **1**:161, 1916.

15. Papanicolaou, G. N.: Observations on the origin and specific function of the histiocytes in the female genital tract. *Fertil. & Steril.,* **4**:472–78, 1953.

16. Rodway, H. E., and Marsh, F.: A study of Hofbauer's cells in the human placenta. *J. Obst. & Gynaec. Brit. Emp.,* **63**:111–15, 1956.

17. Waldeyer, W.: Bemerkungen über den Bau der Menschen-und Affen-Placenta. *Arch. f. mikr. Anat.,* **35**:1–51, 1890.

William Fetherston Montgomery and the Tubercles of the Areola

The various bodily changes wrought by pregnancy, which serve even today as the usual criteria for diagnosis, comprised the physician's sole means of confirming a suspicion of the gravid state before modern biologic tests for pregnancy were developed and the roentgen ray was adapted to this purpose. The selective softening of the uterine isthmus, which comprises the basis of Hegar's sign; the altered coloration of the vulvovaginal mucosa, now known as Chadwick's sign; and the alternating phases of contraction and relaxation of the myometrium, associated with the name of Braxton Hicks, are among the principal phenomena of early pregnancy endowed with diagnostic significance. In characteristic fashion physicians have differed in their evaluation of these pregnancy signs; some have placed their principal reliance on the alterations in the breasts. Foremost among the latter group was William Montgomery, who described in great detail the external changes in the mammary apparatus during pregnancy and stressed their diagnostic importance in a volume entitled *An Exposition of the Signs and Symptoms of Pregnancy,*[1] published in London in 1837.

Montgomery was well aware of the value imputed by others to the color change in the vagina and alleged by some to be an invariable accompaniment of early pregnancy, for he wrote in his preface, after a limited experience, that "while in some . . . its existence was very obvious, in others it was so slight as to be scarcely, if at all perceptible." To the pregnancy changes in the breasts, on the other hand, especially those localized in the areolas, he

212

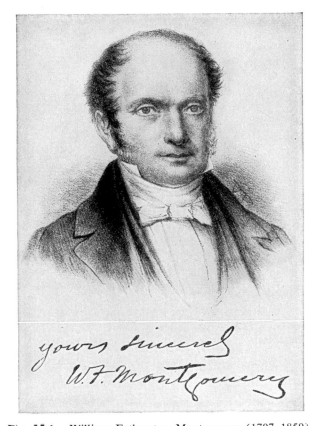

Fig. 25-1. William Fetherston Montgomery (1797–1859).

attached the greater significance, stating: "I wish here to repeat, that my confidence in the condition of the areola as a diagnostic mark of pregnancy is not only unabated, but very much increased by further observations."

MONTGOMERY'S DESCRIPTION OF BREAST CHANGES

Montgomery's chapter on "Mammary Sympathies," containing his description of the breast changes of pregnancy, has never been improved upon. The symptomatic fullness and general enlargement of the organ drew only his passing notice, whereas he dealt with the areola in minute detail, considering its size, color, texture, and, most important, the intra-areolar papillae previously identified with the name of Morgagni but now better known as the *tubercles of Montgomery*. He wrote:

A condition of fullness of the breasts may be natural to the individual, or it may take place at the turn of life, when the menses becoming naturally suppressed, the person grows at the same time fatter, and the breasts under such circumstances become full, and are not infrequently painful,—which circumstances concurring are often improperly considered in the light of cause and effect, and irritability of the stomach being at the same time experienced, the woman believes herself pregnant. There is, however, one of those changes which, if carefully observed, is of the utmost value as an evidence of pregnancy, which, according to my experience, can alone produce it—I allude to the altered condition of the areola.

The alteration which takes place in that part of the breast which immediately surrounds the nipple, and is called the areola, appears to me not to have received that degree of notice which its importance merits, as being one of the most certain external indications of pregnancy, arising from the operation of sympathy. On this, however, as on many other points connected with this investigation, a very marked difference of opinion exists; for while some suppose, with Denman, that the alteration in the areola "may be produced by any cause capable of giving to the breasts a state resembling that which they are in at the time of prenancy;" while others of equal authority maintain the opinion of Smellie and William Hunter, who regarded it as the result of pregnancy only; an opinion in which I entirely concur, and think I shall be able to show that much of the discrepancy of opinion on this subject has arisen from want of sufficient care in observing, and accuracy in describing the essential characters of the true areola.

Most of those who have noticed this change, appear, from their observations on it, to have attended to only one of its characters—namely, its colour, which is, in my opinion, the one of all others most liable to uncertainty.

A notable exception, acknowledged by Montgomery, was Roederer (1727–1763), who had published the following brief statement in his *Elementa Artis Obstetriciae* [5] in 1753, antedating Montgomery's description by 84 years:

Menstruorum suppressionem mammarum intumescentia insequitur, quocirca mammae crescunt, replentur, dolent interdum, indurescunt: venae earum coeruleo colore conspicuae redduntur, crassescit papilla, inflata videtur, color eiusdem fit obscurior; similem colorem induit discus ambiens, qui in latitudinem maiorem expanditur, paruisque eminentiis, quasi totidem papillulis, tegitur. Lympha lactea ad mammae pressionem profluit. [Enlargement of the breasts follows suppression of the menses; as a result of which the breasts increase in size, are refilled, sometimes become painful, and grow hard. Their veins, blue in color, become conspicuous again, the nipple swells, as if blown up, and its color becomes darker. The areola, marked by a similar color, enlarges to a greater diameter, and contains small protuberances, as if covered all over with tiny nipples. On pressure of the breast, milky fluid flows forth.]

Montgomery's account, fuller and more precise than any previous, stressed the following as a constant and particularly noteworthy condition of pregnancy:

. . . a soft and moist state of the integument, which appears raised and in a state of turgescence, giving one the idea that, if touched by the point of the finger, it would be found emphysematous; this state appears, however, to be caused by infiltration of the subjacent cellular tissue, which, together with its altered colour, gives us the idea of a part in which there is going forward a greater degree of vital action than is in operation around it; and we not infrequently find that the little glandular follicles or tubercles, as they are called by Morgagni, are bedewed with a secretion sufficient to damp and colour the woman's inner dress. These changes do not take place immediately after conception, but occur in different persons after uncertain intervals: we must therefore consider, in the first place, the period of pregnancy at which we may expect to gain any useful information from the condition of the areola. I cannot say positively what may be the earliest period at which this change can be observed, but I have recognised it fully at the end of the second month, at which time the alteration in colour is by no means the circumstance most observable, but the puffy turgescence (though as yet slight) not alone of the nipple but of the whole of the surrounding disk, and the development of the little glandular follicles are the objects to which we should principally direct our attention, the colour at this period being in general little more than a deeper shade of rose or flesh colour slightly tinged occasionally with a yellowish or light brownish hue.

Proceeding then with a more detailed consideration of the areolar papillae, Montgomery wrote:

In the centre of the coloured circle the nipple is observed partaking of the altered colour of the part and appearing turgid and prominent, while the surface of the areola, especially that part of it which lies more immediately around the base of the nipple, is studded over and rendered unequal by the prominence of the glandular follicles, which, varying in number from twelve to twenty, project from the sixteenth to the eighth of an inch. . . . [See frontispiece.]

These follicles or tubercles of the areola, although by many considered merely as sebaceous glands, have really a much more important character, and more intimate connexion with the peculiar structure and function of the breasts, and hence might naturally be expected to display an active sympathy in any condition of the system which called into action the peculiar function of these organs, which is the secretion of milk for the support of the new being, for which purpose certain previous changes in the glands and ducts are necessary. Now it appears that these areolar tubercles are intimately connected with the lactiferous tubes, some of which can be traced into them and opening on their summit,* so that in pregnant women a sero-lactescent fluid may be often distinctly perceived issuing from them, and in nurses they have been observed to pour forth drops of perfect milk. . . . It appears . . . that each of these follicles is, in common with the nipple and surrounding areola, furnished with very small sebaceous glands which lie around its base, the ducts of which, from one to four in number, are found opening on the surface of the tubercle.

* Morgagni, G. B.: *Adversaria Anatomica Omnia.* Padua, 1719, Part I, pp. 10–11; Table 4, Fig. 2.

The specificity of the areolar changes for the diagnosis of pregnancy, wrote Montgomery, exceeds their sensitivity:

The areola does not always, in pregnant women, present all the characters I have described as belonging to it, nor does the perfection of its distinctive characters seem to depend so much on the degree of change and increase of vital activity in the breasts, as on some constitutional peculiarity; for I have repeatedly observed the ordinary mammary changes take place with great energy, so that the breasts themselves were greatly altered, and yet the areola exhibit little or no change, and *vice versa* the areolar signs are sometimes very distinct and perfect when the breasts are otherwise but slightly affected. I have seen it at the time of labour presenting the dark circle alone without the prominence of the glandular follicles, but never saw an instance of their development in conjunction with the other changes already described, without the occurrence of pregnancy: their absence, therefore, ought not to decide our opinion against the existence of that condition, though their presence would be with us a very convincing proof of previous conception. . . .

In the parous patient, however, especially if recently pregnant or nursing, the areolar changes may mislead the inexperienced observer, as Montgomery cautioned:

If a woman has been pregnant before, and particularly if she has suckled or is nursing, it may embarrass our investigation. . . . In some persons of fair complexion especially, this colouring matter is removed in some time after delivery, and the breast resumes its virgin appearance; in others the colour remains permanent, and there is even a slight prominence of the little glands to be observed sufficient to deceive an inexperienced eye.

Fetal death in utero, Montgomery pointed out, like termination of the pregnancy, also results in regression of the distinctive alterations in the areola:

Should the fetus be blighted, the characters of the [areola] will soon decline and fade away in common with the other changes previously effected in the breasts. . . . The areolar tubercles also shrink and are no longer bedewed with their sero-lactescent moisture.

MONTGOMERY'S LIFE

William Fetherston Montgomery, one of Ireland's most distinguished obstetricians, was born in 1797 and died in Dublin, December 21, 1859.[3,4] He received his education in the University of Dublin, winning a scholarship for his classical attainments in 1820, his A.B. in 1822, and his A.M. and M.B. in 1825. Montgomery became a licentiate of the King and Queen's College of Physicians, a fellow in 1829, and subsequently its president; but it was not until 1852, after he had been in practice for 27 years, that he took his M.D. degree. Early in his professional career Montgomery, like William Smellie, set himself up as a teacher of midwifery, giving lectures in his house to large classes of students. It was chiefly through his efforts that a chair of midwifery was established in the College of Physicians, and Montgomery had the distinction of occupying it for the first 30 years. Shortly before his death he was elected as one of 13 honorary fellows of the Obstetrical Society of London. He was never Master of the Rotunda, however. Together with Francis Barker he published *Observations on the Dublin Pharmacopoeia of 1826,* used for many years as a standard text by the medical students in the University of Dublin. Montgomery is best known for his *Exposition of the Signs and Symptoms of Pregnancy* and for his essay, *On the Spontaneous Amputation of the Foetal Limbs in Utero,*[2] which is bound together in the same volume with the former.

In this essay Montgomery expounded his view, widely held for many ensuing years, that certain fetal malformations are the result of intrauterine amputations caused by constricting bands of coagulated lymph. He wrote:

Within the last few months a child, of a month old, was brought to me from the county of Westmeath, in consequence of its having been born deprived of the left hand: on examination, I found the fore-arm of that side presenting, a little above the wrist, the appearance of a perfectly well-formed stump, as it would be found after amputation by the surgeon's knife; with this difference, however, that the mark of cicatrix did not extend across the stump but was confined to a small circular depression in its centre; the child was otherwise quite perfect and healthy. Unfortunately, I could not obtain any information as to whether the hand had been found at the time of delivery, or not; the poor woman having been attended only by an ignorant country midwife. . . .

I feel almost convinced, that the removal of limbs in this way is by no means so uncommon an occurrence as the paucity of cases hitherto recorded would, at first sight, lead us to conclude; but the reason appears to me to be this; when the separated portion of limb was not accidentally discovered, the imperfection seems to have been considered quite as a matter of course, and without further examination, as arising from imperfect development, or monstrosity; and, consequently, no search was made for the deficient part; and, even if search was made, the amputated member might have been so small, as to escape undiscovered, involved in the membranes, or buried in coagula, even though the child, to which it belonged, had attained considerable size, because, its separation may, as we have seen, take place a long time previous to birth. . . .

With regard to the theories which have been advanced to account for such accidents as that which we have been considering: some, regarding them as the effects of mental emotions in the mother, or of accidents encountered by her, have attempted to support their views by details which Haller truly designates as "adeo fabulosa ut fidem auferant:" those who attributed this phenomenon to gangrene, did so from theory, and have received no support for their opinions, even from the facts which they have themselves recorded; for it is expressly mentioned, that the parts affected seemed otherwise healthy, were not discoloured, and, at the point of division, were either partially, or entirely healed over. The explanation which facts, fortunately, enabled me to offer does not depend on conjectural reasoning, or theoretical speculation, for its support, but its proof may be "oculis subjecta fidelibus" by the mere inspection of the parts, which are preserved in my museum. And with regard to the nature of the process by which the solution of continuity is effected and the foot or other part amputated, it appears to be strictly that of disjunctive atrophy, and in a great degree similar to that, by which, the separation of the funis from the umbilicus is accomplished.

REFERENCES

1. Montgomery, W. F.: *An Exposition of the Signs and Symptoms of Pregnancy, the Period of Human Gestation, and the Signs of Delivery.* Sherwood, Gilbert, & Piper, London, 1837.

2. Montgomery, W. F.: On the spontaneous amputation of the foetal limbs in utero. *Ibid.,* pp. 321–35.

3. Obituary. *M. Times & Gaz.,* **19**(n.s.):664–65, 1859.

4. Obituary. Dr. Montgomery. *Lancet,* **1**:24, 1860.

5. Roederer, J. G.: *Elementa Artis Obstetriciae in Usum Praelectionum Academicarum.* Göttingen, 1753, p. 62.

Clinical Signs,
Tests, and Rules

PART II

Alfred Hegar: Hegar's Sign and Dilators*

Scientific discoveries and inventions, although built upon the earlier labors of others, are usually credited to him who first proclaims his findings to the world or records his work in the published press. Yet medical history contains numerous instances of misplaced credit for priority in original observations. A possible inequity in obstetric terminology is embodied in Hegar's sign, universally recognized as an early indication of pregnancy.

HEGAR'S SIGN

Hegar's sign, a selective softening of the uterus in the region of the lower segment, resulting in an increased mobility between the cervix and the corpus, was actually described first by C. Reinl, one of Hegar's assistants, who published this observation (Fig. 26-2) in 1884 [8] as a new and certain diagnostic sign of pregnancy:

Apart from the general disturbances in the sense of well-being, amenorrhea, changes in the breasts and external genitalia, alterations in the consistency of the enlarging uterine corpus and the cervix, we have no further diagnostic signs for the early months of pregnancy.

The discovery of a new sign should therefore be of particular value, since some

* This chapter originally published in *Obst. & Gynec.,* **6**:679–83, 1955; reprinted by permission. Copyright © 1955, by the American Academy of Obstetrics and Gynecology.

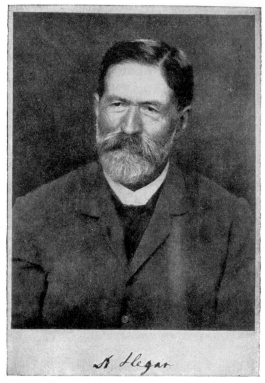

Fig. 26-1. Alfred Hegar (1830–1914). (Reproduced from *Arch. f. Gynäk.*, **103**, Heft II, 1914.)

of the above-mentioned local changes are often absent or are only present in slight degree, or, in multiparas, are not always reliable.

Last winter, in Professor Hegar's gynecology clinic, I had the opportunity of acquainting myself with a new and excellent sign of the early months of pregnancy.

This consists in the demonstration of an unusual softness, flexibility, and thinning of the lower uterine segment, that is, of the part directly above the insertion of the uterosacral ligaments.

This finding is not only demonstrable when the rest of the uterus feels firm, as is often the case, but also very definitely when it is soft and elastic.

Also, in the latter case it is always possible to compress the lower uterine segment, to actually thin it out with the finger, and so to differentiate it from the upper part of the uterus, while it still clearly differs in consistency from the cervix below. The pliability and laxness of these parts can be so extensive that one may be in doubt as to whether any connection exists between the cervix and the larger abdominal or pelvic mass.

We know of no condition which can produce findings similar to pregnancy; solid tumors certainly do not, and hemato- and hydro-metra present no diagnostic

Pränumerationspreis

Mit Postversendung

Recensions-Exemplare und Inserate, die
mit 10 kr. oder 30 Pfg. die gespaltene Petitzeile
berechnet werden, sind an die Verlags-Buch-
handlung zu adressiren.
Manuscripte dagegen sind an die Redaction
II. Brodnergasse 8 zu senden.

Prager
Medicinische Wochenschrift

REDACTION

Prof. Dr. **Friedr. Ganghofner,**
für den Verein deutscher Aerzte in Prag.

Prof. Dr. **Otto Kahler,**
für den Centralverein deutscher Aerzte in Böhmen.

Verlag von **F. Tempsky in Prag.**

IX. Jahrgang.   25. Juni 1884.   Nro. 26.

I. Aus der gynäkologischen Klinik des Hr. Geh. R. Prof. Dr. A. Hegar in Freiburg i. Br.

Ein neues sicheres diagnostisches Zeichen der Schwangerschaft in den ersten Monaten.

Von

Dr. C. Reinl in Franzensbad.

Ausser den consensuellen Störungen im Allgemeinbefinden, dem Ausbleiben der Menstruation, den Veränderungen an den Brüsten, äussern Genitalien, Consistenzveränderungen des vergrösserten Uteruskörpers und Cervix besitzen wir kein weiteres Zeichen für die ersten Monate der Schwangerschaft.

Die Auffindung eines neuen Zeichens dürfte daher immerhin vom Werthe sein, da ein Theil oberwähnter localer Veränderungen oft fehlt oder nur in geringerem Grade ausgesprochen, oder bei Personen mit wiederholter Schwangerschaft nicht gehörig verwerthbar ist.

Im Verlaufe des letzten Winters bot sich mir nun Gelegenheit, an Hr. Geh. R. Hegar's gynäkolog. Klinik ein neues, vorzügliches Zeichen der Gravidität in den ersten Monaten kennen zu lernen.

Dasselbe besteht in dem Nachweis einer ungewöhnlichen Weichheit, Nachgiebigkeit und Verdünnung des unteren Uterinsegmentes, d. h. des Abschnittes unmittelbar oberhalb der Insertion der Ligamenta sacro-uterina.

Diese Beschaffenheit besagter Partie ist nicht allein nachweisbar, wenn sich der übrige Körper, wie dies durchaus nicht selten, fest und hart anfühlt, sondern auch dann noch deutlich ausgesprochen, wenn sich dieser weich und elastisch präsentirt.

Auch im letzteren Falle ist dann immerhin die Möglichkeit vorhanden, den unteren Uterinabschnitt zusammenzudrücken, gewissermassen mit dem Finger auszuziehen und so selben von den oberen Partien zu unterscheiden, während sich nach unten der consistentere Zapfen des Cervix deutlich abhebt. Die Nachgiebigkeit und Schlaffheit jener Partie kann so weit gehen, dass man in Zweifel gerathen kann, ob überhaupt eine Verbindung des Halses mit der grösseren Schwellung in abdomine oder pelvi bestehe.

Wir wissen nun keinen Zustand, der ähnliche Verhältnisse darbieten könnte, wie die Schwangerschaft, feste Geschwülste wenigstens nicht, und bieten Haemato- und Hydrometra, überdies keine diagnostischen Schwierigkeiten. Es ist daher unser Zeichen für die differenzielle Diagnose der Schwangerschaft gewiss vortrefflich zu verwerthen.

Die Ursache dieser markanten Erscheinung ist wohl darin zu suchen, dass das untere Uterinsegment als die dünnste Partie des ganzen Körpers durch die Schwangerschaft succulent, aufgelockert, verdünnt und hochgradig elastisch werden muss, da man, wie dies leicht ausführbar, im Stande ist, den Uterus nach oben schiebend, diese Partie zwischen die touchirenden und palpirenden Finger zu fassen, und selbe so zu sagen zerdrücken und gewissermassen mit den Fingern verdünnen kann.

Ein Fehlen dieses Befundes schliesst jedoch keineswegs das Vorhandensein einer Gravidität aus, da es leicht denkbar ist, dass bei bedeutenden chronischen Infarct Schwangerschaft bestehen kann, ohne dass dies Verhalten des untern Uterinsegmentes sehr deutlich nachweisbar ist.

Ich gebe im Nachstehenden eine Reihe von an der Freiburger Klinik beobachteten Fällen:

1. Frau R. von Hardtheim, 33 J. II p.

Letzte Periode Ende October 1883.

Status vom 29. Jänner 1884:

Brüste gut entwickelt aber sehr schlaff, Montgomerische Drüsen stark vorspringend, Warzen und Warzenhof nicht turgescent, bei Druck sehr wenig helles Colostrum.

Bauch aufgetrieben, starker Fettpolster; Linea alba nur mit einer Spur von Pigmentirungen versehen. Schleimhaut des Introitus nur leicht bläulich, Scheidengewölbe dagegen stärker blau verfärbt.

Vaginalportion in der Umgebung des Muttermundes, besonders an der vorderen Lippe, deutlich blau, allein sonst blass, mässig geschwellt, cylindrisch.

Der Uteruskörper hat die Grösse eines kleinen Kindskopfes und ist auffallend hart anzufühlen.

Untersucht man per anum und dringt direct hinter der Schoossfuge nach hinten und unten, drückt sich so den Hals dem im Mastdarm eingeführten Finger entgegen, und giebt man das obere Ende des Halses, während die Geschwulst in die Höhe gehoben wird, so hat man das Gefühl, als wenn der Uterushals nach oben aufhöre, und die obere Schwellung etwas für sich sei.

Doch überzeugt man sich bald, dass da, wo der Hals aufhört, etwas Weiches beginnt, und wenn man nun die Schwellung herunterdrückt, ist es wieder der Zusammenhang unverkennbar und man fühlt deutlich, dass der consistentere Hals in eine weiche ausgebreitete Masse übergeht, die dann wieder mit der oberen härteren Schwellung zusammenhängt.

26a

Fig. 26-2. The initial description of Hegar's sign, by C. Reinl, in June, 1884. (Reproduced by permission of Státní Zdravotnické Nakladatelství, Prague.)

difficulties. Our sign can therefore be used with confidence for the differential diagnosis of pregnancy.

This remarkable development results from the fact that the lower uterine segment becomes the most attenuated and elastic part of the entire uterus during pregnancy; therefore, as one can easily demonstrate, it is possible, after displacing the uterus upward, to grasp the lower segment between the fingers of the vaginal and abdominal hands, compress it, and completely thin it out.

Absence of this sign does not, however, exclude pregnancy by any means, for one can easily imagine that with chronic infarction of the lower uterine segment pregnancy could occur without this change being demonstrable.

It is not clear, from this account, whether Reinl discovered this sign of pregnancy himself or whether it was pointed out to him by Hegar. It was the latter, however, who taught and publicized it until it eventually came to bear his name, while Reinl's possible role in the discovery has been completely overshadowed by the celebrated name of his master. Hegar's own paper [1] on the subject, with illustrative diagrams, did not appear until 1895, 11 years after Reinl's. In it he acknowledged Reinl's priority of publication, but strongly implied that recognition of the significance of the pregnancy change in the lower segment was his (Hegar's):

Fortunately we have still another diagnostic aid, which is based on the compressibility of the lower uterine segment. I was led to this while reading an article by A. Martin in which he describes hypertrophy of the cervix, as a result of which the connection between the soft lower uterine segment and the cervix can only be demonstrated with difficulty.

Martin, whose paper was published in 1881,[6] had reported seven cases, regarding them as unusual, in which he observed a peculiar hypertrophy of the supravaginal part of the cervix during pregnancy. He discussed the possible diagnostic significance of this change when present but seemed uncertain of its practical clinical value.

Credit for Hegar's sign should therefore probably be divided among three men: Martin, who first called attention to the selective pregnancy change in the lower uterine segment; Reinl, who stressed the specificity of this change and its value for the early diagnosis of pregnancy, and first published on it; and Hegar, who later popularized it.

HEGAR'S CERVICAL DILATORS

Hegar is also remembered today for the curved metal cervical dilators (Fig. 26-3) that bear his name. The development of this type of instrument represented a great advance over the laminaria tents formerly used to dilate the cervix, often with severe parametritis resulting. The first recorded reference to Hegar's dilators was published in 1879 in an article by Tchoudowski,[10] who had seen the dilators in use while visiting Hegar's clinic in the summer of that year. Hegar's own description of the dilators appeared for the first time in the second edition of his textbook on operative gynecology,[3] published with Kaltenbach as coauthor in 1881:

We have used this method of dilatation many times in recent years and found it to be very satisfactory. That it has not been generally adopted as yet is probably due in large measure to unsatisfactory technique and imperfect instruments. One must have a large number of dilators at hand, each one of which that is intro-

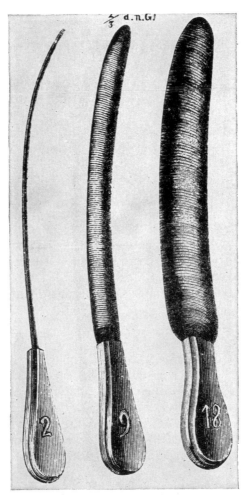

Fig. 26-3. Hegar's original dilators, as illustrated in the second edition of his *Die Operative Gynäkologie*, published in 1881.[3] (Reproduced by permission of Ferdinand Enke, Stuttgart.)

duced having only a slightly greater diameter than the previous one. This is essential at least for difficult cases. We have therefore had solid, cylindrical dilators made out of ebonite with conically tapering ends. They are about 12 to 14 cm long, in addition to a flattened handle, which is about 5 cm long. The smallest dilator is 2 mm in diameter. The rest are graduated in diameters which increase progressively only 1 mm at a time. The increase in circumference is therefore about 3 mm. It is even better to order dilators which increase only 0.5 mm at a time. At least the dilatation will then be easier in difficult cases. For gynecologic purposes, namely for manipulation of the uterus, a dilator with a 16- to 17-mm diameter suffices. Even the first phalanx of a thick index finger can then be inserted into the uterine cavity. Even more marked dilatation can easily be achieved with larger dilators, which we have provided for up to a diameter of 26 mm for gynecologic purposes. For obstetric purposes, for example for use with placenta previa, larger dilators are sometimes necessary. For injections into the uterine cavity, cauterizations with silver nitrate or nitric acid, use of the curette, introduction of a small polyp forceps, etc., 6- to 12-mm dilators suffice. Likewise for cervical stenosis or with the view of stretching the canal to somewhat more than its usual lumen.

In the notes accompanying this description of the dilators, reference is made to graduated metal dilators previously described by others, the earliest description of similar instruments being attributed to Peaslee. Peaslee, while professor of diseases of women, in Dartmouth College, had published in 1870[7] a description of his set of five steel dilators, ranging from ⅛ to ⁵⁄₁₆ in. in diameter. Each dilator had a bulb 1¾ in. from its uterine end, to prevent "needless intrusion into the uterine cavity." This author, in turn, had called attention to a description by Kammerer[5] in the previous year of a similar type of dilator. The principle of progressive cervical dilatation by graduated metal sounds had thus been described in the literature ten years before Tchoudowski's publication first announcing Hegar's dilators.*

HEGAR'S LIFE

Alfred Hegar was born in Darmstadt, Germany, January 6, 1830, the son of a general practitioner. He studied in Giessen, Heidelberg, Berlin, and Vienna, receiving his medical degree in 1852. After a brief stint as a military surgeon he returned to practice in his home town, where he soon established himself as a busy obstetrician. He began to write on the pathology of pregnancy in the early 1860's, and his studies on early abortion were so well received that they led to his appointment, in 1864, as Spiegelberg's successor

---

* Graduated dilators of tin or lead, hollow at one end and mounted on long wooden handles, were actually described long before, in the writings of Hippocrates; these dilators being used principally to permit the introduction of various medicaments into the uterine cavity (Ricci, J. R.: *The Development of Gynaecological Surgery and Instruments.* Blakiston Co., Philadelphia, 1949, p. 13).

as professor of obstetrics and gynecology at Freiburg, where he remained for 40 years until his retirement in 1904. During this period he helped establish the *Oberrheinische Gesellschaft für Geburtshilfe und Gynäkologie,* and in 1898 he founded and served as editor of the *Beiträge zur Geburtshilfe und Gynäkologie.* When the Universitäts-Frauenklinik was opened in Freiburg in 1868, Hegar was made its first chief. He had the reputation of working himself, as well as his assistants, very hard, often starting his schedule of operations as early as 5 A.M. He died on August 5, 1914, at the age of 85.[9]

In addition to the early sign of pregnancy and the cervical dilators with which his name is associated, Hegar distinguished himself in several other spheres. He achieved renown for his diagnostic prowess and was said to possess an unusually well-developed tactile sense. He was an ardent disciple of Semmelweis and was one of the first to implement the latter's principles of antisepsis. Hegar was a pioneer in the early studies on genital tuberculosis in women. He was probably best known among his contemporaries for his work in operative gynecology. Early in his career his reputation for the successful repair of urinary fistulas became widespread, and women from all parts of Europe sought him out for the correction of this affliction. He devised a perineorrhaphy operation which also bears his name, and was the first in Germany to perform myomectomy. In the treatment of uterine fibroids, however, he is better known for his ovariectomies and for his demonstration that this operation resulted in shrinkage of the tumors and cessation of bleeding. Although McDowell of Kentucky had performed ovariectomy many years before (1809), Hegar (July, 1872) was probably the first to remove normal ovaries to create an artificial menopause, an operation he resorted to frequently in the treatment of dysmenorrhea as well as bleeding uterine fibroids.

A bibliography of Hegar's writings, compiled by his son, was published in 1915,[4] and in 1930 a *Festschrift*[2] appeared in commemoration of the hundredth anniversary of his birth.

REFERENCES

1. Hegar, A.: Diagnose der frühesten Schwangerschaftsperiode. *Deutsche med. Wchnschr.,* **21**:565–67, 1895.

2. Hegar, A.: *Zum Gedächtnis.* Speyer & Kaerner, Universitäts-Buchhandlung, Freiburg I. B., 1930.

3. Hegar, A., and Kaltenbach, R.: *Die Operative Gynäkologie,* 2nd ed. Enke, Erlangen, 1881, pp. 87–89.

4. Hegar, K.: Bibliographie von Alfred Hegar. *Monatschr. f. Geburtsh. u. Gynäk.,* **42**:543–46, 1915.

5. Kammerer, J.: On the treatment of uterine catarrh. *Am. J. Obst.,* **2**:185–207, 1869.

6. Martin, A.: Zur Kenntniss der Hypertrophia colli uteri supravaginalis. *Ztschr. f. Geburtsh. u. Gynäk.,* **6**:101–9, 1881.

7. Peaslee, E. R.: Intra-uterine medication: its uses, limitations, and methods. *New York State J. Med.*, **11**:465–84, 1870.

8. Reinl, C.: Ein neues sicheres diagnostischen Zeichen der Schwangerschaft in den ersten Monaten. *Prag. med. Wchnschr.*, **9**:253–54, 1884.

9. Sonntag, E.: Alfred Hegar. *Arch. f. Gynäk.*, **103**:II Heft, 1914.

10. Tchoudowski, M.: De la dilatation du canal cervical (d'après Hegar). *Arch. Tocol.*, **6**:737–55, 1879. (Reprinted from *Gaz. méd. de Strasbourg*, 1879.)

James Read Chadwick and CHAPTER

His Pregnancy Sign 27

Recognition of the color change in the vulvovaginal mucosa during pregnancy, and its utilization as a diagnostic sign, was long withheld from practitioners of obstetrics because of the limitations imposed upon their examinations. Respect for the patient's modesty not only precluded inspection of the genitalia but required that even the manipulations necessary for delivery be carried out under the protective cover of a sheet or other suitable drape.

Neither the precise date nor the actual discoverer is known of what is now designated as Chadwick's sign, but it is probable that this phenomenon was first recognized either in the routine examination of Parisian prostitutes or German syphilitic patients, sometime before 1836, for in both of these clientele categories the physician was freed of restriction in visualizing the patient's genitalia.

One of the earliest references to the altered appearance of the vaginal mucosa in pregnancy appears in the second edition of *De la Prostitution dans la Ville de Paris*,[6] published by Parent-Duchatelet in 1837. Since the author died early in 1836, he must have learned of this pregnancy sign not later than 1835. Wrote Parent-Duchatelet:

Examination of the genitals of prostitutes led M. Jacquemin to the discovery of a new sign of pregnancy, which may become of great use in the field of legal medicine. This sign consists of a violet coloration, sometimes like wine dregs, which the whole mucous membrane of the vagina acquires in this condition. The

229

sign is so obvious that M. Jacquemin is never misled by it and for him it alone suffices, apart from the other signs of pregnancy, to make the diagnosis. I have been witness to curious tests to which M. Jacquemin subjected himself to prove to his colleagues how accurate one can be on this point. . . . M. Jacquemin was able to determine the state of the mucous membrane in 4500 pregnant women.

The M. Jacquemin to whom Parent-Duchatelet assigned credit for this discovery was apparently Étienne Joseph Jacquemin (1796–1872), chief physician to the prison in Mazas. Although Jacquemin published a number of articles on medicolegal topics, he failed to record personally the observations he imparted to Parent-Duchatelet on the pregnancy changes in the vagina. Priority for recognition of this sign has been erroneously credited by some to the well-known French obstetrician Jean Marie Jacquemier, who was a contemporary of Jacquemin's, but the record is quite clear in this respect. In the former's textbook of obstetrics,[3] as a matter of fact, which was published in 1846, he specifically mentioned Jacquemin as the discoverer of the sign.

While Parent-Duchatelet's book was in preparation there appeared in the Danish Journal for *Medicin og Chirurgie* for 1835 a letter from a Dr. Sommer, reporting some of his observations while visiting in Berlin. The following excerpt is taken from the German translation of Sommer's letter, published in the *Berliner Medicinische Central-Zeitung,* January 14, 1837: [7]

Imagine, at my very first visit I saw an assistant in Kluge's wards examining the vagina of a syphilitic woman, whereupon he immediately pronounced her to be pregnant. I was completely astonished. In answer to my question as to how this diagnosis was possible, Professor Kluge explained to me that a bluish coloration of the vagina was present, extending to the cervical os, and this was an infallible sign of pregnancy, provided that no varices were present. According to his assertion, this coloration begins as early as the fourth week of pregnancy, or rather at the time when the menstrual period would have begun if conception had not occurred. This coloration increases up until delivery and disappears with the lochia. However, Kluge was not content with this mere assertion; he showed me several pregnant women concerning whom there was no doubt, for they were between the fifth and ninth months of pregnancy, and I thus saw with my own eyes, through a vaginal speculum, the presence of the bluish coloration. He told me (although he had not yet published anything on the subject) that for years he had used this sign as infallible, except when the aforementioned condition [varices] is present.

However, an appended note to Sommer's letter, by the Danish editor, indicated that this sign was already known in his country, but no clue is given as to the identity of its discoverer.

As in the case of Hegar's sign, therefore, credit for Chadwick's sign must

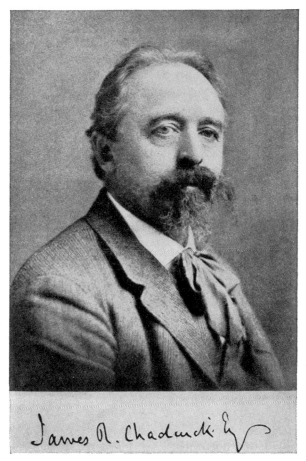

Fig. 27-1. James Read Chadwick (1884–1905). (Courtesy of American Gynecological Society.)

be divided, for it is no longer possible to determine who first recognized its value for the diagnosis of pregnancy. Although neither published on it, Jacquemin in France and Kluge in Germany were obviously using the sign at the same time, probably unbeknown to each other. If all the facts were available, perhaps some Danish physician, now unknown, could also qualify for a share of the credit.

CHADWICK'S DESCRIPTION OF PREGNANCY SIGN

Chadwick did not enter on the scene until 50 years later, when he presented his paper, "The Value of the Bluish Coloration of the Vaginal Entrance as a Sign of Pregnancy," [2] before the American Gynecological Society. This, the first definitive study of the subject, aroused widespread interest and gained eponymic distinction for its author. During the preceding half century, various textbooks had referred to the sign, but usually with an incorrect explanation of its mechanism and reservation as to its practical value. The following statement, which appeared in all three editions of Leishman's *System of Midwifery,*[4] is typical. Referring to the vaginal examination in pregnancy, Leishman wrote:

> There is clear evidence here also of increased activity of the circulation, corresponding to that which we have found to exist in the internal genital organs. It takes the form, in this situation, of a venous engorgement, which is due, in part at least, to obstruction, caused by pressure of the gravid womb, and is indicated by a more or less livid color of the mucous membrane—very different from the rose color of the unimpregnated state. This ocular examination of the parts, although it may thus reveal a sign which is far from being the least important, is, for obvious reasons, a method of research which cannot be generally adopted in the practice of midwifery, so that we have to depend here upon the results which are afforded by an examination conducted, under the bedclothes, by the finger.

Chadwick's paper, published in 1887,[2] reported a systematic clinical investigation of the subject in 20 pages of text, accompanied by a color plate to illustrate the blueness of the introitus with the labia spread apart. His findings were based upon the examination of about 6000 patients, over a period of ten years. The intensity and distribution of the altered color were recorded for 337 patients, 281 of whom were pregnant and 56 not pregnant, and the following conclusions were reached:

1. That its absence is not to be accepted as evidence that pregnancy does not exist, especially in the first three months, when satisfactory evidence is most needed.
2. That from (and including) the second month, this color is generally present, and often of such character as to be diagnostic.

Chadwick's description of the tinctorial change was concise and accurate and his interpretation sound. He wrote:

> The color begins as a pale violet in the early months, becomes more bluish as pregnancy advances, until it often assumes finally a dusky, almost black, tint; this last is familiar to every obstetrician. It is not due to pigmentation, but to an hypertrophy of the venous plexuses in the mucous membrane of the vagina (or a dilatation of the minute veins), induced by the afflux of blood to the uterus under the stimulus of pregnancy. The predominance of the veins in this location could alone account for the bluish color; moreover, when, toward the end of pregnancy, the color is most intense, varicose veins are plainly visible in the labia and in the legs.

With increasing experience with this sign, Chadwick soon learned that inspection of the introitus alone sufficed:

Almost all speak of the violet color as seen on the collum uteri, on the whole extent of the vagina, and consequently require the use of a speculum; now, while I do not claim that the change is not perceptible throughout the whole extent of the vagina and collum uteri, I do maintain that it is equally manifest at the introitus vaginae when the labia are simply separated by the fingers. After satisfying myself on this point by numerous investigations with the speculum, I was consequently able to dispense with that instrument, and thus render the sign more generally and easily applicable.

When Long and Evans, in 1920, described their placental sign in the rat,[5] a diagnostic sign of pregnancy resulting from the leakage of minute quantities of extravasated blood from the implantation site in the uterus into the vagina, they mentioned a reddish discoloration of the ventral vaginal wall, extending to the cervix, as the earliest detectable pregnancy change in this species. This finding in the rat, although not correlated by the authors with the vaginal changes in the human, strikingly corresponds with an observation by Chadwick:

In scrutinizing the color of this part in a large number of women I early discovered that, while in the majority the bluish tinge appeared over the whole vaginal entrance, there was a fair proportion in which the violet tint was confined to the anterior wall of the vagina, just below the urinary meatus, whence it shaded off into the normal pink color laterally. This, when distinctly perceptible, I soon found to be, in my practice, an absolutely sure sign of pregnancy. There were, furthermore, a very few in whom the blue tint was universal, but more accentuated on the posterior wall of the vaginal entrance, which I found was valueless as a sign of pregnancy, unless the color was quite deep. The recognition of this peculiar localization of the blue tint on the anterior wall as a sure sign of pregnancy I feel is the most important new point in this communication.

The widely held belief that the vascular changes in the pregnant vagina resulted from mechanical obstruction to the venous drainage by increased intrapelvic pressure Chadwick refuted in no uncertain terms:

Do fibroid or ovarian tumors ever give rise to this color by pressure or otherwise, as asserted by most writers on this topic? I answer most emphatically, *No.* I have had a large number pass under my observation during the past ten years, and have examined them with special care, invariably with a negative result. I must fain believe that the contrary opinions expressed have not been based upon observations, but upon the transmitted authority of the earlier writers, whose statements were made to accord with the theory that the blue color was due to stasis of blood from pressure upon the larger veins by the pregnant uterus, whence they inferred that the same was likely to result from the pressure of the uterus enlarged by a fibroid. I see no reason for believing that the change of color at such times is, in the slightest degree, due to pressure, but attribute it exclusively to the great afflux of blood caused by the necessity of nourishing the fetus.

CHADWICK'S LIFE

James Read Chadwick, born in Boston, November 2, 1844, attended the Boston public schools and Harvard College, from which he graduated in 1865. After a trip abroad he returned to Harvard for his medical studies, receiving his degree in 1871. He then married Katherine M. Lyman, the daughter of one of Boston's outstanding gynecologists, with whom he later pioneered in founding the American Gynecological Society. As was the fashion in his day, Chadwick then continued his postgraduate education in Europe, spending two years in Berlin, Vienna, Paris, and London, studying gynecology chiefly. Soon after his return to Boston in 1873 he was appointed gynecologist in the outpatient department of the Boston City Hospital. He later opened a private gynecologic dispensary, where he instructed the Harvard medical students after his appointment on the faculty. Chadwick was the first secretary of the American Gynecological Society and served as its president in 1897. In 1890 he organized the Harvard Medical Alumni Association, which he likewise served as president for its first four years. A bibliography of Chadwick's writings is appended to Burrage's obituary of him.[1] He was a great bibliophile, and in 1875 inspired the founding of the Boston Medical Library, in which he succeeded in interesting many fellow members of the profession, including Oliver Wendell Holmes. To this interest Chadwick devoted a tremendous amount of time and energy, often spending his Sundays and holidays in the library, sorting and cataloguing the books and arranging for the suitable disposal of duplicates. Holmes referred to him as "the untiring, imperturbable, tenacious, irrepressible, all-subduing agitator, who gave no sleep to his eyes, no slumber to his eyelids, until he had gained his ends, who neither rested nor let rest until the success of his project was assured." Cremation was another of Chadwick's great interests. In 1892 he reorganized the New England Cremation Society, later serving as its president. Because of his efforts to popularize and dignify this procedure he has been called "the father of cremation in New England." He died at his summer home in Chocorua, New Hampshire, September 23, 1905.

REFERENCES

1. Burrage, W. L.: James Read Chadwick, M.D. (1844–1905). *Tr. Am. Gynec. Soc.*, **31**:437–45, 1906.
2. Chadwick, J. R.: The value of the bluish coloration of the vaginal entrance as a sign of pregnancy. *Tr. Am. Gynec. Soc.*, **11**:339–418, 1887.

3. Jacquemier, J.: *Manuel des Accouchements et des Maladies des Femmes Grosses et Accouchées.* Baillière, Paris, 1846, Vol. 1, p. 215.

4. Leishman, W.: *A System of Midwifery.* Henry C. Lea, Philadelphia, 1873, p. 156. Second American edition, 1875, p. 158. Third American edition, 1879, p. 154.

5. Long, J. A., and Evans, H. M.: A characteristic sign of pregnancy in the rat detectable from the 13th to the 16th day. *Anat. Rec.,* **18**:249, 1920.

6. Parent-Duchatelet, A.-J.-B.: *De la Prostitution dans la Ville de Paris,* 2nd ed. Baillière, Paris, 1837, Vol. 1, pp. 217–18.

7. Sommer: *Berl. med. Centr.-Ztg.,* **6**:34–38, 1837.

Selmar Aschheim, Bernhard Zondek, Maurice Friedman, and Their Pregnancy Tests

From the time of Hippocrates (ca. 460–370 B.C.) many distinguished physicians, including Avicenna (ca. 979–1037) and Savonarola (ca. 1384–1462), as well as quacks, proclaimed their ability to diagnose pregnancy from the characteristics of the woman's urine. It is said that the ancient Egyptians, as early as the fourteenth century B.C., resorted to the urine for diagnosing fetal sex as well as confirming the suspicion of pregnancy. Grains of wheat and barley, in separate bags, were moistened daily with the woman's urine. Germination of either indicated pregnancy: the wheat, a male child; the barley, a female. In medieval England great favor was enjoyed by a cult of "piss-prophets," who professed to be able to recognize every manner of ailment, in addition to pregnancy, from their examination of the urine.[13] This form of medical exploitation was vigorously attacked in 1637 by Thomas Brian, himself a reformed and repentant piss-prophet, in a remarkable little book,[7] only five known copies of which remain. "Urina est meretrix, vel mendax: The urine is an Harlot, or a Lier," wrote Brian. "It were farre better for the Physician to see his Patient once than to view his Urine twenty times."

In this exposé of medical quackery Brian recorded the following letter from a Reverend J. H. to "his cunning Aesculapius," inquiring whether his wife be pregnant, together with the piss-prophet's answer, "darkning the judgment of the learned, and making a specious shew of a falsely assumed knowledge." Wrote the importunate Reverend:

236

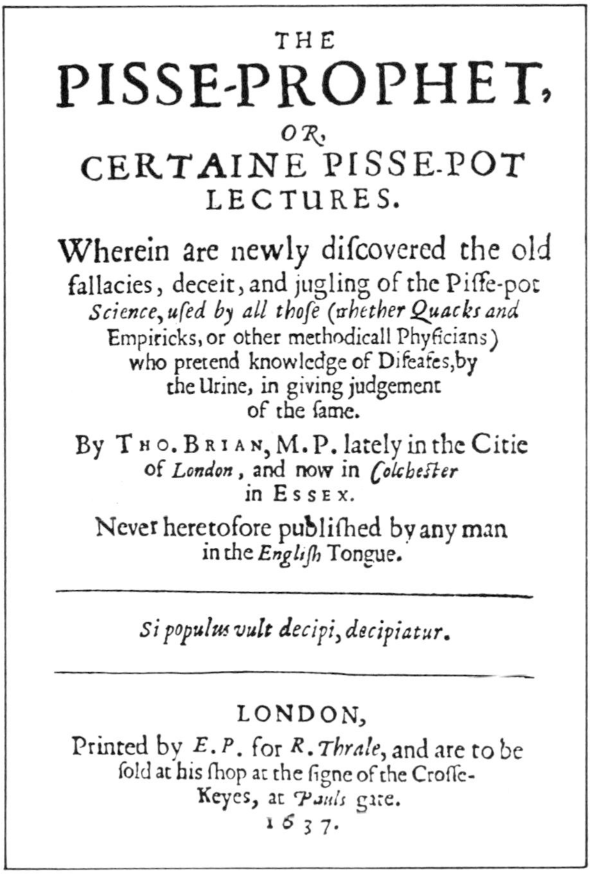

THE

PISSE-PROPHET,

OR,

CERTAINE PISSE-POT
LECTURES.

Wherein are newly difcovered the old
fallacies, deceit, and jugling of the Piffe-pot
Science, ufed by all thofe (whether Quacks and
Empiricks, or other methodicall Phyficians)
who pretend knowledge of Difeafes, by
the Urine, in giving judgement
of the fame.

By T ʜ ᴏ. B ʀ ɪ ᴀ ɴ, M. P. lately in the Citie
of *London*, and now in *Colchefter*
in E s s ᴇ x.

Never heretofore publifhed by any man
in the *Englifh* Tongue.

Si populus vult decipi, decipiatur.

LONDON,

Printed by *E. P.* for *R. Thrale*, and are to be
fold at his fhop at the figne of the Croffe-
Keyes, at *Pauls* gate.
1 6 3 7.

Fig. 28-1. Title page of an early-seventeenth-century book exposing the quackery of diagnosis from the urine.

Worthy Master Doctour, my kind love salutes you &c. My wife being neither sicke nor well, goes up and down the house, but is very puling: she hath a very nauseous stomach, loathes meat, and if she eate any thing (which is very little, or of some very strange dish) she is ready to vomit it up againe: she hath now twice missed (which she orderly enjoyed before) the naturall benefit of her monthly evacuation: ever since which time, that shee had them last, she hath been thus ill: and for the same cause, that she hath missed them, she suspects that she may be with child, or else is thus ill for want of them: I have here sent you her Urine, and desire you to vouchsafe to looke upon it, and to resolve us whether she be with child, or what other infirmity she doth labor of, that we may (if shee be not with childe) prevent a worse danger in time: I pray returne your answer in writing; and so with my best wishes for your owne wel-fare, that others may fare the better for you, I bid you fare-well, and rest

Your wel-wishing friend, J. H.

The piss-prophet, gratuitously proffering facetious marital counsel together with his diagnosis, answered:

Reverend Sir, my best respects to your selfe and your wife, do kindly resalute you both: Your wife (you write) is neither sick nor well; you may then shift your hands of her, if you doe not like her, and tell her that you promised only to keepe her in sickness and in health: but however (good Sir) I am sorie, as she is not sicke, that she is not well, but not so much as otherwise I should be, because your kindnesse hath caused this neutrality of being neither sicke nor well. Her nauseous-nesse of stomach, loathing of meat, and vomitting after, it will shortly cease, and the disease (which now troubles her stomach) will some seven moneths hence, be gotten into her armes. In the meane time it were not amisse for her to take something to corroborate her stomach, which she may very safely doe. I have viewed her water, and can say no more than I have done, unlesse to speak more plainely. I say . . . she is with child, and that almost a quarter gone, God send her a happy deliverance, when the time shall come, and (till then, and ever) health, and so prayes,

Your assured loving friend, H. P.

A growing body of insurgents soon joined ranks with Brian in his attack on "uroscopy," the euphemism for urinary examination practiced in Eliza-bethan times. Thomas Willis,[16] for example, wrote in 1684:

For as much as we cannot search into the most intimate parts of the sick Body, as it were a Vessel shut up, judgment is sought from the infused liquor, washing all its parts and taking from many some little parcels. For neither more certainly do the acidulous or spaw-waters, shew the nature of the hidden Mine, through which they are strained, than Urines give testifications of the divers manners of dyscrasies of our Bodies, and their habitudes. Wherefore the Con-templation of this Excrement, (as vile as it is) hath grown to a Science, and hath exercised the ingenuities of the most excellent Physicians, both Ancient and Mod-ern. . . . The Common People are egregiously deceived, and still pertinaceously will be deceived, whilst they imagine the knowledge of every Disease, and the prog-nostication of it cannot be found out, but by inspecting the Urine; and esteem a Physician of little worth unless he undertakes to divine from the Urinal as from a Magical Glass. But indeed, as to what belongs to the Precepts, and Rules whereon the reason of Judgment by Urine doth depend, there are many collected by diligent observation, that are extant, and from thence establish'd with good Reason and Judgment: yet for as much as the signification of Urines is by some too largely extended to particular Cases, very many uncertain things interwoven, and some obnoxious to deceit, and others plainly false; therefore who shall con-fidently pronounce concerning the business of the Sick, by the judgment only of the Water, deserves rather the name of a jugling Quack, than of a Physician.

During the eighteenth and nineteenth centuries urinary diagnosis of preg-nancy lay in disrepute, except for brief periods when newly described preg-

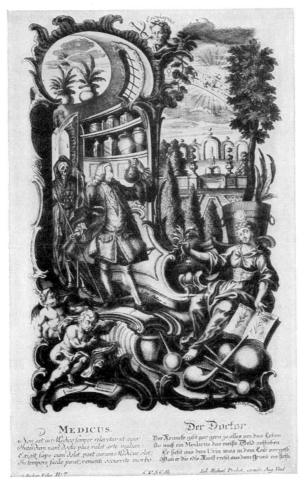

Fig. 28-2. Urinary diagnosis as conceived by artist in seventeenth-century Augsburg. (Author's collection.)

nancy tests gained attention. On July 7, 1831, for example, Jacques Louis Nauche [12] created quite a stir with his report on the Kyesteine pellicle before the Societé de Médecine Pratique of Paris. The word Kyesteine (pronounced kē-ês′ tē-ĭn) is derived from a Greek word meaning conception.[11] "By allowing the urine of pregnant or lactating women to stand for some time," Nauche claimed, "in 30 or 40 hours a deposit takes place of white, flaky, pulverulent grumous matter, *being the caseum or peculiar principle of milk formed in the breasts during gestation*. The precipitation is more readily procured by adding a few drops of alcohol to the urine."

Similar observations were soon reported by Tanchou [14] in support of Nauche's discovery. Added Tanchou:

From the second to the sixth day one sees little opaque bodies rise to the surface of the liquid, and they gradually collect to form a layer covering the whole surface. This is the *Kyesteine.* This layer is rather firm, so that a large part of it can be lifted up at its edge if care is taken. It is whitish, opaque, granular, and can only be compared to the greasy layer that floats to the top of cooled fatty soup. . . . The Kyesteine appears to exist in the woman's urine from the first month to term.

This test was immediately hailed by *The Lancet* as "a new and highly valuable mode of detecting pregnancy," but the literature contains a surprising dearth of subsequent references to it. In an effort to evaluate the Kyesteine test I have observed the formation of this urinary pellicle but have failed to demonstrate either its constancy or its specificity for pregnancy.

THE ASCHHEIM-ZONDEK TEST

In contrast to the poorly controlled or frankly fraudulent methods of urinary diagnosis of pregnancy that preceded, Aschheim and Zondek [3,4,5,6] in 1928 announced a sensitive and specific test based on the presence of gonadotrophic hormone in the urine of pregnant women. This epochal discovery won immediate and universal acclaim, and although their original procedure has since undergone countless modifications, urinary tests for pregnancy, irrespective of technique, are still commonly designated generically as "A–Z tests."

These pioneer gynecologic endocrinologists described the original procedure as follows:

The tests are carried out on infantile mice, three to four weeks old and weighing 6–8 gm. . . . Five infantile mice are used for each urine examination. The urine must be tested on several mice because an animal may die from the injection, but more important, because not all animals react alike. . . . *The pregnancy reaction* [hemorrhagic ovarian follicles or corpora lutea] *is positive if it is positive in only one animal and negative in the others.* . . .

Our test is carried out with morning urine, the first morning specimen. This urine has the optimal concentration. . . . It must be collected in a clean bottle. If the urine is to be sent away, or if it cannot be tested immediately, a preservative must be added. . . . Before the test is begun the reaction of the urine must be determined. If it is alkaline or neutral, acetic acid is added until it is weakly acid (to litmus). The resulting precipitate is filtered off, and the clear filtered urine always used. . . . The urine is injected in 6 parts, divided over 48 hours. . . .

The urine is injected subcutaneously into the infantile animals in the following amounts:

Animal 1: 6 times 0.2 cc
Animal 2: 6 times 0.25 cc
Animal 3: 6 times 0.3 cc
Animal 4: 6 times 0.35 cc
Animal 5: 6 times 0.4 cc

Only the ovarian findings are of significance for the pregnancy reaction. . . . The infantile animals are all killed together on Friday forenoon if the test began on Monday. . . . They are killed with illuminating gas. . . . In the great majority of cases the diagnosis is made by macroscopic examination of the ovaries. If one is not certain, if one does not recognize the blood spot or the corpus luteum definitely, then the ovaries must be sectioned serially. They must be fixed in Zenker's solution. Formalin fixation is unsatisfactory because the resulting shrinkage of the cells can produce pictures leading to erroneous conclusions.

The first report by Aschheim and Zondek was based on their urinary examination of 315 pregnant, nonpregnant, and sick women. They stated:

We have examined 78 cases of pregnancy. In 76 cases the reaction was definitely positive, in one case it came out positive only in retesting, and in one case the reaction was equivocal. It should be noted that we could tell whether or not a pregnancy existed five days after the missed menses. . . .

Among the 236 controls there were—aside from the 16 endocrinopathies and the 22 cancer cases [a number of which gave false positive reactions]—the various phases of the menstrual cycle, benign tumors (myomas, cysts), and inflammatory conditions. In addition there were normals who were definitely not pregnant. In these 198 control cases the reaction was positive twice. . . . The reaction thus has a precision that one cannot hope to surpass with a biologic method.

Twenty tests on puerperal urine showed that the reaction was usually negative after eight days postpartum, occasionally after five. The authors added:

In pathologic pregnancy . . . one case was positive in which the fetus had been dead for three days. One case was negative eight days and another three weeks after fetal death, corresponding to the reactions with puerperal urine. Two cases of hydatidiform mole were positive. In one of them 0.1 cc of urine gave a positive reaction. . . . In the second case 0.05 cc of urine sufficed. Of the urines tested after abortion two were positive on the fifth day, one was still positive on the eighth day; in the other cases the reaction was negative after six days. . . .

We are often asked: Is a tubal pregnancy present? That is not the proper question. What one means, of course, is: Is the pregnancy alive or dead? This question is hard to answer. The reactions will be similar to those in abortions. In general one will be able to assume, when the reaction is negative in a clinically diagnosed tubal pregnancy, that the pregnancy is no longer intact and no biologic contact exists between the ovum and the hypophysis.

Aschheim and Zondek made the understandable error, later rectified, of attributing the pregnancy reaction to anterior pituitary hormone rather than chorionic gonadotrophin. "We cannot demonstrate," they wrote, "any specific substance for pregnancy, for the anterior pituitary hormone is formed in every organism. The only thing characteristic of pregnancy is the tremendous increase in the anterior pituitary hormone and its heavy excretion in the urine." Although demonstrating the high concentration of gonadotrophin in placental tissue, they failed to recognize the hormone's placental origin. They reported:

We have discovered . . . that the placenta contains large quantities of hormone. A positive reaction is obtained from the implantation of about 0.1 gm of fresh human placenta, especially from the early months, so the placenta must contain several thousand units. We could show further that pregnancy is characterized by a colossal flooding of the entire organism with anterior pituitary hormone, the anterior lobe reaction being produced by the injection of 0.5–1.0 cc of pregnancy serum. The demonstration seems especially important, however, that in pregnancy, indeed immediately after conception, the anterior pituitary produces the hormone explosively and the excess concentration is excreted into the urine. This excretion is so characteristic that we have based our biologic test for pregnancy on the demonstration of the anterior pituitary hormone in 1–2 cc of urine.

ASCHHEIM'S LIFE

Selmar Aschheim was born October 4, 1878, in Berlin, Germany.[8] After completing his studies in the universities of Berlin, Freiburg, Munich, and Hamburg, he entered the practice of obstetrics and gynecology. At the same time he worked in the gynecologic pathology laboratory of the Charité Hospital under Robert Meyer. In 1912 Aschheim was appointed director of the laboratory, and in 1931 he was elevated to the rank of professor in the University of Berlin. During these years he conducted various investigations on the physiology of reproduction, and demonstrated the cyclic fluctuations in the glycogen and lipid content of the human endometrium. Most noteworthy, however, were his studies with Zondek on the pituitary-ovarian relations in the mouse, which led to the development of their pregnancy test. With the advent of Hitler, Aschheim was forced to leave the University of Berlin in 1936. He found ready asylum and ultimate citizenship in France, was soon made director of research at the National Center of Scientific Research, and later became director of the laboratory of the Maternité in Paris. A bibliography of his writings is appended to his published remarks [1] on the occasion of his seventy-fifth birthday, celebrated by his colleagues in Paris in 1954.

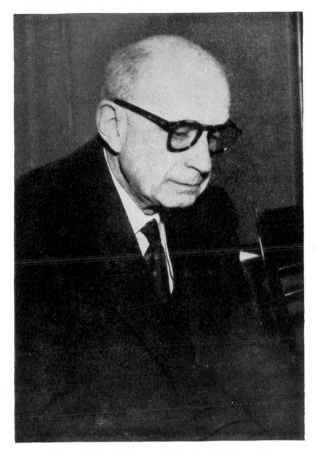

Fig. 28-3. Selmar Aschheim (1878–).

ZONDEK'S LIFE

Bernhard Zondek was born July 29, 1891, in Wronke, Germany. He attended medical school at the University of Berlin and in 1919 was made assistant in obstetrics and gynecology in the Charité, where he was ultimately promoted to associate professor in 1926. Three years later he was appointed director of the Department of Obstetrics and Gynecology in the Berlin-Spandau Hospital, but was forced to leave Germany in 1933 because of Nazi persecution. The following year he was made professor of obstetrics and gynecology in the Hebrew University–Hadassah Medical School in Jerusalem and director of its Hormone Research Laboratory. His books include *Die Hormone des Ovariums und des Hypophysenvorderlappens* (1931 and 1935), *Clinical and Experimental Investigations on the Genital Functions and their Hormonal Regulation* (1941), and *The Antigonadotropic Factor* (1942). Zondek's principal scientific achievements are outlined in a special issue of

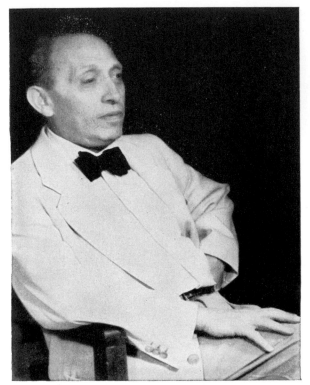

Prisma, Jerusalem

Fig. 28-4. Bernhard Zondek (1891–   ).

Acta Endocrinologica [15] dedicated to him in celebration of his sixtieth birthday in 1951.

THE FRIEDMAN TEST

The rabbit normally ovulates only under the stimulation of coitus. M. H. Friedman was studying the mechanism of ovulation in this species when his attention was arrested by the newly reported discovery of Aschheim and Zondek [2] that the urine of pregnant women contains a gonadotrophic substance simulating the secretion of the anterior pituitary in its effect on the mouse ovary. Applying this observation to the rabbit, Friedman proceeded to develop the pregnancy test known by his name, popularly as the "rabbit test." He wrote in his preliminary report: [9]

In a series of female rabbits in which a previous laparotomy had shown the presence of normal follicles and the absence of corpora lutea, the intraperitoneal injection of 12 cc. of urine from a pregnant woman, twice daily for 4 days, resulted in the appearance of fresh corpora lutea in the ovaries of each of the 7 rabbits so treated. Similar treatment of 9 rabbits with the urine of non-pregnant women was without effect. . . . The clear differentiation between the effects of urine of pregnant women, and the urine of non-pregnant women, and the ease with which these effects can be seen by purely gross examination, justifies further study on a statistical basis to determine whether or not this procedure will be of clinical use in the diagnosis of pregnancy.

Illness interrupted Friedman's research temporarily, but by 1931 he had acquired sufficient experience with the rabbit test, in collaboration with Maxwell E. Lapham,[10] to justify its recommendation as "a simple, rapid procedure for the laboratory diagnosis of early pregnancies." It soon became the most widely used pregnancy test in the United States. As originally outlined by the authors:

The materials and equipment necessary for the performance of the proposed test are: (1) an ordinary bedpan specimen of urine, (2) a five c.c. syringe, and (3) an unmated mature female rabbit. The urine is injected intravenously thrice daily for two days in 4 c.c. doses. Forty-eight hours after the first injection the rabbit is killed. If the ovaries contain either fresh corpora lutea or large bulging corpora hemorrhagica, the reaction is positive and the patient who furnished the sample is presumably pregnant. If the ovaries contain neither corpora lutea nor corpora hemorrhagica, but only clear, unruptured follicles, regardless of their size, the reaction is negative.

The Friedman test was further simplified by later experimenters, who reduced the test dose to a single intravenous injection of 10 cc of morning urine and the waiting period to 24 hours. Moreover, experience revealed the feasibility of using the same rabbit for repeated tests, with suitable intervening rest periods to allow for ovarian regression after a positive reaction. The Friedman test remains unsurpassed as a sensitive and reliable method for diagnosing pregnancy and tumors containing chorionic elements.

FRIEDMAN'S LIFE

Maurice Harold Friedman was born October 27, 1903, in East Chicago, Indiana. All of his higher education was obtained at the University of Chicago, where he received his B.S. in 1924, his Ph.D. (after working in physiology under A. J. Carlson) in 1928, and his M.D. in 1932. After an internship at the Michael Reese Hospital in Chicago he served until 1938 on the faculty of the University of Pennsylvania Medical School, first as an instructor and later as assistant professor of physiology. During this period he demonstrated the direct action of gonadotrophin on the ovary by injecting pregnancy urine extracts into ovarian follicles, with the resultant formation of functional

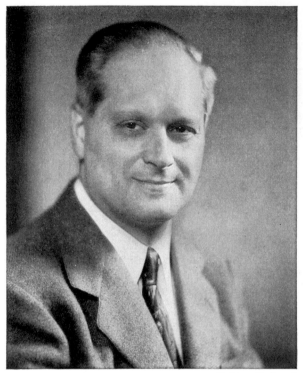

Fabian Bachrach

Fig. 28-5. Maurice Harold Friedman (1903–).

corpora lutea. He also extracted a substance with gonadotrophic activity from the leaves of immature alfalfa and oats. He subsequently joined the research staff of the U.S. Department of Agriculture's Experimental Station at Beltsville, Maryland, but with the outbreak of World War II he transferred his activities to the National Research Council, studying the physiologic effects of acceleration and the circulatory changes during dive bombing. From 1942 to 1946 he carried out various clinical assignments with the U.S. Army Air Forces. After the war Friedman entered the private practice of internal medicine in Washington, D.C., where he holds an appointment as assistant professor of medicine in Georgetown University and serves as attending physician to several of Washington's hospitals, as well as a member of the Board of Trustees of the National Symphony Orchestra.

REFERENCES

1. Aschheim, S.: Réponse de M. le Pr. S. Aschheim. *Ann. d'endocrinol.*, **15**:247–52, 1954.
2. Aschheim, S., and Zondek, B.: Hypophysenvorderlappenhormon und Ovarialhormon im Harn von Schwangeren. *Klin. Wchnschr.*, **6**:1322, 1927.

3. Aschheim, S., and Zondek, B.: Schwangerschaftsdiagnose aus dem Harn (Durch Hormonnachweis). *Klin. Wchnschr.*, **7**:8–9, 1928.

4. Aschheim, S., and Zondek, B.: Das Hormon des Hypophysenvorderlappens. Darstellung, chemische Eigenschaften, biologische Wirkungen. *Klin. Wchnschr.*, **7**:831–35, 1928.

5. Aschheim, S., and Zondek, B.: Die Schwangerschaftsdiagnose aus dem Harn durch Nachweis des Hypophysenvorderlappenhormons. I. Grundlagen und Technik der Methode (B. Zondek). *Klin. Wchnschr.*, **7**:1404–11, 1928.

6. Aschheim, S., and Zondek, B.: Die Schwangerschaftsdiagnose aus dem Harn durch Nachweis des Hypophysenvorderlappenhormons (S. Aschheim). II. Praktische und theoretische Ergebnisse aus den Harnuntersuchungen. *Klin. Wchnschr.*, **7**:1453–57, 1928.

7. Brian, T.: *The Pisse-Prophet, or Certaine Pisse-Pot Lectures.* R. Thrale, London, 1637.

8. Courrier, R.: Allocution de M. Robert Courrier, Secrétaire perpétuel de l'Académie des Sciences. *Ann. d'endocrinol.*, **15**:243–46, 1954.

9. Friedman, M. H.: Effect of injections of urine from pregnant women on ovary of the rabbit. *Proc. Soc. Exper. Biol. & Med.*, **26**:720–21, 1929.

10. Friedman, M. H., and Lapham, M. E.: A simple, rapid procedure for the laboratory diagnosis of early pregnancies. *Am. J. Obst. & Gynec.*, **21**:405–10, 1931.

11. Marshall, M.: The Kyesteine pellicle. An early biological test for pregnancy. *Bull. Hist. Med.*, **22**:178–95, 1948.

12. Nauche, J. L.: [Translated from *Lancette franc.*] *Lancet*, **2**:675–76, 1830–1831.

13. Schullian, D. M.: Piss-pot science. *J. Hist. Med.*, **10**:121–23, 1955.

14. Tanchou: Recherches sur la Kiesteine, substance signalée par M. Nauche dans l'urine des femmes enceintes. *Lancette franc.*, **12**:89–91, 1839.

15. Westman, A.: Professor Bernhard Zondek on the occasion of his sixtieth birthday. *Acta endocrinol.*, **7**:1–5, 1951.

16. Willis, T.: *Practice of Physick.* London, 1684.

Gerhard Leopold and   CHAPTER
the Leopold Maneuvers   29

The obstetric examination consists of two essential parts, the external and the internal, each of which provides information unobtainable by the other. Cognizant of the hazards of indiscriminate vaginal examination of the parturient, most obstetricians, in the routine conduct of labor, perform their pelvic palpations per rectum instead, resorting to the vaginal approach only on specific indication. Refinement of the abdominal examination, a belated development in the history of obstetrics, was likewise stimulated by the dread of puerperal infection and by the newly acquired understanding of its pathogenesis in the latter part of the nineteenth century. Until then the obstetric examination was predominantly vaginal.

A brief plea for external palpation was made as early as 1818 by Schmitt,[11] who wrote: "The abdominal examination is of the greatest importance for diagnosis and therefore should never be omitted in the examination of pregnant patients; indeed it is often far more revealing and decisive than the internal examination, and only rarely does it disappoint the examiner who relies upon it." Nevertheless, midwives and medical practitioners alike continued to employ vaginal examinations almost exclusively in their observation and management of labor.

A significant contribution to the art of abdominal palpation and manipulation was Pinard's monograph of 1878,[10] which dealt with external version and a technique for evaluating the cephalopelvic relation, and devoted 50 pages of text and illustrations to methods of determining the intrauterine

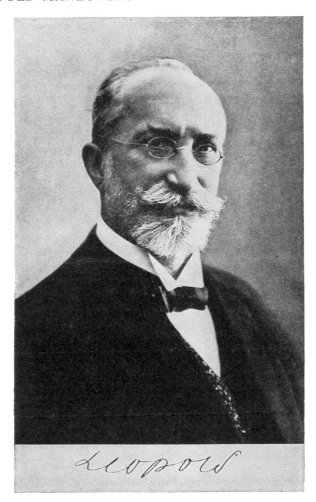

Fig. 29-1. Christian Gerhard Leopold (1846–1912). (Reproduced from *Arch. f. Gynäk.*, **95**:I, 1912.)

orientation of the fetus. Pinard's approach concentrated on suprapubic palpation of the maternal abdomen, to reveal the degree of engagement of the presenting fetal part and the side of the cephalic prominence.

About a decade after Pinard's publication an intensive educational crusade was launched by Gerhard Leopold and his colleagues, including his distinguished father-in-law, Credé, urging abdominal palpation as a substitute for the internal examinations routinely practiced by midwives and physicians on their parturient patients. Leopold apparently recognized the hazards of vaginal examination and developed his technique of abdominal palpation sometime between 1886 and 1890; for the fourth edition of his *Lehrbuch der Hebammenkunst* (Credé and Leopold),[3] published in the former year, contains only a brief chapter on the obstetric examination, with but scant attention to external palpation and no mention at all of the four palpatory maneuvers with which his name is now associated. Credé, however, had already begun to point out the risks of intravaginal examination in labor, in his *Gesunde und Kranke Wöchnerinnen*,[2] published the same year.

THE LEOPOLD MANEUVERS

In 1890 a paper by Leopold and Pantzer [7] appeared, stressing the limitations of the internal examination as well as its dangers as a causative factor in puerperal infection, and deprecating in the strongest terms the intravaginal manipulations commonly employed by midwives to expedite labor. In this paper the maneuvers of Leopold were outlined briefly and their significance emphasized as a means of reducing the number of internal examinations in labor. The description of the external examination, presented in greater detail in the fifth edition of the Credé-Leopold textbook published two years later, found such favor that it was reprinted in separate form [4] at the instigation of the Royal Saxon Minister of the Interior, for the guidance of medical students, midwives, and physicians. Edgar soon published an English translation, from which the following excerpts are taken:

During the examination it is proper to cover the face of the person loosely with some light clean linen, about one yard square. This is to be done especially when idle students stand about as spectators. . . .

The examiner warms both hands and places them flat, gently but firmly on the abdomen in order to determine clearly its distention and circumference; the size, shape, firmness, and mobility of the uterus; and the quantity of the liquor amnii.

After that, partly by a gentle to-and-fro pressure of both hands, partly by a careful tapping, the individual parts of the fetus, their size, attitude, presentation and position, movements and mobility, are sought to be ascertained. In order to perform this external examination accurately and thoroughly, the following well-tested four manipulations should be made use of, and in the following order. . . .

First Manipulation.—The hands approach each other at the finger tips, then the palms of the hands are laid across the abdomen of the woman. After that the palms slide gently and uniformly upward over the entire pregnant uterus as far as the fundus, thus defining its position in relation to the navel and ensiform cartilage. This manipulation determines at the same time whether the child lies vertical or transverse, whether the head or breech lies in the fundus, the size of the child, and how far pregnancy has advanced.

Second Manipulation.—Both extended hands move from the ensiform cartilage to the sides of the abdomen and are laid flat one on each side of the uterus. One hand will feel the small parts, the other the long, large cylinder which corresponds to the child's back. In this manipulation the finding of the child's back is facili-

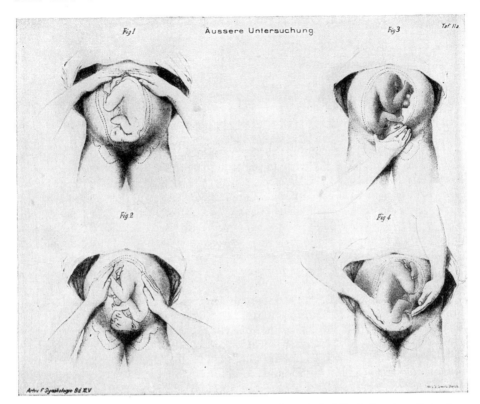

Fig. 29-2. Illustrations from paper of Leopold and Spörlin,[8] showing their four maneuvers in abdominal palpation. (Reproduced by permission of *Archiv für Gynä-kologie.*)

tated by placing one hand flat on the median line of the abdomen and pressing the uterus gently backward. Thereby the liquor amnii is pressed toward one side, and the child's back toward the other, nearer to the abdominal walls, [where it] can thus be felt very easily with the other hand.

Third Manipulation.—The right or left hand spreads its fingers as wide apart as possible, and with the thumb and tip of the middle finger seizes the presenting part of the child just above the pelvic inlet. In order to be able to properly seize the head already engaged in the pelvic inlet in primiparae, it should be sought in the direction of the pelvic cavity with the tips of the thumb and middle finger. In multiparae the hand and finger tips are held more horizontally in order to seize the head which now stands higher in the uterus. For facilitating this manipulation in multiparae especially, the other hand, lying upon the fundus of the uterus, presses against the presenting part of the child. If the presenting part is hard and round, it can only be the head which feels like a hard ball and may be moved hither and thither. The breech appears much softer and more uneven.

If the presenting head or breech is felt uncommonly covered, indistinct, and somewhat softer than usual, the suspicion is justified that the placenta lies in the lower uterine segment. If no presenting part can be detected, the head should be sought in the side of the uterus. This effort will usually succeed if the uterus is gently palpated with short strokes of the fingers of one hand. The head will then make short jerking movements.

The third manipulation is of great value in all cases where the presenting part, head or breech, remains either in or above the pelvic inlet. If, however—as often occurs in primiparae during the last few weeks of pregnancy or in the course of labor—the presenting part is found already in the cavity or outlet of the pelvis, then the

Fourth Manipulation is of importance. In this it is best for the examiner to stand *at the side of the bed,* his back turned toward the face of the parturient. The finger tips of both hands now enter slowly and gently from above along the sides of the pelvis into its cavity. Should the tension of the abdominal walls render this manipulation difficult, it may be greatly facilitated by causing the parturient to draw her thighs somewhat upward, to place her heels together, and to separate her knees. When the head is low, one feels distinctly that a hard, round part of the child fully occupies the pelvis, and the more prominent fore-head on one side can be readily distinguished from the less prominent nape of the neck on the opposite side. . . .

The external examination, always best undertaken in the intervals between the contractions, must naturally often be repeated during the course of labor. For it informs us whether the descent of the presenting part into the pelvis corresponds with the strength and frequency of the pains; it demonstrates any excessive distention of the bladder, and calls attention to dangerous conditions, such as constriction of the uterus, gradually ascending upon its body, after long, violent uterine action; or the painful, excessive tension of the round ligaments which can be felt as thick, sensitive cords on both sides of the bladder, even in the interval between the pains. . . .

During the stages of expulsion, the descent of the head through the pelvis should be followed by means of the fourth manipulation of the external examination, the foetal heart-sounds should be carefully listened to, and the bulging of the pudenda and perinaeum noted; but any unnecessary internal examinations should be avoided.

Credé died shortly before the text on the obstetric examination was completed, but Leopold's evangelistic fervor persisted. From the lecture platform as well as in his writings [6,8] he continued to inveigh against the hazards of internal examination and to preach the virtues of his four manipulations, universally known ever since as Leopold's maneuvers.

LEOPOLD'S LIFE

Christian Gerhard Leopold was born February 24, 1846, in Meerane, Saxony, the only son of the local physician.[1,9] His preliminary studies took him first to Dresden, then Meissen, before he entered the University of Leipzig in 1865. After receiving his medical degree five years later Leopold volunteered for a period of military service with the German Army in the Franco-Prussian War (1870–1871). He then embarked on a long study tour, which encompassed Breslau, Vienna, London, and Edinburgh, and brought him into contact with many of the outstanding obstetricians and surgeons of the day, including Spiegelberg, Billroth, Carl Braun, and Spencer Wells. In 1873 Leopold was made assistant to Credé, whose daughter he later married, and in 1877 he was appointed instructor of midwives in the Leipzig Frauenklinik. In 1883 he succeeded Winckel as chief of the Dresden Lying-in Institute, which he reorganized and built up into one of the leading centers for obstetric training in Europe, and where he carried out a number of important anatomic and physiologic studies on the problems of reproduction. His scientific writings led to more than 120 publications, almost all of which appeared in the *Archiv für Gynäkologie,* which he edited after Credé's death in 1892. Leopold was the first in Germany to perform ovariectomy vaginally, and in 1882 he did the first classical cesarean section in that country with survival of both mother and child. He demonstrated external migration of the ovum in the rabbit by obtaining intrauterine pregnancies in does mated following the removal of one ovary and the contralateral tube.[5] In 1903 Leopold founded the Royal Clinic for Women in Dresden, where his reputation as a lecturer attracted over 1800 physicians from all parts of the world. The title of Privy Councillor was bestowed upon him by the King of Saxony. Leopold died of a heart attack while vacationing in Bärenburg, September 12, 1912.

REFERENCES

1. Bumm, E.: Gerhard Leopold. *Arch. f. Gynäk.,* **95**:I–IV, 1912.

2. Credé, C. S. F.: *Gesunde und Kranke Wöchnerinnen.* A. Felix, Leipzig, 1886.

3. Credé, C. S. F., and Leopold, G.: *Lehrbuch der Hebammenkunst,* 4th ed. Hirzel, Leipzig, 1886, pp. 54–60.

4. Credé, C., and Leopold, G.: *Die geburtshülfliche Untersuchung.* Hirzel, Leipzig, 1892. Published in English by Edgar, J. C.: The obstetric examination. A short guide for physicians, students of medicine, midwives and students in midwifery. . . . *New York J. Gyn. & Obst.,* **2**:1129–44, 1892.

5. Leopold, G.: Die Überwanderung der Eier. *Arch. f. Gynäk.,* **16**:24–44, 1880.

6. Leopold, G.: Exploratio externa. *Compt. rend. XII Cong. Int. Méd. Moscow Aug. 7 (19) – 14 (26) 1897.* Section XIII (Obst. & Gynec.). Moscow, 1898, pp. 110–13.

7. Leopold, G., and Pantzer, M. E. C.: Die Beschränkung der inneren und die grösstmögliche Verwerthung der äusseren Untersuchung in der Geburtshülfe. Vierter Beitrag zur Verhütung des Kindbettfiebers mit einem Rückblicke auf das Jahr 1889. *Arch. f. Gynäk.,* **38**:330–66, 1890.

8. Leopold, G., and Spörlin: Die Leitung der regelmässigen Geburten nur durch äussere Untersuchung. *Arch. f. Gynäk.,* **45**:337–68, 1894.

9. Obituary: Gerhard Leopold, M.D. *Boston M. & S. J.,* **165**:777–78, 1912.

10. Pinard, A.: *Traité du Palper Abdominal au point de vue obstétrical et de la Version par Manoevres externes.* H. Lauwereyns, Paris, 1878, pp. 110–59.

11. Schmitt, W. J.: *Sammlung zweifelhafter Schwangerschaftsfälle nebst einer kritischen Einleitung über die Methode des Untersuchens zum Gebrauche für angehende Geburtshelfer.* F. Wimmer, Vienna, 1818, p. 12.

Otto Spiegelberg and His Criteria of Ovarian Pregnancy

Union of egg and sperm normally occurs in the distal third of the fallopian tube, the wedded zygotes continuing their journey to the uterine cavity before implanting and establishing a nesting place for the dividing ovum. Nidation elsewhere than the endometrium is potentially hazardous to the mother and usually fatal to the conceptus. One of the least common domiciles for the fertilized ovum is the ovary itself.

Most ovarian pregnancies probably follow in the wake of a pre-existing tubal nidation and result from the secondary attachment of the trophoblast to the surface of the gonad after the extrusion of the conceptus from its primary implantation site within the fallopian tube. More rarely the fertilized ovum takes root initially in the substance of the ovary, the stigma in the ruptured follicle presumably having admitted the ambient sperm without permitting egress of the larger egg. Gynecologists have long maintained a proper skepticism toward primary ovarian pregnancy; authentic cases are exceedingly scarce.

Published expression was given to this skepticism in 1877 by Cohnstein,[1] who listed four requirements that had to be satisfied before an alleged case of ovarian pregnancy could be accepted as genuine. Cohnstein's criteria were: (1) absence of a separate ovary on the corresponding side; (2) connection of the gestation sac with the uterus by means of the elongated and thickened ovarian ligament, with enclosure of the sac between both leaves of the broad ligament; (3) nonstratified structure of the sac's capsule, cylindrical epithelium

255

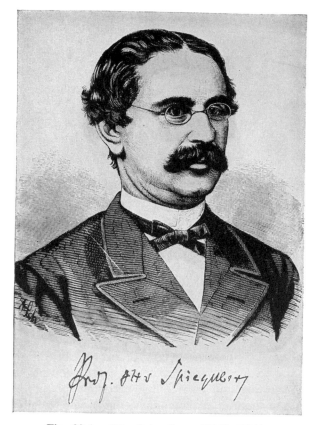

Fig. 30-1. Otto Spiegelberg (1830–1881).

lining its inner surface, and a direct connection of its wall with the fibers of the tunica albuginea; and (4) distinct ovarian tissue in the immediate vicinity of the ovum.

SPIEGELBERG'S CRITERIA

The problem was considered anew the very next year by Otto Spiegelberg,[5] who took issue with some of Cohnstein's criteria, added one of his own, and formulated a revised codification, widely accepted and persisting to this day as the criteria of an ovarian pregnancy, Spiegelberg's criteria. Referring to Cohnstein's requirements, Spiegelberg wrote:

Not all of these findings are necessary; indeed, some are not even likely to be present. An ovary that contains a pregnancy is topographically an ovarian tumor, like a cystoma; and surely no one would maintain that such a tumor need be enclosed between both leaves of the broad ligament. Cylindrical epithelium initially present on the inner surface of the gestation sac would probably disappear with the latter's further growth and with the development of the placenta. A nonstratified structure of the capsule would probably depend on chance factors, for it does not necessarily result from the structure of the ovarian stroma and can be present in the most diverse forms of extrauterine pregnancy. And finally, a connection between the fibrous fasciculi of the albuginea and the wall of the gestation sac can be considered only if another part of the ovary and its associated albuginea are intact and can be demonstrated in continuity.

There thus remain only the following conditions necessary for the assumption of the ovarian character of a gestation sac: (1) the absence of a separate ovary on the same side; (2) ovarian elements in the wall of the sac, indicating the use of the former structure in the formation of the latter; (3) connection of the sac with the uterus by the ovarian ligament; and finally, a requirement not mentioned by Cohnstein, (4) noninclusion of the fallopian tube in the formation of the gestation sac, presenting a topographic relation on the affected side identical or similar to that occurring with large ovarian tumors.

SPIEGELBERG'S LIFE

Otto Spiegelberg was born in Peine, Hannover, Germany, January 9, 1830.[2,3,4,6] He obtained his early education in Hildesheim and Brunswick before entering the study of medicine in the University of Göttingen, where he received his degree in 1851. Under the guidance of von Siebold, his professor, Spiegelberg acquired an early love for obstetrics. Sensing his student's academic potentialities, von Siebold took him along on visits to the lying-in hospitals of Berlin, Vienna, and Prague. Spiegelberg returned to Göttingen inspired by the distinguished professors he had met and eagerly embarked on a teaching career, as lecturer in obstetrics and assistant to von Siebold. In 1855 he made an extensive tour through the British Isles, with prolonged visits at the teaching clinics of London, Edinburgh, and Dublin. This trip had a profound effect on Spiegelberg, who had already acquired an excellent knowledge of the English language, and upon his return to Göttingen he began to use chloroform for obstetric anesthesia and to incorporate many of the British methods into his teaching and practice, which was growing rapidly. In 1860 he was named extraordinary professor in the university, and the following year was called to Freiburg im Breisgau as ordinary professor and director of the gynecology clinic. Here he remained until 1864, when he accepted a similar invitation to Königsberg, but the very next year he moved on to Breslau to become director of the Gebär-und Frauenklinik. In 1878 he declined a call to the University of Strassburg, and as a token of gratitude for his decision to remain in Breslau, was appointed Rector magnificus of the university and given the title of Geheimer Medicinalrath. Prior to 1865 Spiegelberg devoted himself predominantly to obstetrics, but thereafter he turned his attention more and more to operative gynecology, stimulated by the recent exploits of the English and American surgeons in the new operation of ovariotomy. He introduced exploratory puncture of abdominal tumors, and soon achieved renown for his fistula repairs and vaginal plastic operations. In 1870 he was called to military service as director of the army hospital at Forbach and was decorated with the Order of the Iron Cross, but after three months was forced to return to Breslau because of failing health. Trips to the Riviera and Langenau brought no improvement, but he nonetheless resumed his teaching, practice, and writing. He died of nephrosclerosis on August 9, 1881.

Spiegelberg was the first to give an accurate description of parovarian cysts, the first to perform curettage of the uterus for retained secundines, one of the first in Germany to apply antisepsis to obstetrics, and one of the first after T. Spencer Wells to enucleate intramural fibroids. In 1872 he devised his colporrhaphia mediana, the forerunner of the Le Fort operation of partial colpocleisis. He was one of the most prolific authors of the nineteenth century in the field of obstetrics and gynecology. In 1858, when only 28 years old, he published a textbook of obstetrics, *Das Compendium der Geburtshilfe,* which was followed by reports of his investigations on ovarian cysts, the development of the ovarian follicle and the formation of the corpus luteum, cervical changes in pregnancy, the mechanism of labor, contracted pelves, ovariotomy, inversion of the uterus, uterine carcinoma, and a host of other subjects. A selected partial bibliography of his writings is appended to Leopold's obituary of him.[4] With Credé he founded the *Archiv für Gynäkologie* in 1870, and for the rest of his life nearly every volume contained contributions by him. Spiegelberg's greatest literary achievement, his *Lehrbuch der Geburtshilfe,* written under the burden of declining health, was received so warmly following its publication in 1878 that he was induced to issue a new edition of it only two years later, shortly before his death.

REFERENCES

1. Cohnstein: Beitrag zur Schwangerschaft ausserhalb der Gebärmutterhöhle. *Arch. f. Gynäk.,* **12**:355–82, 1877.

2. Dohrn, R.: *Geschichte der Geburtshülfe der Neuzeit.* Part 1 (1840–1860). Pietzcker, Tübingen, 1903, pp. 99–101.

3. Hirschfeld, J.: *Galerie Berühmter Kliniker und Hervorragender Aerzte unsere Zeit.* Moritz Perles, Vienna, 1877.

4. Leopold, G.: Otto Spiegelberg. Nekrolog gesprochen in der Gesellschaft für Geburtshülfe in Leipzig am 17. October 1881. *Arch. f. Gynäk.,* **18**:347–58, 1881.

5. Spiegelberg, O.: Zur Casuistik der Ovarialschwangerschaft. *Arch. f. Gynäk.,* **13**:73–79, 1878.

6. Wiener, M.: Otto Spiegelberg. *Am. J. Obst.,* **15**:445–48, 1882.

Thomas Stephen Cullen and Cullen's Sign

CHAPTER

31

Extrauterine pregnancy is notorious for its protean clinical manifestations. Curiously, its one diagnostic sign that has been dignified with an eponymic designation is among the rarest phenomena associated with this disorder. Most obstetricians and gynecologists fail to encounter it, Cullen's sign, in a lifetime of practice.

That bluish discoloration of the umbilicus could occur in cases of hemoperitoneum might possibly have been predicted before it was actually observed by Cullen in a patient with a ruptured tubal pregnancy. At the 1905 meeting of the Southern Surgical and Gynecological Association, Joseph Ransohoff, a Cincinnati surgeon, read a paper on rupture of the common duct. The ensuing leakage of bile into the peritoneal cavity resulted in umbilical jaundice—the icteric counterpart of the cyanosis of Cullen's sign. The patient was a male, aged 53 years. Ransohoff reported: [4]

On inspection of the abdomen attention was called to a marked jaundice of the umbilicus. The navel was of a distinct saffron-yellow color in strong contrast with the rest of the skin over the abdomen.

At operation large quantities of free bile were found in the peritoneal cavity. Ransohoff continued:

I wish here to call attention to a sign . . . to which I believe attention has never before been directed. It is the localized jaundice of the umbilicus. Although

259

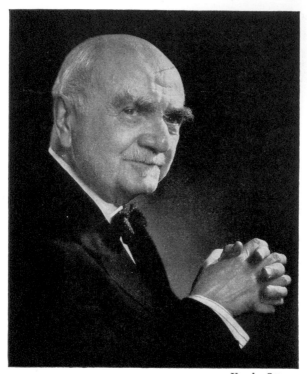

Karsh, Ottawa

Fig. 31-1. Thomas Stephen Cullen (1868–1953).

a single case is not usually sufficient to warrant the assumption that something new has been observed, this feature was so marked that I cannot refrain from believing that further observation will give to this localized jaundice some value as a sign of free bile in the peritoneal cavity. . . . It makes itself manifest first in the integument of the navel, because this part is thinner than the rest of the abdominal wall.

CULLEN'S ACCOUNT OF UMBILICAL DISCOLORATION

While Thomas Cullen was collecting material for his encyclopedic volume, *Embryology, Anatomy, and Diseases of the Umbilicus,*[1] which was published in 1916, he came across Ransohoff's report, and naturally included a reference to it. Any item, once recorded by Cullen, remained indelibly inscribed thereafter in his memory as well. Two years later, therefore, when he encountered a patient in whom ruptured ectopic pregnancy was suspected, bluish discoloration of the umbilicus emboldened him to make the diagnosis, which was confirmed subsequently at laparotomy. Cullen described this case in 1919, in a special collection of papers dedicated to Sir William Osler on the occasion of his seventieth birthday.[2] Reported Cullen:

For three weeks [the patient] had had pain in the right lower abdomen with intermittent attacks of abdominal distention. One week after the onset of the trouble the umbilical region suddenly became bluish black . . . although there had been no injury whatsoever in this region. Pelvic examination was very unsatisfactory on account of the marked abdominal distention.

[At examination under anesthesia on March 27, 1918] with the patient asleep the uterus was found to be slightly enlarged. To the right of the uterus was a freely movable mass about 8 cm. long by 5 cm. broad. I was instantly reminded of a case reported by Dr. Joseph Ransohoff. . . . Bearing Dr. Ransohoff's case in mind I dictated the following note prior to opening the abdomen: "The bluish black appearance of the navel unassociated with any history of injury, together with the mass to the right of the uterus, makes the diagnosis of extrauterine pregnancy relatively certain, although the patient has not missed any period and although there has been no uterine bleeding." On opening the abdomen I found it filled with dark blood, and attached to the fimbriated end of the right tube was an extrauterine pregnancy. . . .

The bluish coloration gradually diminished in intensity during the patient's sojourn in the hospital prior to operation, and disappeared completely within a few days after operation. The gradual change in color that took place in the umbilical region reminded one strikingly of the changes in color that occur in a black eye resulting from a blow.

I record this case in order that subsequent ruptured extrauterine pregnancies may be examined for this sign. Whether it will prove to be of common occurrence or very rare, I cannot say, but we shall naturally expect it only where there is free blood in the abdomen and shall probably be more likely to encounter it in thin individuals. [Cullen's color plate, prepared by Max Brödel, is reproduced in the frontispiece.]

CULLEN'S LIFE

Thomas Stephen Cullen was born November 20, 1868, in Bridgewater, Ontario, Canada, the son of a minister.[3,5] His birthplace, later renamed Actinolite, exists now only as a ghost town. When young Cullen was 13, his family moved to Toronto, where he immediately began to manifest the vigor and determination that were to characterize his whole life, getting up at 3:30 A.M. every weekday to deliver newspapers before school. He entered Jarvis College in 1883 and the University of Toronto medical school three years later, graduating in 1890 with the M.B. degree. Recipient of the silver medal, he stood second in his class only to Lewellys Barker, who became his lifelong friend and whom he followed to Johns Hopkins, where each achieved distinction in his own fields, Barker in anatomy, neurology, and endocrinology, and Cullen in gynecology.

Following graduation from medical school, Cullen interned for a year at the Toronto General Hospital; and it was a fortuitous meeting here with Howard A. Kelly, professor of gynecology at Johns Hopkins, that cast the die for Cullen's future. Kelly, on a fishing vacation in Canada, had stopped off en route for a brief visit in Toronto; and while there was asked to perform an operation. Cullen, who had the good fortune to assist the distinguished gynecologist from Baltimore, was so impressed with the brilliance of the latter's performance that he decided then and there that he must pursue his training under this master surgeon. Cullen succeeded in getting an appointment as intern in the new Johns Hopkins Hospital, which he began after a preliminary period in Welch's pathology laboratory. Soon engulfed by the enthusiasm that permeated this new medical institution, Cullen stayed on, found Baltimore to his liking, and decided to make his future there. In 1893 he was granted a six months' leave of absence, and with a $600 loan from Kelly he took off for Göttingen to visit the laboratory of Johannes Orth. Upon his return to Baltimore, Cullen was put in charge of gynecologic pathology at the hospital; and in 1895 he was appointed instructor in gynecology. It was during this period that he carried out the studies that led to his correct interpretation of adenomyoma of the uterus, the origin of which the great von Recklinghausen had ascribed previously to the Wolffian body. In 1896 Cullen attained the coveted residency in gynecology, and upon its completion entered private practice and was promoted to the position of associate in Kelly's department. Rising through the ranks he eventually succeeded Kelly, becoming the second professor of gynecology at Johns Hopkins. From its inception until his retirement in 1939 Cullen taught every class that graduated from the medical school. I had the honor of being in his last class of students, and still recall his unrestrained delight at our last meeting, when we presented him with an elaborate cake molded realistically into the form of a myomatous uterus flanked by pus tubes and bearing the inscription *"Toujours la même chose,"* his invariable comment on encountering this combination in the operating room.

As chief gynecologist of the Johns Hopkins Hospital, Cullen was the first to establish the requirement of a year's training in pathology before a candidate could qualify for the gynecologic residency. His interest in pathology continued throughout his professional life and is mirrored in most of his publications, especially his books, *Cancer of the Uterus* (1900), *Adenomyomata of the Uterus* (1908), *and Myomata of the Uterus* (published with Kelly in 1909). In these, as in all his writings, Cullen was most meticulous and exacting, as to format and illustrations, as well as content. It is estimated that he spent in excess of $50,000 of his personal funds to achieve the highest possible standards for his publications. Recognizing the genius of Max Brödel, Cullen was primarily responsible for keeping him in Baltimore and establishing the first department of art as applied to medicine.

Like his father, Cullen was an irrepressible evangelist. Once convinced of the merits of a cause, his efforts on its behalf never relented. His perseverance, self-confidence, and talent in dealing with people, coupled with his wide civic as well as professional interests, led him into many new ventures, a host of controversies, and a succession of important positions. Risking the criticism of the medical profession, he stimulated the first public campaign in the United States for the control of cancer, by planning and endorsing a series of articles for the *Ladies' Home Journal* and other popular magazines. He challenged the decision of the Board of Trustees to combine the departments of obstetrics and gynecology at Johns Hopkins, and successfully resisted its efforts in this direction. Despite the board's firm commitment to John Whitridge Williams that his department of obstetrics would be combined with that of gynecology under a single head, the board and Williams were both forced to capitulate to Cullen's skillfully organized opposition. For many years Cullen served on the Board of Trustees of the American Medical Association, and in 1914 was made chairman of its Section on Obstetrics, Gynecology, and Abdominal Surgery. He also served at various times as president of the Baltimore City Medical Society, the Medical and Chirurgical Faculty of Maryland, and the Southern Surgical Association. In 1929 he was made a member of the Maryland State Board of Health and was later appointed chairman of the Chesapeake Bay Authority. Conservation of the bay's dwindling oyster population became a labor of love, for Cullen had developed a fondness for the famed bivalve even before coming to Baltimore. One of his chief nonmedical interests lay in Baltimore's great library chain, the Enoch Pratt Free Library, whose Board of Trustees he served for a time as president. Cullen died on March 4, 1953, at the age of 84. Baltimore has never had a more devoted and loyal adopted son.

REFERENCES

1. Cullen, T. S.: *Embryology, Anatomy, and Diseases of the Umbilicus together with Diseases of the Urachus.* W. B. Saunders Co., Philadelphia, 1916.
2. Cullen, T. S.: Bluish coloration of the umbilicus as a diagnostic sign where ruptured extrauterine pregnancy exists. *Contributions to Medical and Biological Research. Dedicated to Sir William Osler, Bart., M.D., F.R.S. In Honour of his Seventieth Birthday, July 12, 1919. By his Pupils and Co-Workers.* Paul B. Hoeber, Inc., New York, 1919, Vol. 1, pp. 420–21.
3. Deaths. Cullen, Thomas Stephen. *J.A.M.A.,* **151**:1218, 1953.
4. Ransohoff, J.: Gangrene of the gall bladder. Rupture of the common bile duct, with a new sign. *J.A.M.A.,* **45**:393–96, 1906.
5. Robinson, J.: *Tom Cullen of Baltimore.* Oxford University Press, London, 1949.

Alfred Spalding and His Sign of Fetal Death in Utero*

CHAPTER

32

Diagnosis of fetal death in utero is one of the most difficult, as well as unpleasant, tasks that the obstetrician is called upon to perform. Life of the fetus can be established with certainty, but diagnosis of its recent death, based as it usually must be on negative evidence such as the absence of fetal movements and heart sounds, is presumptive. In cases of suspected fetal demise early diagnosis is made, therefore, by evaluation of secondary phenomena, each of which may suggest the true state of affairs but none of which provides crucial evidence. Even the biologic tests for pregnancy, based on the presence of chorionic gonadotrophin in the body fluids, cannot be relied upon, unless negative, because of the varied duration of gonadotrophic activity after fetal death. Wrote Dewees [3] in the early-nineteenth century:

In many instances it would be highly important, could we determine with certainty, that the child was dead while in utero—it would serve to abridge the sufferings of the mother, and sometimes would spare the accoucheur a deep drawn sigh; but this is a matter of great difficulty, as well as oftentimes of great moment to decide. All the commonly enumerated signs have been known to fail, and even when many of the strongest were united.

Evory Kennedy, in his volume [6] on obstetric auscultation, added:

* Parts of this chapter originally published in *Bull. Sloane Hosp. for Women,* **2**:109–14, 1956; reprinted by permission. Copyright © 1956, by The Sloane Hospital.

How frequently have children been destroyed or dragged mutilated into the world, by the practitioner acting upon the supposition that the child was dead, and having recourse to instruments of destruction, when, but for this error in prognosis, the forceps or lever might have been used with safety, and the child's life preserved? On the contrary, how often have practitioners fallen into the opposite error, and had recourse to the forceps or lever, to the imminent risk, nay, in some cases, to the certain destruction of the parent, with a view to preserve the child's life, when it was already dead. Again, in what a much greater proportion of cases than either of the former has the more cautious practise of trusting to the natural efforts, with a view to preserve the lives of both mother and child, been blindly had recourse to, and in this way, the practitioner vainly sat by the bed-side of his patient for hours, or even days, after its death, expecting the birth of a living child, until at length the life of the mother has also in many cases fallen a sacrifice to this unavailing and mischievous delay, when timely interference might have preserved her, and could have been attended with no injury to the innocent cause of her destruction.

Obstetricians and midwives have struggled with this problem from the very earliest times, but with no real progress until the new science and technology of the twentieth century permitted the application of new techniques. Obstetric texts of the seventeenth, eighteenth, and nineteenth centuries bear striking resemblance to Röslin's famous early-sixteenth-century volume, *Der Swangern Frauwen und Hebamen Rosegarten,* in their listing of the signs and symptoms of fetal death. The following passage is taken from the first edition of Thomas Raynold's English translation from the German, published in 1545 as *The Byrth of Mankynde:* [8]

Sygnes then that the byrth is dead in the mothers wombe be these. i. Fyrste yf the mothers breastes do sodenly slake. . . . ii. If it move it self no more beynge wunt before to steare. iii. If when the mother torneth her fro the one syde to the other, she feale it falling fro the one side to the other lyke a stone or a dead wayght. iiii. Yf her belly and navyll begyn to wexe colde, whiche before was wunt to be temperately hote. v. Yf any stynckynge and fylthye humours flowe from the matrice, and chiefly after sume fell disease. vi. Yf the womans eyes were holowe, and that her color change fro whyte to swart and dunne colour, and that her eyes and nose were astoned, and have not theyr ryghte use, and her lyppes were wan. vii. Yf beneth the navyll and about the secreate partes she feale great thronge and payne, the color of her face changynge into wursse and wursse, otherwise then it was wunt to do. viii. Yf she have appetyte to eate such thynges, the whiche be agaynst nature, & not wunt to be eaten or dronken. ix. Yf she be in her slepe vexed with payne and terryble dreames. x. Yf she be payned continually with the strangurye, or yf she enforce her selfe muche to the stole, and with al her power, and yet can not do any thynge. xi. Yf her brethe begyn to stynke, the whiche thynge lyghtly happeneth two or thre dayes after the byrth be dead. xii. Yf her handes put into very warme water, and then layde on the womans belly, & the chyld steare not, is a figure that it is deade.

Of all these sygnes nowe the more that come together of them at one tyme and in one person, the surer maye ye be that the byrthe is deade, the which beyng ones dead, all diligence muste be had that it maye be expelled out of the womans body.

In 1872 Cohnstein [1] proposed a test for distinguishing between the quick and the dead fetus in utero, based on the temperature differential between the cervix and the rest of the maternal body; but this test lacked both reliability and appeal, and never attained any measure of professional acceptance.

Increased mobility of the skull bones had been noted long before as a sign of fetal death; but neither could this be relied upon, as Denman pointed out in his *Introduction to the Practice of Midwifery:* [2]

The original connexion of the bones of the head is such as to allow of their being pressed close to, or over, each other with safety to the child; yet when this has been long dead, and their natural connexion destroyed, they may sometimes be perceived to be loose and distinct. The loose state of the bones of the *cranium* is frequently such as to leave no doubt of the death of the child, as well as the abrasion of the cuticle or the falling off of the hair; but proofs of things self-evident are not wanted in practice, but such as will guide us in doubtful cases.

Roentgenography has made possible the twentieth century's principal contribution to the problem. Widely relied upon in continental Europe as a sign of death of the fetus is the persistence of its position, without change, in repeated roentgenograms (Naujoks' sign). More popular in the United States has been the x-ray appearance of overriding of the cranial bones of the fetus in utero. Although generally known as Spalding's sign, credit for its discovery should be divided with D. A. Horner, for he and Spalding independently came upon this phenomenon at about the same time and, interestingly enough, published their observations in successive issues of the same journal; Spalding in June, 1922,[10] Horner in July, 1922.[5] Each had previously reported his discovery orally before a formal body of his peers, as indicated in footnotes to their papers; Horner to the Chicago Gynecological Society, December 16, 1921, Spalding to the Society of the Alumni of the Sloane Hospital for Women, April 28, 1922. Horner's four months' priority in the reading of his paper was not enough to offset Spalding's advantage of a month in publication. Spalding's name has been perpetuated among the eponyms of obstetrics, while Horner's contribution has long since been forgotten. Such are the vagaries of fame! Wrote Horner:

In my review of the literature I have not come across the utilization of the X-ray in the diagnosis of intra-uterine death. However, during the past year in 3 cases where foetal death was suspected, X-ray revealed overriding of the skull

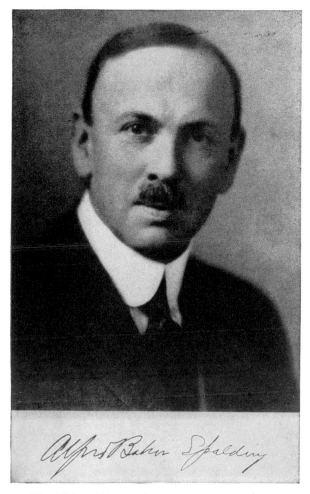

Fig. 32-1. Alfred Baker Spalding (1874–1942).

bones with asymmetry of the head. This to me indicated foetal death and the subsequent clinical course bore out my belief. Therefore, overriding of the skull bones with cephalic asymmetry are signs of foetal death and are the only positive signs of intra-uterine death.*

Horner's observations, it will be noted, were reported along with a discussion of other uses of roentgenography in obstetrics, and attention was attracted principally to his claims for the x-ray in the diagnosis of cephalopelvic disproportion. This may account in part for his failure to receive a proper share of recognition for his codiscovery of the fetal death sign.

* By permission of *Surgery, Gynecology and Obstetrics.*

SPALDING'S DESCRIPTION OF FETAL DEATH SIGN

Spalding's paper, on the other hand, was devoted exclusively to this sign, which he therefore reported in greater detail. Like Horner, Spalding recorded three cases, and also like Horner, he was unaware of the other's observations. Thus wrote Spalding:

In the Women's Clinic of Stanford University we have, during the past few months, made positive diagnoses of intra-uterine death by the aid of X-ray pictures of the foetal skull, and from a review of the literature this seems to be an original observation.

It seems that very shortly after intra-uterine death, the brain tissue shrinks, which produces a typical overlapping of the foetal skull bones. This overlapping of the foetal skull bones seems to be pathognomonic of the condition of the intra-uterine death and gives a picture quite different from the overlapping produced by molding.

With the X-ray, the decreased size of the foetal head from the postmortem shrinking can be determined because the cranial bones remain nearly the same size and shape. As the head shrinks, the bones overlap at times to an astonishing distance. The radius of curvature of the shrunken head becomes obviously smaller than that of the unchanged cranial bones. When both the above changes are noted in the X-ray picture it seems justifiable to conclude that the child is dead and such has been our experience in the X-ray study of 21 babies *in utero*. In this series, 3 babies were dead and presented the typical findings; 18 were alive, of which 17 showed no changes in the X-ray picture of the foetal head and the suture lines. One baby showed marked overlapping of the skull bones due to molding caused by a long first stage of labor, but in spite of this overlapping, the skull bones showed no disproportion in relation to the bulk of the contents of the skull.*

Spalding is also remembered eponymically in conjunction with an operation for uterine prolapse, in which both the cervix and corpus are amputated and the remaining small segment of the uterus is interposed between the bladder and anterior vaginal membrane.[9] Just as Horner's role in the discovery of the sign of fetal death three years later was to be overlooked, Spalding's operation for prolapse attracted little attention following its description in 1919, perhaps because overshadowed by the purely anatomic part of his paper. As a result, Spalding's operation remained almost completely ignored until an identical procedure was devised by E. H. Richardson, a fellow member of the American Gynecological Society who, unaware of Spalding's earlier description, published his operation as an original contribution in 1937.[7] Only then was Spalding's priority recalled. The operation is now known, quite properly, as the Spalding-Richardson operation, to Spalding belonging the credit for its conception, and to Richardson credit for its rediscovery and rescue from oblivion.

* By permission of *Surgery, Gynecology and Obstetrics*.

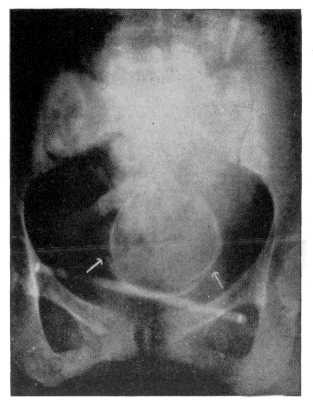

Fig. 32-2. An illustration from Spalding's paper [10] describing his sign of fetal death in utero. (By permission of *Surgery, Gynecology and Obstetrics*.)

SPALDING'S LIFE

Alfred Baker Spalding was born in Atchison, Kansas, July 19, 1874.[4] He entered Stanford University in 1892, a classmate of Herbert Hoover, graduating with his A.B. degree four years later; whereupon he enrolled in the College of Physicians and Surgeons of Columbia University in New York. After receiving his M.D. in 1900, Spalding spent a year as house surgeon in the General Memorial Hospital, now the Memorial Center for the Treatment of Cancer and Allied Diseases, and the following year as assistant resident in the Sloane Maternity Hospital, later known as the Sloane Hospital for Women, and now a unit in the Columbia-Presbyterian Medical Center. Declining an invitation to continue his career at Sloane, he chose instead to return to California as instructor in obstetrics in the University of California. Rising through the academic ranks of that institution, he attained the position of full professor in 1909. During this period he played a key role in the founding of the San Francisco Maternity Hospital, which he served as medical director from 1904. In 1911 Spalding left the University of California for a year of travel and study of gynecologic pathology in Austria and Germany; but it was not until his return to San Francisco that he resigned his post at the University of California to assume the chair of obstetrics at Stanford University, where he accomplished the merger of the San Francisco Maternity Hospital with the School of Medicine and established the residency system of postgraduate training. Spalding has been characterized as a "somber, serious man whom God had failed to bless with a funny bone." During his last years he suffered from a profound depression, which caused him to relinquish his private practice and resign his position in the university in 1934. Living alone in melancholy retirement, he died on November 26, 1942.

REFERENCES

1. Cohnstein: Vom Leben und Tod der Frucht. *Arch. f. Gynäk.,* **4**:547–49, 1872.

2. Denman, T.: *An Introduction to the Practice of Midwifery.* William Fessenden, Brattleboro, Vt., 1807, p. 265.

3. Dewees, W. P.: *A Compendious System of Midwifery, Chiefly Designed to Facilitate the Inquiries of Those Who May be Pursuing This Branch of Study,* 4th ed. Carey & Lea, Philadelphia, 1830, p. 602.

4. Emge, L. A.: Alfred Baker Spalding, 1874–1942. *Tr. Am. Gynec. Soc.,* **68**:287–90, 1945.

5. Horner, D. A.: Roentgenography in obstetrics. *Surg., Gynec. & Obst.,* **35**:67–71, 1922.

6. Kennedy, E.: *Observations on Obstetric Auscultation, with an Analysis of the Evidences of Pregnancy, and an Inquiry into the Proofs of the Life and Death of the Foetus in Utero.* J. & H. G. Langley, New York, 1843, pp. 250–51.

7. Richardson, E. H.: An efficient composite operation for uterine prolapse and associated pathology. *Am. J. Obst. & Gynec.,* **34**:814–27, 1937.

8. Röslin, E.: *The Byrth of Mankynde, Otherwyse Named the Womans Booke. Newly Set Furth, Corrected and Augmented. Whose Contentes Ye Maye Rede in the Table of the Booke, and Most Playnly in the Prologue. By Thomas Raynold, Phisition.* London, 1545.

9. Spalding, A. B.: A study of frozen sections of the pelvis with description of an operation for pelvic prolapse. *Surg., Gynec. & Obst.,* **29**:529–36, 1919.

10. Spalding, A. B.: A pathognomonic sign of intra-uterine death. *Surg., Gynec. & Obst.,* **34**:754–57, 1922.

Max Hühner and the Postcoital Test

CHAPTER

33

Evaluation of the male factor in the investigation of barren matings requires a qualitative appraisal of the semen and a quantitative estimate of its sperm concentration; but until the middle of the nineteenth century the husband's biologic responsibility in procreation was believed to hinge solely on his ability to consummate the act of coitus and deposit his effluvium within the vagina. Virility was synonymous with fertility. This notion was dispelled only after the application of the microscope to the study of sterility. In addition, the effect of the female environment, the vaginal fluid and cervical mucus, on the newly discharged spermatozoa came under scrutiny, and the study of sperm survival within the female genital tract assumed transcendent importance, providing a composite index of the male's ability to deliver a functional ejaculate at the proper site and of the amicability or hostility of the female secretions.

As part of a systematic study of the various body fluids in 1844, Donné[2] included an examination of the vaginal secretions. He called attention to the acidity of the vaginal fluid in contrast to the alkaline reaction of the cervical mucus; and in the microscopic examination of the former in a patient who had been admitted to the hospital the preceding night, he noted the presence of spermatozoa. This was probably the first time that the male cells had been demonstrated in fluid recovered from the vagina.

The survival time of spermatozoa within the female genital tract has been the subject of great interest and investigation since then. In 1861 Percy[7]

271

reported his finding of living sperm cells in the cervical mucus of a patient eight and one-half days after her last coitus, and insisted that "I would stake my reputation on her honor"; but the reader cannot fail to note that the husband had been absent from the city during this entire period. When Haussmann [3] studied the problem of sperm survival systematically in 1879 by examining the cervical mucus of 20 women at various intervals after coitus, he observed some motility as late as five and one-half days, but this consisted only of a type of lateral motion, in the manner of a pendulum, and not the darting and thrashing characteristic of the vigorous sperm cell.

The postcoital examination first came into the clinical limelight through the writings of the intrepid J. Marion Sims,[10] who did not hesitate to publicize his experiments at the risk of offending professional morality and in the face of the sharpest criticism from many of his colleagues. Speaking of sperm survival Sims wrote:

> I have examined the semen many times with the view of determining this point . . . and think I can safely say that spermatozoa never live more than twelve hours in the vaginal mucus. But in the mucus of the cervix they live much longer. At the end of twelve hours, while all are dead in the vagina, there are but few dead ones to be found in the cervix. When the cervical mucus is examined from thirty-six to forty hours after coition, we shall ordinarily find as many spermatozoa dead as alive. But my observations on this point could not, under the nature of things, be accepted as the rule, for they were all made upon those who were, or had been, the subjects of uterine disease in some form or other. . . . I saw no reason why many of these active spermatozoa [removed from the cervix 40 hours after coitus] should not have lived for a still longer time. Many of them lived six hours after their removal. This was in July.

The use of the microscope in the diagnosis and treatment of sterility was carried forward by Sims's son, Harry, whose report to the American Gynecological Society in 1888 [9] detailed the essentials of the postcoital test of today's practice. Young Sims explained:

> A drop or two of the semen taken from the vagina, or from the cervical canal soon after coition, and placed under the microscope will show the presence of zoösperms in great abundance if the semen is normal and fit for procreation. But if these are wanting, then fecundation is impossible. . . . When the male is capable of performing the sexual act even feebly and unsatisfactorily, if we find the seminal fluid in a normal state and full of living spermatozoa, we may take it as proven that the fault does not lie with the male; and we proceed to inquire into the aptitude of the female for conception.

Referring to the postcoital examination as a guide to the efficacy of treatment of cervical inflammations in sterility cases, Sims added:

During the progress of the treatment of such cases the vaginal and cervical mucus should occasionally be examined by the microscope several hours after intercourse. By the condition in which you find the spermatozoa it will be easy to determine whether the case is improving or at a standstill. When the secretions are abnormal the zoösperms will all be found dead, but as the case progresses toward complete recovery the zoösperms will be seen to become more and more lively, and for a longer time after intercourse, until, at last, when the condition is normal, I have found living spermatozoa in the cervical mucus as much as thirty hours after coitus. . . .

Additional reports on the postcoital examination of spermatozoa, based on small series of cases, were made in 1909 by Runge,[8] who stressed the importance of the posterior vaginal vault as a receptacle for the semen, and the following year by Natanson and Königstein,[6] who disputed this view. In clinical practice, however, most gynecologists and urologists based their evaluation of the male's fertility on an examination of a condom specimen of his semen.

HÜHNER'S POSTCOITAL EXAMINATION

In 1913 a book by Max Hühner appeared, entitled *Sterility in the Male and Female,*[4] in which he reported in minute detail the results of a large number of postcoital examinations and stressed their value in sterility investigation. As a result, the procedure was soon adopted by a large segment of the profession and has since been known as the *Hühner test.*

Concerning the condom examination Hühner wrote:

I desire . . . to protest most emphatically against a method which is almost universally in vogue for determining responsibility in sterility in any particular case, and that is, the placing of the decision upon the presence or absence of live spermatozoa found in the condom after connection. This test is not at all reliable, except in a negative sense. If spermatozoa are always *absent* in the semen found in the condom, we can say that the sterility is due to the male; but if found present and alive, even in large numbers, we cannot, *on this evidence alone,* absolve the husband from responsibility. The husband may be suffering from a marked hypospadias or epispadias, in which case the condom specimen would be filled with normal spermatozoa, but on account of the abnormal position of the meatus (unless the cervix be also placed in a peculiar position), the stream of semen is directed away from the genital orifice of the female or even, in particularly bad cases, may not be ejaculated into the vulva at all, but entirely outside the genitals. He may be suffering from premature emissions . . . and still, in such a case again, the condom specimen might be all that can be desired. In certain cases of stricture of the urethra, the seminal fluid is not at all ejaculated, but dribbles out *after* coitus . . . and here again the condom would show normal spermatozoa.

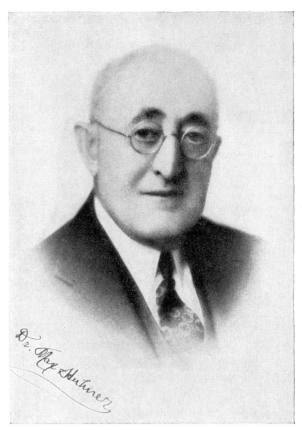

Fig. 33-1. Max Hühner (1873–1947). (Courtesy of New York Academy of Medicine.)

The postcoital examination is simplicity itself. As Hühner explained:

All that is necessary is for the woman to come after coitus, the sooner the better . . . and [she] is placed in the regular gynecological position; a bivalve speculum is inserted, the cervix is seen, and with an ordinary platinum loop on a glass rod a particle of mucus from within the cervical os is placed on the glass slide and examined under the microscope. In normal cases we will at once see many live spermatozoa. This is all there is to it; yet what a wealth of information is obtained from this few minutes examination! We need not care whether the husband has stricture, old epididymitis, hypospadias or what not, or whether, as many women complain, the husband is somewhat impotent by premature ejaculation. . . . Similarly we need not listen to the wife's complaint that *all* the semen runs out of her immediately after coitus, for we know that enough spermatozoa are in the cervical canal for purposes of impregnation. . . . We have seen that in the vagina the spermatozoa begin to lose their motility 10 to 15 minutes after coitus, and most of them are dead by the end of the first hour; therefore, except in unusual cases, only those spermatozoa which are directly thrown upon the cervix during coitus ever reach the uterus proper.

Hühner thus aligned himself with Natanson and Königstein in opposition to Runge's concept of the posterior vaginal vault as a *receptaculum seminis*. The merits of the question have never been settled to everyone's satisfaction, however, and many gynecologists still counsel the supine position, with elevation of the hips, to facilitate conception after coitus or artificial insemination.

In his investigation of the sterile couple Hühner examined specimens of mucus from various levels of the female genital tract, from the vulva to the uterine cavity. He wrote:

I admit that when we find live spermatozoa all along the genital tract we cannot scientifically assert that, when the sound or loop is withdrawn and rubbed on the slide, the spermatozoa thereon came from the uterine fundus. But if we make several examinations from the various parts of the genital tract, and find no or only dead spermatozoa in the vulva, vagina and various parts of the cervix and then push our sound easily up into the fundus and find live spermatozoa there, we can practically say, that the spermatozoa found came from the fundus. . . . And this condition is not the exception, but the rule. The longer after coitus the examination is made the less likely are we to find live spermatozoa, or, indeed any spermatozoa at all outside of the uterus and cervix. . . . It is only those that are protected in the interior of the cervix and body of the uterus that remain alive for several days . . . any spermatozoa found several days after coitus must have come from the uterus, for even if found in the vagina they were extruded from the uterus with the uterine mucus. . . .

From this postcoital examination of the infertile couple Hühner drew the following conclusions:

If live spermatozoa are found in the cervical mucus we can at once absolve the husband from all responsibility. If dead spermatozoa are found in the cervical mucus it is safer to get a condom specimen to see whether the spermatozoa came out dead, or whether they were killed after they had entered the female by the secretions of the latter's genitals. . . . If after careful examination we find spermatozoa in the cervix but never beyond the internal os or angle of flexion in an anteverted uterus, we may conclude that the flexion is the cause of the sterility as far as can be determined. . . . [This idea, once popular among gynecologists, has since been abandoned.] If no spermatozoa at all are found in any portion of the genital tract, or only dead ones in the vagina, but none at all in the cervix, the fault may be either with the husband or the wife. . . . As long as no spermatozoa are found in the cervix it is always advisable to examine the husband, no matter what we find in the condom specimen.

HÜHNER'S LIFE

Max Hühner, a New York urologist, was born in Berlin, Germany, on June 30, 1873, and graduated from the College of Physicians and Surgeons of Columbia University 20 years later.[1,5] He served on the staff of Bellevue Hospital for many years, and from 1923 to 1925 was assistant surgeon in the genitourinary clinic of the Mount Sinai Hospital. His major work, *Sterility in the Male and Female,* reported the first large-scale scientific study of the behavior of human spermatozoa in the female, based on more than 500 examinations and experiments. His second book, *A Practical Treatise on Disorders of the Sexual Function in the Male and Female,* published in 1916, went into three editions and a Spanish translation, and was followed in 1937 by another volume, *The Diagnosis and Treatment of Sexual Disorders in the Male and Female, Including Sterility and Impotence.* Hühner was the first to resort to testicular aspiration in the study of male sterility resulting from azospermia. He died of heart disease on November 8, 1947, at the age of 74.

REFERENCES

1. Deaths. Max Hühner. *J.A.M.A.,* **136**:485, 1948.
2. Donné, A.: *Cours de Microscopie Complémentaire des Études Médicales, Anatomie Microscopique et Physiologie des Fluides de l'Economie.* Baillière, Paris, 1844, pp. 291–305.
3. Haussmann, D.: *Ueber das Verhalten der Samenfäden in den Geschlechtsorganen des Weibes.* A. Hirschwald, Berlin, 1879.
4. Hühner, M.: *Sterility in the Male and Female and its Treatment.* Rebman, New York, 1913.
5. Kagan, S. R.: *Jewish Contributions to Medicine in America from Colonial Times to the Present,* 2nd ed. Boston Medical Publishing Co., Boston, 1939, pp. 678–79.
6. Natanson, K., and Königstein, H.: Ueber das Verhalten der Spermatozoen im weiblichen Genitaltrakt bei Effluvium seminis. *Wien. klin. Wchnschr.,* **23**:820–22, 1910.
7. Percy, S. R.: A fact for medico-legal science. *Am. M. Times,* **2**:160, 1861.
8. Runge, E.: Beitrag zur Aetiologie und Therapie der weiblichen Sterilität. *Arch. f. Gynäk.,* **87**:572–85, 1909.
9. Sims, H. M.: Sterility, and the value of the microscope in its diagnosis and treatment. *Tr. Am. Gynec. Soc.,* **13**:291–307, 1888.
10. Sims, J. M.: *Clinical Notes on Uterine Surgery. With Special Reference to the Sterile Condition.* Hardwicke, London, 1866, p. 385.

I. C. Rubin and
Uterotubal Insufflation*

CHAPTER

34

A myriad of factors affect conception, but only a few are understood sufficiently to merit investigation in the routine clinical study of infertility. Of transcendent importance are the anatomic pathways that must be pursued by the egg and sperm until their nuptial tryst in the fallopian tube and by the fertilized ovum in the subsequent journey to its uterine haven. Tubal obstruction is one of the commonest causes of infertility and one of the few demonstrable barriers to conception amenable to correction. "A plug of hardened mucus of the most insignificant character—the merest débris of the Fallopian secretion—may cut off an illustrious race, or change a dynasty." Thus wrote Tyler Smith [11] more than one century ago, when he proposed catheterization of the oviducts with a curved metal tube and fine whalebone bougie.

Before World War I the office diagnosis of tubal patency or obstruction depended on the clinical acumen of the physician, and was hence subject to frequent error. Discussing diseases of the adnexa as a cause of sterility in the female, Howard Kelly [3] wrote:

This is an interesting group of cases belonging to a class which are peculiarly difficult to investigate on account of the inaccessibility of the organs, namely, those cases in which the sterility is due to disease of the uterine tubes or the ovaries. It

* This chapter originally published under the title "I. C. Rubin, a Gynecologic Eponym," in *J. Mt. Sinai Hosp.,* **25**:221–28, 1958; reprinted by permission. Copyright 1958, The Mount Sinai Hospital.

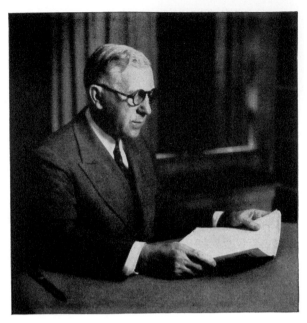

Fig. 34-1. Isidor Clinton Rubin (1883–1958).

is because it is difficult to get at these organs and therefore to obtain an accurate knowledge of their condition that they are frequently forgotten in the clinical examination.*

Some gynecology texts of the late-nineteenth century failed even to mention the fallopian tubes in their discussion of female sterility. As Rubin later wrote: [8]

The determination of patency of the fallopian tubes has hitherto been possible only by direct inspection and palpation obtained by laparotomy. Physical examination was wholly inadequate because it still left the question of patency a matter of speculation. This is especially true when, as in certain instances, the tubes are sealed tight at their fimbriated end, although no distention of the lumen is present. In other instances it is hard to diagnose occlusion of the tube due to hydrosalpinx when the walls are flaccid. Some tubes are closed by adhesions secondary to a peritonitis that arises outside of the gynecological domain. No matter how clear the history, the question as to whether such a tube is patent or not is always a matter of doubt. The same holds true in cases in which the tube may be occluded by a tumor.

The problem had already been outlined by Carey [1] in similar terms:

* From Howard Kelly, *Medical Gynecology,* 1908. Courtesy of Appleton-Century-Crofts, Inc.

In taking up the question of sterility in the individual case we can seldom feel that our diagnosis is accurate or any prognosis warranted because of our inability to determine if the tubes are obstructed. An occasional case presents a history of tubal infection with signs of diseased adnexa so evident that a temporary unfavorable prognosis is warranted. Other frank lesions may be present which prevent fertility. More frequently, however, we are consulted by the patient who has no reason to suspect pelvic disease and in whom we find no gross lesion. . . . If in this large group of causes of sterility we can now bring to bear definite knowledge regarding the patency of the tubes, the most important single factor is determinable so far as the woman is concerned. An intelligent prognosis may be given.

Independently of each other Carey and Rubin [5,6] carried out experiments in 1914, the results of which were published almost simultaneously, outlining the uterine and tubal lumens with the radiopaque silver colloid, collargol. This substance proved objectionably irritating to the tissues, however, and was soon abandoned in the search for a suitable method for testing tubal patency.

Air insufflation of the fallopian tubes was first suggested in 1849, by the *Revue Médico-Chirurgicale de Paris,*[4] in an editorial on Tyler Smith's catheterization procedure. The reviewer wrote:

After all, even if catheterization proves impossible, should the therapeutic idea be lost, and could one not try to open up the tube by means of an injection of water or air as is done with the eustachian tube? Liquid injections that have sometimes been made into the tube have caused serious accidents; but these were irritating injections, and pure water would not necessarily produce the same effect. There should be no objection to starting with injections of air, which, as experimentation has shown, can be made into the serous cavities without the least inconvenience.

RUBIN'S ACCOUNT OF TUBAL INSUFFLATION

Not until 70 years later, on November 3, 1919, was tubal insufflation, the first Rubin test, actually performed, oxygen being used as the test medium. As Rubin later [9] recalled this experiment:

The quantity was measured roughly by gauging the number of bubbles passing through the wash bottle per minute. The intrauterine pressure was not controlled by a manometer; the gas was allowed to enter the peritoneal cavity until a moderate amount of visible abdominal distention resulted. . . . Theoretically we expected to see the abdominal wall rise in case the oxygen gas succeeded in gaining access through open tubes into the abdominal cavity. Those were indeed tense moments as [the physicians] . . . who happened to be present, were observing this first patient through whose uterus I ventured to insufflate oxygen. The actual rise of the abdominal wall was corroborated by everyone present. This constituted

4. The toxic property is not destroyed in the ordinary process of sterilization by boiling (from one-half to one hour), is not soluble in water or removable by irrigation, appears in toxic amounts in arsphenamin, neo-arsphenamin and dilute sodium hydroxid solution merely on passing them through a new tube en route from container to vein, and is not apparently associated with the mechanically removable debris from the inner surface of the tube.

5. The reaction induced by this agent, as obtained by the use of new tubing for intravenous injection of the substances mentioned, consists of chills coming on from thirty to sixty minutes after injection, with nausea, vomiting, diarrhea, a sharp rise of temperature, sweating, severe headache and lumbar cramps, emotional disturbance amounting at times almost to hysteria, and subsequent profound prostration.

6. The reaction can be induced in typical form in dogs.

7. The identity and toxicology of the poisonous principle are under investigation.

NONOPERATIVE DETERMINATION OF PATENCY OF FALLOPIAN TUBES IN STERILITY

INTRA-UTERINE INFLATION WITH OXYGEN, AND PRODUCTION OF AN ARTIFICIAL PNEUMOPERITONEUM

PRELIMINARY REPORT *

I. C. RUBIN, M.D.

NEW YORK

The value of oxygen in conjunction with the roentgen ray as an aid in the diagnosis of obscure abdominal conditions has been demonstrated in a number of recent publications. No ill effects have accompanied or followed the pneumoperitoneum produced by inflation of the abdominal cavity with oxygen gas. The tolerance of the peritoneum for oxygen even in large volume, and the fact that its presence can be detected by fluoroscopy and roentgenography have led to its use as a diagnostic procedure in determining patency of the fallopian tubes. If the gas injected into the uterus under certain measurable pressure would pass into the fallopian tubes, it ought to reach the general peritoneal cavity. In patients with patent fallopian tubes the gas would establish an artificial pneumoperitoneum identical with that produced when injected by direct abdominal puncture. In patients with occluded tubes no such result could be obtained.

Accordingly, experiments were carried out on extirpated uteri with the adnexa intact. In the first experiment it was readily seen that oxygen passed into the uterine opening of the tubes and then escaped through the fimbriated end. When the tubes were ligated or were occluded by pathologic processes, this did not follow. After determining the amount of gas required for our purposes, the first clinical application of the intra-uterine oxygen inflation was made, Nov. 3, 1919, at Mount Sinai Hospital. It was successful in proving the patency of the fallopian tubes in this first patient. The abdomen became visibly distended and the pneumoperitoneum was confirmed by the roentgeno-

* From the Second Gynecological Service and X-Ray Department of Mount Sinai Hospital.

graphic examination. The symptoms associating the gas inflation by way of the uterus were the same as those described for the method by direct abdominal puncture.

Encouraged by the result of the first trial, I tested it out in a series of thirty-five cases of sterility in which there were different clinical histories and physical findings. In this first series it was our endeavor to find out the limits of application, the quantity of gas to be employed, the time and rate of flow, and the reliability of the oxygen injected as a diagnostic procedure. In the second series of twenty cases, estimations were made on pressure. This has proved a valuable adjunct. Altogether, fifty-five patients were examined by means of oxygen inflation of the uterus. There were absolutely no untoward symptoms or sequelae. The patients with two exceptions were ambulatory, and were allowed to go home from within a few minutes to a half hour after examination. Two cases were from the hospital wards. The patients were all followed up and carefully examined for complications, none of which have to the present writing appeared.

In some cases the result confirmed our clinical diagnosis of probably closed or patent tubes. In a number of cases the tubes were proved to be open when we had reason to suspect they were closed by disease, while in others the tubes were demonstrated to be occluded when we had believed them to be normal. The method had practically the value of an exploratory laparotomy for purposes of determining the continuity of the lumen of the fallopian tubes. The two possible dangers, namely, embolism and infection, are more theoretical than actual.

Embolism from oxygen introduced into the uterus in a stream of discrete bubbles never occurs, and infection need never occur if the cases are not acute and are properly selected. In fifty-five cases which form the basis of this preliminary report, there were no symptoms even suggestive of a possible peritoneal irritation, although some of them had presented gross pathologic conditions before the examination was made. These questions, with the case histories, will be more fully discussed in a future communication.

261 Central Park West.

Children's Year: Looking Backward and Forward.—In thirty-eight states the Children's Year child welfare committees have planned to "carry on" with the cooperation of the Children's Bureau; in thirty states child hygiene divisions have been established, and in sixteen states child welfare commissions have been appointed. The end of Children's Year was marked by an international child welfare conference in Washington, at which minimum standards were drawn up, discussed in eight regional conferences throughout the country, and put into final form by an advisory committee formed for that purpose. These standards cover the fundamental needs of maternity and infant care; of the preschool and school child; of the child in need of special care; of the child at work; and of the economic and social bases for these standards. The standards for the protection of maternity and infancy are already crystallized in the Sheppard-Towner maternity bill now in Congress. This bill would make available to all mothers public health nurses, accessible hospital care and medical attention; consultation centers; teaching and practical demonstration in hygiene of maternity and infancy, and the household arts essential to the well-being of mother and child. One hundred and thirty-four children's health centers were established in fifteen states; in nine other states they were reported but the actual number not given.

Fig. 34-2. Rubin's first report[7] on uterotubal insufflation. (Reproduced by permission of *The Journal of the American Medical Association*.)

first-hand proof that the oxygen actually passed through the tubes and into the peritoneal cavity. Nevertheless it was deemed necessary to establish the presence of the oxygen gas in the abdominal cavity by subjecting the patient to fluoroscopy and radiography. In every respect the x-ray evidence was the same as that which was obtained when oxygen had been introduced into the peritoneal cavity by direct abdominal puncture.

The patient, having been insufflated with several liters of oxygen, was comfortable in the recumbent posture, but we noticed that she had great epigastric distress and severe shoulder pains when she stood up before the radioscopic screen. She was kept on her back for a little while and, as she was ambulatory, she was brought home about one hour later and put to bed with the foot of the bed elevated. This gave her tolerable comfort. The discomfort rapidly disappeared so that at the end of the third day she was able to report to the x-ray department complaining only of slight uneasiness in the shoulder regions. A small amount of oxygen was still present under the diaphragm. The patient became gravid within two months after the insufflation and was delivered of a full-term baby.

Rubin reported his discovery in a preliminary note to *The Journal of the American Medical Association* [7] and presented the results of his further experiments before the Section on Obstetrics, Gynecology, and Abdominal Surgery of the AMA on April 29, 1920.[8] His description of the technique:

The cervix is exposed by means of the speculum; the vagina is carefully wiped clean and the cervix is cleansed dry and painted with tincture of iodin. If there is any uncertainty regarding the direction of the uterine cavity, it may be determined by passing the sound. The cervix is steadied with tenaculum forceps grasping its anterior lip. The oxygen, which has been released from the tank and regulated, is now allowed to pass from the water bottle through the glass and rubber connecting tubing to which the metal cannula is attached. By pinching the rubber tubing near the cannula one can make sure that all the joints are air tight. The mercury immediately rises in this case. . . . This is a very important point to be observed. Having made certain of the pressure, the air valves in the manometer are opened and the catheter is then inserted into the uterine cavity to a point well beyond the internal os. This is done so that there is no immediate escape back along the cervical canal and out into the vagina. The rubber urethral tip, placed ordinarily from 1½ to 2 inches away from the cannula tip, is then fitted into the external os, insuring better obturation. This is not essential in the nulliparous intact cervix, but is required in the irregular patulous external os resulting from previous operations or from lacerations attending childbirth. The air valves are now closed. Within a few seconds after the oxygen enters the uterine cavity, the pressure as noted in the mercury manometer will rise; within from one half to three quarters of a minute in the patent cases the mercury reaches its maximum point. It then fluctuates for a few seconds or drops rather sharply from 10 to 30 points, maintaining the last level more or less for the rest of the time. There may be a slight audible escape of oxygen from the external os in the cases of patent tubes, but as a rule there is none until the cannula is removed, when slight regurgitation is present.

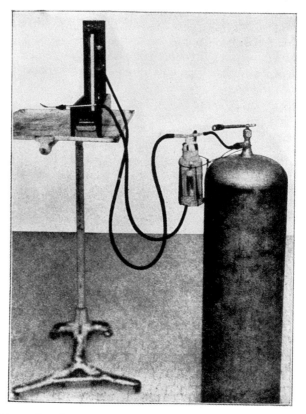

Fig. 34-3. Illustration from Rubin's second report,[8] showing the apparatus used in his early tests of tubal patency. (Reproduced by permission of *The Journal of the American Medical Association.*)

In the nonpatent cases, the pressure usually rises steadily for three quarters of a minute to a minute or longer, and then drops sharply as the gas regurgitates into the vagina. As the time required for sufficient oxygen to pass into the abdomen where it can be detected by fluoroscopic examination is one and a half minutes, the cannula is not withdrawn till this time limit is reached. If the pressure reaches 200 mm. in one minute, it is well to open one of the air valves (needle valve) to prevent it from mounting higher. In all our patent cases this high level was not reached. . . .

With the manometer attached to the water bottle we can decide, knowing the rate of flow beforehand, how much we wish to inject into the abdomen. From the moment the pressure falls, we allow the gas to flow for from one-half to one minute. . . . In the positive cases the pressure need not exceed 40 mm. The average pressure is from 60 to 80; occasionally the pressure rises to 100 or more before the oxygen will pass through the uterine ostium of the fallopian tubes. When the pressure reaches 150 or more, the likelihood is that the tube lumen is closed completely or stenosed, but not necessarily in every case. A pressure of 200 is tolerably certain to be due to closed tubes.

Rubin soon discovered that carbon dioxide was preferable to oxygen as the insufflating agent, for the former, being resorbed more rapidly, caused less discomfort and eliminated the danger of embolism. He also introduced a number of modifications in his apparatus, the most notable being a kymographic attachment for better interpretation of the functional status of the fallopian tubes.

No innovation is ever without its detractors. History has proved how wrong was John Polak, then professor of obstetrics and gynecology in the Long Island College of Medicine, when in his discussion of Rubin's paper he predicted that the method would fail to achieve general use, and stated that in cases of suspected tubal obstruction "it would be safer to do abdominal section than to inflate the tubes or uterus with gas." On the contrary, tubal insufflation was enthusiastically adopted by others, and in one of the early papers confirming the value of the procedure Furniss [2] gave it the designation of "Rubin test," by which it has since been known. Many gynecologists regard it as the twentieth century's most important contribution to the clinical study of female infertility.

RUBIN'S LIFE

Isidor Clinton Rubin was born in Friedrichshof, Germany, January 8, 1883. He migrated to the United States at an early age and was educated at the College of the City of New York, which subsequently honored him with its Distinguished Alumnus Award. He studied medicine in the College of Physicians and Surgeons of Columbia University, and after graduating in 1905 served for three years on the house staff of the Mount Sinai Hospital. The following year was spent in Schottländer's laboratory of gynecologic pathology in Vienna's II Universitäts-Frauenklinik. Upon his return to New York Dr. Rubin was made associate pathologist and adjunct gynecologist at the Beth Israel Hospital, and from 1934 to 1937 he served as director of its gynecologic service. In 1916 he was also appointed to the visiting staff of the Mount Sinai Hospital, where he ultimately rose to the rank of attending gynecologist (1937–1945). During this period he held the title of clinical professor of obstetrics and gynecology at the College of Physicians and Surgeons, his alma mater. He was elected president of the New York Obstetrical Society in 1928 and served the American Gynecological Society in a similar capacity in 1955–1956. In addition to his book, *Uterotubal Insufflation* (1947),[10] he published *Symptoms in Gynecology* (1923) and, together with Josef Novak, a three-volume text, *Integrated Gynecology* (1956). In 1947 a special number of the *Journal of the Mount Sinai Hospital* noted the Rubin test's twenty-fifth anniversary. The American Society for the Study of Sterility commemorated Dr. Rubin's seventy-fifth birthday with a special issue of *Fertility and Sterility* (Vol. 8, No. 6, 1957). He died of a heart attack July 10, 1958, while attending the International Cancer Congress in London.

REFERENCES

1. Carey, W. H.: Note on determination of patency of fallopian tubes by the use of collargol and x-ray shadow. *Am. J. Obst.*, **69**:462–64, 1914.

2. Furniss, H. D.: The Rubin test simplified. *Surg., Gynec. & Obst.*, **33**:567–68, 1921.

3. Kelly, H. A.: *Medical Gynecology.* D. Appleton & Co., New York, 1908, p. 347.

4. Revue critique: Du cathétérisme de la trompe de Fallope *pour remédier à la stérilité*, par le docteur Tyler Smith. *Rev. méd.-chir. de Paris*, **5**:113–14, 1849.

5. Rubin, I. C.: Röntgendiagnostik der Uterustumoren mit Hilfe von intra-uterinen Collargolinjektionen. *Zentralbl. f. Gynäk.*, **38**:658–60, 1914.

6. Rubin, I. C.: X-ray diagnosis in gynecology with the aid of intra-uterine collargol injection. *Surg., Gynec. & Obst.*, **20**:435–43, 1915.

7. Rubin, I. C.: Nonoperative determination of patency of fallopian tubes in sterility. Intra-uterine inflation with oxygen, and production of an artificial pneumoperitoneum. Preliminary report. *J.A.M.A.*, **74**:1017, 1920.

8. Rubin, I. C.: The nonoperative determination of patency of fallopian tubes by means of intra-uterine inflation with oxygen and the production of an artificial pneumoperitoneum. *J.A.M.A.*, **75**:661–67, 1920.

9. Rubin, I. C.: The beginnings of uterotubal insufflation. *J. Mt. Sinai Hosp.*, **10**:231–37, 1943.

10. Rubin, I. C.: *Uterotubal Insufflation.* C. V. Mosby Co., St. Louis, 1947.

11. Smith, W. T.: The new uterine operation. On a new method of treating sterility, by the removal of obstructions of the fallopian tubes. *Lancet*, **1**:603–5, 1849.

George Papanicolaou, Walter Schiller, and Uterine Cancer Detection

More than 26,000 women die in the United States every year from cancer of the uterus. Despite the recent extension of the surgical attack against this disease and the continuing improvement in radiation therapy, the greatest immediate hope for combating this frightful mortality lies in earlier case detection, for early treatment of uterine cancer almost guarantees cure.

THE PAPANICOLAOU SMEAR

Mass screening by the vaginal smear technique has provided one of the most promising approaches to this problem. In the city of Memphis, for example, where 25,000 women were examined by this method and retested a year later, early cancer was overlooked at the first examination in less than 0.2 per cent. In the words of the reporting investigators,[17] "the number of false negatives is so small, the likelihood of their being missed in the second examination is so slight, and the cancer in these is so early that these persons can receive effective treatment when the cancer is detected the second year." Fifty-nine per cent of the cervical cancers thus brought to light were clinically unsuspected.

Cancer diagnosis by the cytologic technique, universally known as the Papanicolaou smear, is based on the continuous shedding of cells, like autumn leaves, from all epithelial surfaces. The rapid proliferation of malignant tissue results in an increased rate of exfoliation and a disproportionate number

285

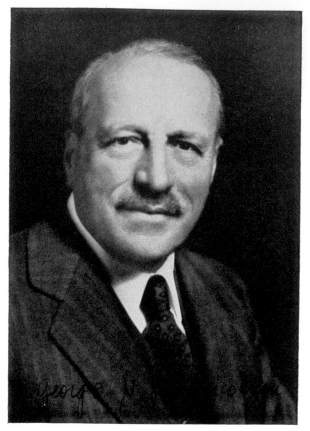

Fig. 35-1.　George Nicholas Papanicolaou (1883–　).

of cancer cells in a sample from the affected membrane. Superficial cancers may thus be detected in their incipient, preinvasive phase, even before the appearance of clinical symptoms. The criteria of malignancy in the shed cells have been arranged in outline form by the method's originator:

I. Structural modifications of cells and their nuclei.
    A. Nuclear changes.
        1. Disproportionate enlargement of the nucleus. . . .
        2. Increase in chromatin content, causing hyperchromasia.
        3. Structural abnormalities such as an aberrant chromatin pattern, elongation, irregularity in outline, deep indentation and furrowing, lobulation and budding.
        4. Enlarged nucleoli or an increase in their number beyond normal variability.

5. Multinucleation, when associated with nuclear atypia.
6. Mitotic activity with abnormal mitotic figures.
7. Marked thickening of the nuclear membrane.
8. Degenerative changes, such as abnormal vacuolation, fading or complete resorption of the nucleus.

B. Cytoplasmic changes.
1. Changes reflected in the staining reaction.
2. Cytoplasmic inclusions such as pigment granules, leucocytes or cellular debris.
3. Atypical vacuolation.

C. Changes of the cell as a whole.
1. Enlargement of cells beyond their normal range.
2. Aberrance in the form of the cell.
3. Degenerative or necrotic changes.

II. Criteria based on the interrelationships of the cells.
1. Irregularity of pattern.
2. Anisokaryosis and anisocytosis.
3. Lack of distinct cell boundaries.
4. Dense grouping and crowding of cells and nuclei.
5. Engulfment of one cell by another.
6. The grouping of cells into characteristic patterns.
7. Pronounced stratification.

III. Indirect criteria.
1. Presence of blood.
2. Excess of lymphocytes.
3. Prominence of histiocytes.
4. Polymorphonuclear leucocytes.*

The literature of the past decade numbers well over 1000 publications dealing with the Papanicolaou smear and its applications; cytologic diagnosis now comprises an essential service of nearly every integrated clinical pathologic laboratory; and even the most reactionary gynecologists have been goaded into use of the smear by importunate patients demanding their annual or semiannual "cancer test."

Only since 1943 has cancer cytology gained any measure of clinical acceptance; yet the origins of the method go back almost a century, when Beale [1] observed tumor cells in the smears of sputum from a patient with carcinoma of the pharynx. Discussing the examination of the vaginal discharge in patients with uterine cancer, he wrote:

* Reprinted by permission of the publishers and The Commonwealth Fund from Papanicolaou, G. N.: *Atlas of Exfoliative Cytology.* Cambridge, Mass.: Harvard University Press, Copyright, 1954, by The Commonwealth Fund.

In cases of cancer of the uterus, we should expect to meet with cancer cells in the discharge, but these are often so broken down as not to be distinguishable; still, when this condition is suspected, the discharge, and also the urine, should be subjected to very careful and repeated microscopic examination. In this investigation, the resemblance of the cells of columnar epithelium from the ureter, to spindle-shaped cancer cells, must be borne in mind, and the student must be careful not to mistake the former for the latter. In many cases it is not difficult to remove a little of the softened cancerous matter upon the extremity of the sponge used in vaginal examinations, when there is a much better chance of meeting with entire cancer cells than in the urine.

A few years later, in his manual of clinical microscopy,[2] Friedlaender repeated: "In carcinoma of the uterus there are frequently found, suspended in the fluid which has exuded from the cancerous ulcer, cellular elements, or even pretty large fragments and shreds, the structure of which as viewed through the microscope assists in establishing the diagnosis." Far in advance of his time, Friedlaender also learned to recognize evidence of pregnancy in the uterine drainage: "Pregnancy alone causes a characteristic change in the cells; even at the beginning of this condition we find in the swollen mucous membrane the familiar large decidual cells, from five to ten times the size of leucocytes, rich in protoplasm, round or polygonal in form, and provided with processes."

Königer, among others, contributed further to the infant science of tumor cytology in 1908 with a monograph on the cellular contents of the serous cavities.[3] He wrote:

The effusions associated with neoplasms contain in many cases tumor elements, the demonstration of which naturally establishes the diagnosis at once. Unfortunately the recognition of the tumor cells often presents difficulties. The following characteristics are to be noted: striking differences in size and shape of the cells, the abundance of vacuoles and fatty droplets in the cytoplasm, definite enlargement of the nucleus and the presence of several nucleoli within it.

Nineteenth-century studies in exfoliative cytology failed to gain general professional acceptance, however. In 1887 von Bergmann correctly named the illness of Kaiser Friedrich III as laryngeal cancer by this method, but Morell Mackenzie, British consultant to the royal medical council, rejected the diagnosis and the Kaiser died with his lesion untreated.

The development of modern cytologic technique began in 1917 with the studies of Stockard and Papanicolaou [18] on reproduction in the female guinea pig. In their efforts to analyze the estrous cycle of this species, they were led to the daily microscopic examination of its vaginal fluid, searching for a phenomenon comparable to the periodic menstrual discharge of the primates. Papanicolaou recalls: [8]

There were moments of real excitement when the examination of the first slides revealed an impressive wealth of diverse cell forms and a sequence of distinctive cytologic patterns by which the vaginal, as well as the uterine and ovarian cyclic morphologic changes and the exact time of ovulation could be accurately determined.

Papanicolaou later referred to this discovery as an example of serendipity, Horace Walpole's term for "the happy accident," for the early objectives were totally unrelated to cancer detection. Only after several years had elapsed and Papanicolaou applied his cytologic technique to the study of the sexual cycle in women did he make his first observation of cancer cells in a smear from the uterine cervix, which he characterized as "one of the most thrilling experiences of my scientific career." His first report on the application of the smear to uterine cancer diagnosis,[6] in 1928, won no clinical acceptance for the technique, however. Cytologic examination of the vaginal fluid seemed an unnecessary addition to the time-tested diagnostic procedures, endometrial curettage and cervical biopsy.

In 1943, after a three-year period of concentrated collaborative experience with the vaginal smear for the diagnosis of gynecologic cancer, Papanicolaou and Traut published their widely heralded monograph, *Diagnosis of Uterine Cancer by the Vaginal Smear,*[9] which acted as "a new tributary flowing into an old stream and helping it to gather new strength to surmount the obstacles which had blocked its further advancement." This report encompassed a variety of physiologic and pathologic states, including the menstrual cycle, puerperium, abortion, ectopic pregnancy, prepuberty, menopause, amenorrhea, endometrial hyperplasia, vaginal and cervical infections, and 179 cases of uterine cancer, 127 cervical and 52 corporeal.

In the cytologic examination of patients with cervical tumors, Papanicolaou and Traut wrote:

The cancer cells found in vaginal smears show a great variety of size and form, more so than those seen in sections of the cancer tissue. This applies more particularly to the highly differentiated types of cervical cancer. The more differentiated cellular elements acquire very unusual and aberrant forms, the identification of which is relatively simple. It is not an exaggeration to say that a cancer of the highly differentiated type can be definitely diagnosed on the strength of a few of these aberrant cells, and sometimes where only one is found. . . . In actual practice it will be seen that the vaginal smear has revealed the presence of practically all the malignant lesions of the cervix which could be detected either clinically or by the use of biopsy diagnosis. In addition, it has revealed a group of early lesions which could not be seen and hence could not be subjected to tissue diagnosis. Some of these were on the portio and others were hidden in the cervical canal. . . . As the group of failures is very small, it may be fairly said that the criteria of malignancy as outlined are reliable and sufficiently characteristic to be of practical importance. . . . For the study of the borderline group of incipient malignancy, the vaginal smear forms an ideal method of approach to a problem which has been neglected necessarily for want of a method.*

The cytologic recognition of endometrial cancer, although not so spectacularly successful as with cervical lesions, likewise proved reliable in most cases. Papanicolaou and Traut explained:

In the diagnosis of adenocarcinoma of the fundus by means of the vaginal smear the most important single indication of abnormality which may be significant of malignancy is the matter of atypical shedding of mucosal cells. Shedding of clumps of endometrial cells at any time except during the normal menstrual flow, prior to the onset of menopause, or a more or less continuous shedding of these cells after menopause is a matter requiring a clinical explanation that should completely rule out malignancy. This concept is of some importance because in the normal cases endometrial cells are only exceptionally found outside of the menstrual phase. Likewise, in benign processes, such as hyperplasia of the endometrium and endometrial polypi, shedding of glandular cells in clumps does not generally occur except at intervals corresponding to menstruation.

The adenocarcinoma of the fundus does not bring about as many intrinsic or characteristic cellular changes as the carcinoma of the cervix. There are a number of reasons why this is true; in the first place, the cells are smaller and, in addition, they are shed in dense clumps which limit analysis to those cells that happen to be advantageously placed with reference to staining and clearing procedures. This is not to say that here and there one does not see the cellular and particularly the nuclear changes so characteristic of malignancy. They do occur, but they are much less prominent than in the carcinoma of the cervix. These are the reasons why greater care and more experience are necessary before reliable opinions concerning malignancy can be made from the evidence furnished by the smear preparation. . . . In general, the diagnosis of an adenocarcinoma presents greater difficulties than the diagnosis of a cervical carcinoma because of two factors: first, the possibility that the cells of the adenocarcinomas may not be carried into the vagina in large numbers and may escape attention due to their smaller size; second, the less pronounced differentiation of the adenocarcinoma cells which makes it more difficult to distinguish them from nonmalignant endometrial cells. Nuclear enlargement, vacuolization of the cytoplasm, and leucocytic invasion may often cause a wrong interpretation. For this reason, more caution should be exercised in the diagnosis of adenocarcinomas. . . . We still adhere to the position that the vaginal smear should usually be considered as an accessory or preliminary method of diagnosis and that the actual demonstration of the malignant cells in the biopsy specimen should be the basis for decision as to the method of therapy.†

The Papanicolaou smear, on scrapings, washings, and exudates, was rapidly extended to the diagnosis of cancer of other organs, including the fallopian

---

* Reprinted by permission of the publishers and The Commonwealth Fund from Papanicolaou, G. N., and Traut, H. F.: *Diagnosis of Uterine Cancer by the Vaginal Smear.* Cambridge, Mass.: Harvard University Press, Copyright, 1943, by The Commonwealth Fund.
† *Ibid.*

tube, ovary, skin, vulva, oral cavity, nasopharynx, antrum, larynx, lung, esophagus, stomach, gallbladder, pancreas, colon, rectum, kidney, urinary bladder, prostate, and breast. The smear's principal value still lies in cancer screening, but it has also been applied with some success to the prediction of radiosensitivity in cervical cancer and to the evaluation of therapy in patients with borderline or frankly malignant lesions.

PAPANICOLAOU'S LIFE

George Nicholas Papanicolaou was born in Coumi, Greece, May 13, 1883. He received his medical degree from the University of Athens in 1904 and his Ph.D. from the University of Munich six years later. After serving as physiologist to the Oceanographical Institute of Monaco, he migrated to the United States in 1913, to become assistant in the Department of Pathology of the New York Hospital and assistant in anatomy at the Cornell University Medical College, where he was ultimately made professor emeritus. All of his subsequent scientific work, devoted almost exclusively to the physiology of reproduction and exfoliative cytology, has been carried out in these two institutions, each of which has named a laboratory in his honor. In addition to his monograph with Traut, he has published *The Sexual Cycle in the Human Female as Revealed by Vaginal Smears* (1933), *The Epithelia of Woman's Reproductive Organs* (with Traut and Marchetti, 1948), *Atlas of Exfoliative Cytology* (1954),[7] and over 100 journal articles. He has received countless honors for his scientific contributions, including the Borden Award, Lasker Award, Passano Foundation Award, the Honor Medal of the American Cancer Society, and the Royal Order of Phoenix, presented to him in 1953 by King Paul of Greece.

THE SCHILLER TEST

Practically all gynecologists still rely on tissue biopsy for the definitive diagnosis of cervical cancer. Microscopic interpretation of the excised sample rarely poses much of a problem to the pathologist; but since his verdict applies only to the tissue submitted, paramount importance is attached to the physician's selection of site for biopsy. In this choice he may be greatly aided by the Schiller test, which permits easy visualization of the suspect area after staining of the cervix with iodine.

In his meticulous studies on the histogenesis and diagnosis of early cervical cancer in 1927 and 1928 [10,11] Schiller lamented the fact that "until today we have no morphologic nor histochemical criterion that applies unequivocally to carcinoma and only carcinoma." His attention was then directed to the observation of Lahm [4,5] and others that anaplastic cells lose their ability to secrete glycogen, which is therefore absent in rapidly growing cancers. After

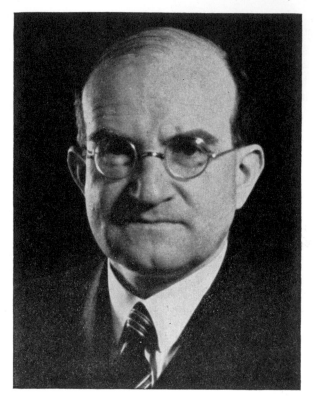

Fig. 35-2. Walter Schiller (1887–   ).

studying the glycogen distribution in many histologic sections of normal and cancerous cervices, Schiller reported: [12]

I have been able to convince myself that the epithelium of the [normal] portio, and even of the taller, vesicular layers of cells, contains large quantities of glycogen. Glycogen is sometimes found in the cytoplasm of the deeper layers also, often almost to the basalis, but only very sparsely and in the form of very fine granules. It is more abundant in the layer of taller cells, especially in the peripheral part of the cytoplasm, whereas the immediate vicinity of the nucleus is usually free of glycogen. This glycogen, which is a physiologic component of normal portio epithelium, is completely lacking in carcinomatous epithelium—that is, in carcinomas of low maturity. Carcinomas of greater maturity sometimes show traces of glycogen in the vicinity of the horny pearls. This cornification only occurs, however, when the carcinomas are older and more advanced and begin to invade. There can thus be no doubt in beginning, superficial carcinomas, as are found in scrapings. The superficial normal layers that overlap the carcinomatous area for a short distance at its oblique line of demarcation almost always contain glycogen also.

Schiller soon applied this phenomenon to the clinical detection of early cervical cancer,[13,14,15,16] the first phases of which may easily escape visual detection in the unstained state until the carcinomatous transformation of the superficial epithelium results in actual ulceration. He said:

The histologic results of glycogen staining in section led me to carry out staining in a macroscopic preparation also and later in the living. . . . If the normal portio or vaginal epithelium is painted with an iodine solution containing potassium iodide, such as Lugol's solution . . . the normal epithelium soon stains a deep dark brown after a few seconds. Pathologic epithelium, especially carcinomatous, does not take up the stain, but instead remains light, or at most slightly yellowish. The pathologic epithelial areas, especially the carcinomatous fields, thus appear as bright spots sharply delimited from the dark-brown-black background. This staining with iodine solution is completed in a few seconds. The process . . . suggests the change in appearance of a photographic plate during development. The coloration soon disappears after a few minutes but can be reversed at will by repeated application of the iodine solution. This is best accomplished with a saturated sponge, which can be left in the vagina for a short time, against the portio.[13] [See frontispiece.]

The Schiller test, like most new procedures, soon came under the attack of critics, who failed to recognize the method's limitations and demanded of it greater specificity than the test could provide. As Schiller carefully pointed out, however:

It is obvious that the method of glycogen staining is specific only in its staining, but not in its failure to stain. That which stains dark brown is normal epithelium; by contrast the unstained squamous epithelium is very often carcinomatous, but it can also be hyperkeratotic epithelium, as we sometimes find in cases of prolapse. . . . This type of horny epithelium contains glycogen only in small amount and is protected by the thick horny layer from the action of the iodine. Also, epithelium altered by inflammation, in which the superficial, glycogen-containing layers are reduced by sloughing to a few cell layers, stains much lighter than the normal portio epithelium. This sort of inflammatory epithelium, however, merges gradually with the normal; it is never bounded from the normal epithelium by a sharp, irregular line, as carcinoma almost always is. . . . Obviously also, the cervical mucosa, which contains only small amounts of glycogen in the mucus, does not take the iodine stain, so that healing erosions and also eversions are not stained by iodine. The cervical mucosa, however, is easily recognized, without special help, by its dark red color and its soft velvety surface. Thus the iodine staining method only serves to distinguish pathologic epithelium from normal epithelium; it is to facilitate the finding of early carcinoma, still confined to the epithelium, and also to determine the boundary of the cancerous area, but not to differentiate an advanced carcinomatous ulcer from an erosion. The reaction provides a convenient means for discovering beginning carcinomas, which develop as spotlike thickenings. . . . The procedure is so simple and can be performed so quickly that it can be carried out in any case without trouble and without significant loss of time. If a sharply demarcated zone in the epithelium remains unstained, then the diagnosis as to whether it is a beginning carcinoma or a harmless epithelial change is determined by histologic examination of the unstained epithelium. If, on the other hand, the whole portio stains uniformly dark brown, then one has the assurance that the portio epithelium is everywhere normal.[13]

Tumor recurrence commonly involves the vaginal vault following unsuccessful excision of a cervical cancer. Surgical failure of this type is usually attributable to incomplete removal of the zone of intraepithelial carcinoma, invisible to the naked eye, which often surrounds invasive tumors. This problem presented an additional field for application of the Schiller test. Schiller wrote:

It had been a constant objective of our clinic to find a method that would permit a definite preoperative delimitation of the cancerous from the noncancerous epithelium in the patient. Biopsies were out of the question, for the cancerous field often extends around the entire vagina, not circularly but by the extension of processes. Determination of the boundary by excision of the line of demarcation would be valid only for the site of excision but not for the rest of the circumference. . . . A very rapid differentiation can be obtained after staining by wiping the portio with a highly diluted solution of sodium thiosulfate or potassium iodide (without free iodine). . . . It can serve in this manner as a control for radical operations: When the vaginal cuff is examined, the excised rim must be surrounded everywhere by a border of darkly stained epithelium. If this is lacking, then the line of excision has gone through carcinomatous epithelium. It is obviously preferable to carry out this control on the patient before operation and thus produce an exact picture of the boundary between the carcinoma and the normal portio or vaginal epithelium.[13]

SCHILLER'S LIFE

Walter Schiller was born in Vienna, December 3, 1887. After receiving his M.D. from the University of Vienna in 1912 he served with a bacteriology unit during the war with Bulgaria, before training in pathology under Weichselbaum. During World War I he headed a medical laboratory of the Austrian Army, variously assigned in Bosnia, Turkey, Palestine, and Russia. Returning to the University of Vienna, he worked in its medical clinic for two years, after which he was made director of laboratories in the II Universitäts-Frauenklinik, under the direction of Kermauner and later Weibel. He came to the United States on a lecture tour in 1936 and the following year was appointed director of laboratories at the Jewish Memorial Hospital in New York. Shortly thereafter he moved to Chicago to accept a similar position at the Cook County Hospital (1938–1944) and later the Women's and Children's Hospitals (1945–1952). He subsequently was made consultant to the Cuneo, Columbus, and Lewis Memorial Hospitals as well. Schiller's numerous scientific publications are devoted chiefly to gynecologic pathology.

REFERENCES

1. Beale, L. S.: *The Microscope in its Application to Practical Medicine,* 3rd ed. Lindsay & Blakiston, Philadelphia, 1867, p. 197.

2. Friedlaender, C.: *The Use of the Microscope in Clinical and Pathological Examinations,* 2nd ed. Translated by H. C. Coe. D. Appleton & Co., New York, 1885, pp. 168–69.

3. Königer, H.: *Die Zytologische Untersuchungsmethode ihre Entwicklung und ihre Klinische Verwerthung an den Ergüssen Seröser Höhlen.* Fischer, Jena, 1908, pp. 99–100.

4. Lahm, W.: Über den Glykogengehalt der Uteruskarzinome und der atypischen Plattenepithelwucherungen im Bereich des Os externum. Vorläufige Mitteilung. *Ztschr. f. Geburtsh. u. Gynäk.,* **93**:356–63, 1928.

5. Lahm, W.: Die biologische Carcinomheilung. *Strahlentherapie,* **28**:779–83, 1928.

6. Papanicolaou, G. N.: New cancer diagnosis. *Proc. Third Race Betterment Conference, January 2–6, 1928.* Race Betterment Foundation, Battle Creek, Mich., 1928, pp. 528–34.

7. Papanicolaou, G. N.: *Atlas of Exfoliative Cytology.* Harvard University Press, Cambridge, 1954.

8. Papanicolaou, G. N.: The evolutionary dynamics and trends of exfoliative cytology. *Texas Rep. Biol. & Med.,* **13**:901–19, 1955.

9. Papanicolaou, G. N., and Traut, H. F.: *Diagnosis of Uterine Cancer by the Vaginal Smear.* Commonwealth Fund, New York, 1943.

10. Schiller, W.: Untersuchungen zur Entstehung der Geschwülste. I. Teil. Collumcarcinom des Uterus. *Virchows Arch. f. path. Anat.,* **263**:279–367, 1927.

11. Schiller, W.: Über Frühstadien des Portiocarcinoms und ihre Diagnose. *Arch. f. Gynäk.,* **133**:211–83, 1928.

12. Schiller, W.: Zur histologischen Frühdiagnose des Portiokarzinoms. *Zentralbl. f. Gynäk.,* **52**:1562–67, 1928.

13. Schiller, W.: Zur klinischen Frühdiagnose des Portiokarzinoms. *Zentralbl. f. Gynäk.,* **52**:1886–92, 1928.

14. Schiller, W.: Jodpinselung und Abschabung des Portioepithels. *Zentralbl. f. Gynäk.,* **53**:1056–64, 1929.

15. Schiller, W.: Early diagnosis of carcinoma of the cervix. *Surg., Gynec. & Obst.,* **56**:210–22, 1933.

16. Schiller, W.: Early diagnosis of carcinoma of the portio uteri. *Am. J. Surg.,* **26**:269–80, 1934.

17. Sprunt, D. H.; Hale, W. M.; Chang, F. C.; Richmond, S. G.; and Erickson, C. C.: Present status of cancer tests. *Science,* **122**:273–74, 1955.

18. Stockard, C. R., and Papanicolaou, G. N.: The existence of a typical oestrous cycle in the guinea-pig—with a study of its histological and physiological changes. *Am. J. Anat.,* **22**:225–83, 1917.

Phenomena of Pregnancy and Labor

PART III

John Braxton Hicks, Bipolar Version, and the Contractions of the Pregnant Uterus*

CHAPTER

36

Turning the fetus in utero remained for many years one of the principal methods of coping with a variety of major obstetric complications. It was frequently resorted to in the management of cephalopelvic disproportion, malpresentation, placenta previa, and even eclampsia; only in the present century has it been supplanted by improved methods of therapy for these conditions.

Until the second half of the last century only one method of version was used, the internal podalic, associated with its well-known limitations and risks. External version was then proposed as a method for changing the polarity of the fetus from head to breech, but its shortcomings proved too great for general acceptance.

HICKS'S DESCRIPTION OF BIPOLAR VERSION

Hicks's (1860) method of combined internal and external, or bipolar, version was received as one of the major contributions to obstetric practice in his generation.† It has been known ever since as the Braxton Hicks version

---

* Parts of this chapter originally published in *J. Obst. & Gynaec. Brit. Emp.*, **63**:268–71, 1956; reprinted by permission.

† A method for converting a shoulder to a cephalic presentation by combined intrauterine and external abdominal manipulation was described in 1854 by M. D. Wright of Cincinnati, who credited the even earlier use of a similar method for correction of shoulder presentations to Professor Flamand of Strasbourg. (Wright, M. D.: *Difficult Labors and Their Treatment*. Jackson, White & Co.'s Mammoth Steam Printing, Cincinnati, 1854.)

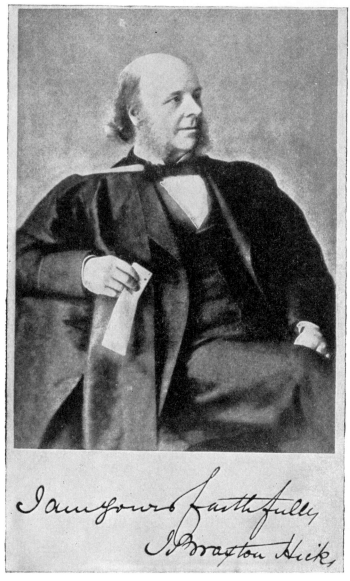

Fig. 36-1.   John Braxton Hicks (1823–1897). (Courtesy of American Gynecological Society.)

and is still resorted to occasionally by a few obstetricians. Hicks's original description: [2]

The method I have found successful, and very easy of application, is conducted thus:—We will suppose the simplest condition, a case where the uterus is passive, membranes unbroken, the liquor amnii plentiful, the os uteri expanded sufficiently to detect the presentation, which is cephalic . . . ; the patient is in the ordinary position, the trunk curved forwards as much as possible, to relax the abdominal muscles. Introduce the left hand, with the usual precautions, into the vagina, so far as to fairly touch the foetal head, even should it recede an inch. (This generally requires the whole hand.) Having passed one or two fingers (if only one, let it be the middle finger) within the cervix, and resting them on the head, place the *right* hand on the *left* side of the breech at the fundus uteri. . . . Employ gentle pressure and slight impulsive movements on the fundus towards the right side, and simultaneously on the head towards the left iliac fossa. In a very short time it will be found that the head is rising and at the same time the breech is descending. The shoulder is now felt by the hand in place of the head . . . ; it in like manner is pushed to the left, and at the same time the breech is depressed to the right iliac fossa. The foetus is now transverse; the knee will be opposite the os, and, the membranes being ruptured, it can be seized . . . and brought into the vagina.

Comparing his new method with external version, Hicks continued:

Before I had read of [external version] . . . I had already employed a method, combining the power possessed by external manipulation with the power and certainty derived from pressure and touch through the cervix, and which . . . appears to be more satisfactory, and more easily managed by those who have not given, nor are able to give, to the external diagnosis of foetal position such care and skill as Professor Carl Esterle; for even Martin, of Jena, insists that by his plan it is necessary—first, that immediate delivery be not called for; second, that there be a capacious pelvis; third, that there be active pains; fourth, that the child be living. From the following remarks and illustrative cases, I think I shall show sufficiently that the method I have employed does not require such conditions. Accepting, then, the valuable fact, that the foetus in utero can be turned without the necessity of the entry of the hand into the uterus, I shall now prove the extensive applicability of the plan I have adopted to labour in its various complications.

Proceeding with a comparison of his method with internal podalic version, Hicks wrote:

In considering, secondly, the general advantages of this operation over the ordinary method, I disclaim all intention of unnecessarily deprecating an exceedingly valuable and ancient operation—one which has saved numberless lives, and one with which, at present, we cannot dispense. Still, if it can be shown that in a considerable number of cases requiring version, the operation can be accomplished as quickly, or even more so, without the necessity of introducing the hand into the uterus, with the exception of one or two fingers passed a little way into the os, I am sure that such a modification of this more or less hazardous operation will recommend itself without any panegyric on my part. For in that case it will readily be perceived that we shall avoid:

1. The addition of the hand, and perhaps arm, to the uterine contents; and the irritation, present and future, caused by it.
2. Entry of air within the uterine cavity.
3. Liability to rupture of the uterus.
4. Much of the pain and distress felt in the ordinary plan.
5. The removal of the coat, and baring the arm of the operator; and, as a minor consideration,—
6. The fatigue and pain endured by the operator while the hand is in utero.

Hicks concluded his paper with mention of the conditions in which his method of combined version could be used to advantage, and appended reports of five cases in which it was employed in the treatment of placenta previa:

From the foregoing remarks, it will be readily seen that it can be applied at the earliest period a malpresentation is detectable. As soon as the finger can enter the cervix, so soon can version be performed, converting all forms into breech presentations. In malpositions of the head, perhaps it may be found capable of improving its position without having recourse to complete podalic version; in puerperal convulsions, diminishing the great risk in such cases from the addition of the hand to the contents of the uterus; in narrow brims when version is decided upon, it will save the pressure upon the os uteri against the projecting parts of the brim. . . . I shall for the present confine myself to the advantages this method gives us in placenta praevia—at least, in every form of partial insertion.

It was this last condition for which the Braxton Hicks method of version proved most valuable, its wide adoption in the management of placenta previa leading to a reduction in maternal mortality from 30 per cent to 5 per cent.[1] In a case of severe hemorrhage, with the cervix dilated only sufficiently to admit one or two fingers, Hicks found:

Anything which gave the practitioner some power of action was to be earnestly welcomed; anything better than to stand with folded arms, incapable of rendering assistance for hours and even days, every moment of which might be carrying the sinking and suffering patient nearer to the grave. . . . Turn, and if you employ the child as a plug the danger is over. Then wait for the pains, rally the powers in the interval and let nature, gently assisted, complete the delivery.

HICKS'S DESCRIPTION OF CONTRACTIONS OF PREGNANT UTERUS

Important as was Hicks's method of bipolar version to the obstetrics of his day, far more basic and enduring was his later description of the contractions of the uterus during pregnancy,[3] now universally known as Braxton Hicks contractions. This classic contribution to obstetric literature is a masterpiece

men downwards, the knees of the fœtus are opposite the os uteri; and if the os is large enough to introduce a finger, the knee can be hooked down and the presentation secured. Thus it is evident that it is merely necessary for the fœtus to assume the above position, where delivery by knee or foot is sought for, or where we wish that the delivery may be at our command. I shall defer alluding to version of cephalic into pure breech presentation till I speak of the method of operation.

The next fact to be borne in mind is that, should the fœtus, either naturally or by the method to be described, present by its back to the os uteri, the case would be very rare in which one side or the other was not the more dependent, and consequently one or the other knee be within finger-reach of the os.

The third fact needful to reflect upon is this, that the shape of the cavity of the fully-developed uterus being oval, with the long axis placed vertically, the tendency of the slight pains towards the end of pregnancy is to place the longer axis of the fœtus in a corresponding direction; or, in other terms, to cause it to present by the head or breech: so that if the fœtus be at any time situated transversely, a slight preponderance of force in either direction will be sufficient to determine the ultimate presentation. It will be thus perceived that, the head being heavier than the pelvic extremity, the natural tendency of a spontaneous rectification will be to head presentation; but at the same time it would have taken but little force to have caused it to rise to the fundus.

Having premised these considerations, we will discuss the other facts as they arise in the application of the above principles, taking for granted that it is admitted possible to turn the fœtus in utero from the outside. The method I have found successful, and very easy of application, is conducted thus:— We will suppose the simplest condition, a case where the uterus is passive, membranes unbroken, the liquor amnii plentiful, the os uteri expanded sufficiently to detect the presentation, which is cephalic, and in the first or fourth position (occiput to left side); the patient is in the ordinary position, the trunk curved forwards as much as possible, to relax the abdominal muscles. Introduce the left hand, with the usual precautions, into the vagina, so far as to fairly touch the fœtal head, even should it recede an inch. (This generally requires the whole hand.) Having passed one or two fingers (if only one, let it be the middle finger) within the cervix, and resting them on the head, place the *right* hand on the *left* side of the breech at

FIG. 1.

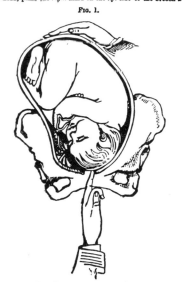

the fundus uteri, as shown at Fig. 1. Employ gentle pressure

and slight impulsive movements on the fundus towards the right side, and simultaneously on the head towards the left iliac fossa. In a very short time it will be found that the head is rising and at the same time the breech is descending. The shoulder is now felt by the hand in place of the head, as in Fig. 2; it in like manner is pushed to the left, and at the same time the breech is depressed to the right iliac fossa. The

FIG. 2.

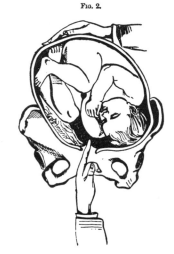

fœtus is now transverse; the knee will be opposite the os, and, the membranes being ruptured, it can be seized, as at Fig. 3, and brought into the vagina.

Having now the labour at command, the case must be treated according to the circumstances which called for turning. In

FIG. 3.

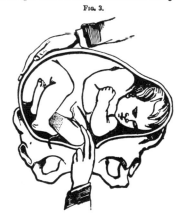

obedience to the law above stated, when the fœtus is placed transversely, a slight impulse will determine the final position of the head. When the leg is seized, therefore, it is advisable

29

Fig. 36-2. A page from Hicks's paper on bipolar version, with illustrative diagrams.

of clinical observation and inductive reasoning. The following paragraphs from it are sequential but not necessarily consecutive:

It was a source of difficulty to the older obstetricians to explain how that, at a certain time, namely, at the full period of pregnancy, the uterus, passive up till then, began all at once to acquire a new power, that of contracting; forgetful that, long before the full period had arrived, the uterus has the power to expel the foetus, and under mental excitement or local stimulation, attempted to do so frequently.

But after many years' constant observation, I have ascertained it to be a fact that the uterus possesses the power and habit of spontaneously contracting and re-laxing from a very early period of pregnancy, as early, indeed, as it is possible to recognize the difference of consistence—that is, from about the third month.

. . . If, then, the uterus be examined without friction or any pressure beyond that necessary for full contact of the hand continuously over a period of from five to twenty minutes, it will be noticed to become firm if relaxed at first, and more or less flaccid if it be firm at first. It is seldom that so long an interval occurs as that of twenty minutes; most frequently it occurs every five or ten minutes, sometimes even twice in five minutes. However, in some cases I have found only one contraction in thirty minutes. The duration of each contraction is generally not long, ordinarily it lasts from two to five minutes. When the uterus is irritable or has been irritated it lasts longer than this; under particular circum-stances . . . it may assume an almost continuous action analogous to that which is noticed after long obstructed labour.

. . . The consistency with which these contractions of the uterus have always occurred to me leaves no doubt on my mind but that it is a natural condition of pregnancy, irrespective of external irritation.

In a general way the pregnant woman is not conscious of these contractions of the uterus, but sometimes she will remark that she has a tumour in her lower abdomen, thinking it a constant thing; but another will observe that she has a swelling sometimes, but which vanishes at other times. But occasionally it hap-pens that the uterus is more than usually sensitive, and that the contractions are accompanied by pain; and then on examination it is found that each pain she complains of is co-incident with a contraction.

. . . We need not, with the cognizance of this intermittent action, any longer wonder how it is that suddenly a new function is given to the uterus at the end of the ninth month; it is already in active exercise, not perceptible to the pregnant woman, though it is to the examining hand. We also find in this frequent contrac-tion an explanation of the change of note in the uterine souffle. Every one con-versant with the sounds of pregnancy has noticed that while listening to the sounds formerly called placental, but now acknowledged to be uterine, the loud sonorous sound has become gradually higher till it is almost a shrill piping musical one. It has puzzled many authors to explain this, but one sees no difficulty in it; the diameters of the uterine sinuses are slowly reduced by the contraction of the walls, the rapidity of the rush of the blood increased, and the pitch of the sound con-sequently heightened. It also explains the phenomenon of "after pains," in which we see a continuation of the same intermittent movements after removal of the exciting cause. . . .

Hicks's views concerning the "effects or uses" of these contractions have not been improved upon to this day:

In the first place, it will provide for the frequent movement of the blood in the uterine sinus and decidual processes, for as the sinuses of the uterus are so much larger than the supplying arteries, the current is more slow in them than in the ordinary systemic veins. The contraction of the walls through which the sinuses meander tends to send the current onward, and to act somewhat as a supplementary heart.

Besides this, it facilitates the movement of the fluid in the intervillal space of the placenta, or in that which is called the placental sinuses. . . .

In the second place, the uterine action adapts the position of the foetus to the form of the uterus. . . .

Hicks also called attention to the value of the contractions in establishing the diagnosis of pregnancy:

For the last six years and upwards I have made use of the intermittent action of the uterus as the principal symptom upon which I have depended in the diagnosis of pregnancy. I am not aware that I have been less successful than others in determining the existence of pregnancy; on the contrary, I have felt myself at an advantage in the possession of an additional sign to make up the deficiency or temporary inapplicability of the others; as, for instance, when external noise prevents the heart sounds from being heard.

HICKS'S LIFE

John Braxton Hicks, one of the most illustrious figures in British obstetrics, was born in Rye, Sussex, in 1823.[1,4,5,6] He studied medicine at Guy's Hospital, where he won many prizes and honors, receiving his M.D. degree in 1851. He then entered general practice in Tottenham in partnership with Mr. W. Moon. Later devoting himself to obstetrics, Hicks was appointed to progressively higher teaching posts at Guy's Hospital, and was finally made obstetric physician to St. Mary's Hospital as well. He held diplomas from the Royal College of Surgeons and the Apothecaries' Society; was a fellow of the Royal Society and the Linnaean Society, a member of the Hunterian Society, of which he was president in 1879, and a founding member of the Obstetrical Society of London, which he served as president in 1871 and 1872. He retired from practice in 1894, and died at the Brackens, Lymington, on August 28, 1897, at the age of 74. His bibliography contains 133 medical titles and 23 other scientific papers on nonmedical subjects, outstanding among the former being his studies on uterine inertia and the state of the uterus in obstructed labor. The name of Braxton Hicks is also associated with a modified cephalotribe, which became the standard instrument of its type in England. The breadth of his interests, which encompassed botany and zoology, is shown by the titles of some of his publications, such as *Lichen Mosses and Unicellular Algae, On Certain Sensory Organs in Insects Hitherto Undescribed,* and *On the Homologies of the Eye and Its Parts in Invertebrates.*

REFERENCES

1. Cullingworth, C. J.: Annual address. *Tr. Obst. Soc. London,* **40**:65–78, 1898.
2. Hicks, J. B.: On a new method of version in abnormal labour. *Lancet,* **2**:28–30, 55, 1860.
3. Hicks, J. B.: On the contractions of the uterus throughout pregnancy: their physiological effects and their value in the diagnosis of pregnancy. *Tr. Obst. Soc. London,* **13**:216–31, 1871.
4. Mundé, P. F.: John Braxton Hicks, M.D., F.R.C.P., F.R.S., London, England. *Gynec. Tr.,* **23**:477–80, 1898.
5. Obituary. John Braxton Hicks. *Brit. M. J.,* **2**:618–19, 1897.
6. Obituary. John Braxton Hicks. *Lancet,* **2**:692, 1897.

Carl Conrad Theodor Litzmann
and Posterior Asynclitism

From 1819, when Naegele [8] suggested that the fetal head normally enters the pelvis in a position of lateral flexion, until precise roentgenographic studies of the labor mechanism were made over a century later, obstetricians warmly debated the question of asynclitism (from the Greek, meaning "to lean together") and its role in the process of engagement. Naegele, as already related (see Chap. 21), maintained that the fetal head normally engages with its sagittal suture inclined posteriorly, an attitude variously designated as anterior parietal presentation, anterior asynclitism, or Naegele's obliquity. Although endorsed by some, the majority of nineteenth-century obstetric authorities rejected Naegele's concept of anterior asynclitism as the normal mode of engagement.

LITZMANN'S DESCRIPTION OF POSTERIOR ASYNCLITISM

Carl Conrad Theodor Litzmann, destined to become one of the most renowned students of the female pelvis, was only four years old when Naegele's monograph on the mechanism of labor was published. A half century later he described the obverse of Naegele's obliquity, namely a variety of engagement in which the sagittal suture approximates the symphysis pubis and the posterior parietal bone presents at the pelvic inlet. This observation was not entirely original with Litzmann, for posterior parietal presentation had already been noted in occasional cases and briefly commented upon by

307

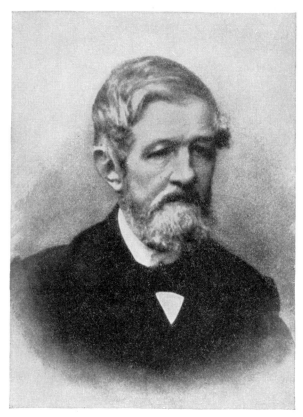

Fig. 37-1. Carl Conrad Theodor Litzmann (1815–1890). (Courtesy of Schleswig-Holstein Landesbibliothek.)

Michaelis,[7] Scanzoni,[9] Hecker and Buhl,[3] Fuhrmann,[2] and others. But it was Litzmann who first described this type of asynclitism in detail and offered an interpretation of its obstetric significance. He erred, however, in his estimate of its infrequency and in emphasizing its abnormalcy. Posterior parietal presentation has since been known as Litzmann's obliquity or Litzmann's asynclitism. In 1871 Litzmann wrote: [5]

In the following pages I propose to discuss an abnormal cephalic presentation, which seems to me not to have received as much attention as its practical importance warrants. I refer to the presentation of the parietal bone toward the promontory, a position I shall refer to simply as posterior parietal presentation. In most textbooks it is completely ignored. . . . But this position of the head is neither so rare . . . nor is it limited to contracted pelves. . . . As examples of this abnormality I consider all cases in which the parietal bone facing the promontory projects into the pelvic inlet to a greater extent or more deeply than does the anterior one. In these cases the head usually lies in the direct transverse; occasionally the sagittal suture is found more in the direction of one of the diagonal diameters. Three grades of the abnormality can be differentiated. In the first grade the sagittal suture deviates about 1.5 cm to 2.5 cm anterior to the midline of the pelvis. In the second grade the sagittal suture lies close behind the upper edge of the pubic symphysis, and the boss of the posterior parietal bone projects directly into the lumen of the pelvic canal. In the third grade only the posterior bone presents, and it can be felt, up to the ear, at or near the promontory. In contracted pelves, but by no means exclusively in the flat forms, I have encountered this position of the head about once in every ten cases; in normal pelves far less often. In a review of the records of 1800 cephalic deliveries, conducted by myself for the most part, I find it noted only 23 times in the normal pelvis, or in 1.2 per cent of the cases; but it had undoubtedly been overlooked more often, with early spontaneous correction. Among these 23 cases, 13 were of the first grade, 9 of the second, and only 1 of the third. In 10 cases the atypical position of the head at the pelvic inlet was discovered six times before and four times after rupture of the membranes. . . . In the 13 cases in which the head had already entered partly into the pelvis, six times before and seven times after the loss of the amniotic fluid, the grade of the abnormality was always less, the second grade being observed in only 2 cases and the third grade not at all. . . .

The conditions under which this abnormal position of the head occurs in the normal pelvis still remain partly obscure to me. Initially and after my first obser-vations on contracted pelves, I was inclined to assume . . . that for its occurrence an unusual degree of uterine relaxation was necessary, involving the whole organ or limited to the lower segment, allowing either the whole fetus to fall forward, or at least an abnormal anterior position of the presenting head in its relation to the pelvic inlet. But 12 of these 23 patients were primigravidas, 8 secundigravidas, and only 3 multiparas, and in only 7 cases was a truly pendulous abdomen or a marked protrusion of the anterior uterine wall over the pubic bones present. In 4 other cases the uterine wall was considered lax, but in 1 case it was remark-ably firm and unyielding. Now in those cases where the abdomen was not pendu-lous, an explanation may be found for the head's rising up over the superior border of the pubic symphysis in a different relation than the uterus, the long axis of the head deviating sharply from the posteriorly directed axis of the pelvic inlet. . . .

The diagnosis of posterior parietal presentation is based essentially on the internal examination. Only so long as it rests in its normal relation above the upper border of the pubic symphysis can the head be felt projecting outward there. With deeper engagement of the posterior parietal bone . . . external palpation becomes progressively less feasible and external examination alone does not even permit one to suspect an abnormal position of the head. On internal examination the sagittal suture is felt, usually in the transverse position, anterior to the midline of the pelvis and more or less near the anterior pelvic wall, and can be followed to the large or small fontanelle, according as the front or back of the head is more deeply engaged. At times the sagittal suture is accessible to the examining finger only with the aid of external suprapubic pressure. Through such pressure the position of the head is momentarily improved, as a rule, the anterior parietal bone is depressed, and the sagittal suture is displaced back toward the midline; but upon release of the pressure the head resumes its previous posi-tion.

The anterior parietal bone is forced into the sagittal suture by the pressure of the upper border of the pubic symphysis, this occurring sometimes in early labor but always upon entry of the head into the pelvis. After the ensuing correction [of the asynclitism] and the complete entry of the parietal bone into the pelvis the depression is not always effaced and is often palpable for a long time in the head of the newborn. If the position of the head does not improve with strong labor contractions, then after drainage of the amniotic fluid a swelling of the head appears, on the posterior parietal bone at first but gradually involving the entire presenting part of the skull and obscuring the sutures and fontanelles. If one sees the patient for the first time in this stage of labor he may easily overlook the abnormal position of the head altogether, for the external examination reveals nothing unusual; and only by inserting half the hand above the pelvic rim to a suture, or fontanelle, or even to the posterior ear, can one avoid an error that may be potentially fatal to mother and child.

The prognosis for delivery is generally favorable in the normal pelvis. The labor contractions almost always succeed in improving the position of the head sufficiently in an anterior direction for its entrance into the pelvis. The anterior parietal bone is gradually forced down behind the pubic symphysis, and as this occurs the sagittal suture approaches the midline of the pelvis and the posterior parietal bone is displaced upward over the promontory. This movement can be facilitated by means of a well-fitting abdominal binder or, after drainage of the amniotic fluid, by posterior suprapubic pressure applied manually during the labor contractions. . . . Progress in labor is out of the question without a change in the position of the head. . . .

Modern roentgenography has amply corroborated Litzmann's principal observations on posterior asynclitism. Indeed, this eccentric presentation of the fetal head at the pelvic brim occurs with far greater frequency than Litzmann suspected, and in its transient form actually comprises a normal part of the birth mechanism. From their stereoscopic studies Caldwell, Moloy, and D'Esopo [1] reported:

In 60 per cent of the cases the head was noted in the transverse or just off the transverse, either slightly anterior or posterior. . . . There is considerable obliquity of the plane of the pelvis and . . . the axis of the uterus or child . . . is not perpendicular to this plane but is posterior to it so that the fetal head actually descends below the promontory before it is met by the symphysis pubis. . . . For descent to occur from this resting position, *the anterior parietal bone must slip behind the symphysis while the posterior parietal remains relatively fixed at or below the promontory.* As it descends in this manner the head tends to fit more and more squarely into the transverse diameter until the usual appearance of the head in midpelvis is noted.

The x-ray studies of these distinguished students of the labor mechanism showed that, instead of synclitic presentation of the head prior to its engagement:

High parietal position of the head is more frequently noted and disproportion is by no means the sole cause. It may be held in this high position by firm soft parts, but its persistence long after the onset of labor is distinctly pathologic. . . . The mechanism described . . . is somewhat similar to the mechanism of the posterior parietal presentation discussed in most obstetric texts with reference to the contracted pelvis. . . . From this investigation we are led to accept this mechanism as the common and usual method of engagement.

LITZMANN'S LIFE

Carl Conrad Theodor Litzmann was born in Gadebusch, Mecklenburg, Germany, October 7, 1815.[10] Educated at home until his seventeenth year, he was then sent to the Lübecker Gymnasium, where his early leanings toward poetry and literature formed the basis of a close friendship with Geibel, the poet. Not until a severe epidemic of typhus had taken the lives of two of his siblings and a teacher residing in his house did Litzmann begin to consider seriously the urging of his father, a physician, to take up the study of medicine. Partly from a sense of filial duty he entered the University of Berlin in 1834, but continued to devote to his literary pursuits all the time he could spare from his medical courses. In the middle of his studies he transferred to the University of Halle, but took private instruction in obstetric surgery from d'Outrepont in Würzburg. After completing his formal education and examinations Litzmann, having developed a strong interest in academic medicine by this time, resisted the importuning of his father to return home and enter general practice, and instead accepted a position as assistant in Niemeyer's obstetric clinic. A few years later he undertook private practice as well, and in 1840 his dissertation, *De Causa Partum Efficiente,* was published. Soon thereafter he began to give lectures in the university on a variety of subjects, including pathologic physiology, neurology, anthropology, forensic medicine, and selected topics in obstetrics. Johannes Müller, under whom he had studied in Berlin, had exerted a profound, stimulating effect on Litzmann, who sought to strengthen the bonds between clinical medicine and the natural sciences. He therefore proved a popular choice as assistant to the professor of theoretic medicine in Greifswald in 1845 and from this position was elevated the following year to the rank of ordinarius.

Litzmann's move to Greifswald brought with it the perennial dilemma of the full-time medical teacher. In Halle he had enjoyed a good income and a comfortable living from his private practice, but his meager salary in Greifswald required so drastic a change in his standard of living, especially since no prospect existed for any significant augmentation through practice, that the minister of health interceded and obtained for Litzmann a salary increase from 300 Thaler (about $215) to 500 Thaler annually. His economic and social position improved somewhat with his promotion, but Litzmann continued to chafe under the restrictions on his teaching. Obstetrics had become his favorite field, but since this subject was covered in its entirety by Berndt, director of the obstetric clinic, Litzmann was not permitted to lecture on it. He was therefore glad to leave Greifswald in 1848 in response to an invitation to Kiel, where he became ordinary professor of obstetrics, gynecology, and pediatrics. The clinical facilities in Kiel proved woefully inadequate, but Litzmann worked there happily for 37 years, in the course of which he succeeded in obtaining a new hospital, built by funds of the Danish King. One of Litzmann's principal pleasures in Kiel derived from his membership in a small literary group who called themselves "Anonyma" and who met one night each week for the reading and discussion of Greek authors and the traditional collation. After his retirement at age 70, Litzmann returned to Berlin, where he died four years later, on February 24, 1890. His biography of Hölderlin, the poet, was in press at the time.

Litzmann became an outstanding teacher of clinical obstetrics in Kiel, and with the introduction of aseptic surgery he began to practice major gynecology as well. He published a paper on the surgical treatment of extrauterine pregnancy in 1880 [6] and was the first to perform a second laparotomy for removal of the placenta in cases of abdominal pregnancy. He served as coeditor of the *Archiv für Gynäkologie;* completed and edited Michaelis' monumental work, *Das Enge Becken;* and published a number of books of his own, including a textbook of obstetrics, one on gynecology, and several monographs on the normal and contracted pelvis.

His *Die Formen des Beckens,*[4] one of the classics of obstetric literature, contains in its very first paragraph one of the most lucid and succinct interpretive descriptions of the female pelvis ever written:

The pelvis fulfills more extensive functions in the female body than in the male. In the female it forms not merely the bony foundation of the trunk . . . to which strong and numerous muscles are attached, but also shelters the largest part of the sexual apparatus in addition to the distal end of the intestinal canal and urinary passages, and thereby assumes great importance in reproduction. In addition to admitting the male organ during coitus, it has to provide space for the whole uterus at the beginning of pregnancy, and later for expansion of the lower uterine segment at least, and at birth a passageway into the outer world for the mature fetus together with its membranes. Nature has understood how to satisfy, in an amazing manner, the diverse and to some degree contradictory demands with which she is thus confronted. She has imparted the necessary firmness to the pelvis with maximal economy in bony substance by giving it an annular shape and supporting its joints with powerful ligaments, but amassing larger concentrations of bone only in the regions exposed directly to pressure. She has placed the canal that opens at the lowermost part of the trunk in such a position that the pelvis can maintain the burden of the abdominal viscera and provide support and purchase for the enclosed organs, by inclining the pelvis anteriorly at a sharp angle to the horizon, bending its axis in a curve convex posteriorly, and covering and finishing its walls with contractile and elastic soft parts; and in this way also achieving adequate capacity and dilatability for the act of birth. However, the space is so proportioned that even a relatively slight deviation from its normal size can interfere with delivery, insofar as a correspondingly more favorable condition in the remaining birth factors does not compensate for the difficulties.

This monograph has become increasingly scarce in the nearly 100 years since its publication, the present author's being one of the few known copies remaining.

REFERENCES

1. Caldwell, W. E.; Moloy, H. C.; and D'Esopo, D. A.: A roentgenologic study of the mechanism of engagement of the fetal head. *Am. J. Obst. & Gynec.,* **28**:824–41, 1934.

2. Fuhrmann, W.: Zur Lehre von der Wendung auf die Füsse bei engem Becken. *Berl. klin. Wchnschr.,* **5**:95–97, 107–10, 119–21, 150–54, 167–70, 1868.

3. Hecker, C., and Buhl, L.: *Klinik der Geburtskunde.* Engelmann, Leipzig, 1861.

4. Litzmann, C. C. T.: *Die Formen des Beckens, insbesondere des Engen Weiblichen Beckens, nach Eigenen Beobachtungen und Untersuchungen, nebst einem Anhange über die Osteomalacie.* G. Reimer, Berlin, 1861.

5. Litzmann, C. C. T.: Ueber die hintere Scheitelbeinstellung, eine nicht seltene Art von fehlerhafter Einstellung des Kopfes unter der Geburt. *Arch. f. Gynäk.,* **2**:433–40, 1871.

6. Litzmann, C. C. T.: Zur Feststellung der Indicationen für die Gastrotomie bei Schwangerschaft ausserhalb der Gebärmutter. *Arch. f. Gynäk.,* **16**:323–401, 1880.

7. Michaelis, G. A.: Ausnahmen von der Regel. *Neue Ztschr. f. Geburtsh.,* **4**:361–89, 1836.

8. Naegele, F. C.: Ueber den Mechanismus der Geburt. *Deutsche Arch. f. d. Physiol.,* **5**:483–531, 1819.

9. Scanzoni, F. W.: *Lehrbuch der Geburtshilfe,* 2nd ed. Seidel, Vienna, 1853, p. 648.

10. Werth, R.: Zum Gedächtnisse Litzmann's. *Arch. f. Gynäk.,* **38**:177–98, 1890.

Ludwig Bandl and Bandl's Ring

CHAPTER 38

Recent technologic advances in the study of uterine contractility during labor have led to renewed appreciation of the essential functional difference between the fundal myometrium and that of the lower uterine segment. Normal labor is characterized by uterine contractions that begin earlier, develop greater intensity, and are sustained longer in the fundus than in the lower segment. This fundal dominance, coupled with the myometrial property of retraction, results in a progressively widening disparity between the upper and lower uterine wall, the former increasing in thickness at the expense of the latter.

In May, 1870, an expectant mother in Austria, despairing of life, committed suicide by drowning herself after labor had begun. Granted permission for an autopsy, Ludwig Bandl, a young graduate student in obstetrics, exposed the pelvic contents by sawing the body sagittally in half after first freezing it solid. Clearly visible was a muscular ring encircling the lower part of the uterus and demarcating the fundus from the lower uterine segment. Bandl spent the next five years in the study of this and related phenomena, his efforts resulting in two major additions to the obstetric literature and a full explanation of the retraction ring between the upper and lower uterine segments, soon to be known as "Bandl's ring."

BANDL'S DESCRIPTION OF RETRACTION RING

The first of Bandl's principal contributions appeared in 1875 in the guise of a monograph on uterine rupture, *Über Ruptur der Gebärmutter*,[1] by far

314

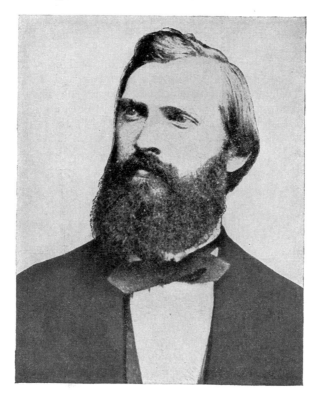

Fig. 38–1. Ludwig Bandl (1842–1892).

the best treatment this important subject had yet received. Here Bandl pointed out for the first time the passive nature of the lower uterine segment in labor, explained the predilection of spontaneous rupture for this part of the uterus, and called attention to the ominous prognostic significance of a pathologic retraction ring. His concept of the mechanism of uterine rupture is well illustrated in a case report taken from his monograph. The patient was a 34-year-old para 5 with a true conjugate of 9 cm.

She came to the hospital at 12:30 A.M., July 28, 1874, 15 hours after rupture of the membranes and 48 hours after the onset of labor. She was extremely exhausted, her pulse was rapid, and her face had the same pained and apprehensive expression that I have always seen in association with uterine rupture. The upper parts of the uterus were uniformly hard, the lower somewhat softer. A shallow, transverse furrow, an inch below the umbilicus, indicated the boundary between the uterine corpus and the cervix. The very attenuated uterus deviated somewhat to the right, and the head and shoulders were partly palpable through the abdominal wall, covered only by a very thin layer. I therefore thought of a beginning rupture. On internal examination I found the face presenting in the first position [L.M.A.], in midpelvis. The cervix, dilated 2.5 cm and a thumb thick, was palpable posteriorly; it was visible, bluish-red, on separation of the labia. After a vain attempt with forceps, I performed craniotomy and extracted an infant weighing 3780 gm.

In my subsequent examination I found the internal os at the level of the umbilicus. The whole cervix was uniformly paper-thin and enormously stretched out, so that it must surely have contained half the infant, while the body of the uterus and the fundus sat on the infant like a cap. The anterior wall of the cervix measured about 20 cm, 4 cm of which was taken up by the intravaginal part; the posterior wall measured 16 cm. . . . The conditions in this case were obviously

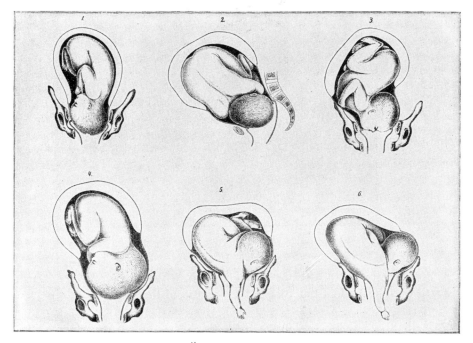

Fig. 38-2. Plate from Bandl's *Über Ruptur der Gebärmutter*,[1] showing normal *(1)* and pathologic *(2-6)* retraction rings.

most favorable for rupture of the uterus, as Plate III, Figure 3 [Fig. 38-2] shows. It would have taken only one or two additional contractions of the uterus or the increased pressure of the physician's hand or an instrument to bring it about. . . .

Discussing the clinical findings that portend uterine rupture, Bandl subsequently added:

Of late I have always succeeded in tracing the development of these relations. The internal os can be seen rising higher and higher and the cervix being stretched out more and more. . . . In a borderline or contracted pelvis, if the head is at a high station with its greatest circumference near the inlet, and the external os is palpable behind the pubic arch and only 2–3 cm dilated, then the internal os is already almost midway between the symphysis and umbilicus. If labor continues . . . pathologic stretching of the cervix occurs, with the uterine musculature extending farther and farther above the infant's head. When the cervix is elongated and stretched over the head (also in shoulder presentation) and the uterine musculature retracts to the opposite side, the conditions for rupture have developed.

In 1876, only a year after the publication of his book on uterine rupture, another monograph by Bandl appeared, attempting to clarify the relations between the uterine corpus and cervix during pregnancy and labor.[2] Confusion and disagreement had characterized pre-existing views. The anatomists of the seventeenth and early-eighteenth century, from de Graaf on, had taught that the cervix remains unchanged to the very end of pregnancy. Baudelocque, on the other hand, held the sharply contrasting view that by the end of pregnancy nothing remains of the cervix but the small ring of the external os; the cervical canal being gone, incorporated into the common cavity of the uterus. In 1839 Kilian, in his textbook of obstetrics,[6] called attention to the shortening and thickening of the vaginal part of the cervix in pregnancy, but his views were lost sight of in the welter of conflicting statements. Isaac Taylor,[8] after a thorough review of the subject in 1862, concluded:

From the investigations made during life, at various periods of pregnancy, at full term, and during the first stage of labor, and on post-mortem examinations, [it appears that] the cervix uteri does not undergo any shortening or expansion of the supra or infra-vaginal portion, but retains its whole length, and only becomes expanded or dilated at the commencement of labor, the cervix serving as an intermediate channel, or canal, between the body of the uterus and the vagina; this dilatation is effected through the combined operation of the softened condition of the neck, and by the pressure of the liquor amnii and the descent of the child's head or body, the internal os being the first to yield. The expansion thus beginning slowly, tends downwards towards the external os, and then the walls of the cervix are gradually expanded and unfolded for the passage or exit of the child; no better or more perfect illustration can be adduced, than the gradual expansion of the horse's anus during an evacuation, and its contraction after an evacuation occurs.

With but a few exceptions, all students of the subject adhered to the belief that the internal os opens only with the onset of labor.

Confusion was compounded by disagreement over the nature of the internal os. Two concepts emerged: (1) that the internal os is characterized by a palpable ridge or ledge at the upper end of the cervical canal (obstetric internal os of Braune); and (2) that it is defined by the upper end of the cervical mucosa (histologic internal os of Müller). Bandl brought both concepts into the same perspective, as he explained the formation of the lower uterine segment:

The pressure of the ovum and the weight of the fetus usually bring about its formation by the eighth lunar month. In primigravidas the process can be detected only by vaginal examination, for in these patients one can usually enter the cavity of the uterus for the first time in the last eight days to three weeks of pregnancy, in a third of the cases only with the onset of labor. The gradual disappearance of the supravaginal part of the cervix and the retraction of its walls to the lower uterine segment can be detected, however, through the walls of the vagina. . . . In such circumstances the upper boundary of the cervical mucosa, Müller's ring, is frequently drawn out by the presenting ovum into a delicate membrane with a very small opening, often scarcely palpable. The term "hymen uteri" is more appropriate than "sphincter uteri" for this line of demarcation. . . .

If one penetrates this opening with his finger he finds that Müller's ring lies at almost the same level as the internal os of Braune under these conditions, but between them the lower uterine segment is already present, thinner walled and softer than the walls of the corpus and cervix. On further descent of the membranes or the presenting part of the fetus a very simple process occurs: the fine-seamed line of demarcation, closed or slightly dilated, is forced outward by the membranes or the fetal part, and the muscle layers of the cervix are transformed into the lower uterine segment. . . . The lower uterine segment grows progressively longer at the expense of the cervix. . . . Now even if the Hippocratic theory is not correct, that the child delivers itself through its own active efforts, the view of the older physicians, Aristotle, Aetius, and Avicenna . . . that the weight of the infant is a factor in labor, contains much truth, for the formation of the lower uterine segment depends upon the pressure of the ovum, and, in slight measure, upon the weight of the infant also. . . . [All obstetricians are aware of the tendency of polyhydramnios and of multiple pregnancy to bring about early development of the lower uterine segment, dilatation of the cervix, and premature labor.]

In multigravidas the formation of the lower uterine segment and the associated changes in the cervix can be detected more easily, because one can often insert a finger into the uterus four to eight weeks from term. . . .

If the cervix admits a finger, but is still intact, then one can readily detect its beginning dilatation and the formation of the lower uterine segment six, eight, or ten weeks before the onset of labor. . . . Above the internal os a small trough forms, becoming large enough in a few days to accommodate a nut. One gets the impression that Müller's ring has dilated, but it actually lies more or less closed in the floor of the little trough; and the longer the walls of the latter grow, the less prominent and palpable Müller's ring becomes. The rim of the little trough moves progressively outward, while being drawn more and more away from the floor and into the lower uterine segment, as a result of softening and elongation. As it moves laterally the rim finally touches the lower end of the corpus, the internal os of Braune. Without any palpable stretching of its walls the little trough thus gets progressively larger, so that the fetal head eventually finds room in it. In this way the upper closed, or slightly dilated, boundary of the mucosal canal is removed progressively farther from the lower boundary of the corpus uteri.

Figure 7 [Fig. 38-3] shows the intact cervix diagrammatically in the dotted

Fig. 7.

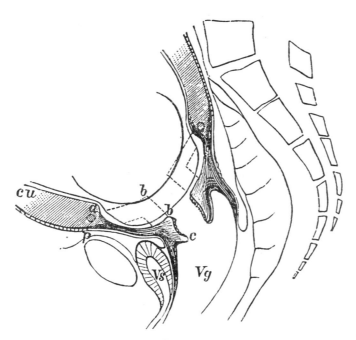

Fig. 38-3. Illustration from Bandl's *Über das Verhalten des Uterus und Cervix in der Schwangerschaft und während der Geburt,*[2] showing his concept of the relations between the cervix and lower uterine segment, *b*, histologic internal os; *a*, retraction ring.

lines, and in the solid lines its relation to the lower uterine segment, as these structures are usually encountered quite readily in multiparas three to four weeks before the onset of labor. . . .

In labor, therefore, the internal os of Braune became the retraction ring to which Bandl devoted a large part of his attention and which is now named for him. Bandl attached special significance to its external abdominal manifestations. He wrote:

No indication is to be found of a boundary in the uterus as long as all factors are working together normally to deliver the infant, for the corpus uteri and the lower segment then comprise a coordinated muscle mass.

If resistance at the pelvic floor is too great, however, manifestations soon appear, indicating that the whole labor mechanism is disturbed and is beginning to function abnormally. Contours of the corpus uteri and of the lower segment become visible and palpable on the abdominal wall. This clearly results from the fact that the stronger corpus uteri contracts its cavity and thickens its walls while emptying a large part of its amniotic fluid and a larger part of the fetus into the weaker lower uterine segment and upper vagina than normally. . . .

After the contours of the corpus and lower segment once become visible, the uterus often begins to deviate during a contraction—usually toward the side opposite from the occiput, while the lower segment rises upward over the pubic inlet. . . . The organ continues to contract even under such conditions . . . but the contractions have acquired a pathologic character; and the forces no longer work toward the expulsion of the fetus, since the components of the forces have become uncoordinated.

BANDL'S LIFE

Ludwig Bandl was born November 1, 1842, in Himberg, Southern Austria.[3] He studied medicine in Vienna under Hyrtl and Carl Braun, and in 1878 was made director of the women's division of the Vienna Poliklinik. Two years later he received an appointment as extraordinary professor of gynecology in the university of the same city. In 1886 he was called to Prague as ordinary professor of obstetrics and gynecology, to fill the chair recently vacated by Breisky. Bandl's colleagues in the United States were saddened, only a few months later, to read his obituary in the *American Journal of Obstetrics*.[4] In a subsequent issue of the same journal, however, the following item [5] appeared:

Prof. Ludwig Bandl, whose obituary appeared in the January number, is not dead, after all. His sudden, unexpected illness (melancholia) soon after his arrival in Prague originated the report of his death, and caused the publication of his obituary in a German contemporary, and from the latter in this Journal. We are much gratified to hear that he is in a fair way to recover and resume his labors, and congratulate him on the unusual distinction of being able to read his own obituary.

A brief note in the *Wiener Medizinische Wochenschrift* [7] added a few details:

The newly named professor of gynecology in Prague, Dr. Bandl, was hard hit by a tragic fate at the beginning of his course of lectures. Bandl feared, it was reported, that he would not measure up to his new and great duties, especially since he would have to compete with the memory of such an outstanding predecessor. Anxiety finally assumed such proportions in this man, who had already been nervous for some time, that when he was to give his inaugural lecture his strength forsook him at the last moment. . . .

Bandl retired to the home of his parents in Krems, but was later admitted to the psychiatric institution in Döbling, where he died on August 26, 1892.

REFERENCES

1. Bandl, L.: *Über Ruptur der Gebärmutter unde ihre Mechanik.* Czermak, Vienna, 1875.

2. Bandl, L.: *Über das Verhalten des Uterus und Cervix in der Schwangerschaft und während der Geburt. Nach klinischen Beobachtungen und anatomischen Untersuchungen.* Enke, Stuttgart, 1876.

3. Dohrn, R.: *Geschichte der Geburtshülfe der Neuzeit.* Part 1 (1840–1860). Pietzcker, Tübingen, 1903, pp. 92–93.

4. Grandin, E. H.: In memoriam. Ludwig Bandl. *Am. J. Obst.,* **20**:46–48, 1887.

5. Item: *Am. J. Obst.,* **20**:224, 1887.

6. Kilian, H. F.: *Die Geburtslehre von Seiten der Wissenschaft und Kunst dargestellt,* 2nd ed. Varrentrapp, Frankfurt-am-Main, 1847, Vol. 1, pp. 173–76.

7. Notizen: *Wien. med. Wchnschr.,* **36**:1488, 1886.

8. Taylor, I. E.: On the non-shortening of the supra and infra-vaginal portion of the cervix uteri up to the end of pregnancy. *Am. M. Times,* **4**:342–47, 1862.

Alexandre Couvelaire and Uteroplacental Apoplexy*

The writer of one of Alexandre Couvelaire's obituaries,[4] in order to emphasize the originality of his subject's observations, stated that even in Germany one would someday speak of the "maladie de Couvelaire." These lines, written about a French patriot shortly after World War II, were intended to stress the importance of Couvelaire's studies on premature separation of the placenta and the universality of the term *Couvelaire uterus*.

In one of his papers on uteroplacental apoplexy,[2] Couvelaire referred to a few previous authors who had already noted, at cesarean section or autopsy, subserosal ecchymoses in the uteri of patients with premature separation of the placenta. The characteristics of the Couvelaire uterus remained unrecognized, however, although this condition was undoubtedly responsible for many of the secondary hemorrhages requiring postpartum hysterectomy in patients with placental abruption. The cataclysmic and extensive hemorrhage into the myometrium, ovaries, broad ligaments, and pelvic peritoneum that occasionally accompany this accident were described for the first time in a detailed case report by Couvelaire in 1911.[1]

* This chapter originally published in *Obst. & Gynec.*, **9**:740–43, 1957; reprinted by permission. Copyright © 1957, by the American College of Obstetricians and Gynecologists.

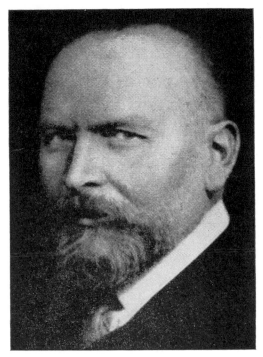

Fig. 39-1. Alexandre Couvelaire (1873–1948). (Reproduced from *Gynéc. et obst.*, **47**:603, 1948.)

COUVELAIRE'S REPORT ON UTEROPLACENTAL HEMORRHAGE

The patient was a 26-year-old primigravida with toxemia of pregnancy who developed signs of retroplacental hemorrhage in the eighth month. Despite artificial rupture of the membranes her condition worsened. The cervix failed to dilate; the uterus, ligneous in consistency, continued to enlarge, and shock rapidly ensued. Although the fetus was known to be dead, as judged by the absence of its heart sounds, Couvelaire undertook to empty the uterus by cesarean section in order to control the retroplacental bleeding. The placenta was found completely separated, the uterine cavity full of blood. Not only was the surface of the uterus covered with subserosal hemorrhages but the myometrium itself, the broad ligaments, and the adnexa appeared to be completely infiltrated with blood. Because of this, Couvelaire elected to perform hysterectomy and bilateral salpingo-oophorectomy. The patient recovered. Couvelaire's description of the specimen employed the term *uteroplacental apoplexy* for the first time and accurately pictured the hemorrhagic extravasations which have been recognized ever since as the characteristic lesion of the Couvelaire uterus.

The lesions observed during the course of the operation and later on histologic examination could not be exactly characterized by the classic term retroplacental hematoma.

The bloody infiltration was not localized at the placenta and decidua serotina. The whole utero-ovarian apparatus seemed covered with blackish splotches. The uterine wall, in the zone of membranous insertion as well as the zone of placental insertion, was the site of a tremendous bloody infiltration separating the muscle bundles and dissociating some of them fiber from fiber [Fig. 39-2]. The ovaries were peppered with a punctiform bloody suffusion. The broad ligaments were infiltrated with blood.

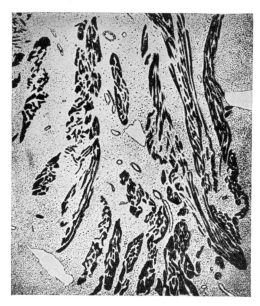

Fig. 39-2. Illustration from Couvelaire's paper.[1] Section of uterus, showing dissociation of muscle bundles by hemorrhage into myometrium. (Reproduction by permission of Masson & Cie, Paris.)

This was indeed a true case of *uteroplacental apoplexy*. One could do no better than to compare the appearance of these lesions with that of ovarian cysts with a twisted pedicle. However, no analogous position of the pregnant uterus was observed during the operation. The uterus was tilted slightly to the right and dextrorotated, as is usual during pregnancy.

Histologic examination did not reveal any lesion in the walls of the blood vessels to explain their bursting.

These lesions made it extremely unwise to conserve the uterus and sufficed in themselves to justify hysterectomy.

Couvelaire concluded his paper with these recommendations:

1. The anatomic state of the uterine wall alone can make hysterectomy necessary.

2. A desire to preserve reproductive function cannot in itself serve as an a priori argument in favor of conservative surgery.

3. Surgery must be rapid and provide the maximum degree of security with respect to hemostasis during and after the operation.

For all these reasons, it seems to me that for the severe cases in which utero-placental hemorrhage clearly dictates surgical treatment, it is wisest to operate by the abdominal route; it is most prudent to perform a Porro cesarean section, an operation which is absolutely indicated when the uterine walls are infiltrated with blood.

For four decades Couvelaire's therapeutic recommendations occupied a prominent place in obstetric practice. In the light of modern knowledge of blood coagulation, however, and with the present-day availability of blood for transfusion, blood substitutes, and fibrinogen, they seem unnecessarily radical. Certain it is that Couvelaire's teachings have saved many maternal lives; it is equally certain that they have been responsible for the needless removal of many uteri.

COUVELAIRE'S LIFE

Alexandre Couvelaire was born in Bourg, France, in 1873, the son of a professor.[6] Early in his professional life he came under the influence of Varnier and later was accepted as an assistant to Pinard. Each of these distinguished French obstetricians exerted a characteristic and permanent influence on the sensitive, impressionable Couvelaire. From Varnier he obtained an appreciation of scientific method and precision of thought; from Pinard, a feeling for the social, humanitarian, and public health aspects of obstetrics.

Couvelaire spent his entire professional life in the Baudelocque Clinic, where he was made chief of clinic in 1901 and from which he did not retire until October 1, 1943. In 1914 he was appointed professor in the University of Paris and was later elected president of the Société d'Obstétrique et de Gynécologie.

In addition to his studies on placental abruption, Couvelaire is best known for the special dispensary he organized, together with Marcel Pinard, for the antisyphilitic treatment of pregnant patients, and for his establishment of a special pavilion for tuberculous women in his obstetric clinic, each of these units long serving as a model. Couvelaire was especially accomplished in obstetric surgery and in 1913 published a magnificently illustrated book, *Introduction à la Chirurgie Utérine Obstétricale,*[3] in which his obstetric teachings are set forth. In addition to his radical therapy for premature separation of the placenta, Couvelaire was one of the pioneers in the use of cesarean section for certain cases of placenta previa.

Couvelaire went into seclusion following the German occupation of France, and after a long illness, died on March 14, 1948.[5] During his active career he was probably the dominant figure in French obstetrics.

REFERENCES

1. Couvelaire, A.: Traitement chirurgical des hémorrhagies utéro-placentaires avec décollement du placenta normalement inséré. *Ann. de Gynéc.,* **8**:591–608, 1911.

2. Couvelaire, A.: Deux nouvelles observations d'apopléxie utéro-placentaire (hémorrhagies rétro-placentaires avec infiltration sanguine de la paroi musculaire de l'utérus). *Ann. de Gynéc.,* **9**:486–95, 1912.

3. Couvelaire, A.: *Introduction à la Chirurgie Utérine Obstétricale.* G. Steinheil, Paris, 1913.

4. Lacomme, M.: Alexandre Couvelaire (1873–1948). *Gynéc. et Obst.,* **47**:603–12, 1948.

5. Lepage, F.: Alexandre Couvelaire (1873–1948). *Paris méd.,* **38**:181, 1948.

6. Portes, W.: Alexandre Couvelaire. *Bull. Acad. nat. méd.,* **132**:341–47, 1948.

Thomas Denman, John Douglas, and Spontaneous Evolution of the Fetus

CHAPTER

40

A transverse lie, or cross birth, comprises the least favorable of all possible positions of the fetus for spontaneous delivery. Unless skilled intervention is forthcoming, the infant has almost no chance of survival; without obstetric help the mother too may perish. The devices often resorted to by ignorant eighteenth-century midwives, in their frantic but futile efforts to rectify Nature's mistake, are well illustrated in one of Smellie's case reports: [8]

In the year 1742, being called to a watchman's wife, the midwife told me, that the waters had come off in a large quantity, on which the arm was forced down into the birth, and the hand appeared without the external parts: she had tried different methods, to make the child . . . withdraw up its hand into the womb, and change itself into the natural position; dipping its hand in a bason of cold water; and also in vinegar and brandy; but finding these trials fail, she had recourse to the last remedy, before any assistance from a man practitioner was thought necessary: she directed the woman's husband to take hold of her legs over his shoulders, and lift up her body three times, with her back to his, and her head downwards; being of opinion, that although the former methods failed of success, this would answer expectation.

SPONTANEOUS EVOLUTION OF DENMAN

In extraordinary circumstances Nature herself, as though reluctant to admit her error, and through the rarest of labor mechanisms, may accomplish the

327

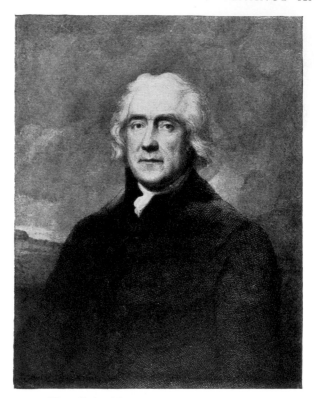

Fig. 40-1. Thomas Denman (1733–1815).

spontaneous birth of an infant who, either because of neglect or obstetric failure, has maintained its uncorrected transverse position within the uterus throughout labor. Such a birth process, termed spontaneous evolution, was first described by Thomas Denman in a letter to a Dr. Simmons, dated December 7, 1783, and published in the *London Medical Journal* the following year.[1] In this note Denman communicated his observations of three cases, in each of which the infant was born dead:

Case I. In the year 1772, I was called to a poor woman in Oxford-street, who had been in labour all the preceding night under the care of a midwife. Mr. Kingston, now living in Charlotte-street, and Mr. Goodwin, surgeon, at Wirksworth, in Derbyshire, who were at that time students in midwifery, had been sent for, some hours before I was called. The arm of the child presenting, they attempted to turn and extract it by the feet, but the pains were so strong as to prevent the introduction of the hand into the uterus. I found the arm much swelled and pushed through the external parts in such a manner, that the shoulder nearly reached the perinaeum. The woman struggled vehemently with her pains, and during their continuance, I perceived the shoulder of the child to descend.

Concluding that the child was small and would pass, doubled, through the pelvis, I desired one of the gentlemen to sit down to receive it, but the friends of the woman would not permit me to move. I remained by the bed-side till the child was expelled, and I was very much surprised to find, that the breech and inferior extremities were expelled before the head, as if the case had originally been a presentation of the inferior extremities. . . .

Case II. In the year 1773, I was called to a woman in Castle-street, Oxford-market, who was attended by a midwife. Many hours after it was discovered that the arm of the child presented. Mr. Burosse, surgeon, in Poland-street, was sent for, and I was called into consultation. When I examined, I found the shoulder of the child pressed into the superior aperture of the pelvis. The pains were strong and returned at short intervals. Having agreed upon the necessity of turning the child and extracting it by the feet, I sat down and made repeated attempts to raise the shoulder, with all the force which I thought could be safely used; but the action of the uterus was so powerful that I was obliged to desist. I then called to mind the circumstances of the case before related, mentioned them to Mr. Burosse, and proposed that we should wait for the effect which a continuance of the pains might produce, or till they were abated, when the child might be turned with less difficulty. No further attempts were made to turn the child. Then every pain propelled it lower into the pelvis, and in little more than one hour the child was born, the breech being expelled, as in the first case. . . .

Case III. January the 2d, 1774, I was called to Mrs. D——, who keeps a toy-shop in Crown-court, Windmill-street. She had been a long time in labour, and the arm of the child presented.

The late Mr. Eustace had been called on the preceding evening, and had made attempts to turn the child, which he had continued for several hours without success. I was sent for about one o'clock in the morning, and on examination found the arm pushed through the external parts, the shoulder pressing firmly upon the perinaeum. The exertions of the mother were wonderfully strong. I sat down while she had two pains, by the latter of which the child was doubled and the breech expelled. I extracted the shoulders and head, and left the child in the bed. . . .

In all these cases, the women were at the full period of utero-gestation, and the children were of the usual size.

Intrigued by the unprecedented sequence of events he had witnessed, Denman began, soon after the first case, to include a discussion of this phenomenon in his lectures; and his aphorisms, printed for the use of his students in 1773, pointed out the circumstances in which "the knowledge of the fact might be rendered useful in practice; but with great circumspection." Similar cases were soon brought to his attention, through personal communications from his colleagues. He said:

Other cases of the same kind have occurred to me, and with the histories of several, varying in the time or manner in which the evolution of the child was made, I have lately been favoured by gentlemen of eminence in the profession.

But these are sufficient to prove the fact, that in cases in which children present with the arm, women will not necessarily die undelivered, although they are not assisted by art.

By 1784 Denman had been informed of about 30 such cases, in addition to the three he had attended personally; and in one, a case of a Dr. Garthshore, the child was born alive. Soon thereafter he learned from Mr. Martineau, a surgeon at Norwich, of another such case with live birth of the infant.[2]

The mechanism of spontaneous evolution is described by Denman, albeit not very precisely, in his *Introduction to the Practice of Midwifery:* [2]

As to the manner in which this evolution takes place, I presume, that after the long continued action of the *uterus,* the body of the child is brought into such a compacted state, as to receive the full force of every returning action. The body in its doubled state, being too large to pass through the *pelvis,* and the *uterus* pressing upon its inferior extremities, which are the only parts capable of being moved, they are forced gradually lower, till the body turning as it were upon its own axis, the breech of the child is expelled, as in an original presentation of that part. Nor has there been any thing uncommon in the size or form of the *pelvis* of those women to whom this case has happened, nor have the children been small, or softened by putrefaction. . . . I believe on the contrary that a child of a common size, living or but lately dead, in such a state as to possess some degree of resilition, is the best calculated for expulsion in this manner. . . .

The time required for the spontaneous evolution of the child, and the facility with which it may be made, will depend upon a variety of circumstances, but chiefly upon the size of the child, the aptitude of its position, the dimensions of the *pelvis,* and the power exerted by the *uterus.* If the child be very large, or much below the common size, the slower I believe will be the evolution, nor can it be made at all without a strong action of the *uterus.*

Most obstetricians have felt that Denman held an unduly optimistic view of the expectation of spontaneous evolution in cases of neglected transverse lie. Indeed, Michael Ryan, in his editorial preface to Denman's *Aphorisms* [3] stated that "he [Ryan] has, on some occasions, differed from the text, as on spontaneous evolution, which all modern Obstetricians consider as the only objectionable and untenable part of Dr. Denman's valuable productions."

DENMAN'S LIFE

Thomas Denman was born in Bakewell, England, June 27, 1733, the third of eight children of the village apothecary.[5,9] At the age of 21 he set out for London, to attend the lectures in anatomy at St. George's Hospital, but his education was interrupted after six months by the exhaustion of his funds.

He thereupon signed on as ship's mate and spent the next nine years roaming the high seas, serving variously as mate and as surgeon on a number of vessels of different types, including fighting ships. In his wanderings he saw much adventure, including the capture of French ships, from the sale of which he shared the proceeds. After participating in the successful siege of Havana in 1762, Denman determined to resume his medical studies, and in 1763 he returned to England, to pursue further lectures in anatomy and midwifery. He entered practice in Winchester but returned to London after four months because of his failure to earn expenses. In 1764, after receiving his medical degree from Aberdeen, he re-entered practice, but again met with little success. While pondering his next move he entered seriously into the study of midwifery and published two papers, an *Essay on Puerperal Fever* and a pamphlet on *Construction and Use of Vapour Baths.* This seems to have been the turning point of his professional career, for he soon found himself in possession of a modest practice and a respectable reputation. In 1769 Denman was appointed physician man-midwife to the Middlesex Hospital, and the following year, in partnership with a fellow student from St. George's Hospital, he bought some second-hand equipment and began to give lectures in midwifery. After the death of William Hunter in 1783, Denman succeeded him as the leading figure in the field and was admitted as first licentiate in midwifery in the Royal College of Physicians. As his practice rapidly grew and the demands for his services increased, he began to limit himself more and more to the role of consultant. Eventually he took his son-in-law, Richard Croft (later Sir Richard), into practice with him. Denman died on November 25, 1815, at the age of 82.

Although his name is attached particularly to spontaneous evolution of the fetus, Denman's description of this rare phenomenon does not rank in importance with some of his other contributions to the science of obstetrics. He gave the first good description of snuffles in congenital syphilis and an early account of membranous dysmenorrhea. He was among the first to suggest that puerperal fever was a contagion and that the physician was responsible for its dissemination. He urged the conservative treatment of eclampsia and warned against forcible efforts at delivery in its management. He was one of the first to resort to premature delivery of patients with contracted pelvis, but never entered into much discussion of this practice, assuming it to be generally known.[7] His most important writings were his *Aphorisms* and his *Introduction to the Practice of Midwifery,* each of which went into many editions. The third edition of the latter has been referred to as "the most splendid work on midwifery in the English language, whether regarded from the point of view of the format, paper, printing and illustrations of the work; the learning and knowledge it exhibits; or the ordered, lucid, and judicial manner in which that knowledge is presented." [9]

Thomas Denman will always be remembered as the most conservative of obstetricians. He neither personally performed nor even witnessed a cesarean section. His obstetric philosophy is clearly expressed in his own words:

> In the most perfect state of society, all just and true knowledge being founded upon observation of the proceedings of Nature, and all sound practice upon the imitation, the practitioner would return to the primitive state; that is, he would do nothing unless it was absolutely necessary for him to act, and then he would act in imitation of Nature. From a retrospective view of the practice of midwifery in all former times, and in all countries, every intelligent person sees, and is ready to acknowledge, that there has been too officious an interposition, and too great a readiness to give assistance in various ways, for the relief of many difficulties attending parturition, which are not only fully proved to require no assistance, but which are also now allowed to be surmounted in a safer and more effectual way by the resources of the constitution. This should certainly put us upon our guard against hasty determinations upon what is possible or otherwise, or upon the use of any means which may be destructive to the child, or injurious to the mother. . . . The abuse of art produces more and greater evils than are occasioned by all the imperfections of Nature.[2]

SPONTANEOUS EVOLUTION OF DOUGLAS

Among the contemporaries of Denman who soon witnessed additional cases of spontaneous birth of an infant from the transverse lie was a young Irish obstetrician, John C. Douglas. Douglas saw his first case of spontaneous evolution in 1810, while a resident-assistant in the Dublin Lying-in Hospital. His observations in two additional cases soon thereafter led him to the publication of a pamphlet in 1811, purporting to correct Denman's views on the subject. Unfortunately, as Douglas later admitted, this paper "was too hastily written and not free from error." The high feeling generated by his tactless statements took long to subside, as evidenced in a commentary by one of Douglas' biographers,[6] written four decades later: ". . . It is to be regretted that the author did not confine himself simply to its announcement. From an exaggerated idea of the practical importance of his discovery, he hazarded some conjectures which incurred severe reprehension, and which would, doubtless, have consigned to oblivion any work of less real merit."

Lesser men than Denman would have taken umbrage at the unbridled criticism contained in Douglas' pamphlet. The gentle, kindly Denman, however, now 78 years old, instead of quarreling, sent Douglas a disarmingly gracious letter, which Douglas published as a preface to the revised version of his essay.[4] "For my own part," wrote Denman, "I am so far from taking offence by any freedom of criticism you have used regarding what I had written on the subject of the evolution, that I feel obliged by what you have said upon it, in terms sufficiently flattering."

By the time of his more temperate and carefully worded report of 1819

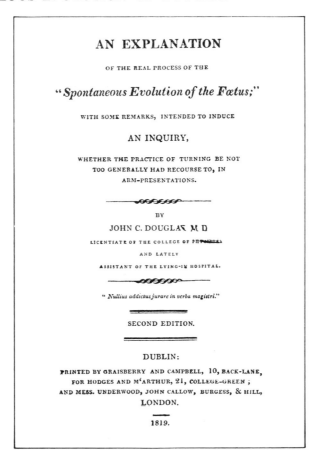

AN EXPLANATION

OF THE REAL PROCESS OF THE

"*Spontaneous Evolution of the Fœtus;*"

WITH SOME REMARKS, INTENDED TO INDUCE

AN INQUIRY,

WHETHER THE PRACTICE OF TURNING BE NOT
TOO GENERALLY HAD RECOURSE TO, IN
ARM-PRESENTATIONS.

BY
JOHN C. DOUGLAS M D
LICENTIATE OF THE COLLEGE OF PHYSICIANS
AND LATELY
ASSISTANT OF THE LYING-IN HOSPITAL.

" *Nullius addictus jurare in verba magistri.*"

SECOND EDITION.

DUBLIN:
PRINTED BY GRAISBERRY AND CAMPBELL, 10, BACK-LANE,
FOR HODGES AND M'ARTHUR, 21, COLLEGE-GREEN ;
AND MESS. UNDERWOOD, JOHN CALLOW, BURGESS, & HILL,
LONDON.

1819.

Fig. 40-2. Title page of Douglas' revised edition of his pamphlet on spontaneous evolution.

Douglas had seen four more cases of spontaneous evolution, making a total of seven. The mechanism of birth as explained by him has since been known as the spontaneous evolution of Douglas. Its essential difference from Denman's mechanism is pointed out in Douglas' own words:

The only inference which I conceive can be drawn from Doctor Denman's theoretical explanation . . . is,—that the shoulder of the child, after having been impacted into the *pelvis* by a series of uterine actions, each successive action forcing it lower and lower; that subsequently, after some indistinct period of time, repetitions of the same propelling power, instead of producing a furtherance of the same effect, should cause another part of the child, namely the breech, to descend, and to occupy the place where the shoulder had been; and, that the shoulder should, by some miraculous effort, at the same moment recede again into the *uterus,* and take possession of the place from which the breech had just been propelled. Or, to speak briefly,—that the breech higher up in the *uterus,* and the shoulder lower down in the *pelvis,* had, by an unexpected uterine effort, changed places.

Now it seems to me incompatible with all received ideas of uterine action to suppose that the *uterus,* when contracting so powerfully as to force down that part of the child which was at its *fundus,* should, at the same moment, form a vacuum, into which another portion, already low down in the *pelvis,* should recede.

The fact however is—that the shoulder and thorax, thus low and impacted, instead of receding into the *uterus,* are, at each successive pain, forced still lower, until the ribs of that side, corresponding with the protruded arms, press on the *perinaeum,* and cause it to assume the same form as it would by the pressure of the forehead in a natural labour. At this period not only the entire arm, but the shoulder, can be perceived externally, with the clavicle laying under the arch of the *pubis.* By further uterine contractions, the ribs are forced more forward, appearing at the *os externum,* as the vertex would in a natural labour; the *clavicle* having been, by degrees, forced round on the anterior part of the *pubis,* with the *acromion* looking towards the *mons veneris.*

In contrast to his brash criticism of Denman, Douglas now showed himself capable of a more balanced evaluation of the problem, adopting an almost conciliatory attitude toward the old gentleman:

. . . In the early stage of such a labour, the trunk of the *foetus* is nearly perpendicular, with respect to the axis of the *pelvis;* but as it descends through the *pelvis,* it gradually approaches to the horizontal; and immediately previous to its expulsion, it lays exactly horizontal, with respect to the *os externum.* So, in fact, there is a process somewhat (although not exactly) similar to the theoretical one of Dr. Denman, but with this *material* difference, that the mechanism of it takes place in the *vagina* and *pelvis proper;* and not, as he conjectured, in the *uterus,* and between the *alae* of the *Ilia.*

Douglas was quite explicit in his description of the mechanism that has come to bear his name. He continued:

But in order to render as clear as possible the successive movements in this astonishing effort of nature, I will endeavor to describe, still more precisely, the situation of the *foetus* immediately prior to its expulsion. The entire of it somewhat resembles the larger segment of a circle; the head rests on the *pubis* internally; the *clavicle* presses against the pubis externally, with the *acromion* stretching towards the *mons veneris;* the arm and shoulder are entirely protruded, with one side of the *thorax* not only appearing at the *os externum,* but partly without it: the lower part of the same side of the trunk presses on the *perinaeum,* with the breech either in the hollow of the *sacrum,* or at the brim of the *pelvis,* ready to descend into it; and, by a few further *uterine* efforts, the remainder of the trunk, with the lower extremities, is expelled.

And, to be still more minutely explanatory in this ultimate stage of the process, I have to state, that the breech is not expelled exactly sideways, as the upper part of the trunk had previously been; for during the presence of that pain, by which the evolution is completed, there is a twist made, about the center of the curve, at the lumbar vertebrae, when both buttocks, instead of the side of one of them, are thrown against the perinaeum, distending it very much; and immediately after, the breech, with the lower extremities, issues forth; the upper and back part of it appearing first, as if the back of the child had originally formed the convex and its front the concave side of the curve.

DOUGLAS' LIFE

John Cuppage Douglas was born in Lurgan, County Armagh, Ireland, June 14, 1778. Following in the footsteps of his father, a medical practitioner, young Douglas was sent to Dublin for his education, and in 1800 received his certification by the Royal College of Surgeons in Ireland. In contrast to Denman, who had served a number of years as a naval surgeon, Douglas was appointed in 1801 as surgeon to the Military Regiment of Foot for the County Tipperary. Two years later he was awarded his medical degree from the University of St. Andrews, and in 1808 was nominated assistant at the Lying in Hospital, beginning a career devoted exclusively to obstetrics for almost 43 years. In his very first year of private practice, however, he had two cases of ruptured uterus, which almost led him to quit the profession. In 1810 he received a medical diploma from Trinity College and was made a licentiate of the King and Queen's College of Physicians in Ireland, and later served as president of this body's association. He died on November 20, 1850. There is no known portrait of him in existence.

Aside from his contribution to our knowledge of spontaneous evolution, Douglas published but two other papers, one on hourglass contraction of the uterus, and another on puerperal fever, in which he called attention to its resemblance to erysipelas. Few obstetricians have achieved as wide a reputation as Douglas by so small a number of literary contributions. Perhaps this itself attests their originality.

REFERENCES

1. Denman, T.: Observations to prove that in cases where the upper extremities present, at the time of birth, the delivery may be effected by the spontaneous evolution of the child. Communicated in a letter to Dr. Simmons, F.R.S. *London M. J.,* **5**:64–70, 301–9, 1784 [1785].

2. Denman, T.: *An Introduction to the Practice of Midwifery.* J. Johnson, London, 1795, Vol. 2, pp. 291–99.

3. Denman, T.: *The Obstetrician's Vademecum; or, Aphorisms on Natural and Difficult Parturition; the Application and Use of Instruments in Preter-*

natural Labours; on Labours Complicated with Haemorrhage, Convulsions, etc. Considerably Augmented, and Arranged According to the Present State of Obstetricy, by Michael Ryan, 9th ed. E. Cox, London, 1836, p. ix.

4. Douglas, J. C.: An Explanation of the Real Process of the "Spontaneous Evolution of the Foetus;" with some Remarks, intended to induce an Inquiry, whether the Practice of Turning be not too generally had Recourse to, in Arm-Presentations, 2nd ed. Graisberry & Campbell, Dublin, 1819.

5. Findley, P.: Priests of Lucina. The Story of Obstetrics. Little, Brown & Co., Boston, 1939, pp. 190–96.

6. McClintock, A. H.: Memoir of the Late John C. Douglas, M.D. Dublin Quart. J. M. Sc., 11:248–56, 1851.

7. Michaelis, G. A.: Das Enge Becken. Ed. by C. T. Litzmann. Wigand, Leipzig, 1851, p. 43.

8. Smellie, W.: A Collection of Preternatural Cases and Observations in Midwifery. D. Wilson & T. Durham, London, 1764, Vol. 3, pp. 238–39.

9. Spencer, H. R.: The History of British Midwifery from 1650 to 1800. John Bale, Sons & Danielsson, London, 1927, pp. 128–42.

Bernhard Schultze, James Matthews Duncan, and Expulsion of the Placenta

CHAPTER

41

The placenta, like a coin, has two readily distinguishable surfaces. Following its separation from the uterus it may be extruded into the vagina with either its smooth, glistening, amnion-covered fetal surface or its coarse, dull, beefy-red maternal aspect presenting at the introitus. The former method of presentation occurs in almost three fourths of all cases of vaginal delivery. For many years students of the birth process considered the presenting surface of the placenta an indication of the process by which the organ became detached from the uterine wall; and a labor record was considered incomplete without a notation regarding the "mechanism" of placental separation. These two "mechanisms" have long been associated with the names of Schultze and Duncan, respectively, who described them, the former designating presentation of the fetal surface of the placenta as physiologic, the latter the maternal surface. Several generations of medical students, to aid their memory in properly distinguishing between the presentations, have employed the alliterative, if somewhat inelegant, terms "shiny Schultze" and "dirty Duncan."

John Harvie [5] recognized the two modes of placental expulsion two centuries ago and presented a simple explanation for the occurrence of each. He wrote:

When the *placenta* is delivered by nature alone . . . in general it comes away inverted; that is, the side which was in contact with the child, comes first; and

337

the side which adhered to the *uterus,* is covered by the membranes; thus the lobular side is rendered smooth, and, of course, slips away with ease, and perfectly whole.

If the *placenta* be seperated with force, and brought away by the hand, the reverse takes place; that is, the lobular side comes away first; which is thence liable to be torn, and some part of it even to be left behind.

The distinguished Baudelocque, in his widely celebrated textbook, *L'Art des Accouchemens,*[1] likewise took note of the varying mechanics of the third stage of labor, according as the fetal or the maternal surface of the placenta presented. Relying somewhat on his powers of imagination, Baudelocque, from this observation, extrapolated the earlier details of placental separation and expulsion. He said:

Separation begins at the center of the placenta at times and at a point on its periphery at others, producing different phenomena in each case. As the center of the placenta is pushed forward in the former case, this mass becomes inverted on itself, so that a bag is formed which fills with blood, and the side covered with membranes and vessels presents. When the placenta begins to separate at the edge farthest from the internal os, it forms a similar bag and presents in the same manner; but not so when separation begins at the lower part of the placenta, especially if this be near the internal os. In the latter case the placenta is rolled up on itself in the shape of a cylinder, in the longitudinal axis of the uterus, so that it presents its curled edge to the examining finger; and its expulsion is always preceded by a little fluid blood.

SCHULTZE'S MECHANISM

The name of Schultze became associated with presentation of the fetal surface of the placenta following the publication of his magnificent atlas of obstetric wall charts in 1865.[7] Figure 44-1 illustrates Schultze's conception of the normal mechanism of placental separation and expulsion. In the volume of explanatory text that accompanied the charts Schultze wrote:

The labor contractions that expelled the fetus brought about such a diminution in size of the uterus, that the placenta was separated to a large extent from the uterine wall. The subsequent contractions and the considerable flow of blood that ensues from the torn vessels of the uterine wall, force the placenta completely off the uterine wall and into the now empty amniotic sac. . . . A strong contraction forces the placenta and the inverted membranes forward, along with much clotted and fluid blood, through the cervix, and often as far as the external genitalia if the retained clots are abundant.

In a second edition [8] of his atlas, published in two parts, in 1888 and 1892, Schultze amplified his explanation of placental expulsion, again stressing the role of the retroplacental hemorrhage from the uterine sinuses in completing

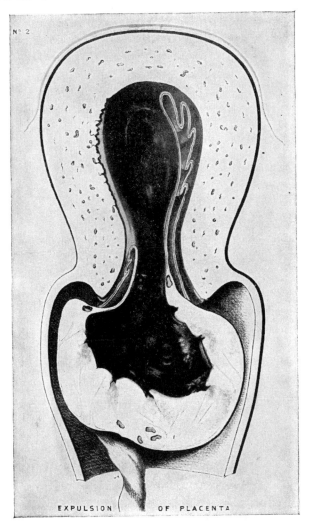

Fig. 41-1. Illustration from Schultze's *Wandtafeln,* showing his conception of the normal mechanism of placental expulsion. (After Duncan.[4])

placental separation, and picturing egress of the organ through the same rent in the membranes through which the fetus emerged, the placenta pulling its attached membranes along, their inner surface showing, like a sock turned inside out.

SCHULTZE'S LIFE

Bernhard Sigmund Schultze was born in Freiburg im Breisgau, December 29, 1827.[2,6] His father and older brother having distinguished themselves as

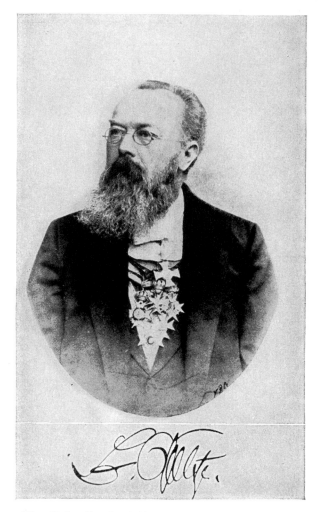

Fig. 41-2. Bernhard Sigmund Schultze (1827–1919).

anatomists, young Schultze embarked along the same line of study, in Greifswald. It was here that he showed a propensity for teaching with diagrams,
charts, and sketches, which he drew himself with great skill and clarity. The
atlas of wall charts that he later published was considered the best collection
of obstetric visual aids since Smellie's *Anatomical Tables*. In 1853 Schultze
transferred to the University of Berlin, where he qualified in obstetrics three
years later. Thereafter he enjoyed a meteoric rise in the academic sphere and
in 1858 was called to the chair of obstetrics in Jena, where he spent the rest
of his life. In 1866 he introduced a method for resuscitating the asphyxiated
newborn by swinging, a procedure known by Schultze's name but no longer

practiced. He also published a book on the subject, *Der Scheintod Neugeborener,* in 1871. Schultze's obstetric textbook, *Lehrbuch der Hebammenkunst,* enjoyed tremendous popularity, going into 15 editions and being translated into several languages. Among his contributions was the demonstration that the remains of the fetal yolk sac are normally incorporated into the placenta. His name is also associated eponymically with the amniotic folds at the site of attachment of the umbilical cord to the placenta. Schultze died in Jena, April 17, 1919, in his ninety-second year, working up to the very end on asphyxia of the newborn.

DUNCAN'S MECHANISM

Schultze's views concerning the separation and expulsion of the placenta became obstetric dogma, but for only a brief period did they remain unchallenged. On March 22, 1871, James Matthews Duncan, whose name had already become one of the most highly respected in British medical circles, rose before the Obstetrical Society of Edinburgh to question the previous teachings on the subject and to propound his own version of the third stage of labor.[4] Said Duncan:

The erroneous belief that the placenta generally descends presenting its foetal surface, seems to me to have arisen from observers not keeping in mind the very great frequency with which the natural mechanism of delivery of this cake is interfered with. I may say, that it is unfortunately the rule to interfere with this part of the natural mechanism of delivery. Such interference, generally carried out as it is by pulling the cord, produces an unnatural mechanism—inversion of the placenta . . . [which] comes to be described as the natural conduct of the delivery. . . .

My own numerous observations satisfy me that the inversion of the placenta, or its folding upon itself transversely to the passage, or the presentation of its foetal surface . . . is a very rare occurrence,—so rare as to debar describers from calling it *a* natural, and still more from calling it *the* natural mechanism. The placenta is folded upon itself during the process . . . but the folds are according to the length of the passage, not transverse to it, as inversion or presentation of the foetal surface imply.

The Schultze mechanism of expulsion was attributed by Duncan to the zealous efforts of the accoucheur to hasten delivery of the placenta. He stated:

When any considerable force is used to deliver the placenta by traction of the cord . . . then indeed, truly, the placenta is inverted, and its edge puckered up purse-like. The insertion of the cord comes first. . . . The placenta is transversely bent on itself, and puckered up; haemorrhage flows to fill up the partial vacuum which is thus produced. The inverted mass forms a firm plug, closely filling the vagina. Traction on this plug is exactly like traction on the piston of a pump. If haemor-

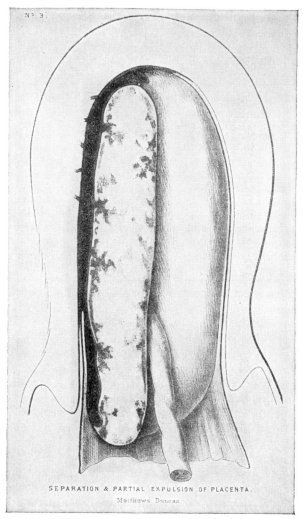

Nᵒ 3.

SEPARATION & PARTIAL EXPULSION OF PLACENTA.

Matthews Duncan

Fig. 41-3. Illustration from Duncan's paper,[4] showing his concept of the normal mechanism of placental expulsion.

rhage does not naturally take place to fill up the void which tends to be formed beyond the placenta, then it is powerfully attracted and induced by the piston-like action of the placenta pulled by the cord. The interior of the uterus, already scarified by the separation of the placenta, requires but this pulling at the cord to be effectively cupped.

Duncan's correlation of the presenting surface of the placenta with the spontaneity of, or forceful interference with, its delivery was thus the precise reverse of Harvie's explanation a century earlier.

To observe the natural mechanism of placental expulsion, Duncan advised:

It is only necessary to watch the process as nature conducts it; that is, in cases in which the practitioner does not try to modify it in any way. This any one can easily do, by wounding or otherwise marking the part presenting at the mouth of the womb, and then after its birth examining the placenta to find out where the wound is. . . . In this way it is easily discovered that the part of the placenta presenting at the os uteri, and subsequently at the os vaginae, is not the foetal or amniotic surface, but the edge of the placenta, or a part very near the edge.

With his characteristic quest for purposeful interpretations Duncan offered the following analysis of the mechanical superiority of his over Schultze's mechanism:

The advantages of the natural mechanism, as I have described it, are obvious. It is true, that after the passage of the bulky child, there is no such necessity for a mechanism of the delivery of the comparatively small placenta, as there is for the passage of the child's head. There is ample room and verge enough for the placenta passing in any way. But the natural mechanism claims respect as the *natural* mechanism, and, moreover, it presents obvious advantages over any other mechanism. Just as the child's head passes through the pelvis so as to dilate the passages as little as may be, or in the manner demanding the least expenditure of force, so also does the placenta. It comes edgeways. If it came inverted, or transversely doubled up, or folded into a cup shape, we should have a body passing that required at least twice as much space as it required if it passes edgeways, and only longitudinally folded. But this is not the only advantage of the natural mechanism.

If the placenta is expelled as Baudelocque describes, and as Schultze depicts, then a loss deserving the name of a haemorrhage is almost as necessary as it is certainly a generally described accompaniment of the process of the expulsion of the placenta. For the placenta has a certain amount of rigidity, and its folding on itself and the forcing of it into a cup-like shape cannot be effected without a hollow space being offered for the reception of blood, or indeed without a certain force being exerted to produce the folding and a vacuum, which force will also tend to draw blood into the said hollow, from the open uterine sinuses which were in opposition to the part folded.

[On the other hand] if the placenta comes edgeways, its uterine surface glides along the surface of the uterus; its foldings, parallel to the length of the maternal passages, are well squeezed together, and little space is offered for the reception of blood flowing from uterine sinuses. The uterine wall keeps close to the folded placenta. The uterus contracts, forces the placenta downwards, and at last its body is nearly globular and empty. There is no haemorrhage worthy of the name. . . . I believe that interference, which, though common, is frequently injudicious, is occasionally the cause of this haemorrhage, which is, therefore, in such circumstances, unjustly laid to the account of the natural mechanism. . . .

DUNCAN'S LIFE

James Matthews Duncan was born April 29, 1826, in Aberdeen, Scotland, where his father was engaged in shipbuilding and mercantile pursuits.[3] Young

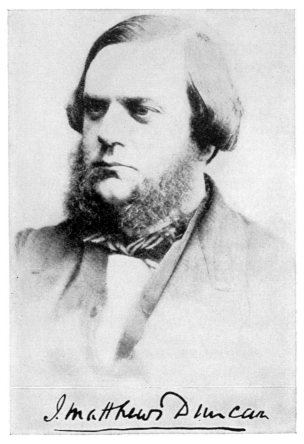

Fig. 41-4. James Matthews Duncan (1826–1890). (Courtesy of American Gynecological Society.)

Duncan was educated in Marischal College of his native city, receiving his M.A. in 1843, when only 17 years old, and his M.D. three years later. He then entered the University of Edinburgh where he, like so many others, was drawn to obstetrics by the inspiring teaching and personality of James Young Simpson. Duncan soon attracted attention through his interest in obstetric pathology, the zeal with which he sought out cases for autopsy among the women of Edinburgh who died during pregnancy or the puerperium, and the thoroughness of his examinations of their viscera. When, after a year of study at the Hôtel-Dieu in Paris, Duncan returned to Edinburgh, Simpson engaged him as his private assistant. This marked the beginning of a long and mutually beneficial association of the two men. Duncan, collaborating with Simpson in the latter's quest for an anesthetic superior to ether for childbirth, was the first person to inhale the vapors of chloroform, on the historic night of November 4, 1847, in Simpson's dining room. In 1848 Duncan received his license from the College of Physicians and entered the private practice of obstetrics in Edinburgh; and in 1853 he began giving a course of lectures, through which he rapidly established his reputation as a teacher of obstetrics.

When the chair of midwifery in the University of Edinburgh fell vacant in 1870 as the result of Simpson's death, Duncan was regarded as the logical successor to this coveted post and, indeed, was favored for it by the majority of the profession. It came as a bitter disappointment to him, therefore, when the Town Council elected A. R. Simpson, Sir James's nephew, to the chair instead. Seven years later Duncan moved to London in response to a call from St. Bartholomew's Hospital, where he assumed the post of physician-accoucheur and lecturer on midwifery. His private practice, as well as his renown as a teacher, thrived in London, the Duchess of Albany being numbered among his fashionable obstetric clientele. In 1881 he was elected president of the Obstetrical Society of London. Because of ill-health, Duncan retired from practice and teaching in June, 1890. He died of a heart attack on September 1 of the same year, while vacationing with his family at Baden-Baden.

Duncan is remembered largely for his obstetric contributions; he remained aloof from the new gynecology that was springing up, and was indeed outspoken in his criticism of the operation of ovariotomy. On obstetric topics, by contrast, he was prolific as well as articulate. His book, *Fecundity, Fertility, and Sterility,* which appeared in 1866, is regarded as the first scientific inquiry into the subject in the English language. Other volumes that appeared under his name include: *On Displacements of the Uterus; A Practical Treatise on Perimetritis and Parametritis; Researches in Obstetrics; Contributions to the Mechanism of Natural and Morbid Parturition;* and *Clinical Lectures on the Diseases of Women.* One of Duncan's most important contributions was his demonstration, in 1879, of the liver necrosis that may result from pernicious vomiting of pregnancy. He was also the first to use the term "missed abortion." The folds of peritoneum on the postpartum uterus are often referred to as "Duncan's folds."

REFERENCES

1. Baudelocque, J.-L.: *L'Art des Accouchemens.* Paris, 1781, Vol. 1, p. 311.
2. *Biographisches Lexikon der hervorragenden Ärzte aller Zeiten und Völker,* 2nd ed. Ed. by W. Haberling, F. Hübotter, and H. Vierordt. Urban & Schwarzenberg, Berlin & Vienna, 1934, Vol. 5, p. 164.
3. Doran, A.: James Matthews Duncan, M.D., F.R.S., Etc. *Am. J. Obst., 23:* 1090–98, 1890.
4. Duncan, J. M.: On the mechanism of the expulsion of the placenta. *Edinburgh*

M. J., **16** (Part 2):899–903, 1871. Also appears as chapter, "The Expulsion of the Placenta," in Duncan's *Contributions to the Mechanism of Natural and Morbid Parturition, Including that of Placenta Praevia*. Adam & Charles Black, Edinburgh, 1875, pp. 246–56.

5. Harvie, J.: *Practical Directions, Shewing a Method of Preserving the Perinaeum in Birth, and Delivering the Placenta Without Violence*. D. Wilson & G. Nicol, London, 1767, pp. 47–48.

6. Küstner, O.: Bernhard Sigmund Schultze—Jena. *Zentralbl. f. Gynäk.*, **43**:393–98, 1919.

7. Schultze, B. S.: *Wandtafeln zur Schwangerschafts-und Geburtskunde*. Günther, Leipzig, 1865, Tafel XVI.

8. Schultze, B. S.: *Wandtafeln zur Schwangerschafts-und Geburtskunde*, 2nd ed. Fischer, Jena, 1888 and 1892.

Bacteria | PART IV

Albert Döderlein and the Bacillus Vaginalis

CHAPTER

42

Maturation of the vagina is a complex phenomenon, which includes morphologic, chemical, and bacteriologic changes. Epithelial hyperplasia, with cornification of the superficial cells, characterizes the first category; increased intracellular glycogen content and acidity of the membrane, the second. The principal bacteriologic alteration at puberty consists in the sudden emergence of a Gram-positive, acid-producing, nonmotile rod, the *Lactobacillus acidophilus* of Döderlein, as the predominant organism of the vaginal flora. The resulting symbiotic relation, between the Döderlein bacillus and its host, prevails throughout the reproductive years of the latter, helping to maintain the integrity of the vagina in the nonpregnant state and to safeguard against ascending infection of the genital tract after childbirth.

In August, 1890, at the tenth international medical congress in Berlin, Albert Döderlein gave a preliminary report of his studies on the bacteriology of the vagina in pregnancy. His definitive monograph,[3] published two years later, laid the foundation for our understanding of puerperal infection of endogenous origin and established the nature, frequency, and cultural characteristics of the vaginal organism that bears his name. Others [2,4,5,8,9] had seen these bacilli in the vaginal fluid before Döderlein, but none had consistently succeeded in culturing them or in defining their position in the vaginal economy. Döderlein's contribution, based on the study of 195 patients in the Leipzig Universitäts-Frauenklinik, was a milestone in the development of gynecic bacteriology.

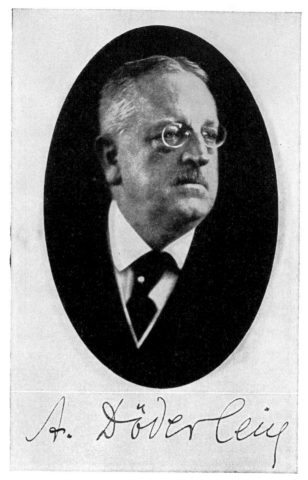

Fig. 42-1. Albert Döderlein (1860–1941).

DÖDERLEIN'S DESCRIPTION OF BACILLUS VAGINALIS

Döderlein's subjects were healthy, pregnant women who had had no previous vaginal examination. He wrote:

The secretion that I designated as normal contains a whitish, crumbly material, having the consistency of curdled milk, without admixture of mucus. This secretion coats the surface and folds of the vaginal membrane with a thin, whitish-gray covering, which can be wiped off easily. Sometimes it is thinner in consistency and larger in amount, about a teaspoonful collecting in the upper end of the speculum.

The reaction of this normal secretion is always intensely acid on blue litmus paper. In this easily demonstrable characteristic lies one of the principal features of the normal secretion. Bacteriologic examination of it reveals the almost exclusive presence of a special kind of bacillus, whose biologic characteristics are to be seen in the vagina as well as in the culture tube.

In his microscopic examination of hundreds of vaginal preparations, Döderlein was struck "again and again by the same picture [Fig. 42-2]: Bacilli of a special kind are seen, in almost pure culture, among the large epithelial cells, this picture being characteristic of the secretion of the healthy vagina."

It was the special cultural requirements of the vaginal bacilli that had so long delayed their proper study. Döderlein's faltering first efforts, like those of the earlier workers, failed:

If one carries some of the normal vaginal secretion, which shows many bacilli microscopically, on to the usual culture media of meat-peptone-gelatin and agar . . . the culture usually fails completely. . . . The most diverse alterations in the culture medium led repeatedly to the same observation, that even the secretions richest in bacteria resulted in scarcely any increase in the organisms.

In contrast to the consistent failure of his predecessors, however, Döderlein's perseverance, coupled with expert bacteriologic counsel, led ultimately to success. He wrote:

After many vain attempts the culture finally succeeded, by the following method, in achieving a typical outgrowth of the organisms. . . . A small amount of the undiluted secretion was transferred on a platinum spatula from the vaginal membrane directly into sterile meat peptone broth with 1 per cent sugar. These bouillon tubes, several of which were inoculated each time from the same pregnant woman, were incubated at 37° C for 24 hours. The tubes were then opened . . . and from each several streak cultures were made on an agar slant. The agar, like the bouillon, contained 1 per cent sugar, and 3 per cent glycerin was added in order to make the culture medium more fluid.

If no contamination of the bouillon occurred at the inoculation . . . then one sees on the agar slant a most delicate pure culture, consisting of individual globules resembling the smallest drops of water [Fig. 42-3].

The culture is most sensitive to drying. If the agar tubes are kept sealed under glass, with an air humidifier also in the incubator, these delicate cultures can be grown successfully. They then increase somewhat in area, rise very slightly above the surface of the culture medium, but always remaining very delicate and transparent. By cultivation in bouillon, many generations can be transplanted successfully; by transplanting the bacilli from one solid culture medium to another of the same they soon assume degenerative forms. . . . Cultivation was also successful in milk and in blood serum, but propagation could not be achieved on potato slices.

These pure cultures of the bacilli showed the greatest sensitivity to temperature, just as they did to drying of the culture medium. Growth failed consistently

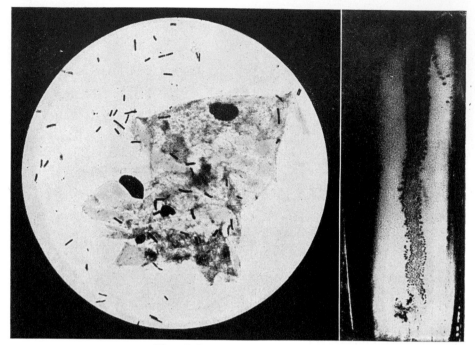

Fig. 42-2   Fig. 42-3

Figs. 42-2 and 42-3. Illustrations from Döderlein's monograph.[3] *Left:* Bacilli in
the vaginal smear of a pregnant woman. *Right:* A slant culture of the vaginal bacilli.
(Reproduced by permission of Georg Thieme, Leipzig, and Prof. Dr. G. Döderlein, Jena.)

in the ordinary gelatin at 25°–27° C. For thriving of the cultures much higher
temperature is necessary, whereupon they develop not only on agar but in the
resulting liquefied gelatin as well. Whether the bacilli themselves liquefy gelatin
cannot therefore be determined.

If the cultures are deprived of oxygen, growth becomes more vigorous rather
than inhibited. The anaerobic cultures also remained alive longer, for in them
evaporation of water could be prevented more effectively than when the air was
not excluded from the culture tubes. The bacilli thus belong to the facultative
anaerobes.

Examined in hanging drops, the vaginal bacilli show no motility. Similarly,
specific staining for cilia by Löffler's method never gave them the appearance of
motile organisms.

With consummate logic and clarity Döderlein next considered his newly
cultured organisms as the source of the vaginal acidity. He observed:

Since the vaginal secretion is not the product of specific glands, and acid-
forming glands are present neither in the cervix nor corpus uteri, the cervical
mucus indeed reacting strongly alkaline . . . an extraneous process must be
invoked to explain the source of the acid in the vaginal secretion.

The secretion of newborn girls provides a clue to this process. This secretion gives only a very weakly acid reaction, whether taken from a living infant or a stillborn. The pale red stain that appears on blue litmus paper disappears after a short time; this is explained by the evaporation of carbonic acid.

In virgins, on the other hand, in whom it was possible to test the reaction of the normal vaginal secretion in eight cases, it was just as strongly acid on blue litmus paper as was the normal secretion of pregnant women. . . .

The only difference between the vaginal secretion of the newborn, on the one hand, and that of the virgin and especially the pregnant woman, on the other, appears to be that the former is free of organisms while the latter always contains a large number of the described bacilli, often in pure culture. The suggestion was therefore made to study the bacilli cultured from the vagina with respect to their fermentation characteristics.

The slight amount of acid that the solution of meat peptone contained was determined each time . . . allowance being made for it in the calculation. After the marked cloudiness occurring in the solution showed how luxuriantly the culture had grown out, the bouillon was boiled to remove the free carbonic acid produced by the yeasts; and after cooling, it was titrated with baryta solution. This showed that the acid had increased considerably in the culture solution, and the sugar was in large part fermented, in all cases in which the purity of the bouillon culture had been established by inoculation on agar before boiling.

To determine the rate of acid production, Döderlein added 10 cc of sugar-containing bouillon to each culture tube inoculated with the vaginal bacilli. He explained:

Two test tubes were taken out of the incubator every 24 hours, and after the free carbonic acid was boiled off, the newly formed quantity of acid was titrated. The averages, expressed in terms of SO_3, were:

in	24	hours,	16 mg
in	48	hours,	25 mg
in	72	hours,	32 mg
in	96	hours,	40 mg
in	120	hours,	50 mg

The last, figured on the basis of 100 cc of solution, corresponds to 0.5 per cent SO_3, which is equivalent to 1.125 per cent lactic acid.

If the tubes remained in the incubator longer than five days, even up to 14 days, the acid content never increased beyond 56.32 mg SO_3, despite an excess of sugar. The acid maximum is not very great, thus showing that the further growth of bacilli cultured from the vagina is inhibited by their own acid. The acid formed by the bacilli in the culture containing added sugar was shown by test to be lactic acid also.

When one considers the facts that the vaginal bacilli produce an acid concentration up to about 0.5 per cent, at which point acid formation ceases; that the acid level of the secretion freshly obtained from the normal vagina likewise goes as high as 0.4 per cent; and that in both cases, in the culture as in the vagina, lactic acid is demonstrable in large amount; then it might properly be assumed that the bacilli and the acid vaginal secretion are dependently related to each other: that the bacilli produce the acid content of the normal vagina. . . .

Döderlein was an intensely practical clinical obstetrician. His primary interest in puerperal infection permeated his entire bacteriologic investigation; indeed, served as its initial stimulus. The effect of the vaginal bacilli on pathogenic organisms therefore engaged much of his attention. It soon became apparent to him that the acid of the vaginal fluid permitted the development of these characteristic bacilli and aciduric yeasts, but by contrast inhibited the growth of saprophytic organisms. He noted:

Bacteriologic examination showed that saprophytic organisms are present only occasionally at most in the normal vaginal secretion, although opportunities for entry of the most diverse types of organisms into the vagina are surely not rare, through coitus, bathing, douching, etc. It should be stressed particularly that I could never demonstrate pathogenic organisms in the normal secretion.

This last statement probably indicates Döderlein's more limited concept of pathogenicity than that of the modern bacteriologist. He continued:

The acid in the normal vagina heightens our obvious interest in the conditions for pathogens introduced into the vagina. The following investigations that I carried out are capable of clarifying the opposing relations between the acid-forming bacilli and the pathogenic microorganisms. First it was important to find out to what extent the acid bacilli inhibit the development of the pathogens.

Several parallel streaks of the vaginal bacilli from a pure bouillon culture were made . . . on an agar medium in a Petri dish. After three days the Petri dish . . . showed distinctly developed streaks of the pure culture of the bacilli. Now streaks of a pure bouillon culture of *Staphylococcus pyogenes* were made on the agar, across the culture of the vaginal bacilli that had already developed. In this experiment, in which the staphylococcus culture was superimposed on the culture of the vaginal bacillus and mixed superficially with it without the delicate culture of the vaginal bacilli being wiped off at the points of contact, the staphylococcus culture failed to grow in the region of the vaginal bacilli . . . while in remote places a thick stand of staphylococci appeared. The staphylococcus thus succumbs in its battle with the vaginal bacillus, despite the favorable culture medium of meat peptone agar.

Döderlein was quick to point out, however, that under these conditions, "the competition of the two organisms is not equal"; and, as he showed in another experiment, if the vaginal bacilli and staphylococci were transferred into bouillon simultaneously, "then the latter were able to overgrow the bacilli to the extent that the vaginal bacilli could no longer be demonstrated 24 hours after streaking on plates." He continued:

> If, on the other hand, the bouillon cultures of the vaginal bacilli were kept for a day or two at 37° C and only then, when they had come to a luxuriant growth and their metabolic products were amply present, inoculated with *Staphylococcus pyogenes aureus*, the result now was that the pathogenic organisms disappeared and the transfer onto other culture media yielded no development of staphylococcus cultures.
>
> This type of experiment . . . proves that the vaginal bacilli, or rather their metabolic products, of which I would consider the acid the most important although not the sole part, act as an inhibiting agent against the development of the staphylococci. This attains its full effect, however, only when the vaginal bacilli are present in predominant concentration, as ought to be the case in the normal vagina of pregnant women. . . .

In an effort to evaluate the cultural conditions in the nonpregnant vagina, Döderlein introduced several cubic centimeters of a pure bouillon culture of *Staphylococcus aureus* into the upper vagina of a virgin, in which previous examination had revealed only the presence of the vaginal bacilli. Serial cultures of the girl's vagina yielded heavy growth of the staphylococci at first. The concentration of this organism diminished progressively, however, and at the end of four days the vaginal culture yielded no further staphylococci. Döderlein's conclusion, slightly modified, seems amply justified: "Never underestimate the power of the vaginal bacilli!"

DÖDERLEIN'S LIFE

Albert Döderlein was born in Augsberg, Germany, July 5, 1860, the son of a military surgeon, the nephew of Ludwig von Döderlein, the Erlangen philologist, and the grandnephew of Johann Christoph Döderlein, the theology professor of Jena. After his preliminary education in the St. Anna Gymnasium in Augsberg, Döderlein entered the University of Erlangen in 1879. His first position after graduation was as assistant to Professor Zweifel, and when the latter was called to Leipzig in 1888 he took his young disciple along. Döderlein's efforts were rewarded by an invitation to Groningen in 1897, but he relinquished this post, after only a few months, for the chair of obstetrics and gynecology in Tübingen. Ten years later, in 1907, he again transferred the site of his activities, this time in response to a call to Munich, where he succeeded Franz von Winckel, who had examined him in obstetrics on his state examinations 23 years earlier. After 1934, when Döderlein was relieved of his duties as director of the Universitäts-Frauenklinik in Munich, he devoted himself to editing the *Archiv für Gynäkologie,* together with G. A. Wagner, and the quiet pursuit of his scientific interests. He died in Erlangen, on December 10, 1941.

Döderlein achieved distinction in three spheres of activity: his bacteriologic investigations, his contributions to operative obstetrics and gynecology, and his work in gynecologic radiotherapy. His qualifying thesis on the presence of yeasts in the lochia, *Untersuchungen über das Vorkommen von Spaltpilzen in den Lochien des Uterus und der Vagina gesunder und kranker Wöchnerinnen,* led to his more extensive studies on the bacteriology of the vagina in pregnancy and his identification with the vaginal bacilli that now bear his name. He introduced rubber gloves into obstetrics, for the prevention of puerperal infection.

Renowned as an operator, Döderlein devised a modification of Gigli's pubiotomy operation for cephalopelvic disproportion, and developed an improved instrument for craniotomy, his *Kephalothryptor.* Always eager to try new things, he was one of the first to use blood transfusion in obstetrics and gynecology. His *Operative Gynäkologie,* written in conjunction with Krönig, enjoyed four editions in rapid succession and was translated into Spanish. His *Handbuch der Geburtshilfe,* published in 1915, was also translated into Spanish.

As one of the first to use radium and roentgen rays for gynecologic cancer Döderlein, representing the clinicians of Germany, was invited to participate in the international radiologic commission established for the study of cancer radiotherapy. In January, 1913, he presented his first case of inoperable uterine cancer, which had undergone impressive regression following radiation treatment. By February, 1929, he was able to report on 1319 cases of cervical and 88 of endometrial cancer that had been treated with radiation exclusively, with results surpassing those previously attained with surgery. He also pioneered in the use of roentgen therapy for climacteric menorrhagia and uterine myomas.

A special number of the *Münchener Medizinische Wochenschrift,* July 4, 1930, was dedicated to Albert Döderlein, on the occasion of his seventieth birthday.[1,6,7]

REFERENCES

1. Albrecht, H.: Albert Döderlein und die Münchener gynäkologische Gesellschaft. *München. med. Wchnschr.,* **77**:1132–36, 1930.

2. Bumm, E.: Ueber die Aufgaben weiterer Forschungen auf dem Gebiete der puerperal Wundinfection. *Arch. f. Gynäk.,* **34**:325–56, 1889.

3. Döderlein, A.: *Das Scheidensekret und seine Bedeutung für das Puerperalfieber.* Besold, Leipzig, 1892.

4. Goenner, A.: Über Mikroorganismen im Sekret der weiblichen Genitalien während der Schwangerschaft und bei puerperalen Erkrankungen. *Centralbl. f. Gynäk.,* **11**:444–49, 1887.

5. Haussmann, D.: *Die Parasiten der weiblichen Geschlechtsorgane des Menschen und einige Tiere.* A. Hirschwald, Berlin, 1870.

6. Mayer, A.: Albert Döderlein: zum 70. Geburtstag. *München. med. Wchnschr.,* **77**:1129–32, 1930.

7. Nürnberger, L.: Albert Döderlein. *München. med. Wchnschr.,* **89**:107–9, 1942.

8. Steffeck, P.: Bacteriologische Begründung der Selbstinfection. *Ztschr. f. Geburtsh. u. Gynäk.,* **20**:339–83, 1890.

9. Winter, G.: Die Mikroorganismen im Genitalkanal der gesunden Frau. *Ztschr. f. Geburtsh. u. Gynäk.,* **14**:443–88, 1888.

Albert Neisser and the Gonococcus

CHAPTER 43

The ravages of gonorrhea produce many of the commonest of gynecologic complaints, including leucorrhea, backache, dysuria, dysmenorrhea, abnormal uterine bleeding, incapacitating pelvic pain, and barrenness; and until recently this infection, acquired at birth, was the most frequent cause of blindness in children. For less than 100 years, however, have the nature and agent of gonorrhea been understood. As late as the early-nineteenth century many physicians even refused to recognize the separate identity of this infection and syphilis, a state of ignorance that remained unaffected by the ill-fated self-inoculation experiment of John Hunter.

Gonorrhea was attributed by some to chilling of the genitals, as from urinating into the night air, or to the intemperate use of alcohol or rich or highly seasoned foods.[14] Its relation to pelvic inflammatory disease was not even suspected until the second half of the nineteenth century. Mauriceau had taught that pelvic inflammation resulted from obstruction to the lochia, while others indicted lacteal suppression and the resultant stasis of milk in the pelvis. Trauma, excessive intercourse, or involuntary abstinence in a "single woman of strong passions" were later listed among the causes of pelvic inflammation. In 1857 the relation between gonorrhea and pelvic inflammatory disease was demonstrated for the first time, from autopsy examinations, by Bernutz and Goupil,[1] who summarized their augmented observations in a book published five years later.[2] They wrote:

358

We thus see that in 99 cases of pelvic peritonitis, 28 or more than one fourth occurred in association with gonorrhea. So large a proportion is attributable in part to the special type of hospital in which we made our observations [l'hôpital Lourcine, which admitted a large number of the poorest class of patients] and this surely reduces the value of our figures, but they still possess indubitable significance. They appear to us not only to exclude the idea of simple coincidence between pelvic inflammation and gonorrhea, but to establish a close relation between these two pathologic conditions, which we have seen together so often.

These observations of Bernutz and Goupil attracted very little attention until ten years later, when Emil Noeggerath, a German gynecologist who had migrated to New York, published a monograph of 125 pages, entitled *Die latente Gonorrhoe im weiblichen Geschlecht*,[10] in which he drew the following conclusions:

1. Gonorrhea usually remains for life in the male as well as the female, despite apparent cure.
2. There occurs a latent form of gonorrhea in man as in woman.
3. Latent gonorrhea can flare up into an acute form in man or woman.
4. Latent gonorrhea in woman manifests itself as acute, chronic, recurrent perimetritis or ovaritis, and catarrh of certain parts of the genital membrane.
5. The wives of men who have ever had gonorrhea are usually sterile.
6. Those who do conceive either abort or bear only one child; only exceptionally do they bear three or four.
7. From the discharge associated with latent gonorrhea an organism may be cultivated analogous to that of the florid discharge in male gonorrhea.

In a reaffirmation of his radical views before the historic inaugural meeting of the American Gynecological Society four years later,[11] Noeggerath insisted:

. . . Gonorrhea in the female is, as a rule, followed by tubal catarrh. It is . . . a peculiarity of gonorrhea to affect the entire tract of the female genital organs, to disappear in some portions of it, to remain for life in others, in the tube among the latter. And, since the majority of females who are married to husbands who have gonorrhea, are, as a rule, in the same condition as if they had gone through an attack of gonorrhea themselves, you find that chronic perimetritis, the effect of salpingitis, is one of the most frequent results of latent gonorrhea. . . . About 90 per cent of sterile women are married to husbands who have suffered from gonorrhea either previous to, or during married life.

The leading figures in American gynecology were neither ready nor willing to accept Noeggerath's new concept, which Fordyce Barker, the presiding officer, characterized as "so startling in the present state of the morals in society." In the ensuing discussion Dr. Trenholme, of Montreal, among others, rose to protest:

On behalf of one half of this continent, at least as far as area is concerned, I feel that I should call for protection from the doctrines of this paper. We, upon our side of the line, look upon it as rather a reproach not to have a large family; and if our Canadian ladies found out that their sterility was dependent upon the former condition of their husbands, I do not know what would take place.

The gynecologists of this era were stymied, of course, by their inability to determine the nature of vaginal discharges. Noeggerath himself admitted:

. . . It is very rare that the discharge itself is of such a character as to enable us to recognize its nature by its quality alone. . . . The secretion in the female looks, in the great majority of cases, exactly like that of a simple cervical endometritis. No means of examination, not even the microscope, under these circumstances, will add to our knowledge. . . . You have to look for circumstantial evidence to pronounce about its nature.

Matthews Duncan, in his lectures on vaginitis,[3] likewise voiced the perplexity that plagued the profession in the diagnosis of leucorrhea:

Is it, in any special case, venereal or not venereal? You will, in practice, often be asked this question, and I advise you never to answer it explicitly. You cannot decide absolutely whether a case is venereal or not. . . . I have seen gonorrhea which was certainly not venereal bear every character of the ordinary venereal disease. I do not say that there is no distinction, but only that the distinction cannot be made out by the practitioner so as to justify him, from his own inquiries into a case, in giving a decided opinion on the subject.

This diagnostic dilemma, superimposed on the concern of most physicians for the patient's sensibilities, appears to have resulted in a general disinclination to pronounce a discharge gonorrheal. Edis, for example, in his *Diseases of Women,*[4] wrote in 1882:

Although the evidence may appear to us convincing, there are often such intricate moral and social complications involved, so many reasons for dissimulation on the part of the patient, and so much difficulty in obtaining proof, that we should be extremely careful in expressing an opinion as to the nature of the disease. Cases will be met with where it is impossible to decide definitely on medical grounds alone, and we should always lean to the side of charity when the question is one of chastity.

In like vein C. C. Lee wrote in Mann's *American System of Gynecology:* [8]

Some years ago, when I had charge of the large venereal wards in the (New York) Charity Hospital, I made very numerous and careful clinical examinations

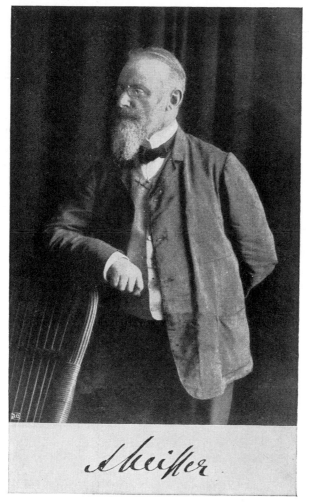

Fig. 43-1. Albert Ludwig Siegmund Neisser (1855–1916). (Reproduced from *Hyg. Med. Tidsk.*, **78**:1401, 1916.)

to test the possibility of this distinction [between venereal and nonspecific vaginitis], with exceptional facilities for such an object. The result was absolutely negative. Since then a like inference has resulted from equally careful observation of my cases in the Woman's Hospital and in private practice. That gonorrhea, either in man or woman, is a "specific" disease, in the proper sense of specificity, I do not believe; nor is it easy to comprehend how any pathologist can hold that view in the light of our present knowledge. That a simple virulent vaginitis can be distinguished from one of "gonorrhoeal" origin I equally disbelieve; and it needs but a moment's reflection to perceive the vast importance of this in its bearing upon the happiness of the families we may be called upon to advise.

NEISSER'S DESCRIPTION OF GONOCOCCUS

As these very words were being readied for publication in America, Albert Neisser, a dermatologist on the other side of the Atlantic, was recording his observations on some minute organisms he had discovered in gonorrheal discharges.* He reported: [9]

If gonorrheal pus is spread out in as thin a layer as possible, allowed to dry, stained by simply pouring an aqueous solution of methyl violet over it, dried again, and examined under high magnification with the illumination dimmed as much as possible, then in addition to the pus cells that appear in the most varied forms with dark violet-blue nuclei and faintly stained cytoplasm, a number of more or less concentrated masses of micrococci are seen at first glance. These have a quite characteristic, typical form, immediately recognizable.

The individual ones are round and strikingly large, and have a strong affinity for methyl violet and dalia. They can also be stained with concentrated solutions of eosin but are then not so striking among the many granules of the pus cells themselves. . . . They remain unstained by methyl green and indulin. Under low-power magnification they appear surrounded by a halo, which probably represents a mucous coat. They seldom appear as individual cells; almost always two micrococci are seen lying close together, so close in fact that they give the impression of one organism resembling an 8, a roll, or a biscuit. The apparent variation in the arrangement of these double forms results chiefly from the method of propagation of the micrococcus. This is readily construed as follows:

(a) The individual micrococcus is round.

(b) It soon develops into an oval, very short little body.

(c) Division begins very quickly by a pinching in the middle, resulting in the appearance of two new micrococci. It cannot be stated with certainty yet whether the majority of micrococci that have attained this roll-like appearance are the result of prolonged cohesion of two individual micrococci or whether multiplication proceeds so rapidly that the individual can seldom be seen in isolated form.

(d) The individual micrococci finally separate and remain apart by a distance corresponding to about the size of a micrococcus.

(e) Each individual micrococcus soon grows out again, but now in a direction perpendicular to the plane of the first division. In this way . . . small groups of four are formed.

These micrococci usually form colonies of 10, 20, or more individuals. . . . In these colonies the micrococci never lie directly against one another but are always separated by larger intervening spaces. Most often the micrococci are situated at the surface of pus cells, rarely on epithelial cells.

In some pus cells containing micrococci the nucleus was missing, and in others

---

* In 1869, exactly ten years before Neisser's publication, Ernst Hallier [5] had mentioned, in a single sentence, his finding of both intra- and extracellular cocci in gonorrheal pus, but this observation had escaped the attention of the medical world.

a diminution of its size was immediately apparent. . . . However, the idea that our micrococci might be the product of nuclear fragmentation must be rejected as out of the question.

This sort of micrococcus has already been seen, by many observers as well as myself, in 35 cases of gonorrhea of varying duration [three days to 13 weeks] that have come to examination; but I could not demonstrate these micrococci in a case of chronic gonorrhea of one and one-half years' duration. It was immaterial whether previous treatment had been given or not. . . .

Every specimen of gonorrheal pus examined by me contained only this one type of bacteria. . . . On the other hand, this micrococcus was absent from all other types of pus, heavily laden with bacteria. . . . It was not present in 13 unselected cases of simple leucorrhea. It was present in large numbers, however, in the purulent vaginal discharge of two young girls who had been abused by a man later shown to be suffering from gonorrhea. I observed the same micrococci typical of male gonorrhea in nine cases of purulent urethritis in women.

These same characteristic micrococci were also present in extraordinary numbers in seven cases of acute purulent ocular blennorrhea of the newborn that I had an opportunity to examine. The duration of the blennorrhea was one day, three days, and three, five, and six weeks. The micrococci were absent in one case, 14 days old, which furnished only very minimal secretion after very energetic treatment. They were likewise absent in all the control cases of simple conjunctivitis. They were present in two cases of gonorrheal ocular blennorrhea in adults. . . .

These characteristic micrococci thus appear to be a constant mark of all gonorrheal affections . . . which has repeatedly allowed me to diagnose the specific gonorrheal nature of pus.

NEISSER'S LIFE

Albert Ludwig Siegmund Neisser was born January 22, 1855, in Schweidnitz, Lower Silesia, the son of Moritz Neisser, who later achieved prominence as a physician and commissioner of health in Breslau and Charlottenbrunn.[6,7,12,13] Young Neisser studied medicine in Breslau and Erlangen, and after receiving his degree in 1877 was appointed assistant to Oskar Simon in the newly established dermatology clinic in the University of Breslau. He announced his discovery of the gonococcus two years later, at the age of 24; and though only 27 years old when Simon died, Neisser was chosen as his successor as director of the clinic. Stimulated by Virchow, Cohnheim, and Robert Koch, Neisser adopted a broad view of dermatology and quickly extended his investigations beyond purely morphologic limits and into the field of general pathology, in quest of etiologic factors. In addition to the spectrum of dermatologic disorders, the problems of tuberculosis, leprosy, gonorrhea, and syphilis remained under continuous investigation by Neisser and his students. A bibliography of the published researches carried out under his direction during his last ten years lists 267 titles.[7]

Neisser had long toyed with the possibility of producing an antiserum against syphilis and had made many unsuccessful attempts to infect animals with the disease, when Metchnikoff and Roux discovered in 1903 that syphilis could be transmitted to monkeys. Neisser immediately had a monkey house built in the garden of his home, where he kept as many as 200 animals, and embarked on a protracted series of experiments. The early results were promising, but the practical disadvantages of large-scale experiments on monkeys in Europe soon became apparent, because of the cost of the animals and their suscepti- bility to disease. Together with an assistant he therefore set out on the first of two personally financed expeditions to Java, where he conducted experi- ments that added greatly to the knowledge of syphilitic infection and the host's reaction to the parasite. Their extensive observations were summarized in Neisser's *Beiträge zur Pathologie und Therapie der Syphilis,* published in 1911. A close friend of Paul Ehrlich, Neisser collaborated in some of the former's investigations on organic arsenicals, tested some of Ehrlich's early preparations in Java, and later helped demonstrate their therapeutic value. Neisser is noted for his early insistence on the administration of mercury con- currently with arsphenamine, a measure that helped reduce the frequency of neurosyphilis, which often developed in patients treated with arsenicals alone. He was also associated with Wassermann's development of his serologic test for syphilis.

With F. J. Pick, Neisser organized the German Dermatological Society in 1888 and was later made its honorary president. In 1902 he founded the German Society for Combating Venereal Diseases, and served as coeditor of its journal as well as the *Archiv für Dermatologie und Syphilis;* and in 1907 he was appointed ordinary professor in the University of Breslau. Two volumes (84 and 85) of the *Archiv,* published that year, were entitled *Festschrift Neisser,* to which over 60 of his pupils contributed original articles. He died July 30, 1916, following an operation for urinary calculi. His name remains immortalized in *Neisseria gonorrhoeae,* the organism he discovered, and in "Neisserian infection," the eponymic euphemism for the disease he did so much to combat.

REFERENCES

1. Bernutz, G., and Goupil, E.: Recherches cliniques sur les phlegmons péri- utérins. *Arch. gén. de méd.,* 9:285–308, 419–32, 1857.

2. Bernutz, G., and Goupil, E.: *Clinique Médicale sur les Maladies des Femmes.* F. Chamerot, Paris, 1862, Vol. 2, p. 140.

3. Duncan, J. M.: Clinical lecture on vaginitis. *M. Times & Gaz.,* 1:685–87, 1880.

4. Edis, A. W.: *Diseases of Women: Including Their Pathology, Causation, Symp- toms, Diagnosis, and Treatment.* Henry C. Lea's Son & Co., Philadelphia, 1882, pp. 427–28.

5. Hallier, E.: Die Parasiten der Infectionskrankheiten. *Ztschr. f. Parasitenk.*, **1**:117–84, 1869.

6. Harrison, L. W.: Neisser and Neisserian principles in venerology. *Brit. J. Ven. Dis.*, **31**:65–73, 1955.

7. Jadassohn, J.: Albert Neisser. *Arch. f. Dermat. u. Syph.*, **123**:XVII–LXIV, 1916.

8. Lee, C. C.: In *A System of Gynecology. By American Authors*. Ed. by M. D. Mann. Lea Brothers, Philadelphia, 1888, Vol. 2, pp. 19–20.

9. Neisser, A.: Ueber eine der Gonorrhoe eigentümliche Micrococcusform. *Centralbl. f. d. med. Wissensch.*, **17**:497–500, 1879.

10. Noeggerath, E.: *Die latente Gonorrhoe im weiblichen Geschlecht*. Max Cohen & Sohn, Bonn, 1872.

11. Noeggerath, E.: Latent gonorrhea, especially with regard to its influence on fertility in women. *Tr. Am. Gynec. Soc.*, **1**(1876):268–93, 293–300 (discussion), 1877.

12. Obituary: Albert Neisser (1854–1916). *Brit. J. Dermat.*, **28**:320–21, 1916.

13. Reenstierna, J.: Albert Neisser. *Hyg. Med Tidsk.*, **78**:1401–7, 1916.

14. Sinclair, W. J.: *On Gonorrhoeal Infection in Women*. H. K. Lewis, London, 1888.

Ovarian Tumors

PART V

Friedrich Krukenberg and

the Krukenberg Tumor *

CHAPTER

44

Gynecologic pathologists differ widely in their criteria for a Krukenberg tumor. Some apply this designation to any metastatic tumor in the ovary. Others reserve the term for secondary ovarian carcinomas that originate in the gastrointestinal tract. A third group limits this diagnosis to metastatic lesions of the ovary with a specific type of mucin-producing epithelium containing the so-called signet-ring cell. All now agree that rarely, if ever, does a Krukenberg tumor originate in the ovary.

KRUKENBERG'S DESCRIPTION OF OVARIAN TUMOR

The tumor that bears his name was described in 1896 by Friedrich Krukenberg as a primary malignant neoplasm of the ovary, in a paper entitled "Ueber das Fibrosarcoma ovarii mucocellulare (carcinomatodes)." [2] This report contained an excellent pathologic description of six cases of a distinctive type of bilateral ovarian tumor, collected over a period of five years in Marchand's laboratory at Marburg.

The first patient was a young woman of 26 years who died with large bilateral ovarian tumors after several weeks' treatment, including multiple thoracic and abdominal paracenteses. At autopsy the right ovary, largely

---

* This chapter originally published under the title "Friedrich Krukenberg and Ovarian Tumors" in *Cancer,* **8**:869–71, 1955; reprinted by permission. Copyright, 1955, by the American Cancer Society, Inc.

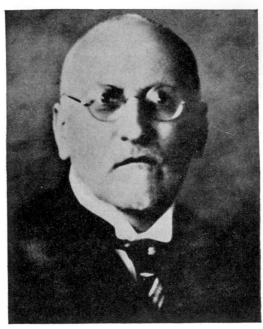

Fig. 44-1. Friedrich Ernst Krukenberg (1871–1946). (Courtesy of National Library of Medicine, Washington, D. C.)

solid, measured 12 cm in its greatest diameter; the left ovary, largely cystic, was only slightly smaller. In addition to the malignant ovarian tumors with diffuse involvement of the peritoneum and pleura, the autopsy findings showed lymphatic dissemination of the tumor to the broad ligaments, tubes, stomach wall, liver, mesentery, pericardium, and mesenteric, retroperitoneal, pleural, bronchial, and axillary nodes. The mucosa of the gastrointestinal tract appeared intact, uninvolved by tumor.

These neoplasms, which Krukenberg believed to be of primary ovarian origin, he described as follows:

Microscopic examination of the tumor elements, which were so widely disseminated in the lymphatics throughout the body, disclosed in large measure such a striking similarity to epithelial cells that the original suspicion seemed thereby to be confirmed that we were dealing with a true epithelial tumor of the ovary, a so-called fibrous carcinoma.

The nature of the cellular elements disseminated in the lymphatics suggested a colloid carcinoma. Study of the primary tumor gave no evidence of the pre-existing epithelial elements that could be regarded as the starting point of the tumor. Among these the following must be considered: the germinal epithelium as such or proliferations of it in the form of Pflüger's tubules, the graafian follicles, and intraovarian tubules of the parovarium. There was absolutely none of the germinal epithelium still visible, and formations that could be interpreted as remains of Pflüger's tubules were present only to a very slight degree. The sparse graafian follicles showed no evidence of proliferation and to some extent even appeared to be in a retrogressive phase; epithelial formations that could be traced back to remains of the Wolffian body in the ovary were not demonstrable; and also no proliferative processes were to be seen in the parovarian tubules in the broad ligament. Even if this negative finding does not definitely rule out a carcinoma, nevertheless the most precise study provides no support for such an assumption. The main part of the tumor formed a very cellular growth, which obviously had resulted from the elements of the connective tissue stroma and consisted in large part of spindle-shaped cells with a fibrous, and in places myxomatous, ground substance. The swollen round cells embedded in it, in lesser or greater amount, could be traced back to a proliferation of the endothelium of either the lymph or blood vessels, but apparently are of the same origin as the spindle-shaped cells. . . .

The clinical histories of the other five patients were lacking, and no information was available concerning the condition of any of their organs except the ovaries. Krukenberg considered the ovarian tumors in all six cases as belonging to one group, because of their similar gross characteristics and almost identical microscopic structure. He wrote:

The described tumors which were designated partly as fibrosarcoma, myxosarcoma, but especially as fibrous carcinoma, comprise representatives of a well-characterized form of solid ovarian tumor that possesses the following peculiarities:

The tumor formation always appears bilaterally, so it seems, occurs as well in youth as in older age, and seems to distinguish itself by its slow growth. As a rule it is associated with ascites.

The neoplasia leads to enlargement of the whole ovary, the form of which is maintained, even though the surface becomes more or less unevenly knobby.

The cut section has, for the most part, a firm and uniformly dense quality, especially near the surface, while in the interior, firm areas alternate with rather myxomatous ones. In places the solid tumor mass is arranged in roundish patches. Larger, smooth-walled cysts may develop as a result of progressive softening of the myxomatous tissue. In places smaller, epithelium-lined cysts also appear, which may be traced back to enlarged follicles.

The histologic structure of the tumor mass shows certain differences, which in their extremes can produce highly variable pictures. The solid parts arise from intense proliferation of the spindle-shaped cells of the ovarian stroma, which changes into a fine fibrillar mesh with spindle-shaped or branching cells in the softer areas.

In the cellular proliferations, round swollen cells with finely vacuolated cytoplasm, often distinctly mucin-containing, appear chiefly in the form of smaller or larger clusters, which [cells] are embedded among the spindle-shaped cells of

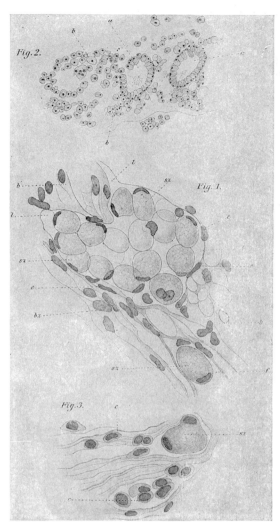

Fig. 44-2. A plate from Krukenberg's paper,[2] the center illustration showing a cluster of the characteristic signet-ring, mucin-containing cells in a lymphatic channel. (Reproduced by permission of *Archiv für Gynäkologie.*)

the stroma and extend into the mesh of the myxomatous part, not infrequently arranged quite individually or here also in little clusters or rows of several cells of epithelial appearance lined up one behind another. . . .

In Krukenberg's interpretive summary of this tumor group one senses a persistent uncertainty, perhaps even a slightly apologetic attitude, on the part of the author:

. . . The peculiar character that is given to the tumor through the appearance of the large swollen tumor cells . . . might then be expressed with the least possible prejudicial addition as "mucocellulare." The great epithelial similarity and the malignancy of the quite pure cell types in the metastases justify the further designation "carcinomatodes."

A Krukenberg tumor is then, according to Krukenberg, an unusual type of primary sarcoma of the ovary, with areas of mucin-producing cells and lymphatic metastases resembling epithelial cells. How different this from any of the current views of the Krukenberg tumor!

KRUKENBERG'S LIFE

Friedrich Ernst Krukenberg was born in Halle, Germany, April 1, 1871, the son of a judge.[1,3] Many members of his family had achieved renown in their own right. His brother, an orthopedic surgeon, is identified with the eponymic, Krukenberg's arm; his maternal grandfather, Professor Keiser, was a close friend of Goethe; and his great-grandfather, Johann Christian Reil, was the neuropathologist after whom the island of Reil is named.

Only the scantiest biographic data are available concerning Friedrich. He studied in Halle and Marburg and later served as assistant to Axenfeld, the physiologist. Krukenberg is best known for his paper on the ovarian tumors with which his name is associated. He died February 20, 1946.

REFERENCES

1. Anon.: Cancer eponyms: Krukenberg tumor. *Cancer Bull.,* **7**:5, 1955.
2. Krukenberg, F.: Ueber das Fibrosarcoma ovarii mucocellulare (carcinomatodes). *Arch. f. Gynäk.,* **50**:287–321, 1896.
3. Norris, J. C.: Krukenberg tumors. *South. M. J.,* **47**:116–20, 1954.

Fritz Brenner and
the Brenner Tumor*

A new type of ovarian tumor, called by its discoverer "fibroma papillare superficiale carcinomatosum ovarii," was described by Orthmann in 1899.[4] A fuller description of this tumor type, under the designation "oophoroma folliculare," together with the addition of three more cases, was given eight years later by Fritz Brenner. This tumor was subsequently popularized by Robert Meyer,[3] who pointed out its association with pseudomucinous cysts, its lack of endocrine function, and its probable origin from Walthard's cell rests. He gave it the name by which it has since been known, the Brenner tumor, it being the only ovarian tumor having no pathologic designation other than its eponym.

BRENNER'S DESCRIPTION OF OVARIAN TUMOR

The first of Brenner's three cases reported in 1907 [1] was that of a 62-year-old woman who had been known to have a small pelvic tumor for at least four years. A sudden spurt in its growth led to the presumptive clinical diagnosis of sarcomatous change in a myomatous uterus, for which operation was undertaken, consisting of subtotal hysterectomy and right salpingo-oophorectomy. The tumor was confined to the right ovary, and a small amount

* This chapter originally published under the title "Fritz Brenner and Brenner Tumors of the Ovary" in *Cancer,* **9**:217–21, 1956; reprinted by permission. Copyright, 1956, by the American Cancer Society, Inc.

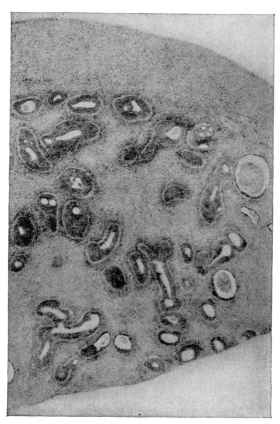

Fig. 45-1. This, together with Figure 45-2, is from Brenner's paper.[1] They show the histologic characteristics of the tumors.

of ascitic fluid was present in the abdominal cavity. The patient died eight days later from intestinal obstruction. Wrote Brenner:

The ovoid tumor [was] almost as large as a man's head . . . completely smooth on its surface. In places several parts project as thick, flat protuberances; the consistency is solid, corresponding somewhat to a moderately firm myoma. On cut surface one distinguishes a thin, firmly adherent capsule from the tumor parenchyma. One sees a solid, gray-yellow tumor mass, which in a few places shows small, smoothly lined cavities up to the size of a cherry, into which the adjacent parts of the tumor encroach as flat projections. In the yellow-gray parenchyma numerous rather light strands of connective tissue form a dense fibrous network, in which are embedded, in the hardened preparation, the smaller round, oval, and elongated, rather depressed areas of softer tissue, concentrated in some places and sparse in others. In many areas they widen into small to pinhead-sized cysts, usually filled with yellow-brown, viscid colloid contents. Occasionally such cysts are as large as a hazelnut and then they usually lie near the surface. The cut surface is avascular and rather moist. The other ovary is small and atrophic. Neither macroscopic nor microscopic changes are to be seen in the uterus.

The other two tumors, both considerably smaller than the first, were discovered at autopsy in elderly women who had died of unrelated causes. Because of the morphologic similarity of the three tumors, the following description by Brenner is applicable to all:

On fixation in formalin all three tumors acquire an unusual degree of hardness. . . .

The tumors . . . show macroscopically an extensive uniformity, differing only in size and in that two of them seem to replace the ovary completely, while the third—without a sharp boundary, to be sure—only forms a solid mass in the ovary itself. Microscopically we find an even more extensive similarity. Almost to the smallest details do they present the same microscopic picture, so that the following description serves for all three tumors. . . .

Epithelial formations are embedded in varying configuration in a rather cellular connective tissue stroma corresponding approximately to the normal ovarian stroma [Fig. 45-1]. Lying here in close approximation and there only individually

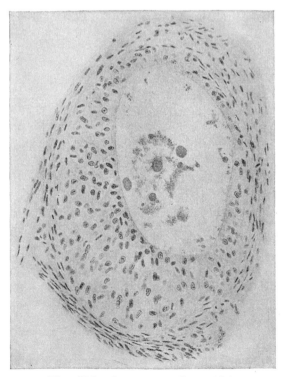

Fig. 45-2. See legend, Figure 45-1.

in the stroma are roundish and elongated groups of rather large, chiefly polygonal cells with nuclei that are not very large but rich in chromatin. In part they form solid pegs in the stroma; more often, however, thick mantles of cells, which surround a cavity. The row of cells enclosing the cavity usually permits an even, sharp, almost membranous boundary to be recognized about the lumen in cross section. This row of cells is usually cylindrical [Fig. 45-2]. In many instances the cell layer next to the cavity is flattened, just as well with the small epithelial complexes, corresponding to about twice the size of a primordial follicle, as with the larger ones. Especially often is the picture that of a thicker layer, composed of several to many rows of cells, gradually flattening out on one side to one or two layers of cells. It is precisely this arrangement that gives the tumor an unusually distinctive appearance under high power. Here and there the epithelial nests near the large spaces sharply bordered by cells, where the cells lie in a thicker layer, contain small vacuole-like cavities, which are sharply delineated from the cells. In the solid cell cords there are also at times several small vacuoles of this kind. The shape of the cavities is in general oval, sometimes round; they sometimes simulate two cavities of the same or different size joined together in different ways. The smallest groups, containing only five to six cells, about the size of a primordial follicle and less cellular than the larger cell complexes, are found in the connective tissue stroma. The somewhat larger ones likewise show small but already sharply demarcated vacuoles, located centrally or eccentrically. Homogeneous globules, a bright yellow with Van Gieson stain, are usually present within the smaller cavities as well as the larger to largest ones; finer globules are also present but these are clearly distinguishable from fibrin clots by their intense color. Small vacuoles, closely surrounded by the cell mantle, show the finest granularity in places, and very occasionally one or two granular, darker-colored, small inclusions. At times one or more typical granular cells also lie in the cavities inside the cell mantle. These epithelial cell nests are surrounded in most places by a concentric arrangement of connective tissue, which is more cellular in the neighborhood of these structures. This arrangement reminds one strikingly of the theca folliculi, in that it usually has a uniform relation to the separating layer of connective tissue. Examination in serial sections shows that the epithelial masses occasionally are isolated spherical or elongated forms, more often, however, sending out rootlike arborizations that remain connected with each other through thin septa or strands. These branchings are best developed in the largest of the three tumors which, as a result, shows in section in many places large epithelial anastomoses, looking like strands of carcinoma at first glance. However, most strongly against the picture of carcinoma, even at lower magnification, is the width of the intervening connective tissue. In no case does the capsule of the tumor show any epithelial penetration. The epithelial formations often extend right up to the capsule, especially in the third tumor. In the second tumor the capsular tissue changes into a broad outer marginal zone showing a uniform course of fibers, in which no epithelial formations lie and which simulates the tunica albuginea [Fig. 45-1]. The larger cystic spaces that are present in places are lined with one or two layers of flat to cuboidal epithelium and also contain the amber-yellow colloidal masses, which are even visible macroscopically.

The vascular network of the tumors is considerable. Nowhere can any relations between the epithelial cords and the blood or lymph vessels be made out. . . .

Brenner had seen no pseudomucinous cystic elements in any of his three tumors, and he was apparently unaware of their microscopic similarity to the epithelial nodules later associated with the name of Max Walthard. It is understandable, therefore, that he related his tumors to abnormal follicular growth, because of the superficial resemblance of the cystic tumor masses to ovarian follicles. He wrote:

Since Pflüger's tubules are said to persist after infancy also, the simplest conception of the origin of these tumors, even if not proven by this alone, would be somewhat as follows: They develop from Pflüger's tubules, which contain no primordial ova. In the menopause the tubules, only partially developed previously, proceed either in the form of belated development or, in the course of the altered conditions caused by involution of the ovaries or other bodily systems, in exuberant growth. This progresses to a moderate ripening of follicle formation, but for the most part without involution of the individual follicles. It is possible that this growth and follicle formation occurs even in earlier periods of life, progressing rather extensively.

In any case, our tumors . . . are to be regarded as distortions of the ovary in which the essential architecture of the ovary is viewed rather broadly.

This formation is best characterized—the combination of a Latin word and Greek ending is not happily chosen in folliculoma—by the name *oophoroma* with which the surname *folliculare* recommends itself.

BRENNER'S LIFE

The only recorded information about Fritz Brenner's life appears in his curriculum vitae in the 1908 registry of publications from German universities.[2] This entry indicates that Brenner was born in Osthofen, Germany, December 16, 1877, and grew up in Frankfurt-am-Main. He obtained his preliminary education at the Weilburg Gymnasium, from which he graduated in 1900. He then studied for two years in Strasbourg, a year in Freiburg-im-Breisgau, and subsequently went to Heidelberg, where he received his medical degree in 1904 and his license on June 23, 1905. His dissertation, excerpted above, was published from the Senckenbergsche Pathologische Institut in Frankfurt, the forerunner of the present pathology institute of the university in that city, where he served as assistant under Eugen Albrecht, who has been described as "the kindest of all beings." One of Albrecht's few surviving students has written me of their master's selflessness and devotion to his assistants, who were made the beneficiaries of his ideas, his spirit, and even his wording. Brenner was one of those privileged to work in this great man's laboratory.

Search of the registry of German physicians [5,6] showed a Fritz Brenner in Dürkheim in 1909 but not in 1910 or subsequently. In the edition for 1910, however, the very year in which Fritz Brenner was dropped from the listing

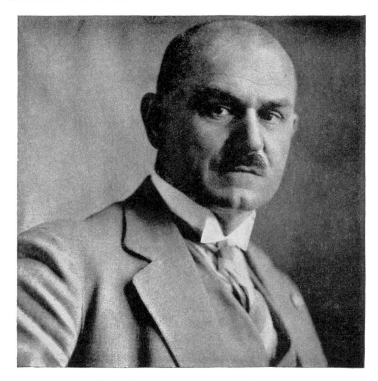

Fig. 45-3.   Fritz Brenner (1877–).

of physicians in Germany, a Dr. Brenner, first name omitted, appeared among the physicians listed in Southwest Africa, then a German colony.[6] This Dr. Brenner, entrusted with official duties (Regierungsarzt) in the seaport of Swakopmund, was presumed to be the object of our search, but conclusive evidence was lacking. The German registry listed Brenner in Swakopmund again in 1913 and again in 1914, but still without an identifying first name. The volumes of this registry for the ensuing years of World War I are missing. The first available postbellum volume, for 1926–1927, failed to list Brenner, but Southwest Africa was no longer under German rule, and Brenner's whereabouts became unknown. Diligent search of the obituary notices in the German medical periodicals, with the skilled help of librarians at the Columbia University Medical Library and the New York Academy of Medicine, was unrewarding.

As we paused for breath in our search, the arrival of Dr. Horst Naujoks, a new resident in our department, suggested a possible redirection of our efforts through his father, Professor Hans Naujoks of the Department of Obstetrics and Gynecology in Frankfurt; for it was from the pathology institute in that city that Brenner had published his thesis. Professor Naujoks had never known Brenner personally and could add nothing to our meager knowledge of him—except the information, obtained through the current director of the pathology laboratory in Frankfurt, that one of Brenner's contemporaries and erstwhile colleagues in Albrecht's laboratory, Dr. Edgar Goldschmid, was the current professor of medical history in Lausanne. Professor Goldschmid was most helpful. Although he had not seen Brenner since 1908, he confirmed our presumption regarding the identity of the Dr. Brenner in Southwest Africa, establishing him as the genuine Fritz Brenner. During a recent visit to Frankfurt, Goldschmid had inquired about old friends, but few survived and none had maintained a continuing contact with Brenner since his departure almost a half century ago. At the conclusion of World War I Brenner had elected to remain in Southwest Africa rather than return to Germany; and he soon became lost to his European contemporaries, his whereabouts and activities unknown.

Professor Goldschmid also succeeded in unearthing a long-forgotten group photograph, taken at a small tea party in the lecture hall of the old Senckenberg Institute in 1907. Fritz Brenner is clearly visible in the group scene, along with ten others, attired in the sartorial elegance of that era.

Still flushed with elation over this vital accession to my file on Brenner, I soon received word from the magistrate of Swakopmund, in answer to my inquiry, again confirming the fact that Dr. Fritz Brenner had been registered there, but stating that he had left for Johannesburg, South Africa, in 1923. I promptly solicited the help of Dr. S. Shippel, in the Department of Obstetrics and Gynecology of the University of the Witwatersrand, who was known to me through his contributions to the *Journal of Obstetrics and Gynaecology of the British Empire,* in the hope of finally tracking down Fritz Brenner. Gratification was exceeded by surprise as I read Dr. Shippel's reply, stating that (1) "the Dr. Brenner you seek is still very much alive and in general practice here in Johannesburg"; (2) the local gynecologists "had no idea that the Brenner of gynaecological history was practicing here amongst us in Johannesburg, and had you not sent me the letter I still would not have known"; and (3) when my letter of inquiry was read to Dr. Brenner "he was very surprised to hear that the tumor he described way back in 1907 was known by his name."

The search for Fritz Brenner is ended. In the pleasant correspondence that I have had with him he has supplied some of the heretofore missing details of his personal and professional life and corrected one or two inaccuracies in previous reports. In 1922, for example, he left Swakopmund for the inland city of Windhoek, the capital of Southwest Africa, and it was not until 1935 that he migrated to South Africa. More significant than these details, however, is his repeated profession of surprise at our interest in his "kleinen Beitrag zur gynäkologischen Pathologie!"

REFERENCES

1. Brenner, F.: Das Oophoroma folliculare. *Frankfurt. Ztschr. f. Path.,* **1**:150–71, 1907.

2. *Jahres-Verzeichnis der an den Deutschen Universitäten erschienenen Schriften; 15. August 1906 bis 14. August 1907.* Behrend & Co., Berlin, 1908, Vol. 22, p. 283.

3. Meyer, R.: Über verschiedene Erscheinungsformen der als Typus Brenner bekannten Eierstocksgeschwulst, ihre Absonderung von den Granulosazell-tumoren und Zuordnung unter andere Ovarialgeschwülste. *Arch. f. Gynäk.,* **148**:541–96, 1932.

4. Orthmann, E. G.: Zur Casuistik einiger seltenerer Ovarial- und Tuben-Tumoren. *Monatschr. f. Geburtsh. u. Gynäk.,* **9**:771–82, Plate VII, 1899.

5. Schwalbe, J. (ed.): *Reichs-Medizinal-Kalender für Deutschland auf das Jahr 1910.* Georg Thieme, Leipzig, 1909, Teil II, p. 393.

6. Schwalbe, J. (ed.): *Reichs-Medizinal-Kalender für Deutschland auf das Jahr 1911.* Georg Thieme, Leipzig, 1910, Teil II, p. 747.

Syndromes | PART VI

Johann Chiari, Richard Frommel, and the Chiari-Frommel Syndrome

Puerperal involution of the reproductive organs embodies the most rapid and striking of all the physiologic growth changes in woman. The rate of return of the uterus especially, from its pregnant to nonpregnant condition, is without parallel. Full gestational enlargement of this organ, requiring 40 weeks, reverses itself completely in little more than a month. Its weight regresses from 1 kg at term to 60 gm at the end of the puerperium, while all its dimensions shrink correspondingly: from 40 cm to 10 cm in length, 25 cm to 5 cm in breadth, and 6 liters to 5 ml in capacity.

As the activity of the mammary apparatus comes into the ascendancy during the puerperium, ovarian function recedes to its ebb. There thus results a period of enforced reproductive rest, which has great adaptive value for both the mother and her nursling; for by preventing early reimpregnation this utero-ovarian hibernation protects the former against the metabolic drain of recurrent gestation and ensures the infant against competitive nutritional demands on its source of sustenance.

After a variable number of months, usually longer in the presence of continued lactation, cyclic ovarian function returns, accompanied by resumption of the menses. The woman's capacity to lactate is also limited, so that even in the face of continuing and urgent suckling efforts by the infant, the breasts eventually go dry. Very rarely, and for reasons still imperfectly understood, the ovaries and uterus fail to rouse from their puerperal slumber, remaining in a state of permanent atrophy, while the mammary glands continue to give forth milk, even without the stimulus of suckling. This aberration of puerperal readjustment is known as the Chiari-Frommel syndrome. Only within very recent years has light been shed on its specific endocrine basis.[4,6]

CHIARI'S DESCRIPTION OF SYNDROME

Attention was first directed to this rare syndrome in 1855 by J. Chiari, C. Braun, and J. Spaeth, who reported two cases in their textbook of obstetrics

II. Anomalien der Grösse.

a. Als abnorme Kleinheit durch ursprüngliche Bildung sind die zwei zuletzt angeführten Fälle anzuführen.

b. Als acquirirte Volumsabnahme des Uteruskörpers beobachteten wir mehrere Male Schrumpfung des Uterus bei chlorotischen Kranken, wobei der Uteruskörper an Dicke der Substanz bedeutend abgenommen, und merklich erschlafft zu finden war. Mit dieser Atrophie waren meist Lageveränderungen nach rückwärts oder vorn, Mangelhaftigkeiten und Beschwerden der menstruellen Function vergesellschaftet.

Zu den acquirirten Uterusatrophien sind noch die im Gefolge des Puerperiums frühzeitig eintretenden Schrumpfungen des Uterus zu zählen, welche mit gänzlichem Aufhören der Menstruation trotz des wenig vorgerückten Alters, und, wie wir diess in den zwei unten näher zu beschreibenden Fällen beobachteten, mit andauernder Milchsecretion in den Brüsten verbunden war:

1. N. N., **36** Jahre alt, verheirathet, hatte vor 8 Jahren ein Mädchen leicht geboren. Sie säugte das Kind mehrere Monate. Seitdem blieb die Menstruation gänzlich aus, die Milchsecretion dauerte aber in dieser ganzen Zeit bald mehr, bald minder stark fort, und die Frau bemerkte, dass sie immer fetter wurde. Die Untersuchung der Brust zeigte beim Drucke wässrige Milchabsonderung. Die Vaginalexploration zeigte die Vaginalportion klein, den Muttermund enge, den Uterus sehr leicht und schlaff. Die Untersuchung der Uterushöhle mit der Sonde wies eine Länge desselben von nicht ganz **2** Zoll nach.

2. N. N., **28** Jahre alt, vor 14 Monaten das erstemal leicht und natürlich entbunden, hatte ihr Kind durch **3** Wochen gesäugt. Hierauf bekam sie **2**mal die Periode in regelmässigen Zwischenräumen, darnach aber, bis zur Zeit der Beobachtung nie mehr. Seitdem klagt sie über Magenschmerzen, die des Tags einigemal, am heftigsten aber bei Nacht eintraten. Auch bemerkt sie zeitweise Milchabsonderung in den Brüsten, was eben zur Zeit der Untersuchung durch Ausdrücken gelblich weisser, dicker Milch constatirt wurde. Die Vaginalexploration zeigte die Vaginalportion geschwunden, so dass der spaltförmig etwas geöffnete Muttermund die Spitze der Scheide bildete; der Uterus erschien beim Heben sehr leicht, schlaff, die Sonde zeigte aber die gewöhnliche Länge.

Schliesslich bemerken wir, dass in beiden diesen Fällen keine

Fig. 46-1. Report of two cases of puerperal atrophy of the uterus with amenorrhea and persistent lactation, in *Klinik der Geburtshilfe und Gynaekologie* by Chiari, Braun, and Spaeth (1855).

and gynecology.[2] Discussing the general subject of abnormalities of uterine size, they wrote:

To the cases of acquired uterine atrophy must be added those of premature shrinkage of the uterus occurring in the course of the puerperium, with complete cessation of the menses despite the patient's youth, and associated with persistent milk secretion in the breasts, as we observed in the following two cases:

N.N., 36 years old and married, had born a daughter with ease eight years previously and nursed the infant for several months. Since that time the patient remained completely amenorrheic, but lactation continued, more or less copiously, during this entire period, and she noticed that she was getting progressively fatter. Examination of the breasts revealed a watery milk secretion on pressure. Vaginal examination showed the portio vaginalis to be small, the cervix narrow, the uterus very light and flabby. Examination of the uterine cavity with the sound revealed its length at not quite 2 inches.

[The second patient, a 28-year-old primigravida] had an easy spontaneous delivery 14 months previously and nursed her infant for three weeks. She then had two normal menstrual periods but none thereafter up to the time of observation. During the interim she complained of gastralgia, which sometimes occurred during the day but was most severe at night. During this period she also noticed milk secretion in the breasts, which could be confirmed at the time of examination by the expression of yellowish-white, thick milk. Vaginal examination revealed absence of the portio vaginalis, so that the slitlike, rather patulous cervix formed the vault of the vagina. The uterus felt very light and flabby to palpation, but the sound showed its length to be normal.

In both these cases no blennorrhea had been present, either at the time of observation or previously. We regard them both as cases of premature senile atrophy of the uterus, which exerted a more or less deleterious effect on the general health, depending on the resistance of the individual.

Although the volume reporting these cases represented the combined efforts of Chiari, Braun, and Spaeth, the senior author alone was responsible for the section on diseases of the uterus. Only his name of the three, therefore, has been associated with the newly described syndrome.

CHIARI'S LIFE

Johann Baptist Vitus Liberalis Chiari was born in Salzburg, Austria, June 15, 1817.[1,9] Upon the completion of the philosophic curriculum in the university there he went to Vienna in 1835 for his medical studies, which culminated in 1841 with the publication of his dissertation, *De Legibus Mechanicus Motus Muscularis*. To round out his clinical training, Chiari spent the next two years in the medical and surgical clinics affiliated with the university. In 1842 he was appointed assistant in obstetrics and in short order developed a reputation for the excellence of his lectures. His interest soon drifted chiefly to gynecology, and in 1847 he received formal accreditation as a surgeon. In 1853 Chiari was called to the chair of obstetrics in the oldest German university, in Prague, but found himself unhappy in this post, despite the

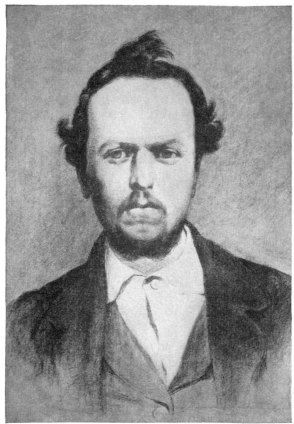

Fig. 46-2. Johann Baptist Vitus Liberalis Chiari (1817–1854). (Courtesy of Dr. Hermann Chiari, Pathologisch-Anatomisches Institut, Vienna.)

authorization he received to lecture on gynecologic as well as purely obstetric subjects. An invitation to return to Vienna the very next year, as professor of obstetrics in the Josephs-Akademie, was eagerly accepted, therefore; but Chiari's short-lived tenure of this coveted chair was abruptly cut off by an attack of Asiatic cholera, of which he died on December 11, 1854. His principal work, *Klinik der Geburtshilfe und Gynaekologie,* was published after his death by his coauthors. A bibliography of his other scientific contributions is appended to his obituary.[9] The family name has been kept alive in the annals of medicine by Chiari's son, Hanns, a pathologist, who coined the term, *salpingitis isthmica nodosa;* and by his grandson, Hermann, currently professor at the Pathologisch-Anatomisches Institut in Vienna.

FROMMEL'S DESCRIPTION OF SYNDROME

Subsequent to the publication of Chiari's two case reports a number of other authors recorded additional examples of puerperal atrophy of the uterus, but without galactorrhea. Among these accounts was a paper by Richard Frommel,[5] published in 1882, which added to the literature 28 such cases, one of which, like Chiari's cases, was associated with persistent lactation. Wrote Frommel:

This patient was 28 years old and had had five normal deliveries, the last of which occurred one and one-half years ago. After delivery the patient lactated for three months, then weaned the infant, whereupon the menses returned and recurred normally for three months. The menses stopped thereafter, and at the same time milk began to drip continuously from both breasts, so that the patient's blouse and clothes were constantly soaked. This condition has now persisted for a year. The uterus was slightly retroverted, 5.5 cm long, rather thin-walled, and both ovaries were very small and atrophic. Abundant milk could be expressed from both breasts in manifold streams. The patient had to wear napkins over her bosom to protect herself from constant soaking. The condition has not yet changed in any respect.

The factors responsible for persistent lactation remained completely obscure until the relatively recent identification of the functions of the anterior pituitary. Frommel regarded puerperal uterine atrophy as the result of mammary activity. He wrote:

If we ask ourselves what sort of etiologic factors produce an effect that could result in such a profound disorder of the uterine tissue, then I believe that an important role must be ascribed to lactation above all. It is a well-known fact that among women who nurse their children, very prompt and complete involution of the uterus and the entire genital apparatus is observed in the puerperium; and because of this all doctors quite properly urge their patients most firmly to nurse their children if at all possible.

The treatment of galactorrhea is still unsatisfactory. We can well sympathize with Frommel, therefore, in his nineteenth-century pessimism toward atrophy of the uterus. He reluctantly concluded:

The prognosis of uterine atrophy in the puerperium must be designated as exceedingly poor. . . . It is a priori clear that the prospect of regeneration of the organ is bad in patients with a flabby, thin-walled uterus and small, atrophic ovaries. The atrophy resulting from prolonged lactation appears likewise to offer no favorable prospects for treatment, at least in our experience.

FROMMEL'S LIFE

Julius Theodor Richard Frommel was born July 16, 1854,* in Augsburg, Germany.[3,7,8,10] After a preliminary education in the famous old gymnasium of St. Anna in his native city, he studied medicine in the universities of Munich,

* Martin [8] gives Frommel's birth date as July 15, 1854.

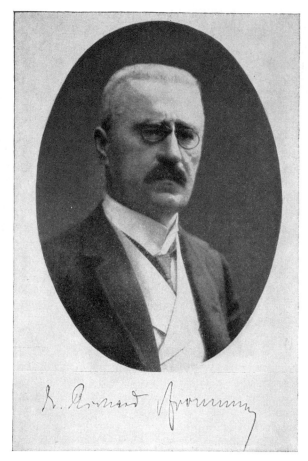

Fig. 46-3. Julius Theodor Richard Frommel (1854–1912).

Göttingen, and Würzburg, receiving his M.D. from the last in 1877. He then devoted himself to postgraduate work in obstetrics and gynecology in Vienna and Berlin, followed by three years as Schröder's assistant in the Universitäts-Frauenklinik of the latter city, during which period he published an important contribution on uterine motility. In 1882 he returned to Munich, where he maintained a private gynecologic hospital until called to the University of Erlangen to succeed Zweifel as professor of obstetrics and director of the Obstetric and Gynecologic Institute in 1887. In Erlangen, Frommel distinguished himself as a teacher, administrator, and ruthless critic of his students and assistants, and published the results of his investigations on the histology of the fallopian tubes, the physiology of the mammary glands, puerperal infection, and uterine cancer. He performed the first successful laparotomy in Germany for ruptured tubal pregnancy. Frommel is also known for his study of the development of the bat's placenta and for a yearbook of obstetrics and gynecology, which he founded and edited for 14 years. In 1901 he resigned his professorship and returned to private practice in Munich; but after a brief period he abandoned this as well, living in retirement until his death from appendicitis on April 6, 1912.

REFERENCES

1. *Biographisches Lexikon der hervorragenden Ärzte aller Zeiten und Völker,* 2nd ed. Ed. by W. Haberling, F. Hübotter, and H. Vierordt. Urban & Schwarzenberg, Berlin & Vienna, 1930, Vol. 2, p. 13.

2. Chiari, J.; Braun, C.; and Spaeth, J.: *Klinik der Geburtshilfe und Gynae-kologie.* Enke, Erlangen, 1855, pp. 371–72.

3. Eversbusch, O.: Richard Frommel. *München. med. Wchnschr.,* **59**:1048–50, 1912.

4. Forbes, A. P.; Henneman, P. H.; Griswold, G. C.; and Albright, F.: Syndrome characterized by galactorrhea, amenorrhea and low urinary FSH: Comparison with acromegaly and normal lactation. *J. Clin. Endocrinol. & Metab.,* **14**:265–71, 1954.

5. Frommel, R.: Ueber puerperale Atrophie des Uterus. *Ztschr. f. Geburtsh. u. Gynäk.,* **7**:305–13, 1882.

6. Greenblatt, R. B.; Carmona, N.; and Hagler, W. S.: Chiari-Frommel syndrome. A syndrome characterized by galactorrhea, amenorrhea, and pituitary dysfunction; report of two cases. *Obst. & Gynec.,* **7**:165–70, 1956.

7. Holzapfel, K.: Richard Frommel. *Zentralbl. f. Gynäk.,* **36**:665–66, 1912.

8. Martin, A.: Richard Frommel. *Monatschr. f. Geburtsh. u. Gynäk.,* **35**:535–37, 1912.

9. Nekrolog. *Wochenblatt der Zeitschrift der k. k. Gesellschaft der Aerzte zu Wien,* **1**:65–68, 1885.

10. Obituary: Julius Theodor Richard Frommel, M.D. *Boston M. & S. J.,* **166**:833, 1912.

Harold Leeming Sheehan and Sheehan's Syndrome

Pregnancy produces two remarkable changes in woman's reaction to hemorrhage. On the one hand, tolerance to acute blood loss is increased by her augmented store of extracellular fluid. On the other, hemorrhagic shock at delivery may result in necrosis of the anterior pituitary, whereas this lesion is never caused by blood loss of whatever magnitude in the non-pregnant. Hypopituitarism in women is usually produced by obstetric factors; yet the obstetrician rarely encounters this condition in its definitive form unless the patient consults him later for her resultant amenorrhea.

The clinical aspects of postpartum hypopituitarism were clearly described one century ago [7] by Sir James Young Simpson in his lecture, "On Super-Involution of the Uterus and Amenorrhoea"; but as the cause and mechanism of this disorder remained obscure to him, he limited his remarks to exposition rather than explanation. He reported the case of a young woman of 20 years of age, who never menstruated after her first delivery:

. . . It was two years subsequent to her confinement that this patient sought admission to our clinical ward, in consequence of amenorrhoea and great constitutional debility. She was then subject to various distressing symptoms in connection with the pelvic organs. . . . The mammae were shrunk and flat; and she was thin, feeble, and anaemic in appearance. On making a vaginal examination, I found the uterus small and mobile, the cervix uteri much atrophied, and its vaginal portion scarcely forming any projection into the cavity of the vagina. The os uteri was so contracted as to admit with difficulty a surgeon's probe. It was dilated by a slender bougie left in it for a few days, and when the sound was subsequently introduced, the uterine cavity was found to be only an inch and a half in length. Various remedial measures were adopted without any very marked effect; and as the uterine symptoms seemed to be only of secondary importance, she was transferred to another ward, where she died in the course of months in a state of prolonged coma.

Generalizing about the patient suffering from "super-involution of the uterus," Simpson added:

Formerly, in all probability, she used to menstruate regularly, and when the term of utero-gestation and the period of lactation have been brought to a close, and her child has been weaned, she wonders why the usual monthly flow does not reappear. She is quieted for the moment by the assurance that, in some cases, the recurrence of the catamenia may be retarded for a time without any ultimate disturbance of the general health. But, as months pass on, and no discharge at all, or only a very imperfect degree of it, returns, unfulfilled expectation grows into alarm, and not unreasonably; for now the breasts tend sometimes to shrink and shrivel up, the subcutaneous adipose matter begins to be absorbed, so that the skin looks withered and wrinkled, and the patient, though still, it may be, young in years, offers often prematurely to assume the aspect of age. The whole system usually sympathises with the change that has been effected in the uterus, just as it does in women who have reached the climacteric period, and in whom the uterus normally ceases from all functional activity; and the appearances which are familiar to you as the normal characteristics of women who have passed that period of life, begin to be abnormally presented by the patient in whom the functional powers of the uterus are destroyed, as a consequence of the morbid process that leads to its atrophy. It results, further, from the morbid condition of the womb, and from its inability any longer to perform its normal functions, that the patient becomes henceforth sterile, and the oppressive idea that she will never have any more family comes to be added to the burden of her other troubles. Most frequently, too, she is in a state of marked constitutional ill health; she is very anaemic; her digestive powers are low; she has frequent headaches; is easily fatigued; and is the subject of general debility, and shows often, also, depression and impaired activity of mind.

Alexander Simpson, nephew of James Young Simpson and the latter's successor to the chair of obstetrics in the University of Edinburgh, likewise interested himself in this unusual and unexplained condition, and in 1883 emphasized its association with hemorrhage in childbirth. He wrote: [6]

My attention was first called to the connexion between flooding and super-involution about five years ago by seeing in my consulting room, in the course of one week, three cases of the disease; and in all the three the patients had suffered from excessive loss of blood. In some cases the hemorrhage is unavoidable or accidental; more frequently it occurs during the third stage or post-partum. . . .

I have in several cases remarked a marked diminution in the intellectual powers, or a thickness and hesitancy of utterance, or unsteadiness of gait, in patients affected with superinvolution.

Simpson erred, however, in assuming the nervous system to be at fault; not until the twentieth century was the role of the pituitary discovered.

Postpartum necrosis of the pituitary was first reported in 1913 by Glinski,[1] who described this pathologic change at autopsy in two patients, one of whom died of sepsis nine days after cesarean section, the other six weeks following abortion in the sixth month of pregnancy. The following year Simmonds [5] described the clinical condition that now bears his name, but which he characterized as "senium praecox," in a woman who died in coma with almost complete destruction of the anterior pituitary 11 years after her recovery from puerperal sepis. Stander [8] later reported the same lesion of the anterior lobe in several patients who died of pernicious vomiting, eclampsia, and chronic nephritis.

Postpartum necrosis of the pituitary is now recognized as the commonest cause of Simmonds' disease, or chronic anterior pituitary insufficiency, in women. At least 60 cases of pituitary necrosis had been reported in the literature before 1937, but not until Sheehan's publication in that year [2] was the obstetric background of this disorder fully appreciated. The clinical syndrome resulting from the pituitary lesion, when traceable to an accident of parturition, is often known, therefore, as Sheehan's syndrome.

SHEEHAN'S DESCRIPTION OF PITUITARY NECROSIS

In a meticulous autopsy study of 59 women who died in the puerperium, Sheehan discovered almost complete necrosis of the anterior pituitary in seven cases and smaller areas of destruction in four. He reported: [2]

The fully developed lesion is a coagulative necrosis with the typical appearances of an infarct and an ischaemic origin appears to be the most reasonable explanation on general pathological grounds. The necrosis centers usually in the antero-inferior part of the anterior lobe in the mid-line and spreads out to involve most of the lobe. The parts which normally escape are the postero-superior angle beneath and in front of the stalk and a very thin layer on the surface; the middle and posterior lobes are unaffected. From about ten days *post partum* the necrosed area is surrounded by a sharply demarcated zone where the alveoli contain large rounded phagocytic cells instead of the normal parenchyma cells. These alveoli collapse and atrophy, leaving a loose meshwork of condensed stroma but with no fibrosis.

Estimating the duration of the lesions from their histologic characteristics, Sheehan concluded:

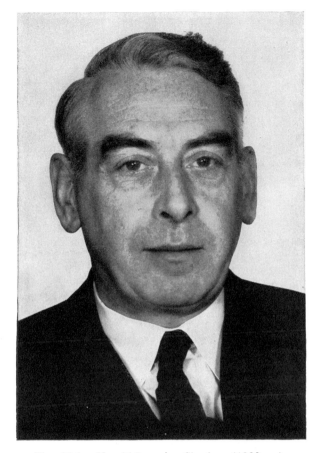

Fig. 47-1. Harold Leeming Sheehan (1900–   ).

. . . The *necroses all appear to date from about the time of delivery.* . . . The age of the thrombi in the sinuses can only be estimated very approximately from the density of the fibrin net, but they too appear to have originated at about the time of delivery.

Sheehan was naturally led by his interpretive dating of the pituitary lesions to an inquiry into the clinical circumstances surrounding the patients' confinement. He found:

[Two] had no haemorrhage at delivery apart from that due to the operation but they were both very gravely ill before delivery, which was by hysterotomy. The other nine cases all had severe haemorrhage at delivery leading to serious collapse; in five of them the cause was retained placenta. . . . There appears to be enough evidence to consider this clinical condition as of possible aetiological importance.

Combining with his own the data gleaned from the scattered cases in the literature, Sheehan concluded:

The occurrence of haemorrhage at delivery in 24 of the 28 cases in which details are available is *prima facie* evidence that it is of aetiological importance, though not necessarily the essential causative factor. This factor appears to be "collapse" produced by the haemorrhage. It is significant that, in the few cases where haemorrhage is not recorded, collapse due to other causes occurred. . . . In the cases of recent and old pituitary necroses the cause of the haemorrhage at delivery was placenta praevia in 3 cases, rupture of the uterus or tube or cervical tears in 4 cases, retained placenta in 9 cases and aneurysm in 1 case; in the others the cause is not indicated.

The predisposition of pregnant women to pituitary necrosis demanded explanation. Sheehan theorized:

The situation of the necroses suggests a peculiar distribution of the blood supply to the anterior lobe during pregnancy. . . . The sudden change from hypertrophy to rapid involution that occurs in the anterior lobe after delivery and the increased coagulability of the blood during parturition and the early puerperium are of course general factors that are probably of importance in this connection.

In a subsequent report [3] Sheehan described more fully the pathologic findings in patients dying of pituitary necrosis. He observed:

The amount of anterior lobe tissue which remains in clinically severe cases is usually less than 10 per cent of the original lobe, and often a great deal less. . . . The cells remaining are usually chromophobe, though some eosinophil and occasional basophil cells may be present. These two factors, the amount and the cellular constitution of the remaining part of the anterior lobe, are presumably of importance in determining the course of the disease.

The thyroid is usually small. It is often between 8 and 13 gm. in weight, as compared with a normal of about 25 gm. The size does not, however, give any clear indication of the severity of the histological involvement. Microscopically, about one-third of the glands show normal appearances or slight atrophy, about one-third show moderate atrophy, and the remaining third a very severe atrophy with extensive fibrosis. . . .

The suprarenals are usually very much below the normal weight. There is nearly always atrophy of the cortex, often so severe that the cortex is described as "as thin as paper." Microscopically, in these severe atrophies there is a loss of the normal layered structure of the cortex which appears to consist mainly of zona fasciculata; the zona glomerulosa and reticularis are very thin and, in places, absent. . . . The medulla is normal except in rare instances. The atrophy of the cortex appears to be a direct result of the pituitary lesion. The pathological appear-

POST-PARTUM PITUITARY NECROSIS

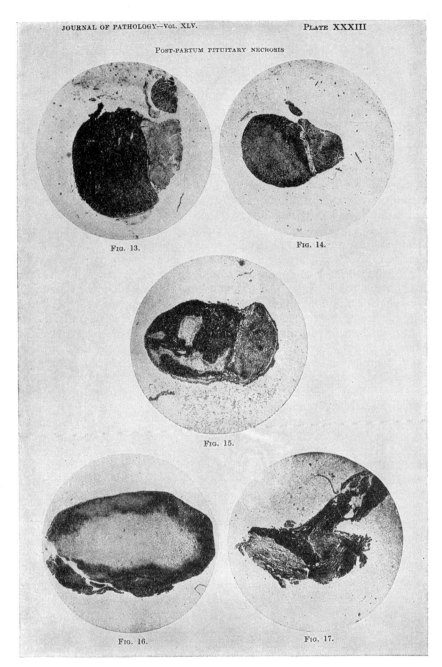

Fig. 13.   Fig. 14.

Fig. 15.

Fig. 16.   Fig. 17.

Fig. 47-2. Illustrations from Sheehan's first paper [2] on postpartum necrosis of the pituitary, showing extent of glandular destruction. (Reproduced by permission of *Journal of Pathology and Bacteriology*.)

397

ances are quite unlike those of the primary atrophy which is so commonly seen in Addison's disease, where the suprarenal shows very gross scarring with small nodules of regenerating cortical cells.

Sheehan's summary of the clinical manifestations of postpartum pituitary necrosis recapitulated the well-known picture of anterior hypopituitarism. In addition he attempted to correlate quantitatively the severity of functional disturbance with the amount of glandular destruction. He wrote:

There will probably be no symptoms with a loss of less than 50 per cent of the gland, the symptoms will be slight with a 60 per cent loss, moderate with a 75 per cent loss, and severe with a 95 per cent loss. The necroses which follow these complicated deliveries vary in size from 1 to about 98 or 99 per cent of the gland, so that there is a possible range of subsequent symptoms from normal health up to evidence of almost complete absence of the anterior pituitary. . . .

In severe cases, there is usually a complete absence of mammary activity during the puerperium; instead of the normal development of swelling and hardness at the fourth day after delivery and the establishment of lactation, the breasts shrink rapidly and remain dry. In patients whose subsequent symptoms of hypopituitarism are only moderate, this condition occurs in only about half the cases. . . .

In the severest cases the ovaries become very atrophic and their functions are completely lost, involving disturbances of menstruation, loss of hormone control of the genital tract, and lack of follicular development. The absence of oestrogenic hormones is characterized by complete genital atrophy, namely superinvolution of the uterine body and cervix, atrophy of the endometrium to a thin layer of epithelium, loss of glycogen in the vaginal epithelium, loss of the acid reaction and Döderlein's bacilli in the vaginal secretion, and shrinkage and a senile appearance of the vagina and vulva. These organic changes are associated with a permanent absence of menstruation or molimina, dating from the delivery. There are sometimes related menopausal symptoms, such as flushing of the face, for a year or two, but these are inconstant. Less severe cases have the permanent amenorrhoea, but not the complete genital atrophy, though the uterus is smaller than normal. In less severe cases still, there is a return of menstruation nine to eighteen months after delivery, but it is scanty and occurs only occasionally at irregular intervals of a few months. . . . Though sterility is, of course, the rule in severe cases, subsequent pregnancy may occur in patients who have had no menstruation since the significant delivery. . . .

In severe cases there is a loss of axillary and pubic hair. This is a gradual process which may be obvious within a few months after delivery, but is rarely complete in less than five years. In less severe cases the hair is only thinned, and the loss is most marked in the axillae and least over the labia. The loss of body hair appears to be a symptom of a severe pituitary lesion. . . .

Most of the patients develop a group of somewhat related general symptoms which may be considered together, asthenia, apathy, and undue sensitivity to cold. While the more severe cases usually show a full development of all three symptoms together, the less severe cases may have various combinations of them; sometimes the physical disturbances are present with little or no psychological change, and sometimes the opposite condition obtains. . . . The asthenia may be of any gradation of intensity. The less severely affected patients are able to do light housework, more severe cases spend most of the day sitting quietly in a chair and may have an unsteady gait, and some patients become so weak that they are confined to bed during the later stage of their illness. . . . It is difficult to assess how far the inability to work is physical and how far mental in origin. . . . There are also various grades of the psychological change, which shows some similarities to the apathy of myxoedema.

In the rare cases in which subsequent pregnancy occurs, Sheehan observed, "the symptoms are permanently cured, probably as a result of hypertrophy of the remaining portions of anterior lobe tissue."

Increasing experience with the syndrome of postpartum pituitary necrosis soon convinced Sheehan that the condition is more prevalent than had hitherto been realized. Indeed, he suggested [3] that "every woman who nearly dies of haemorrhage or collapse at delivery develops a large pituitary necrosis, and it can be accepted that any patient who does die from these causes at delivery would have developed a pituitary necrosis if she had lived long enough." The previously presumed rarity of the condition Sheehan attributed to its usually remaining undiagnosed. He explained:

The patient does not bother to seek medical care. Her only concern is to keep warm and to be left undisturbed in her mental torpor and physical inertia.

. . . In many of the severe cases the patient is dull and not sufficiently interested to discuss her symptoms. She makes only vague complaints about weariness and weakness and cold. Quite commonly she does not bother to mention any of the significant points in her history, such as that her illness began after a delivery at which she nearly died of hemorrhage, that she has had amenorrhea since then, and that she lost her pubic and axillary hair within the next couple of years. She is usually dirty and wearing too many clothes, and the house is in a state of neglect. In these difficult conditions even the best doctor is naturally discouraged from making a detailed investigation, and diagnosis easily gives place to symptomatic therapy. The doctor notices that she is pale so he prescribes iron and when this proves to be without effect, he tries liver therapy. When this in turn is found useless, he notices that her face is rather puffy, her skin dry and her eyebrows thin, so he prescribes thyroid. This treatment is of no more value, and the patient gradually drifts out of medical care again. At this stage she may develop delusions and be transferred to a psychiatric hospital, where the interests of the staff are naturally focussed rather more on the mental than the physical aspects.[4]

Sheehan has estimated that "in each 10,000 of the population there are about two severe cases and seven lesser cases of hypopituitarism due to postpartum necrosis." With modern methods for combating blood loss and shock, obstetricians must regard Sheehan's syndrome, like death from postpartum hemorrhage, as a wholly preventable accident of parturition.

SHEEHAN'S LIFE

Harold Leeming Sheehan was born in Carlisle, England, August 4, 1900. After graduating in medicine from Manchester University in 1921, he spent six years in general practice in his home town, the following seven years as lecturer in pathology at his alma mater. Sheehan came to the United States in 1934 for advanced study as a Rockefeller research fellow at the Johns Hopkins Medical School for one year, upon the completion of which he was made director of research in the Glasgow Royal Maternity Hospital. In 1946 he was appointed professor of pathology in the University of Liverpool. His principal fields of investigation have included renal physiology, shock, the pathology of pregnancy, and experimental diabetes.

REFERENCES

1. Glinski, L. K.: Anatomische Veränderungen der Hypophyse. *Deutsche. med. Wchnschr.,* **39**:473, 1913. (Abstracted from *Przegl. lekarski,* No. 1.)
2. Sheehan, H. L.: Post-partum necrosis of the anterior pituitary. *J. Path. & Bact.,* **45**:189–214, 1937.
3. Sheehan, H. L.: Simmonds's disease due to post-partum necrosis of the anterior pituitary. *Quart. J. Med.,* **8** (n.s.):277–309, 1939.
4. Sheehan, H. L.: The incidence of postpartum hypopituitarism. *Am. J. Obst. & Gynec.,* **68**:202–23, 1954.
5. Simmonds, M.: Ueber Hypophysisschwund mit tödlichlem Ausgang. *Deutsche med. Wchnschr.,* **40**:322–23, 1914.
6. Simpson, A. R.: Superinvolution of the uterus. *Edinburgh M. J.,* **28** (Part 2): 961–68, 1883. Oliver & Boyd, Ltd., Edinburgh.
7. Simpson, J. Y.: *Clinical Lectures on the Diseases of Women.* Ed. by A. R. Simpson. D. Appleton & Co., New York, 1872, pp. 597–611.
8. Stander, H. J.: Hemorrhagic retinitis in vomiting of pregnancy. *Surg., Gynec. & Obst.,* **54**:129–33, 1932.

Joe Vincent Meigs and Meigs's Syndrome

CHAPTER

48

Malignant tumors of the ovary are notorious for their insidious development. In a large proportion of cases the first symptoms result from the associated ascites, which usually signifies peritoneal dissemination of the tumor. The additional presence of fluid in the chest, suggesting pleural involvement, almost always portends a hopeless prognosis for the patient. Serous effusions may occasionally develop in the pleural and peritoneal cavities from benign abdominal tumors also, especially ovarian fibromas. The pathogenesis of these effusions in patients with benign neoplasms is poorly understood, but removal of the offending tumor results in abrupt cessation of the process and rapid resorption of the residual fluid from the serous cavities.

The combination of ovarian fibroma, ascites, and hydrothorax was first reported in 1866 by Otto Spiegelberg,[14] in a 38-year-old woman who died of peritonitis several days after undergoing abdominal paracentesis. Thirteen years later Cullingworth [1] recorded a similar case of a patient who died with fibromas of both ovaries, ascites, and bilateral pleural effusions. Although the benignancy of the ovarian tumors had been established by microscopic examination, Lawson Tait, influenced by the serous effusions, refused to accept the proposed diagnosis in his discussion of the case and characterized the lesions instead as "solid fibroid cancer of both ovaries."

Further documentation of this phenomenon was provided by Demons [2] at a meeting of the Surgical Society of Paris on December 21, 1887. He reported:

401

Mrs. B., whom I saw recently, presented a cyst of the right ovary together with a large bilateral pleural effusion. The presence of the latter complication made her physician think that the patient had multiple cancerous tumors. He performed several thoracenteses on each side, but the fluid kept accumulating very quickly and the patient's health deteriorated rapidly. I performed ovariotomy. The bilateral effusion disappeared as if by magic and never recurred. Mrs. B., threatened by approaching death, recovered completely and is in excellent health today.

Fascinated by this case, the vigilant Demons soon succeeded in adding several similar ones to his experience. He related:

I have encountered pleural effusions of greater or lesser magnitude on one or both sides of the chest in a rather large number of women with ovarian cysts. It is important to recognize this complication, just as much from the viewpoint of diagnosing the principal disease as from the veiwpoint of therapy and prognosis. . . . In contrast to simple hydrothorax or pleural effusion resulting from secondary tumors of the lung . . . I interpret this as an entirely different phenomenon . . . pleural effusions in women with common ovarian cysts that do not recur after extirpation and do not metastasize. . . . I have already observed this complication nine times among 50 patients examined, such a proportion that I cannot accept the possibility of simple coincidence. . . .

When the effusion is unilateral it does not always occupy the side corresponding to the side of the abdomen where the ovarian tumor originated. . . . The fluid was pale yellow and transparent, at least in the one case in which thoracentesis was performed. . . . Several patients had more or less pronounced ascites at the same time. . . . Some presented edema of the lower extremities.

I believe that the pleural effusions occur in the following manner: The abdominal tumor disturbs the circulation of the abdominal lymphatic vessels and this disturbance extends across the diaphragm into the pleural lymphatics. Whatever the explanation may be, it is important to distinguish these pleural effusions, which are dangerous only because of the quantity of their fluid, from the much more serious effusions that result from a secondary tumor of the lungs or from cancerous infection. The slow growth of the abdominal tumor, the characteristics of the tumor itself, the absence of the signs of cachexia, the absence also of any hemoptysis, and the nonsanguineous nature of the pleural effusion are the basis of differential diagnosis. . . . In every case I have seen the effusion resorb rapidly after ovariotomy, without any special medication having been given for it.

In the discussion that followed Demons' presentation, Terrillon stated that he also had seen a case of pleural effusion in a patient with an ovarian cyst; Bouilly reported two such cases, one with an ovarian cyst and one with a solid ovarian tumor, in both of which the effusions resorbed spontaneously after ovariectomy; and Verneuil maintained that any abdominal tumor may produce pleural effusion.

Demons added to these observations three cases of ovarian fibroma associated with ascites and hydrothorax, which he reported to the French Surgical

Congress in 1902; [3,4] but just as he had overlooked the earlier case reports of Spiegelberg and Cullingworth, his own observations escaped the attention of contemporary and later gynecologists for many years. Lawson Tait,[15] for example, was apparently unaware of Demons' experience when he reported a case of his own in 1892. Wrote Tait:

I have determined in my own mind to discourage all operative proceedings in cases where, as well as abdominal disease, there was ascitic effusion with well-marked pleural effusion on both sides, especially if the latter were determined by aspiration to be of a sanguinolent character, on the ground that the certainty of these cases being malignant was almost absolute, and as the probability was that the pleural lining was infected as well as the peritoneal surface, no hope could be entertained of relieving them by any operation. I have now, however, to place on record a case which shows that such a conclusion may be quite erroneous.

The patient, aged 36, first consulted Tait in January, 1890, with the complaints of abdominal swelling, productive cough, and dyspnea. Tait reported:

On examining the chest, the left side was absolutely dull nearly up to the clavicle . . . the intercostal spaces were increased and bulged . . . and the heart was displaced to the right. . . . There were all the physical signs of ascitic effusion free in the peritoneal cavity. In addition there could be felt on deep pressure through the fluid a large rounded solid tumour, apparently moored in the pelvis and floating freely in the ascitic fluid. As the breathing was much distressed the left pleural cavity was aspirated and ninety-five ounces of blood-stained serum removed. A few days after the tapping of the left side fluid was discovered in the right pleura, and was similarly removed. . . . The diagnosis of malignant disease of the peritoneum with secondary infection of the pleural surfaces was made. I declined to operate on the abdominal tumour, and the patient returned home to die.

About a fortnight after returning home her left pleura was again tapped, and eighty ounces of pale yellowish fluid removed. . . . In February, 1890, the abdomen was tapped, and eleven quarts of pale yellow thin ascitic fluid removed. From this time until February, 1891, her abdomen was tapped over thirty times, from eight to fourteen quarts of thin clear yellowish fluid being removed at each operation.

At laparotomy on March 5, 1891, Tait found and removed a fibroma of the right ovary weighing 2 lb 2 oz, curing the patient. Enunciating one of the tenets of modern gynecology, he concluded:

The lesson in this case is a very valuable indication that no set of conditions in the abdomen, however apparently unfavourable, are sufficient to justify us in an absolutely unfavourable condemnation in any particular case. Looking back upon my experience of pleural effusion as complicated by abdominal disease . . . I think that probably my general impression that it is a very fatal complication, especially when the fluid is of a bloody character, is correct; and if half of the

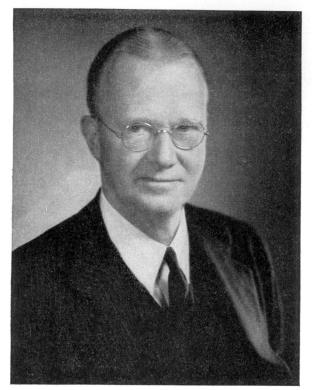

Fig. 48-1. Joe Vincent Meigs (1892–   ).

cases had been submitted to abdominal section, simply for the purpose of exploration and removing the bulk of fluid the likelihood is not great that permanent benefit would have accrued in many of them; but if one of the lives had been saved by
the discovery of a mistake, I think it would have quite justified the performance
of the incision in all the rest. . . . The striking results obtained in this case by
the correction of my initial mistake have gone a long way to confirm me in the
advisability of extending the principles of exploration and confirmatory incisions
in abdominal disease to an almost universal application.

Individual case reports rarely make a lasting impression. Tait's experience
too, soon forgotten, failed to be recalled by similar cases later reported by
others. Again in 1934, for example, Salmon,[13] without reference to the earlier
literature, recorded an isolated case of ovarian fibroma and one of uterine
fibroids, each associated with ascites and pleural effusion; and Meigs, in the
section on fibromas of the ovary in his book, *Tumors of the Female Pelvic
Organs,*[5] included the notation:

Three patients with large cellular tumors had been in the medical ward, where
because of fluid in the chest a diagnosis of tuberculosis had been made and their

chests tapped. Paracentesis had been done more than three times in each case. One had multiple abdominal taps. . . . An abdominal tumor was finally discovered and operation advised. A fibroma was found in each instance with fluid in the abdomen; the tumor was removed and the patient promptly recovered . . . and had no reaccumulations of fluid within the abdomen or chest.

This combination of clinical phenomena, still not recognized as a distinct syndrome, awaited the aggressive and persistent interest that Meigs was to supply. In 1936, at a meeting of the American Association of Obstetricians, Gynecologists and Abdominal Surgeons, he reported seven cases,[11] four (including the three he had mentioned earlier) being from his own hospital, the other three from other clinics. In the report of an additional case of ovarian fibroma with ascites and hydrothorax, soon added by Rhoads and Terrell,[12] the authors suggested the term "Meigs's syndrome." With a spate of subsequent papers on the subject [6,7,8,9,10] Meigs seems to have clinched his claim to this designation.

MEIGS'S ACCOUNT OF ASCITES AND HYDROTHORAX

From his earliest reports Meigs, like other students of the syndrome, has struggled with an explanation for the effusions. He wrote with Cass: [11]

The reason for the presence of fluid in the abdomen and chest in such cases is not clear. The ascites has been ascribed for many years to irritation of the peritoneum by the hard tumor mass. It is possible that such irritation might cause abdominal fluid, but it does not seem possible to explain fluid in the chest by such reasoning. Both fluids are part of the same process, for removal of the tumor of the ovary caused the chest fluid to disappear also. It might be imagined that fluid from the abdomen could get into the chest cavity by direct extension, but anatomically this does not appear to be possible. The chest cavities are hollow boxes, and if there were any communication with the area below the diaphragm there ought to be some difficulty with the normal process of respiration. If the tumor were malignant and had metastasized to the chest it would be easy to understand the presence of fluid, but no such pathology is present. Ascites can be caused by metastatic tumor with secretory areas in the tumor, such as is present in the papillary cystadenoma of the ovary. It may be due to a general renal or cardiac failure. Inflammatory processes, such as peritonitis and especially tuberculous peritonitis, are often accompanied by abdominal fluid. Portal obstruction is known to cause ascites in certain cirrhoses of the liver. But how to explain the presence of abdominal fluid by a freely movable tumor of the ovary is difficult enough without having to explain the presence of fluid in the chest and its cure by removal of such a tumor. The fluid is probably a transudate, and thus it would seem to be due to some pressure or obstruction, but how a pelvic tumor could cause sufficient pressure to permit the accumulation of quarts of fluid is difficult to explain. Lack of drainage of the right chest by the azygos vein may play a part, but in one case the fluid was in the left chest and in another in both. These facts exclude the possibility of an azygos obstruction at least being the only etiological factor. . . . If in some way an opening might be found in the chest cavity that would allow free communication with the abdomen, the hydrothorax would be explained, but it is doubtful if there is any such communication. After much discussion with surgeons and pathologists interested in thoracic disease, and with internists, it has been impossible to give any logical etiology that can withstand all criticism.

The pathogenesis of the peritoneal and pleural effusions still remains unexplained.

With the growing recognition that ascites and hydrothorax may develop secondarily to any of a large variety of pelvic tumors a number of recent authors have attempted to liberalize the pathologic criteria for Meigs's syndrome. Meigs himself, however, insists on limiting the syndrome to cases in which the tumors are ovarian, "fibrous, hard, solid, and benign." His definition of the condition lists four requirements:

As the *first* characteristic we must have a fibroma or a fibroma-like tumor [including thecomas, granulosa cell tumors, and Brenner tumors]; *second,* this tumor must be accompanied by ascites. . . . The fluid may be of very great or of small amount, but it must be there. *Third,* there must be fluid in the chest. This fluid is most often found in the right thoracic cavity but can occur in the left, and even in both sides. . . . *Fourth,* the removal of the benign ovarian solid tumor must relieve the patient of her ascites and chest fluid. . . . It is not necessary that the fluid always be clear and yellow; it can be bloody or serosanguineous, but this is not common.[8]

Meigs's syndrome remains unsurpassed as a clinical complex in which the apparent gravity of the patient's condition preoperatively contrasts so sharply with her prognosis after treatment.

MEIGS'S LIFE

Joe Vincent Meigs, born in Lowell, Massachusetts, October 24, 1892, was destined to add fresh luster to a long-established medical name. His father and maternal great-grandfather were well-known New England physicians. He is distantly related to the eloquent Charles D. Meigs of Philadelphia, the latter being the grandson of our subject's fourth great-grandfather. After obtaining his A.B. from Princeton in 1915 and his M.D. from Harvard in 1919, Joe Meigs embarked on a career in gynecology. In 1927 he was appointed gynecologist to the Pondville State Cancer Hospital of the Massachusetts Department of Public Health, and subsequently became director of gynecology at the Vincent Memorial Hospital, Massachusetts General Hospital, and Palmer Memorial Hospital as well. Since 1942 he has held the title of clinical professor of gynecology in the Harvard Medical School. A fellow of the American Gynecological Society and a founder and president of the

Society of Pelvic Surgeons, he has also served as president of the Boston Surgical Society and the Boston Obstetrical Society. Meigs is best known for his revival of interest in the surgical treatment of cervical cancer. In addition to his book, *Tumors of the Female Pelvic Organs* (1934), he has edited a volume on *Surgical Treatment of Carcinoma of the Cervix* (1954) and, together with Somers Sturgis, three editions of *Progress in Gynecology*.

REFERENCES

1. Cullingworth, C. J.: Fibroma of both ovaries. *Tr. Obst. Soc. London,* **21**:276, 288, 1879 [1880].

2. Demons, A.: Épanchements pleurétiques compliquant les kystes de l'ovaire. *Bull. et mém. Soc. d. chirurgiens de Paris,* **13**:771–76, 1887. Masson & Cie, Paris.

3. Demons, A.: Sur un point de l'évolution clinique des fibromes de l'ovaire et les ligaments larges. *Assoc. franç. de chir., Quinzième Congrès de chir.* Paris, 1902, pp. 739–40.

4. Demons, A.: Fibromes des ovaires et des ligaments larges. *Rev. de chir., Paris,* **26**:680, 1902.

5. Meigs, J. V.: *Tumors of the Female Pelvic Organs.* The Macmillan Co., New York, 1934, pp. 262–63.

6. Meigs, J. V.: Fibroma of the ovary with ascites and hydrothorax. A further report. *Ann. Surg.,* **110**:731–52, 1939.

7. Meigs, J. V.: Fibroma of the ovaries with ascites and hydrothorax (a new syndrome). In *Frank Howard Lahey Birthday Volume.* Charles C Thomas, Publisher, Springfield, Ill., 1940, pp. 331–38.

8. Meigs, J. V.: Fibroma of the ovary with ascites and hydrothorax—Meigs' syndrome. *Am. J. Obst. & Gynec.,* **67**:962–87, 1954.

9. Meigs, J. V.: Pelvic tumors other than fibromas of the ovary with ascites and hydrothorax. *Obst. & Gynec.,* **3**:471–86, 1954.

10. Meigs, J. V.; Armstrong, S. H.; and Hamilton, H. H.: A further contribution to the syndrome of fibroma of the ovary with fluid in the abdomen and chest, Meigs' syndrome. *Am. J. Obst. & Gynec.,* **46**:19–33, 1943.

11. Meigs, J. V., and Cass, J. W.: Fibroma of the ovary with ascites and hydrothorax. *Am. J. Obst. & Gynec.,* **33**:249–67, 1937.

12. Rhoads, J. E., and Terrell, A. W.: Ovarian fibroma with ascites and hydrothorax (Meigs's syndrome). Report of a case. *J.A.M.A.,* **109**:1684–87, 1937.

13. Salmon, U. J.: Benign pelvic tumors associated with ascites and pleural effusion. *J. Mt. Sinai Hosp.,* **1**:169–72, 1934.

14. Spiegelberg, O.: Mittheilungen aus der gynäkologischen Klinik von Otto Spiegelberg. I. Fibrom des Eierstockes von enormer Grösse. *Monatschr. f. Geburtsk. u. Frauenk.,* **28**:415–25, 1866.

15. Tait, L.: On the occurrence of pleural effusion in association with disease of the abdomen. *Med.-Chir. Tr.,* **75**:109–18, 1892.

Irving Stein, Michael Leventhal, and the Stein-Leventhal Syndrome; Henry Turner and Turner's Syndrome

CHAPTER

49

With the discovery of the endocrine function of the ovary in the early-twentieth century, gynecologists redirected their attention from uterine malposition as a cause of female disorders to this new and more fertile field for speculation and therapy. Hypo- and hyperovarian dysfunctional states were postulated, albeit poorly defined, for which a wide range of therapeutic measures, from galvanism to castration, were empirically prescribed, to combat an even greater variety of presumed gynecologic ailments, ranging from insomnia to narcolepsy and from frigidity to nymphomania. As abdominal surgery rapidly developed, the ovary fell easy prey to the intrepid and enterprising gynecologist, who explored, biopsied, needled, resected, transected, excised, suspended, and transplanted the organ for all sorts of indications, real or fancied, limited only by his zeal and ingenuity and the patient's submissiveness. Like the appendix and tonsil, the human ovary has been sacrificed by the ton to therapeutic fashion, often with little benefit or to the frank detriment of the patient.

Except for the normal lag in gonadal secretion during prepuberty and the physiologic ebb during lactation and after the menopause, most states of ovarian dysfunction have resisted clinical diagnosis and classification. Amenorrhea, genital atrophy, and increased urinary excretion of gonadotrophin point to hypoestrogenism but tell nothing of its possible causes. Increased and perverse ovarian function still evade certain recognition. Nonetheless, a few syndromes have been widely recognized, in which disordered action of the ovaries plays an essential role.

408

An organ's size may belie its activity. Enlargement of the thyroid, for example, is often associated with hyperthyroidism, but the largest glands, their follicles distended with colloid, are usually the least active. In the ovary, similarly, functional status cannot always be predicted from size alone. Even histologic section of the ovary may provide only scant interpretable information as to the nature and level of the organ's activity. The gross and microscopic pattern, together with the clinical findings in the patient, however, occasionally suffice for assignment of her condition to an established syndrome. While adding little to our immediate understanding, such grouping of similar cases offers improved prognostic accuracy and permits the use of therapeutic experience as a guide to treatment.

Consistent morphologic aberrations typify the ovaries in two syndromes of primary interest to the gynecologist. In one, the Stein-Leventhal syndrome, the ovaries are characteristically enlarged and cystic, but their functional status is conjectural. In the other, Turner's syndrome, the rudimentary ovaries appear functionless by every criterion. Differing widely from each other in most essentials, both syndromes find common ground in the gynecologist's office, where the afflicted seek relief from their amenorrhea and sterility.

THE STEIN-LEVENTHAL SYNDROME

It has long been recognized that obese women commonly suffer from amenorrhea or menstrual irregularity or excess, and that hirsute women are often infertile. Yet not until 1935 was a specific ovarian derangement associated with these complaints and an effective method of treatment proposed for their alleviation. In that year Stein and Leventhal read a paper [7] at the meeting of the Central Association of Obstetricians and Gynecologists describing seven cases of the syndrome that has since been known by their names. They reported:

In the series of patients which we observed with bilateral polycystic ovaries and amenorrhea the ovaries were found to be from two to four times the normal size and while they often maintained their original shape, they were sometimes distinctly globular. In one case, they were flat and soft, the so-called "oyster ovaries." The ovarian cortex was found to be hypertrophied in all of the cases and the tunica thickened, tough, and fibrotic.

The cysts were follicle cysts, near the surface, and almost entirely confined to the cortex, and they contained clear fluid. There were from twenty to one hundred cysts in each ovary, varying in size from 1 mm. to about 1.5 cm., but rarely larger. The color of the ovary was oyster gray with bluish areas where the cysts were superficial and appeared on the surface as sago-like bodies. On section, the variation in size of the cysts and the clear fluid contents were revealed. Corpora lutea were sometimes absent and when found, they were very small and deeply placed.

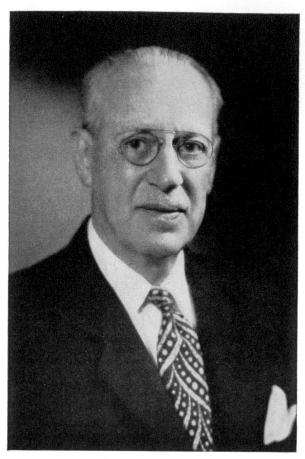

Fig. 49-1.   Irving Freiler Stein (1887–   ).

The uteri in these patients were either normal in size or smaller and firmer than normal. The remaining changes observed were those involving the secondary sex characteristics. The breasts presented no characteristic changes except in cases of long-standing amenorrhea when they were small, firm, and pale.

In some patients, there was observed a distinct tendency toward masculinizing changes. A typical rhomboid hairy escutcheon, hair on the face, arms, and legs, and coarse skin was noted. No voice changes have been observed by us. The external genitals in most patients were normal, but in some, the labia minora were markedly hypertrophied. Libido is apparently not affected by the changes noted in the ovaries.

Wedge resection of the ovaries, the recommended treatment for this condition, was adopted by the authors after their fortuitous observation that several amenorrheic patients menstruated shortly after ovarian biopsy. The *modus operandi* of this procedure as curative therapy is still obscure, however. Stein and Leventhal reported:

We have resected from one-half to three-fourths of each ovary by wedge resection, thereby removing the cortex containing the cysts, and have sutured the hilus with the finest catgut. The immediate results have been entirely satisfactory. All of the patients recovered uneventfully, and were discharged from the hospital from the ninth to the thirteenth postoperative days. Uterine bleeding occurred on the third to the fifth postoperative day and menstruation occurred monthly thereafter in every case. Our first patient, operated upon four years ago, has given birth to two children since operation.

The ovary guards well the secrets of her innermost workings. Even the most careful microscopic study of resected wedges has failed to provide a satisfactory explanation of the patient's symptoms or her relief by operation. Said Stein and Leventhal:

The pathologist is unable to conclude from a study of the sections taken from the ovaries in our patients that amenorrhea was a symptom. He can demonstrate no anatomic structure or characteristic change in the ovary which enables him to describe the clinical picture. The only consistent pathologic finding is the presence of follicle cysts lined by theca cells. . . . The fact remains, however, that when we remove the cystic portion of the ovaries which to all appearances are the same as those observed in patients with uterine bleeding, normal function is restored to the sex apparatus.

The etiology of the ovarian changes in the Stein-Leventhal syndrome remains just as mysterious as their relation to its other manifestations. The authors' suggested explanation reflects the current endocrine concept of gonadal control:

It is unlikely that polycystic ovaries are congenital for the condition develops as a rule after the patient has menstruated more or less regularly for a period of years. The amenorrhea is usually secondary. It is also unlikely . . . that the multiple cyst formation is explained on the basis of inflammatory change. That hormones play a role in the polycystic change in the ovaries is extremely plausible in the light of our present-day conception of sex physiology. Whether it results from an excessive production of anterior pituitary sex hormones or not is debatable.

It is reasonable to assume that a *mechanical* factor operates actually to produce the most significant symptoms, namely: amenorrhea and sterility. The overproduction of cystic follicles which crowd the ovarian cortex but which do not rupture on the surface of the ovary, together with the presence of a thickened tunic, prevents the immature follicles from ripening and reaching the surface. It is possible that some of these follicles develop, and being impeded in their pathway to the surface of the ovary, may rupture into the cysts.

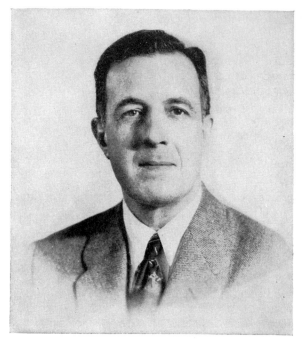

Fig. 49-2.   Michael Leo Leventhal (1901–   ).

STEIN'S LIFE

Irving Freiler Stein was born in Chicago, September 19, 1887. He received his B.S. degree from the University of Michigan in 1910 and his M.D. from Rush Medical College two years later. After completing his internship at the Michael Reese Hospital in Chicago he joined its Department of Obstetrics and Gynecology, in which he subsequently rose to the rank of senior attending. He also holds the title of associate professor emeritus, in the Department of Obstetrics and Gynecology of Northwestern University. He has served as president of the Chicago Gynecological Society and the American Society for the Study of Sterility.

LEVENTHAL'S LIFE

Michael Leo Leventhal was born in Chicago, November 16, 1901. He graduated from the University of Chicago with the B.S. degree in 1922, and received his medical degree from Rush Medical College in 1924. Beginning with his internship, he has maintained a continuing affiliation with the Michael Reese Hospital, attaining the position of attending obstetrician and gynecologist. During World War II he served with the U.S. Army in evacuation hospitals in Africa, Sicily, and Italy.

TURNER'S SYNDROME

The mammalian embryo, although endowed with the rudiments of both male and female reproductive tracts, normally possesses only pure male or pure female gonads, almost never both. Nearly as rare as true hermaphrodism is congenital absence, or aplasia, of the sex glands, a developmental error often associated with multiple somatic defects.

Congenital absence of the ovaries was reported in 1923 by Olivet[5] in a 38-year-old woman 148 cm in height, with small, flat breasts and scant axillary and pubic hair. Fibrous whitish thickenings were found in the middle of either broad ligament, but no typical ovarian tissue. Pich[6] added three additional cases of ovarian agenesis in 1937, but not until more than a decade later was attention sharply focused on the congenital somatic abnormalities frequently associated with this deficiency. At the annual meeting of the Association for the Study of Internal Secretions in 1938 Turner read a paper entitled, "A Syndrome of Infantilism, Congenital Webbed Neck, and Cubitus Valgus,"[8] which he summarized in these words:

Infantilism with webbing of the neck and deformity of the elbow (cubitus valgus), occurring in the same individual is extremely rare, and to the author's knowledge, has not been previously described. This unusual phenomenon was observed exclusively in seven female patients, aged 15 to 23 years. Among the characteristic signs were retardation in growth and sexual underdevelopment. Webbing of the skin of the neck was slight to marked. Absence or fusion of the cervical vertebrae was not demonstrated, and the shortening of the neck was merely apparent, due to the webbing, and not real. The posterior hair margin extended well down on the neck. Deformity of the elbow, consisting of an increase in the carrying angle, or cubitus valgus, was constantly present. Movements of the head and arms were not hindered. Facial asymmetry, dorsal scoliosis, and other deformities, mirror movement, difficulty in breathing and swallowing, shortness of breath, or mental retardation were not present in this group of patients.

Laboratory examinations of the blood and urine showed findings that were entirely within normal limits. Roentgenograms of the skull, cervical spine, elbows, wrist, and pelvis showed no abnormalities with the exception of demineralization and evidence of delayed union of the epiphyses in 6 cases. Treatment with pituitary growth hormones has been unsatisfactory. There was definite genital development following administration of the anterior pituitary gonadotropic hormone in the two cases treated.

The original description of this syndrome, which soon came to be known as "Turner's syndrome," encompassed, let it be noted, only its clinical manifestations, without reference to the status of the gonads. Not until four years later, with the publication of a paper by Albright, Smith, and Fraser,[1] was the constancy of the elevated follicle-stimulating hormone excretion pointed out, this observation suggesting primary ovarian failure and leading to the

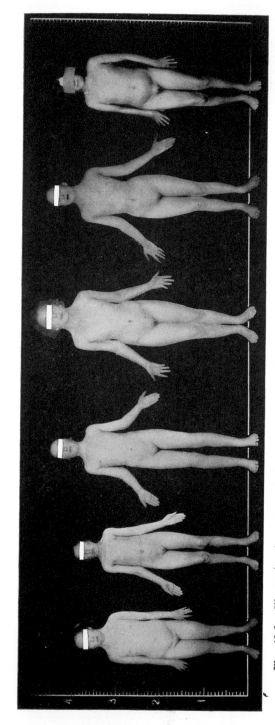

Fig. 49-3. Illustration from Turner's first paper on gonadal dysgenesis. (Reproduced from Turner, H. H.: A syndrome of infantilism, congenital webbed neck, and cubitus valgus. *Endocrinology,* **23**:567, 1938. Charles C Thomas, Publisher, Springfield, Ill.)

alternate designation, "ovarian dwarfism." Turner,[9] however, considers this term "one of convenience rather than scientific accuracy . . . no author has clearly explained the *modus operandi* by which primary hypogonadism may result in eunuchoid tallness in one instance and dwarfism or short stature in another." He has continued to urge [10] that the syndrome be defined by the following purely clinical criteria: "short but not dwarfed stature, in an amenorrheic or at least hypogonadal girl, in the absence of a history of potentially castrating disease, with any one, or more, of certain congenital anomalies apparent at first glance, and often with visceral, skeletal or other anomalies detectable in clinical study." The syndrome is distinguished from hypopituitary dwarfism by the shorter stature, complete absence of axillary and pubic hair (even after estrogen therapy), asthenia, greater retardation of bone age, and especially by the absence of urinary follicle-stimulating hormone in the latter condition.

Among the manifold congenital anomalies commonly associated with ovarian agenesis, coarctation of the aorta is of special interest because of its predilection for males. Webbed neck, it may also be noted, was first described [4] in a male. How then to reconcile the frequent occurrence of these malformations among girls with Turner's syndrome?

Sex determination, long considered the simplest of all diagnoses, occasionally presents a complex problem. Four distinct criteria must be reckoned with; namely, somatic sex (body habitus and secondary sex characters), psychologic and behavioral sex, histologic (gonadal) sex, and genetic (chromosomal) sex. In doubtful cases the last is considered the ultimate biologic determinant of the individual's "true" sex. Experiments with rabbit, rat, and mouse embryos [3] have shown that castration during early development results in somatic females irrespective of their genetic sex. This discovery suggested the possibility that patients with Turner's syndrome may in fact be genetic males whose testicular development was stunted during embryogenesis. Not only has this suggestion been supported by chromosomal studies,[2] which have revealed a male chromatin pattern in most (but not all) cases, but by "ovarian" histologic sections as well, which have shown clusters of epithelioid cells closely simulating the Leydig cells of the normal testis.

This explanation, however, fails to illuminate many facets of gonadal dysgenesis, such as the female chromatin pattern in some individuals with Turner's syndrome, their short stature, the normal male habitus of most persons with congenital testicular aplasia, and the female chromosomal picture in patients with Klinefelter's syndrome (testicular tubular aplasia).

Since patients with Turner's syndrome are somatically and behaviorally female, their treatment lies in estrogenic replacement. Explained Turner:

The administration of estrogens results in growth of the breasts, enlargement and rugation of the vagina, growth of the uterus from barely palpable to juvenile

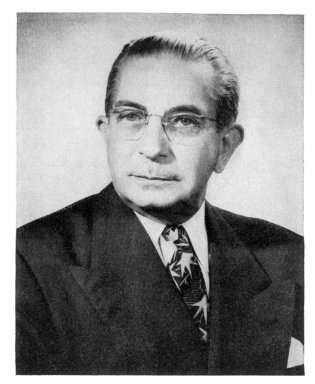

Fig. 49-4.   Henry Hubert Turner (1892–   ).

and' greater size, and the appearance of [more] axillary and pubic hair. These effects on the breasts and growth of hair are permanent, while those on the pelvic organs may recede somewhat if treatment is discontinued. The patients do not grow appreciably under treatment. Provided it is made clear that sterility exists and will not be alleviated, it is possible to produce all the exterior womanly features, to the gratification of these patients, who may then attain marital happiness. Such improvement is maintained after suitably prolonged and intensive treatment, while the increase in the size of the uterus can be minimized since that organ will serve no functional purpose in any event. The estrogenic therapy of this syndrome is, within these limits, wholly satisfactory.[10]

TURNER'S LIFE

Henry Hubert Turner was born in Harrisburg, Illinois, August 28, 1892. After receiving his collegiate and part of his medical education at St. Louis University, he transferred to the University of Louisville, where he graduated in medicine in 1921. Upon completing his residency training at the Louisville City Hospital in 1924 he was appointed instructor in medicine at the University of Oklahoma and promoted later to associate professor. From 1947 to

1949 he was also associate dean of the medical school. Since joining the Oklahoma faculty he has served as chief of the Endocrine Clinic of the University Hospital and as consulting endocrinologist to it and the Children's Hospital, as well as visiting physician to other hospitals in Oklahoma City. He has held the presidency of the American Therapeutic Society, the Oklahoma State Medical Association, the Oklahoma City Clinical Society, and the Oklahoma City Academy of Medicine.

REFERENCES

1. Albright, F.; Smith, P. H.; and Fraser, R.: A syndrome characterized by primary ovarian insufficiency and decreased stature. *Am. J. M. Sc.,* **204** (n.s.):625–48, 1942.

2. Grumbach, M. M.; Van Wyck, J. J.; and Wilkins, L.: Chromosomal sex in gonadal dysgenesis (ovarian agenesis): Relationship to male pseudohermaphrodism and theories of human sex differentiation. *J. Clin. Endocrinol.,* **15**:1161–93, 1955.

3. Jost, A.: Problems of fetal endocrinology: The gonadal and hypophyseal hormones. *Rec. Progr. Hormone Res.,* **8**:379–418, 1953.

4. Kobylinski, O.: Ueber eine flughautähnliche Ausbreitung am Halse. *Arch. f. Anthropol.,* **14**:343–45, 1883.

5. Olivet, J.: Über den angeborenen Mangel beider Eierstöcke. *Frankfurt. Ztschr. f. Path.,* **29**:477–91, 1923.

6. Pich, G.: Über den angeborenen Eierstockmangel. *Beitr. z. path. Anat. u. z. allg. Path.,* **98**:218–63, 1937.

7. Stein, I. F., and Leventhal, M. L.: Amenorrhea associated with bilateral polycystic ovaries. *Am. J. Obst. & Gynec.,* **29**:181–91, 1935.

8. Turner, H. H.: A syndrome of infantilism, congenital webbed neck, and cubitus valgus. *Endocrinology,* **23**:566–74, 1938. Charles C Thomas, Publisher, Springfield, Ill.

9. Turner, H. H.: "Ovarian dwarfism." In *Progress in Gynecology.* Ed. by J. V. Meigs and S. H. Sturgis. Grune & Stratton, Inc., New York, 1946, pp. 134–37.

10. Turner, H. H.: Ovarian agenesis and rudimentary ovaries. In *Progress in Clinical Endocrinology.* Ed. by S. Soskin. Grune & Stratton, Inc., New York, 1950, pp. 340–50.

Positions | PART VII

Friedrich Trendelenburg and the Trendelenburg Position*

Proper positioning of the patient is essential for any operation. The *sine qua non* for pelvic laparotomy is the Trendelenburg position, which lowers the head and chest and elevates the hips, allowing the intestines to gravitate toward the diaphragm and thereby facilitating exposure of the pelvic viscera. The history of this inclined position dates back to antiquity. It has been described and its merits independently rediscovered probably more times than any other contribution to the annals of surgery. From the time of Celsus (ca. 40 B.C. to 20 A.D.) and for the next millennium the inclined position was used in the treatment of abdominal injuries, when eviscerated intestines had to be replaced within the peritoneal cavity. The position was described anew by Paul of Aegina (ca. 660 A.D.), and again by Abulcasis in the eleventh century.[6]

In the ensuing years of the Middle Ages patients were placed in a semi-inverted position for both the manual reduction and surgical repair of abdominal hernias. The chapter on hernias in the famous manuscript of Roger and Roland [15] succinctly describes this position and states its purpose: "In primis ergo patiens collocetur in banco, caput et humeros habens depressos, ut tota intestina descendant ad pectus, coxas vero et crura teneat elevata." This work, variously known as *Practica Chirurgiae* or *Post mundi fabricam,* the latter from the first three words of the preface, was probably written in

* This chapter originally published in *Surg., Gynec. & Obst.,* **105**:114–19, 1957; reprinted by permission. Copyright, 1957, by The Franklin H. Martin Memorial Foundation.

the latter part of the twelfth century. Produced originally by Roger of Salerno, the manuscript was re-edited in 1252 by his pupil, Roland of Parma (1170–1264). Subsequent generations have identified it, the first Italian work on surgery, by the names of both Roger and Roland. Roger is also credited with being the first occidental to recognize the value of iodine, in the form of sea-sponge ashes, in the treatment of goiter.[1]

Among the several later authors who recommended an inclined position for the patient was Caspar Stromayr, a surgeon and ophthalmologist of Lindau im Bodensee. Stromayr's remarkable manuscript of 1559 [17] deals

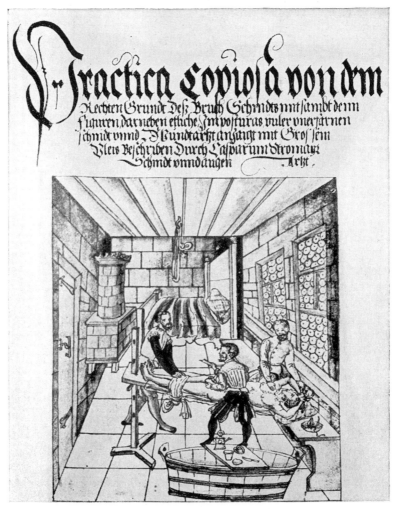

Fig. 50-1. Illustration from Caspar Stromayr's manuscript of 1559,[17] showing inclined position of patient for herniorrhaphy.

largely with hernias. Profusely illustrated with color plates, each accompanied by a caption in old German verse, this manuscript provides both verbal and pictorial evidence (Figs. 50-1, 50-2) of the author's use of the head-down position.

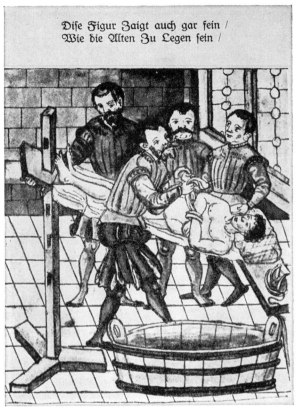

Dise Figur Zaigt auch gar fein /
Wie die Alten Zu Legen fein /

Fig. 50-2. Another illustration from Caspar Stromayr's manuscript of 1559.[17]

The inverted position was mentioned again in 1707, in a letter from Abraham Cyprian,[2] a Dutch surgeon, to Thomas Millington. In reporting an operation for a case of advanced tubal pregnancy Cyprian wrote:

J'avois même pour plus grande precaution afin d'empecher que les boyaux ne descendissent, placé la malade en sorte que les parties superieures du corps étoient un peu abaissées, et la pauvre femme a même presque toujours demeuré dans cette même situation jusqu'a ce qu'elle a été tout afait guerie, pour éviter une hernie.

At one time professor of surgery in Francker, Cyprian later settled in London, where he reputedly performed 1400 lithotomies in 12 years.

Percival Pott,[14] in the middle of the eighteenth century, again pointed out the value of the inclined position in the reduction of hernias. Wrote Pott:

The posture of the body, and the disposition of the lower limbs, may be made very assistant in this operation, when the difficulty is considerable; the nearer the posture approaches to what is commonly called standing on the head the better, as it causes the whole packet of small intestines to hang, as it were, by the strangulated portion, and may thereby disengage it. . . .

Elevation of the pelvis achieved gynecologic recognition in 1815 by Gutberlet,[5] who suggested a pillow under the patient's hips as an aid to hysterectomy:

Man giebt nun der Kranken auf einem Tische oder erhöhten Bette eine horizontale Lage, bey welcher das Becken durch einen unterlegten Polster etwas erhöht wird; durch diese Lage schon wird bey der nachfolgenden Ausschneidung der Gebärmutter der Andrang der Gedärme in das Becken verhütet.

More pronounced tilting of the patient's body was used by Freund,[3] in 1878, when he performed his celebrated total abdominal hysterectomy for uterine cancer.

Trendelenburg began to experiment with the inclined position in Rostock in 1880, for the repair of vesicovaginal fistula and other operations within the bladder. Four years later, in 1884, Trendelenburg's rediscovery of this surgical adjunct was reported by one of his assistants, Willy Meyer,[10] who later migrated to the United States and achieved distinction on his own as one of the leading surgeons in New York City. Meyer's paper contains an interesting woodcut (Fig. 50-3) showing Trendelenburg's early method of maintaining the elevated pelvic position. An attendant, standing at the foot of and with his back to the operating table, supported the patient's flexed knees throughout the operation. In a later publication, in 1890, Trendelenburg compared this to the technique of the ancients in their treatment of hernia, but it is not clear whether he was aware of the centuries of previous experience when he first began to use the position, ten years earlier.

Meyer explained the Trendelenburg posture and its advantages as follows:

It is easy to understand how the viscera, because of their weight, fall back toward the diaphragm. The opened bladder gapes, just as the vagina in the lateral Sims position, thus permitting not only a completely unobstructed view into its interior, but also, after retraction of the edges of the abdominal wall and bladder by means of broad, blunt retraction hooks, . . . the easiest introduction of the instruments necessary for extirpation and other manipulations. The vicinity of the trigone, which is the commonest site of bladder tumors, is thus also especially accessible to both observation and instrumentation. With the operating table placed as usual, and with its foot end opposite the window, the light then falls directly from the window onto the posterior inferior part of the bladder, thus

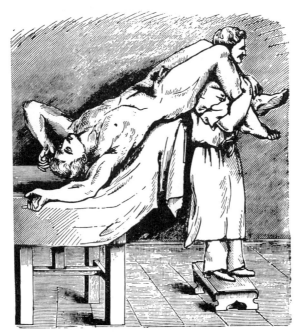

Fig. 50-3. Woodcut from Willy Meyer's paper of 1884,[10] which first described Trendelenburg's use of the elevated pelvic position. (Reproduced by permission of *Archiv für Klinische Chirurgie.*)

illuminating not only the internal urethral orifice, but also very thoroughly the region of the ureteral orifices. Observations can thus be made that are impossible in the usual dorsal position. We could often see during our operations how the urine spurted in a little jet from the ureteral orifices, we could introduce sounds upward into the ureters and ascertain their accessibility and width, etc. Furthermore, not to be minimized is the fact that the blood can now drain continuously toward the part of the bladder that is usually of less interest to us at this time . . . the operative field thus remaining relatively free of blood. In most cases this can not be achieved in the usual dorsal position. A lake of blood and urine tends to collect precisely here, at the trigone.

No displacement of the organs nor any other disturbances at all result from the respiratory movements in this position, since the abdominal excursions are noticeable only up to about the midpoint between the umbilicus and symphysis. . . . How unusually free is the access then even to the deepest reaches of the posterior bladder wall. . . .

This position is best designated as the "elevated pelvic position."

TRENDELENBURG'S DESCRIPTION OF ELEVATED PELVIC POSITION

Trendelenburg's personal comments on the elevated pelvic position, published in 1890 [19] in association with his report of vesicovaginal fistulas repaired

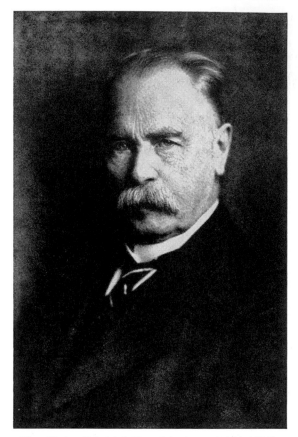

Fig. 50-4.   Friedrich Trendelenburg (1844–1924).

by the abdominal approach, stressed the value of this posture for delicate intravesical procedures. He wrote:

The elevated pelvic position has afforded us a means of operating under direct vision within the bladder with equal or greater ease than within the vagina. Thus nothing could be more natural than a transvesical attack on fistulas that cannot be managed successfully from the vagina. . . .

If the patient is placed on the operating table so that the pubic symphysis forms the highest point of the trunk and the long axis of the latter forms an angle of at least 45° with the horizontal, the abdominal organs . . . fall into the concavity of the diaphragm. The intestines fall out of the true pelvis as far as the atmospheric pressure will permit. In thin individuals with the rectus muscles relaxed under deep anesthesia, the anterior abdominal wall in the hypogastric region exerts an actual sucking action on the pelvic cavity. . . .

If a longitudinal or transverse incision is now made in the hypogastric region, as for lithotomy, and the rectus muscles and their posterior sheath are split, the air then enters the prevesical space at once, often with an audible sound. The peritoneum falls away and an extensive cavity is formed in the prevesical interstitial space, into which the light shines readily and in which the anterior wall of the bladder and the reflected fold of the peritoneum can be seen.

Trendelenburg quickly recognized the advantages of the elevated pelvic position for intraperitoneal as well as intravesical operations. He wrote:

We work in the full light of the window, like the artist at his easel, without having to stoop . . . and without being burdened by protruding loops of bowel. . . . No one who has ever removed a myomatous uterus or an adherent ovarian cyst in this way will readily revert to the old procedure. The tumor falls out of the pelvis . . . as far as the intrapelvic connections permit. All the ligaments to be divided are put on a stretch and the blood drains away from the operative field. The intestines, which remain bunched together in the epigastrium, cause no concern as long as no vomiting occurs. . . .

After the tumor is removed, a surprising view is obtained of the entire true and false pelves; the iliac and hypogastric vessels are seen pulsating, the course of the ureter is observed, and any small bleeding vessels can be picked up and ligated. . . . The elevated pelvic position is of great advantage in myomectomy, especially in difficult cases with intraligamentous extension of the tumor.

The improved exposure afforded by the position led Trendelenburg to recommend total hysterectomy in preference to the subtotal variety in cases requiring removal of the uterus. He said:

The operation is made so easy that panhysterectomy is carried out instead of supravaginal amputation. . . . This procedure, because of its safety and simplicity, surpasses the usual supravaginal hysterectomy. All steps of the operation can be carried out under visual control by use of the elevated pelvic position; blood loss is slight, and the elastic tourniquet for the uterus therefore unnecessary.

Utilizing Sims's discovery that when the pelvis is elevated the opened vagina aspirates air, Trendelenburg soon adapted his position for visualization of the vagina and rectum. He explained:

It is an excellent means of rendering the interior of the vagina or rectum accessible to the eye. Both cavities . . . gape widely as soon as their orifice is held open with the fingers, a short speculum, or some similar device. . . . With a manometer it can be demonstrated that the pressure in the lower abdominal cavity becomes negative when the elevated pelvic position is assumed. One need only connect a rubber tube to a catheter previously introduced into the bladder. Several experiments showed the pressure to be +1 cm of water with the body in the horizontal position, while with the pelvis elevated the pressure fell to −6 to −8 cm.

The term "Trendelenburg position" was first used in 1888 by Mendes de Leon,[9] who reported his experience with this posture for a variety of pelvic laparotomies and for gynecologic examination of patients with tympanites.

The name found immediate acceptance in a paper by Lange [8] the following year and now enjoys universal recognition in surgical terminology.

Trendelenburg noticed facial edema in many of his patients maintained in a steeply inverted position, and soon obtained roentgenographic evidence of dilatation of the right side of the heart during inversion at a 45° angle. He therefore recommended never using this extreme posture for more than five to ten minutes without interruption, and cautioned against using it at all for the obese or patients with congestive heart disease.[11]

In historic perspective Trendelenburg made two principal contributions to the operative posture that bears his name: (1) popularization of the position, and (2) invention of a metal operating table fitted with padded shoulder braces and specifically designed to maintain elevation of the patient's hips and flexion of the knees.

TRENDELENBURG'S LIFE

Friedrich Trendelenburg was born in Berlin, May 24, 1844.[4,7,12,13,16,18,20] His father, Adolf Trendelenburg, who was professor of philosophy in the university, taught him Latin and arithmetic at home, while his mother instructed him in English, his aunt in grammar. After completing his formal schooling in the Joachimsthal Gymnasium, he entered the medical school of the University of Berlin, but spent part of his time in Edinburgh and Glasgow, studying anatomy, embryology, and physics. After graduation in 1866, Trendelenburg entered military service for the next two years, working as surgeon in the hospitals in Gorlitz and Kiel. His thesis in ancient Indian surgery, entitled *De Veterum Indorum Chirurgia,* was published in 1867. From 1868 to 1874 he served as assistant to von Langenbeck, with whom he helped found the German Society of Surgeons in 1872; and in 1898 Trendelenburg was elected its chairman. In 1874, at the age of 30, he was made director of the surgical ward in the Friedrichshain Hospital in Berlin, and the following year was called to the University of Rostock as ordinary professor of surgery. Here he remained until 1882, when he accepted a similar position at the University of Bonn. In 1895 he responded to an invitation to the University of Leipzig, where he occupied the chair of surgery until 1911. He then retired to Nikolassee, a southwest suburb of Berlin, where he died of a malignant tumor of the lower jaw, December 15,* 1924, in his eighty-first year. His autobiography, *Aus Heiteren Jugendtagen,* was published shortly before his death.

Entering the practice of surgery soon after the introduction of antisepsis and general anesthesia, Trendelenburg found fertile fields for his wide interests

---

* Some of Trendelenburg's biographers have given December 16 as the date of his death.

and boundless energy. He performed the first gastrotomy for stricture of the esophagus in Germany and was one of the first to ligate the hypogastric veins for puerperal pyemia. His fields of special interest included orthopedic, vascular, and plastic surgery. To the last he made noteworthy contributions on exstrophy of the bladder, harelip, and cleft palate. He also published a monograph on trigeminal neuralgia.

Trendelenburg's name is associated with an impressive list of eponymics in addition to the Trendelenburg position, for which he is best known. These include a cannula, a sign, a symptom, a test, and four operations. The Trendelenburg cannula, a tube fitted with an inflatable rubber collar, was designed to prevent the aspiration of blood after tracheotomy. The Trendelenburg sign, of congenital dislocation of the hip, consists of falling rather than elevation of the gluteal fold on the sound side when the patient stands on the affected leg and raises the other. Trendelenburg's symptom is the waddling gait resulting from paralysis of the gluteal muscles. The Trendelenburg test determines the competency of the venous valves in patients with varicosities of the leg. The four operations named for Trendelenburg consist of (1) a method of excision of varicose veins, (2) ligation of the great saphenous vein to prevent reflux into varicosities, (3) surgical removal of a pulmonary embolus, and (4) the insertion of an ivory peg into the knee joint for the correction of a slipping patella. A *Festschrift* (Vol. 129) of the *Deutsche Zeitschrift für Chirurgie* was published in Trendelenburg's honor in 1914, on the occasion of his seventieth birthday.

REFERENCES

1. Brown, A.: *Old Masterpieces in Surgery, being a Collection of Thoughts and Observations Engendered by a Perusal of Some of the Works of our Forbears in Surgery.* Privately printed. Omaha, 1928, pp. 43–51.

2. Cyprian, A.: *Lettre d'Abraham Cyprianus, Docteur en Medecine, & cy-devant Professeur en Anatomie & en Chyrurgie dans l'Academie de Franequer. Raportant l'Histoire d'un foetus humain de 21. mois, détaché des trompes de la Matrice, sans que la mere en soit morte. Écrite à Mr. Thomas Millington, Chevalier, Medecin Ordinaire du Roy & Président du College des Medecins de Londres.* Roger, Amsterdam, 1707, p. 9.

3. Freund, W. A.: Eine neue Methode des Exstirpation des ganzen Uterus. *Samml. klin. Vorträge,* **133** (Gynäk. No. 41): 911–24, 1878.

4. Friedrich Trendelenburg. *Medical Classics,* **4**:922–88, 1940.

5. Gutberlet, M. J.: Ueber die Methode, die krebshafte Gebärmutter auszurotten. *J. f. Geburtsh., Frauenzimmer-u. Kinderkr.,* **1**:228–43, 1815.

6. Iff, W.: *Beitrag zur Geschichte der Beckenhochlagerung,* **41**:153–66, 1937.

7. Körte, W.: Zum Gedächtnis Friedrich Trendelenburgs. *Arch. f. klin. Chir.,* **134**:i–vi, 1925.

8. Lange, F.: Zur Blasennaht beim hohen Steinschnitt und zur Werthschätzung

der Trendelenburg'schen "Beckenhochlage" bei Operationen im Becken. *Med. Monatschr.,* **1**:1–9, 1889.

9. Leon, M. de: Ein neues Untersuchungsverfahren. *Centralbl. f. Gynäk.,* **12**: 337–38, 1888.

10. Meyer, W.: Ueber die Nachbehandlung des hohen Steinschnittes sowie über Verwendbarkeit desselben zur Operation von Blasenscheidenfisteln. *Arch. f. klin. Chir.,* **31**:494–525, 1884.

11. Meyer, W.: Der Siegeszug der Beckenhochlagerung. *Deutsche Ztschr. f. Chir.,* **129**:306–20, 1914.

12. Payr, E.: Zum Tode F. Trendelenburgs. *München. med. Wchnschr.,* **72**:568–69, 1925.

13. Perthes: Friedrich Trendelenburg. *Deutsche med. Wchnschr.,* **51**:279–80, 1925.

14. Pott, P.: *A Treatise on Ruptures,* 2nd. ed. Hawes, Clarke, & Collins, London, 1763, pp. 62–63.

15. Roger and Roland: *Glossulae Quator Magistrorum super Chirurgiam Rogerii et Rolandi.* Ed. by C. Daremberg. Naples & Paris, 1854, pp. 186–87.

16. Sauerbruch: Friedrich Trendelenburg. *Deutsche Ztschr. f. Chir.,* **190**:I–IV, 1925.

17. Stromayr, C.: *Die Handschrift des Schnitt-und Augenarztes Caspar Stromayr in Lindau im Bodensee. In der Lindauer Handschrift (P. I.—46) vom 4. Juli 1559.* Reproduced by W. von Brunn. Idra-Verlagsanstalt, Berlin, 1925, p. 55.

18. T. S. W.: "Trendelenburg position." *Am. J. Surg.,* **10**:586, 1930.

19. Trendelenburg, F.: Über Blasenscheidenfisteloperationen und über Beckenhochlagerung bei Operationen in der Bauchhöhle. *Samml. klin. Vorträge,* **355**(Chir. 109):3373–92, 1890.

20. Wilms, M.: Friedrich Trendelenburg zum 70. Geburtstag. *Deutsche med. Wchnschr.,* **40**:1071–72, 1914.

Gustav Adolf Walcher
and the Hanging-Legs Position

CHAPTER

51

The positions assumed by women in labor are so varied and their imputed value and significance subject to such dispute that at least two full-length monographs [11,17] have been devoted to the subject. Observed Engelmann: [11]

According to their build, to the shape of the pelvis, [the parturients of different peoples] stand, squat, kneel or lie upon the belly; so also they vary their position in various stages of labor according to the position of the child's head in the pelvis. . . . Primitive peoples have solved this problem by virtue of their instinct.

Engelmann mentioned 16 different postures for parturition among various races, and Ploss and Bartels [26] subsequently expanded this list to 40. In an effort to learn *the* natural position, Naegele surreptitiously observed an untutored young primigravida, left alone during labor in a room containing a bed, chair, sofa, and obstetric chair. He watched her assume every possible position and finally give birth while tossing about on the bed.

A scientific interpretation of posture in labor was first offered in 1854 by J. Matthews Duncan [9] on the basis of anatomic observations by Zaglas.[33] Wrote Duncan:

It has hitherto been customary to regard the articulations of the pelvis in man as virtually immovable, and to describe in the female at the time of parturition

431

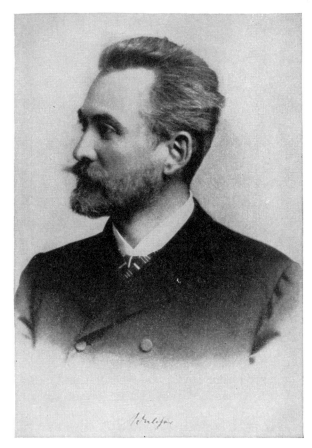

Fig. 51-1.   Gustav Adolf Walcher (1856–1935).

cases where motion evidently takes place as morbid in their character. But Mr.
Zaglas has lately pointed out that in man there is a distinct motion of the ossa
innominata in an antero-posterior direction, or upon an imaginary line passing
tranversely through the second sacral vertebra from one side to the other. In other
words, the sacrum may be described as having a nutatory motion upon this
imaginary transverse axis, the promontory of the sacrum advancing downwards
and forwards, while its apex moves in a contrary direction, and *vice versa.* In the
downward motion of the promontory, which in the non-pregnant is to the extent
of about a line, the brim of the pelvis is diminished to the same extent in its conjugate diameter, while the corresponding upward motion of the apex of the bone
to the extent of about two lines puts the sacro-sciatic ligaments on the stretch, and
enlarges the dimensions of the outlet. By observations on the living and on the
dead subject, Mr. Zaglas has shown that in the erect position the sacral promontory
is not in the position of greatest projection into the brim of the pelvis, but the
reverse, and consequently that the apex is in its forward position diminishing the

outlet, and relaxing the sacro-iliac ligament. When the body is bent forward, on the other hand, the base of the sacrum is protruded, into the brim, the apex is tilted upwards, the sacro-sciatic ligaments put on the stretch, and the outlet of the pelvis consequently enlarged. These movements take place ordinarily in both man and woman, but in her they are of greatest interest and importance in the function of parturition. . . .

That the alteration of the dimensions of the brim and outlet by these movements is not insignificant but the reverse, is a proposition which every obstetrician will confirm. . . . Now in the course of the first stage of labour, while the head is pressing into the brim, the human female is generally standing, sitting, or lying on her back, or in an easy position. But as soon as the head has descended into the pelvis and impinged upon the sensitive vagina, then forcing efforts accompany the pains. These forcing efforts consist, in great part, of powerful contractions of the anterior abdominal muscles, the effect of which, especially the action of the two recti muscles, will be to tilt up the symphysis pubis, thus throwing the promontory forwards, contracting the brim, and enlarging the outlet, and diminishing the angle of inclination of the pelvis. To all these changes the position usually assumed by the female in the second stage of labour will contribute. For . . . the simple bending of the body forwards has for its effect the tilting upwards of the apex of the sacrum and enlarging of the outlet. And it is a curious fact, that a woman in her forcing pains, in the second stage, is found to draw up her legs, and bend her body forwards, thus inducing changes in her pelvis which facilitate the advance of the child in that stage.

Thus was revived, in modified form, the ancient concept of pelvic expansion during labor.

WALCHER'S DESCRIPTION OF POSTURE FOR PARTURITION

Apparently unaware of Zaglas' studies and their obstetric interpretation by Duncan, Gustav Walcher 35 years later independently rediscovered the mobility of the pelvic articulations in pregnancy. By allowing the legs of the parturient to hang from the edge of the table, in the position that immediately became associated with his name, Walcher observed significant enlargement, varying from 8 to 13 mm, in the diagonal conjugate of six patients with contracted pelves. In his brief report,[29] translated herein from the German, he anticipated harsh criticism but the immediate response of the profession was generally receptive and friendly. Wrote Walcher:

I am well aware that with this thesis I shall precipitate among many of my colleagues an immediate storm of indignation, because the unorthodox ideas expressed herein will be interpreted as a revival of old ignorance. He who probes further, however, will be placated!

If a patient in advanced pregnancy, with her pelvis contracted in the antero-posterior diameter, is placed on the examining table with her knees held as close as possible toward the trunk and with the upper part of her body somewhat elevated, the promontory is reached most easily, the diagonal conjugate measuring, for example:

Fröschl	para I	26 yr	10.2 cm
Bröckel	II	40	10.3
Stockburger	IV	36	10.2
Heckel	I	18	10.4
Bischoff	IV	32	10.2
Hetzler	III	29	9.7

If a pillow is now placed under the pelvis and the legs are allowed to hang down as far as possible over the examining table [the Walcher position], the promontory can be felt retreating as the knees are lowered. The diagonal conjugate now measures:

Fröschl	11.1 cm, making a difference of	9 mm
Bröckel	11.6	13
Stockburger	11.0	8
Heckel	11.2	8
Bischoff	11.5	13
Hetzler	10.5	8

Upon elevating the knees and removing the pillow the original measurements are obtained again.

While one is able to reach the promontory while the knees are drawn up, in cases of moderate pelvic contraction, he is no longer able to do so when the legs are extended.

The diagonal conjugate thus varies about a centimeter in many cases (with the exception of ankylosed pelves; but I offer no opinion on this subject, for although I made these observations in all cases that I examined on this point, the numbers are still too small).

Measuring the conjugata vera exactly with a graduated rule in a patient who died of eclampsia, I found a difference of 8 mm.

In the future determination of the degree of pelvic contraction, both measurements should be taken into consideration.

It is unimportant to go further into the explanation and consequences of these facts today; they almost speak for themselves. I shall complete the experiments and report on them in more detail later. I hope that some of my colleagues will be interested enough to do the same.

DISCUSSION OF WALCHER POSITION

Unbeknown to Walcher, the natives of a certain rural district in Germany had long before employed a position for delivery that produced a similar effect on the pelvic joints. According to Hohl,[15] the parturient's husband stood behind her, with each labor pain lifted her upward and backward, and held her in this hanging position, suspended from his arms.

Any method of enlarging the pelvic inlet was bound to win the critical attention of nineteenth-century obstetricians, for the methods then available for coping with cephalopelvic disproportion were only partially satisfactory. The Walcher position was therefore selected as one of the principal topics for discussion at the International Obstetric and Gynecologic Congress held in Amsterdam in 1899,[5] most of the speakers supporting Walcher's observations. On the basis of subsequent experiments on cadavers and live subjects Walcher's position soon received the warm endorsement of a host of investigators,[10,18,20,21,30] who resorted to this position in cases of contracted pelvis, for version and extraction, and in the management of face and breech presentations. Jarcho [16] even reported roentgenographic evidence, obtained from Bay Jacobs, that in eight of ten patients with contracted pelves, the true conjugate was increased between 0.3 and 2.1 cm by a change from the dorsal recumbent to the Walcher position.

A critical minority of obstetricians, on the other hand, reported dissenting experience with the Walcher position. Both Varnier [28] and Paul Bar [1] measured only minimal or no increases in the anteroposterior diameter of the pelvic inlet in cadavers subjected to hyperextension, and in more recent roentgenographic studies Young [32] and Brill and Danelius [3] found only insignificant changes in the superior strait resulting from the assumption of the Walcher position by obstetric patients. The latter authors observed a slight shortening of the obstetric conjugate with the patient in the flexed, or lithotomy, position, and ascribed the apparent lengthening attributed to the Walcher position merely to the recovery of this shortening. In possible explanation of the clinical value imputed to hyperextension, they further noted considerable change in the pelvic angle of inclination, favoring engagement of the fetal head, and also a significant stretching of the rectus muscles. Since the power of a muscle increases with its tension at rest, they suggested that the resulting augmentation of the abdominal muscular force might also aid in bringing the head into the pelvic inlet.

Disputes over priority arose shortly after Walcher's publication. Indeed, this aspect of the problem attracted as much attention and stimulated more heated discussion at the Amsterdam congress of 1899 than the actual value of the Walcher position, Walcher himself insisting that before the publication of his paper "no one in the world had any idea that through this position of a pregnant woman the measurement of her pelvic conjugate could be influenced."

It is nonetheless clear that an identical position had been used by physicians and midwives in the management of certain obstetric difficulties centuries before Walcher. Abulcasis (936–1013) probably gave the first description of this position, and Avicenna (979–1037) soon thereafter advocated it for the delivery of obese patients, to facilitate exposure of the vulva.[12]

In the Middle Ages it was customary for women to be delivered on the birth chair, whose wooden seat was cut out in the manner of a commode. In Scipio Mercurio's famous Italian textbook of obstetrics, however, the hanging-legs position is clearly described and illustrated, for difficult births and the correction of abnormal fetal positions. *La Commare*,[24] which was first published in 1595 and went into 19 later editions, shows the equivalent

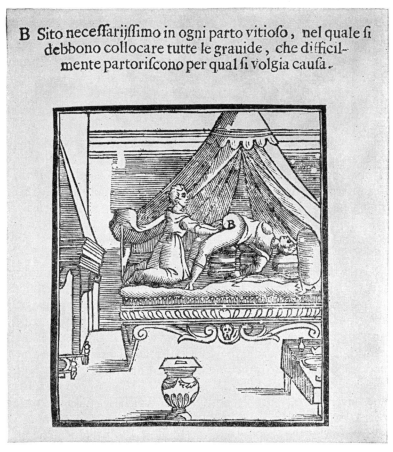

Fig. 51-2. Woodcut from Mercurio's *La Commare*,[24] showing the recommended position for the patient in cases of dystocia, to facilitate manipulation by the midwife.

of the Walcher position in a woodcut (Fig. 51-2) under the caption: "Position essential in every abnormal delivery, in which all pregnant women must be placed who give birth with difficulty from any cause whatsoever." The text, accompanied by an illustration of an occiput posterior presentation, explains:

. . . The patient is placed on the bed supine but with the head flexed so that she is comfortable, several pillows or soft cushions under her shoulders being built up proportionately to the buttocks, so that a gentle inclination is achieved from the buttocks to the head. The midwife then takes her position on her knees between the patient's legs, lubricates her hands with . . . oils or decoctions, contemplates the parts thoroughly, and having determined the position of the child's head, begins to rub gently and push toward the patient's umbilicus. . . . Now the patient will remain in this position . . . until the midwife has brought the child to the middle of the abdomen and out of the narrow passage to which it had progressed and where it was almost fixed. [The fetal position being corrected, the pillows were gradually removed from under the patient's buttocks as the midwife guided the fetal head back into the pelvis.]

Sebastiano Melli, professor of surgery in Venice, redescribed the same position in his *La Comare* [23] more than a century after Mercurio. He, like Avicenna, advised it for excessively obese patients, to help retract the abdominal panniculus, and for the midwife's manipulations in correcting an abnormal position of the fetus. His woodcut (Fig. 51-3) "shows the position in which the midwife must put the parturient when the fetus occupies an abnormal or undesirable position," as illustrated by the fetuses with shoulder and face presentations. After the combined internal and external manipulations, described in the text, the patient was returned to the birth chair.

Most obstetric textbooks of the late-nineteenth and early-twentieth century [2,6,8,10,13,14,19,27,31] advocated Walcher's position for cases of mild cephalopelvic disproportion, for delivery of the aftercoming head, and for high forceps extraction. A few European texts [4,25] still recommend it in selected cases. In American obstetrics, however, the Walcher position has been completely abandoned. DeLee taught it in all seven editions of his textbook [7] but added:

My results, curiously, have been better by the use of the exaggerated lithotomy position, which is theoretically contraindicated because it contracts the inlet. The thighs force the uterus up, correcting the pendulous belly so common with contracted pelvis; the uterus and child are straightened out, the former being thus allowed to act with more directness, and the latter being brought into better position over the inlet.

Greenhill, in his subsequent edition of the DeLee book, denied that the Walcher position had any value.

Similarly, Williams, in the first six editions of his *Obstetrics*,[31] advised:

If engagement fails to occur after complete dilatation of the cervix, the patient should be placed in Walcher's position for as long a time as she will bear it. In many cases this procedure will bring about a lengthening of the anterior posterior diameter of the superior strait sufficient to permit engagement.*

* From J. W. Williams, *Obstetrics. A Text-Book for the Use of Students and Practitioners,* 1st Edition, 1903. Courtesy of Appleton-Century-Crofts, Inc.

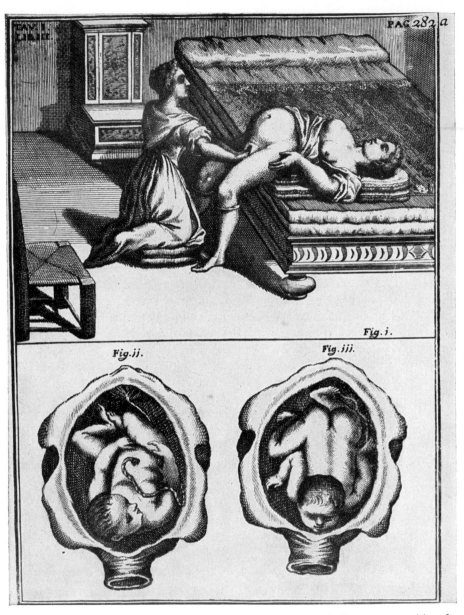

Fig. 51-3. Illustration from Melli's *La Comare*,[23] showing the proper position for the obese patient and for correction of abnormal fetal positions.

In Stander's next three revisions of the text, however, he wrote that "in our experience . . . this is so rarely successful that we have abandoned the use of the Walcher position." The tenth and eleventh editions, edited by Eastman, fail even to mention it. The hanging-legs position, practiced intermittently for over 1000 years, is once again receding into oblivion.

WALCHER'S LIFE

Gustav Adolf Walcher was born November 21, 1856, in Ellwangen, Germany.[22] After completing his formal studies in Leipzig, Berlin, and Tübingen, he served as assistant under von Bruns and then under Säxingen in the Tübingen Frauenklinik, where he qualified in 1886 with his dissertation on uterine prolapse, "Senkung und Vorfall." The following year he was made director of the Württemberg School for Midwives in Stuttgart, a position he held for the next three decades. Here he carried out studies on the shape changes in the fetal skull in relation to its position during labor. He also became known as an ardent advocate of breast feeding and the author of the maxim, "Stillfähigkeit ist Stillwille" (To desire to nurse is to be able to nurse). Walcher's name is also associated with a cervical dilator designed by him. In September, 1918, he retired to his country estate in Ellwangen, where he died June 30, 1935.

REFERENCES

1. Bar, P.: Influence de la position de la femme sur la forme, l'inclinaison et les dimensions du bassin. *L'Obstétrique,* **4**:529–41, 1899.

2. Berkeley, C., and Bonney, V.: *The Difficulties and Emergencies of Obstetric Practice,* 2nd ed. Blakiston Co., Philadelphia, 1915, p. 591.

3. Brill, H. M., and Danelius, G.: Roentgen pelvimetric analysis of Walcher's position. *Am. J. Obst. & Gynec.,* **42**:821–35, 1941.

4. Browne, O.: *A Manual of Practical Obstetrics,* 2nd ed. John Wright & Sons, Bristol, 1948, p. 221.

5. *Compt. rend. Congrès périod. internat. Gynéc. et d'Obstét. 3e session.* Amsterdam, August, 1899. Scheltema & Holkema's Boekhandel, Amsterdam, 1900, pp. 258–344.

6. Davis E. P.: *A Treatise on Obstetrics for Students and Practitioners.* Lea Brothers, Philadelphia & New York, 1896, p. 211.

7. DeLee, J. B.: *The Principles and Practice of Obstetrics.* W. B. Saunders Co., Philadelphia, 1913, pp. 716–17; 7th ed., 1938, p. 809; 9th ed. (ed. by J. P. Greenhill), 1947, p. 655.

8. Dorland, W. A. N.: *A Manual of Obstetrics.* W. B. Saunders Co., Philadelphia, 1896, pp. 454–55.

9. Duncan, J. M.: The behaviour of the pelvic articulations in the mechanism of parturition. *Dublin Quart. J. M. Sc.,* **18**:60–69, 1854.

10. Edgar, J. C.: *The Practice of Obstetrics Designed for the Use of Students and Practitioners of Medicine,* 2nd ed. Blakiston Co., Philadelphia, 1904, pp. 427, 938.

11. Engelmann, G. J.: *Labor Among Primitive Peoples. Showing the Development of the Obstetric Science of To-day, from the Natural and Instinctive Customs of All Races, Civilized and Savage, Past and Present,* 2nd ed. J. H. Chambers, St. Louis, 1883.

12. Graham, H.: *Eternal Eve. The History of Gynaecology and Obstetrics.* Doubleday & Co., Inc., New York, 1951, p. 107.

13. Herman, G. E.: *Difficult Labour. A Guide to its Management for Students and Practitioners.* William Wood & Co., New York, 1911, p. 410.

14. Hirst, B. C.: *A Text-Book of Obstetrics.* W. B. Saunders Co., Philadelphia, 1898, p. 484.

15. Hohl, A. F.: *Lehrbuch der Geburtshülfe mit Einschluss der Geburtshülflichen Operationen und der Gerichtlichen Geburtshülfe.* Engelmann, Leipzig, 1862, p. 444.

16. Jarcho, J.: The value of the Walcher position in contracted pelvis with special reference to its effect on the true conjugate diameter. *Surg., Gynec. & Obst.,* **49**:854–58, 1929.

17. Jarcho, J.: *Postures & Practices During Labor Among Primitive Peoples. Adaptations to Modern Obstetrics With Chapters on Taboos & Superstitions & Postpartum Gymnastics.* Paul B. Hoeber, Inc., New York, 1934.

18. Jewett, C.: The management of face presentation. *Tr. Am. Gynec. Soc.,* **19**: 76–81, 1894.

19. King, A. F. A.: *A Manual of Obstetrics,* 9th ed. Lea Brothers, Philadelphia & New York, 1903, pp. 338–40.

20. Klein, G.: Zur Mechanik des Ileosacralgelenkes. *Ztschr. f. Geburtsh. u. Gynäk.,* **21**:74–118, 1891.

21. Küttner, O. von: Experimentell-anatomische Untersuchungen über die Veränderlichkeit des Beckenraumes Gebärender. *Beitr. z. Geburtsh. u. Gynäk.,* **1**:211–28, 1898.

22. Mayer, A.: Gustav Adolf Walcher. *Zentralbl. f. Gynäk.,* **59**:2705–6, 1935.

23. Melli, S.: *La Comare Levatrice Istruita nel suo Uffizio Secondo le Regoli più certe, e gli Ammaestramenti più Moderni.* Nella Stamperia di Carlo Palese, Venice, 1766, pp. 238, 247–53, 282. (Identical illustration and instructions appear in 1721 edition.)

24. Mercurio, S.: *La Commare O' Raccoglitrice.* Venice, 1703, pp. 118–21.

25. Naujoks, H.: *Winters-Naujoks Lehrbuch der Operativen Geburtshilfe,* 3rd ed. Urban & Schwarzenberg, Munich & Berlin, 1951, p. 72.

26. Ploss, H., and Bartels, M.: *Das Weib in der Natur- und Völkerkunde,* 8th ed. Th. Grieben's Verlag, Leipzig, 1905, Vol. 2, pp. 169–71.

27. Polak, J. O.: *Manual of Obstetrics,* 2nd ed. Physicians & Surgeons Book Co., New York, 1922, p. 113.

28. Varnier, H.: La symphyséotomie. *Ann. de gynéc. et d'obst.,* **48**:189–272, 1897.

29. Walcher, G.: Die Conjugata eines engen Beckens ist keine konstante Grösse, sondern lässt sich durch die Körperhaltung der Trägerin verändern. *Centralbl. f. Gynäk.*, **13**:892–93, 1889.

30. Wehle, J.: Die Walcher'sche Hängelage und ihre praktische Verwerthung bei geburtshülflichen Operationen. *Arch. f. Gynäk.*, **45**:323–36, 1894.

31. Williams, J. W.: *Obstetrics. A Text-Book for the Use of Students and Practitioners.* D. Appleton & Co., New York & London, 1903, pp. 10–11, 631; 7th ed. (ed. by H. J. Stander), 1936, p. 1036.

32. Young, J.: Relaxation of the pelvic joints in pregnancy: Pelvic arthropathy of pregnancy. *J. Obst. & Gynaec. Brit. Emp.*, **47**:493–524, 1940.

33. Zaglas: Mechanism of the pelvic articulations. *Month. J. M. Sc.*, **13**:289–91, 1851.

James Marion Sims, the Sims Position, and the Sims Speculum*

CHAPTER

52

"A sadder situation can hardly exist than that of a woman afflicted with a vesicovaginal fistula. A source of disgust, even to herself, the woman beloved by her husband becomes, in this condition, the object of bodily revulsion to him; and filled with repugnance, everyone else likewise turns his back, repulsed by the intolerable, foul, uriniferous odor. As a result of the seepage from the opening, whether large or small, the usual retention of the urine in the vaginal folds makes it even sharper and more pungent. The labia, perineum, lower part of the buttocks, and inner aspect of the thighs and calves are continually wet, to the very feet. The skin assumes a fiery red color and is covered in places with a pustular eruption. Intolerable burning and itching torment the patients, who are driven to frequent scratching to the point of bleeding, as a result of which their suffering increases still more. In desperation many tear the hair, which is coated at times with a calcareous urinary precipitate, from the mons pubis. The refreshment of a change of clothing provides no relief, because the clean undergarment, after being quickly saturated, slaps against the patients, flopping against their wet thighs as they walk, sloshing in their wet shoes as though they were wading through a swamp. The bed does not soothe them, because a good resting place, a bed, or a horsehair mattress, is quickly impregnated with urine and gives off the

* This chapter originally published in *Bull. Sloane Hosp. for Women*, 3:86–99, 1957; reprinted by permission. Copyright © 1957, by The Sloane Hospital.

most unbearable stench. Even the richest are usually condemned for life to a straw sack, whose straw must be renewed daily. One's breath is taken away by the bedroom air of these women, and wherever they go they pollute the atmosphere. Washing and anointing do not help; perfumes actually increase the repugnance of the odor, just as foul-tasting things become even worse when coated with sugar. This horrendous evil tears asunder every family bond. The tender mother is rejected from the circle of her children. Confined to her lonely little room, she sits there in the cold, at the open window, on her wooden chair with a hole cut in its seat, and may not cover the floor with a carpet even if she could. Indifference overtakes some of these unfortunates; others give themselves over to quiet resignation and pious devotion. Otherwise they would fall victim to despair and would attempt suicide." Thus wrote Dieffenbach [1] in 1836 in his vivid portrayal of the grim plight of women with vesicovaginal fistulas. The lot of such unfortunates was scarcely equaled by any other disaster to which women are subject.

From the earliest days of recorded medical history physicians have struggled with the problem of vesicovaginal fistula, exhausting their ingenuity in an effort to reclaim these social outcasts. Intravaginal sponges and all sorts of urinary receptacles, rings, bags, and tubes, were tried and found wanting. A host of surgical procedures, including cauterization, suturing, skin grafting, and obliteration of the vagina, likewise ended in almost invariable failure.

In what is generally considered the first text on operative gynecology, published in 1663, Hendrik van Roonhuyze [12] wrote of an operation for the cure of vesicovaginal fistula, with the aid of a speculum:

You may also come to the knowledg of it by applying the *speculum vaginae,* having therewith somewhat widen'd the body, so that you may plainly see with your eyes, and feel with your fingers the rupture; as we shall hereafter explain in the Cure. . . . The Operation it self is performed in manner following: The Patient is laid on a Table, towards a good light, and have the upper part of the body covered, and the lower part secured with swathing bands, as is usual in the case of cutting persons of the Stone. This done, 'tis necessary with all speed to widen the body by means of a *speculum vaginae,* according as occasion shall require; and then to make raw and bloody the edges of the ulcerated *vagina,* where with the lacerated part it is joyned to the bladder, and as little as is possible to approach the bladder: For the *vagina* is first by the ulceration, and then by the edges so united to the lacerated Bladder, by the providence of nature, that being but a very little and duly taken off, and stitched together again, the cure may be performed with great ease.

It is not clear that van Roonhuyze actually attempted repair himself, and one can only surmise what must have been the results of such early operations; for almost two centuries later surgeons continued to write despairingly of their efforts to close vesicovaginal fistulas. Velpeau, for example, in his *Operative Surgery,* [18] lamented:

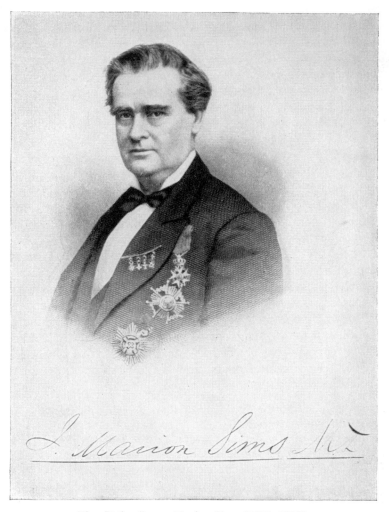

Fig. 52-1. James Marion Sims (1813–1883).

To abrade the borders of an opening when we do not know where to grasp them, to shut it up by means of needles or threads when we have no point apparently to sustain them, to act upon a movable partition placed between two cavities hidden from our sight, and upon which we can scarcely find any purchase, has appeared to be calculated to have no other result than to cause unnecessary suffering to the patient.

Dieffenbach [1] spoke of his own operation with almost the same pessimism: "If it fails . . . as is usually the case, it can be repeated as often as the will and physical condition of the unfortunate patient permits." After another decade of disheartening experience, Dieffenbach wrote again in 1845: [2]

At last I was filled with hope of being able to conquer the grim enemy, when, after what seemed to be the most successful operation, a needle hole or fistula the size of a probe end appeared and resisted the most diligent efforts [to close it]. I saw openings the size of a small pea, after cutting, sewing, and cauterizing, attain the circumference of a large pea; a hole the size of a Groschen [small coin] become twice the size of a Groschen; one of four times a Groschen's size, eight times its size—then I quit. I operated on one woman 18 times and still did not cure her. I tried everything on whole rooms full of these unfortunates, gathered together from all regions, and after exhausting every possibility, cured only a very few.

Until the middle of the nineteenth century progress in surgery was greatly hampered by ignorance of asepsis and the absence of anesthesia. Attempts to repair vesicovaginal fistulas were further impeded by difficulties of exposure, inadequate instruments, and faulty suture materials.

In 1845 J. Marion Sims, a young American surgeon who insisted on washing his hands thoroughly before operating, began his experiments on the now legendary slaves, Anarcha, Betsy, and Lucy, victims of vesicovaginal fistulas. After repeated, fruitless attempts, about 40 in number, to cure these wretched creatures, Sims ultimately succeeded with the aid of silver sutures and the improved exposure provided by the knee-chest position and a vaginal speculum now named for him. Sims's technique, triumphantly reported in January, 1852,[14] and soon mastered by his associate, Nathan Bozeman, initiated a new era in the history of gynecology, which now offered real hope to women suffering from this scourge. In a review of the subject 14 years later Schuppert [13] wrote:

The progress so lately made in the operation for the cure of vesico-vaginal fistula is mainly due to the exertions of Sims and Bozeman . . . to the application of a proper speculum to get easy access to the fistulas, and the use of metallic sutures, and we may safely assert that since in the two cities of New York and New Orleans more cures of that loathsome disease have been accomplished than in the whole of Europe.

THE SIMS POSITION

Previous attempts at fistula repair had been carried out in most cases with the patient lying on her back. But, as Sims was frank to acknowledge, Chelius, and probably Velpeau too, unbeknown to him, had been using the knee-chest position for this operation prior to Sims's publication. Completely overlooked by Sims were the reports by Gosset [3] in 1834 and von Metzler [10] in 1846, of the successful use of this position in the repair of vesicovaginal fistulas. Sims later narrated [15] his accidental discovery of its value while manually correcting a retroversion of the uterus:

To replace the dislocated organ, the patient (covered with a sheet) was placed on the knees with the pelvis elevated, and the thorax depressed. . . . My middle finger is more than half an inch longer than the index, but it could not be used without its fellow; and thus the two were passed, and in a few seconds I could not touch the uterus, or even the walls of the vagina, and the fingers were swept around as it were "in empty nothingness," which was to me at the moment a most puzzling mystery. . . . While I stood doubting and wondering, my patient, now easy, threw herself down on her side, producing thereby a sudden escapement of air from the vagina; and thus the whole mystery of the accidental reduction of the dislocated uterus was explained on the principle of atmospheric pressure. . . . When the patient was in the position described, there . . . [was] a natural tendency of the pelvic viscera to gravitate towards the epigastric region . . . [allowing] the air to rush into the vagina under the palmar surface of the fingers, where, by its mechanical pressure of fifteen pounds to the square inch, this canal was dilated like a balloon . . . and I said to myself, "If by this position the atmospheric air can be made to dilate the vagina to such an extent, even with a force strong enough to reduce a dislocated uterus, why will not the same principle allow me to explore this region, and examine accurately any injury, or disease to which it may be liable?" Full of the thought I hurried home—and the patient (with vesico-vaginal fistula) . . . was placed in the position described, with an assistant on each side to elevate and retract the nates. I cannot, nor is it needful to describe my emotions, when the air rushed in and dilated the vagina to its greatest capacity, whereby its whole surface was seen at one view, for the first time by any mortal man. With this sudden flash of light, with the fistulous opening seen in its proper relations, seemingly without any appreciable process of ratiocination, all the principles of the operation were presented to my mind. . . . And thus in a moment, in the twinkling of an eye, new hopes and new aspirations filled my soul, for a flood of dazzling light had suddenly burst upon my enraptured vision, and I saw in the distance the great and glorious triumph that awaited determined and persevering effort. . . . I thought only of relieving the loveliest of all God's creation of one of the most loathsome maladies that can possibly befall poor human nature. . . . Full of sympathy and enthusiasm, thus all at once I found myself running headlong after the very class of sufferers that I had all of my professional life most studiously avoided.

The knee-chest or *Sims position,* as used in his early operations for fistula repair, was described in Sims's historic paper [14] of 1852:

In order to obtain a correct view of the vaginal canal, I place the patient upon a table about 2½ by 4 feet, on her knees, with the nates elevated, and the head and shoulders depressed. The knees must be separated some 6 or 8 inches, the thighs at about right angles with the table, and the clothing all thoroughly loosened, so that there shall be no compression of the abdominal parietes. An assistant on each side lays a hand in the fold between the glutei muscles and the thigh, the ends of the fingers extending quite to the labia majora; then, by simultaneously pulling the nates upwards and outwards, the os externum opens, the pelvic and abdominal viscera all gravitate towards the epigastric region, the atmosphere enters the vagina, and there, pressing with a weight of 14 lbs. upon the square inch, soon stretches this canal to its utmost limits, affording an easy view of the os tincae, fistula, &c. To facilitate the exhibition of the parts, the assistant on the right side of the patient introduces into the vagina the lever speculum . . . and then, by lifting the perineum, stretching the sphincter, and raising up the recto-vaginal septum, it is as easy to view the whole vaginal canal as it is to examine the fauces by turning a mouth widely open, up to a strong light. . . . This method of exhibiting the parts is not only useful in these cases, but in all affections of the os and cervix uteri requiring ocular inspection. The most painful organic diseases such as corroding ulcer, carcinoma, &c., may be thus exposed without inflicting the least pain, while any local treatment may be instituted without danger of injuring the healthy structures. By this method, also, a proper estimate, anatomically, can be had of the shape and capacity of the vagina; for where there is no organic change, no contraction, and no rigidity of it from sloughs, ulcers, and cicatrices, and where the uterus is movable, this canal immediately swells out to an enormous extent, thus showing its great expansibility.

During the next few years Sims found that the objectives of the knee-chest position could also be provided, and with less discomfort to the patient, by having her lie on her side, in what has come to be known as the *lateral Sims position*. He reported: [15]

In the great majority of cases the patient may lie on the left side, while the operation will be executed with equal facility to the surgeon, and, of course, more ease to the patient.

In this position the thighs are to be flexed at about right angles with the pelvis, the right a little more than the left. The left arm is thrown behind, and the chest rotated forwards, bringing the sternum quite closely in contact with the table, while the spine is fully extended, with the head resting on the parietal bone.

The patient being thus rolled over as much as possible on the front, the assistant standing at her back, elevates with the left hand the right side of the nates, while the right holds the speculum which draws up the perineum, allowing the pressure of the atmosphere to dilate the vagina so as to bring every part of it into view. This position permits the use of anaesthetics if desired, but I never resort to them in these operations, because they are not painful enough to justify the trouble, and risk attending their administration.

THE SIMS SPECULUM

The vaginal speculum is one of the oldest and most frequently modified of all medical instruments. Ricci [11] has made a chronologic listing of 614 models, from the year 97 A.D. to 1940. The speculum designed by Sims was fashioned initially from a pewter spoon. Although neither original with him nor extraordinary, it is still known as the *Sims speculum*. As explained by Sims: [14]

When introduced and held properly, it causes no pain whatever. It is well enough to have two or three of different sizes, so as to be prepared for any case.

The one ordinarily used by me is about 2½ inches from . . . where it supports the sphincter, to its terminal extremity. . . . Its concavity . . . serves to reflect a strong light down on the vagino-vesical septum, the seat of fistula. Its breadth . . . is about ⅞ ths of an inch, widening a little as it approaches the end, making it somewhat in the shape of a duck's bill. The handle is made strong and unyielding, because a considerable degree of leverage has to be exercised by it. The curve . . . being cushioned to prevent its hurting the forefinger, fits accurately over it. The whole instrument is made of German silver, the concavity being highly polished for reflecting the light. . . .

These simple instruments [including a small spatula retractor], with this position and a good light, are all that are necessary for obtaining an accurate view of the parts. If the vagina and outlet are ordinarily capacious, a good strong northern light, of a clear day, from a large solitary window, is all-sufficient. But if this canal has been narrowed by cicatrices after extensive sloughs, or from other causes, then sunlight is absolutely necessary for every stage of the operation from first to last.

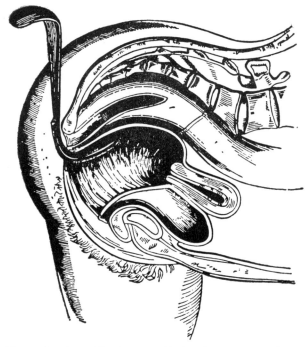

Fig. 52-2. Illustration from Sims's paper,[14] showing his vaginal speculum in place, with the patient in the knee-chest position.

For this purpose, a small table is placed near a window admitting the sunlight. An assistant, sitting by, adjusts on the table a glass . . . some eight or ten inches in diameter, so as to throw the rays of light into the vagina, which, passing to the right of the operator, and striking the concave surface of the bright speculum, are reflected down on the anterior vaginal paries, making everything perfectly distinct.

Although Sims was to receive credit for this speculum, an almost identical instrument of polished silver had already been used in fistula repairs by von Metzler.

SILVER SUTURES

Sims had tried a variety of suture techniques and materials, chiefly silk, in his unsuccessful attempts to repair the fistulas of the long-suffering Anarcha, Betsy, and Lucy, to whom he later [15] paid tribute: "Had they faltered, then would woman have continued to suffer from the dreadful injuries produced by protracted parturition, and then should the broad domain of surgery not have known one of the most useful improvements that shall forever hereafter grace its annals." Sims referred here to silver sutures, with which he found the ultimate solution to fistula repair.

So enchanted was he with the virtues of this new suture material that he chose "Silver Sutures in Surgery" as the topic of his Anniversary Discourse before the New York Academy of Medicine on November 18, 1857.[15] To this body of physicians he boasted intemperately and with misguided patriotism:

So far as it concerns my experience, personal narrative, claims as a discoverer, or defence against aggression, I have a right to declare them openly "from the housetops" . . . I declare it as my honest and heart-felt conviction, that the use of *silver as a suture is the great surgical achievement of the nineteenth century.* . . . For my country I claim the honor of this imperishable discovery, and seize this auspicious occasion to place permanently upon record a history of its origin and progress. . . . Many of you already know that it was not the result of mere accident, but of long, laborious and persevering effort, based upon the immutable principles of science, and forming one of the most beautiful examples of inductive philosophy. . . . Wishing to impress upon the profession its importance and value in general surgery, as well as in injuries from protracted parturition, I shall necessarily be compelled to draw largely and somewhat minutely upon my past experience . . . to place for ever beyond cavil my claims and agency in this discovery. . . . After nearly four years of fruitless labor, silver was fortunately substituted for silk as a suture, and lo! a new era dawns upon surgery. . . . I know that posterity will do me full justice . . . as the discoverer and propagator of a great principle that shall live as long as surgery is cultivated as a science, or practised as an art . . . whose brilliant surgical achievements have so often been the object of envy and detraction.

Continuing in the same immodest vein, Sims predicted:

The next eight years will not find an educated physician anywhere who will dare to use silk sutures, for the silver thread will become as essential to the dressing case as the needle itself; and if I may be allowed to venture a prediction, I will say that fifty years hence the statistics of our hospitals will show a vast improvement in their bills of mortality after great operations, and this improvement will be due mainly to the use of silver as a suture. . . . My language is in nowise extravagant; and I shall yet live to see the day, when the whole profession of the civilized world will accord to this simple discovery the high position of being the most important contribution as yet made to surgery of the present century. . . . The only thing at all comparable to it is Etherization; and in practical results of permanent benefit it is absolutely contemptible, when compared with those from the universal use of silver sutures in the broad domain of general surgery.

Overlooked or deliberately ignored by Sims were the experimental use of silver ligatures by Levert [8] in Alabama and the successful repair of a vesico-vaginal fistula with silver wire by Gosset [3] in England, both a quarter century earlier. Even the perforated lead shot, for which Sims claimed credit in fixing his sutures in position, had been used several years before, by Crampton and Cusack, in the surgical repair of cleft palate.[13] Indeed, as aptly stated by Graham,[4] "all the essentials for a cure of vesico-vaginal fistula were known and had been used, either singly, or in the wrong combination," before Sims made his triumphant entry on the stage of gynecologic surgery. It was Sims's genius to apply these methods and principles with new skill and perseverance, achieving a record of success hitherto unequaled.

SIMS'S LIFE

James Marion Sims, the first of eight children and "the father of American gynecology," was born in Hanging Rock, Lancaster County, South Carolina, January 25, 1813.[5,7,9] As a boy he aspired to become a clerk in the village general store, but instead entered the College of South Carolina, under the urging of his parents and to bolster his qualifications for the affections of Theresa, daughter of Dr. Bartlett Jones, the community's leading physician. Sims, whose father was in constant debt to the Joneses, failed to win their approval as a companion for their daughter, but she finally became Sims's wife nonetheless, serving as a bastion of support to him throughout the turbulent years of his later life.

Perseverance and stubbornness are but variants of a single trait. The same qualities that were to bring Sims honor without measure and the acclaim of the entire medical world, almost prevented his graduation from college. Convinced that he was unable to write compositions, he steadfastly refused to submit the required number, despite the urging of his classmates and an adamant faculty that refused to waive this requirement for graduation. Only through the ruse of another student, who forged Sims's name to compositions of his own, did Sims receive his A.B. in 1832. He then began the study of medicine in the office of Dr. G. Churchill Jones, in Lancaster, South Carolina, enrolled in the Medical College of Charleston two years later, and ultimately transferred to Jefferson Medical College in Philadelphia, where he graduated in 1835. Returning to Lancaster, he entered practice at the age of 22, but soon moved to Mount Meigs, Alabama, after the unfortunate death of his first two patients. Another move, to Montgomery, followed five years later, and here Sims rapidly developed a large surgical practice, successfully performing new operations for clubfoot and strabismus, and beginning his work toward the cure of vesicovaginal fistula. Seeking relief from the dysentery that had plagued him for several years and seriously undermined his health, he moved with his wife and six children to New York in 1853, where he had previously found the climate and water favorable to his condition and where he soon regained his vigor.

His name now well known as a result of his published success in fistula repair, Sims set out to establish a gynecologic hospital, the first of its kind in America. After overcoming the initial apathy to this bold concept he succeeded in 1855 in founding a small hospital for women at 83 Madison Avenue, the forerunner of the famous Woman's Hospital of the State of New York. He served as surgeon-in-chief to this institution, where he attained great renown, until 1862, when he took up residence in Europe, dividing his time between London and Paris for the next six years and accumulating honors and wealth. As the tension between the Northern and Southern states mounted, Sims, sympathetic toward the latter, had found his position increasingly untenable in New York. While in Europe he served temporarily as surgeon-in-chief of the Anglo-American Ambulance Corps in the Franco-Prussian War.

In 1871, the passions fanned by the Civil War having cooled, Sims returned to New York and resumed his activities at the Woman's Hospital, but now only as a member of the newly created medical board (with Emmet, Peaslee, and Thomas) rather than in his former role of surgeon-in-chief. Chafing under the loss of some of his erstwhile authority, he soon became embroiled in controversy with the hospital's board of managers over their policy of refusing admission to cancer cases and over their attempts to limit the number of visitors in his operative clinics. So vigorously did he wage his attack against the board that he was finally forced to resign in 1874, at the age of 61, from the institution he had founded. Eloquent in his appeal for medical facilities for patients suffering from cancer, Sims lost little time in establishing a separate hospital, which has gradually evolved into the present Memorial Center for Cancer and Allied Diseases.

Remorseful over the arrogance and rigidity that caused his ejection from the Woman's Hospital and over his belligerence to its managers, Sims was reinstated as a member of the consulting board several years later; but shortly thereafter he died, on November 13, 1883, and was buried in Greenwood Cemetery, New York City. A statue (Figure 52-3) to Sims's memory, initially erected in Bryant Park in 1894, was moved in 1936 to its present location on the edge of Central Park, opposite the New York Academy of Medicine.

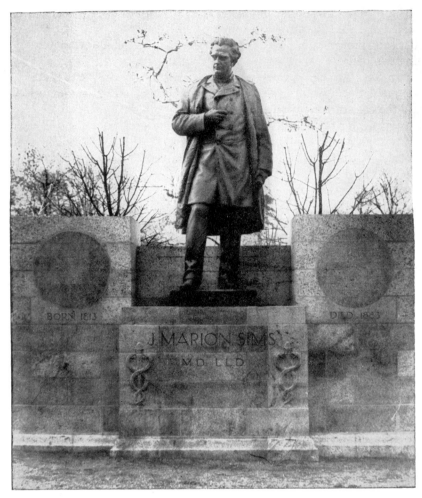

Fig. 52-3. Sims's statue in Central Park, New York City.

Sims was the recipient of countless European decorations as well as domestic honors. In 1875 he was elected president of the American Medical Association, and five years later he served as president of the American Gynecological Society. A bibliography of his biographies [7] lists 73 titles. An autobiography, edited by his son, Harry, was published in 1884. His only other book, *Clinical Notes on Uterine Surgery,*[16] written during his stay in Europe, dealt at length with the management of sterility. In it he concurred in the prevailing, but mistaken, notions "that menstruation is the sign of ovulation; that it is preparatory to the reception of the ovum; that the ovum reaches the cavity of the uterus in from two to ten days after menstruation; and . . . that the uterus itself is the normal seat of conception." Despite these erroneous ideas, Sims succeeded in one of his numerous attempts at artificial insemination, perhaps the first such success since John Hunter's (before 1780), although Sims's patient subsequently miscarried in the fourth month.

In this volume Sims also reported his studies of sperm survival in the vagina and cervical mucus. His staid British colleagues were shocked, however, by such invasion of the nuptial chamber by a physician; and the *Medical Times and Gazette* castigated him in its review [17] of the book:

I do not hesitate to say . . . that all mental, or moral, or hygienic, or medicinal influences are ignored. . . . With regard to the discovery of the total expulsion of the fertilising liquid from the vagina, and to the dabblings in that canal with speculum and syringe under the circumstances described, we can but express our unfeigned regret that Dr. Marion Sims has thought proper to found an odious style of practice on such (*im*)pure assumption. At any rate, if such practices were to be considered the "business of the Physician," there are a good many of us who would quit Physic for some other calling that would let us keep our sense of decency and self respect. Better let ancient families become extinct than keep up the succession by such means.

On a later page of the same journal a contributor [6] twitted Sims in verse:

Say, what is man? An atom at the first,
    Waiting its nuptial atom in the womb;
Too oft, alas, by fate untimely curst,
    In place of fostering home, to find a tomb.
Grieved at the thought, a tear thine eye bedims,
Great son of Aesculapius, Marion Sims.

Sims, should these fail, thou still wilt cherish hope
    To find some other cause that breeds the ill,
With learned digit, searching microscope,
    Or peering speculum, exploring still;—
Nay, wizard-like, ethereal sleep wilt shed,
To win thy point, e'en o'er the nuptial bed.

REFERENCES

1. Dieffenbach, J. F.: Ueber die Heilung der Blasen-Scheiden-Fisteln und Zerreissungen der Blase und Scheide. *Med. Zeitung,* **5**:117–20, 121–24, 173–75, 177–80, 1836.

2. Dieffenbach, J. F.: *Die Operative Chirurgie.* F. A. Brockhaus, Leipzig, 1845, Vol. 1, pp. 572–73.

3. Gosset, M.: Calculus in the bladder.—Incontinence of urine.—Vesico-vaginal fistula. Advantages of the gilt-wire suture. *Lancet,* **1**:345–46, 1834.

4. Graham, H.: *Eternal Eve. The History of Gynaecology and Obstetrics.* Doubleday & Co., Inc., New York, 1951, p. 442.

5. Harris, S.: *Woman's Surgeon: The Life Story of J. Marion Sims.* The Macmillan Co., New York, 1950.

6. H. L.: Ode to Dr. Marion Sims. *M. Times & Gaz.,* 1:216, 1866.

7. James Marion Sims. *Medical Classics,* 2:662–712, 1938.

8. Levert, H. S.: Experiments on the use of metallic ligatures, as applied to arteries. *Am. J. M. Sc.,* 4:17–23, 1829.

9. Martin, H.; Ehrlich, H.; and Butler, F.: J. Marion Sims—pioneer cancer protagonist. *Cancer,* 3:189–204, 1950.

10. Metzler, J. von: Behandlung der Harnröhren—und Blasenscheidenfisteln mittelst erprobter, leicht ausführbarer Operationsmethoden. *Prag. Vierteljahrschr. f. d. prakt. Heilk.,* 10(2):126–54, 1846.

11. Ricci, J. V.: The vaginal speculum and its modifications throughout the ages. *Tr. Gynaec. Dept. City Hosp., 1948–1949.* New York, pp. 1–55.

12. Roonhuyze, H. van: *Heel-konstige Aanmerkkingern Betreffende de Gebreekken der Vrouwen.* T. Jacobsz, Amsterdam, 1663. English translation: *Medico-Chirurgical Observations. Englished out of Dutch by a careful hand.* M. Pitt, London, 1676, pp. 125–36.

13. Schuppert, M.: *A Treatise on Vesico-Vaginal Fistula.* Daily Commercial Bull. Print., New Orleans, 1866.

14. Sims, J. M.: On the treatment of vesico-vaginal fistula. *Am. J. M. Sc.,* 23(n.s.): 59–82, 1852.

15. Sims, J. M.: *Silver Sutures in Surgery. The Anniversary Discourse, before the New York Academy of Medicine . . . November 18, 1857.* Samuel S. & William Wood, New York, 1858.

16. Sims, J. M.: *Clinical Notes on Uterine Surgery, with Special Reference to the Management of the Sterile Condition.* Hardwicke, London, 1866.

17. The Cure of Barrenness. *M. Times & Gaz.,* 1:148–51, 1866.

18. Velpeau, A. A. L. M.: *New Elements of Operative Surgery.* First American from last Paris ed. Translated by P. S. Townsend. Samuel S. & William Wood, New York, 1847, Vol. 3, Part 2, p. 848.

Instruments | PART VIII

William Smellie and His
Obstetric Instruments

CHAPTER

53

In contrast to the frequent, almost routine, resort to operative procedures in most deliveries today, previous generations of obstetricians regarded operative intervention not as a nicety of practice but rather as a grave and hazardous undertaking, fraught with dangers for mother and child and justified only by urgent obstetric indications. Looking back 200 years, to the middle of the eighteenth century, we find an attitude of the utmost conservatism prevailing in the use of obstetric instruments, which were then very limited in scope and variety and confined largely to the hands of specialists in the art. Referring to the forceps, William Smellie wrote in the preface to his *Collection of Cases and Observations in Midwifery,*[4] published in 1754:

. . . In my private practice, I have very seldom occasion for the assistance of that or any other instrument; but I have often been called in by other practitioners, to cases in which I have had opportunities to use it with success.

The forceps and fillet were contrived with a view to save the child, by helping along the head in extraordinary cases, when nature was exhausted, and to prevent, as much as possible, the use of sharp instruments, when the mother's life was in danger. But if these expedients are used prematurely, when the nature of the case does not absolutely require such assistance, the mischief that may ensue will often overbalance the service for which they were intended. . . .

Until Smellie's time, operative obstetrics consisted largely in destructive procedures on the fetus. During the first 13 years or more of his practice Smellie's instruments comprised a blunt hook, straight crotchet, and a per-

457

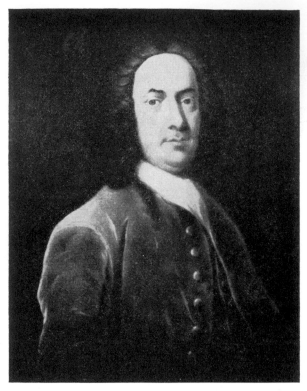

Fig. 53-1. William Smellie (1697–1763). (Courtesy of Royal College of Surgeons of Edinburgh.)

forator, all destructive. Cesarean section had not yet been made safe for the living woman, the obstetric forceps was still in its early stages of development and had not yet achieved wide acceptance, and version was rarely employed by the midwives and general practitioners. Mutilating operations on the fetus thus remained one of the principal methods of dealing with the mechanical difficulties of labor.

Against this background emerged the genius of William Smellie, whose name was to become associated with a number of major advances in clinical obstetrics, and is still eponymically identified with the instruments of his invention. Of these his forceps has been superseded by more efficient models, and the crotchet has fallen into disuse. The Smellie scissors, on the other hand, remains an important part of today's arsenal of destructive instruments.

SMELLIE'S DESCRIPTION OF HIS INSTRUMENTS

The considerations that led to Smellie's development of his own forceps he described as follows:

For my own part, finding in practice, that by the directions of Chapman, Gifford, and Gregoire at Paris, I frequently could not move the head along without contusing it, and tearing the parts of the woman . . . I began to consider the whole in a mechanical view, and reduce the extraction of the child to the rules of moving bodies in different directions: in consequence of this plan, I more accurately surveyed the dimensions and form of the *Pelvis,* together with the figure of the child's head and the manner in which it passed along in natural labours; and from the knowledge of these things, I not only delivered with greater ease and safety than before, but also had the satisfaction to find in teaching, that I could convey a more distinct idea of the art in this mechanical light than in any other. . . . From this knowledge, too . . . I have been led to alter the form and dimensions of the forceps . . . so as to avoid the inconveniences that attend the use of the former kinds.

Smellie's short forceps rivaled Levret's as the most efficient instrument of its kind in the mid-eighteenth century. It was initially made of iron, a few later models of wood, and finally of iron covered with leather. With Smellie's subsequent invention of the lock for the articulated blades and his adoption of the pelvic curve, independently conceived at about the same time by Levret and Benjamin Pugh, the forceps assumed the essential characteristics of the conventional-type instrument in current use. In Smellie's experience, only 10 out of 1000 labors required forceps intervention.

The crotchet, a very old instrument of destruction, consisted in essence of a sharp hook, which was used in difficult labors to impale the head of the dead fetus, usually in conjunction with craniotomy, or to rip open the fetal abdomen preliminary to evisceration. Smellie's curved and double-articulated crotchet was a great improvement over the single straight instrument he had used in his early years of practice. The idea of a double instrument with a cephalic curve he probably got from Mesnard, improving upon it by crossing the handles and adding a lock. The new crotchet increased the power of the weapon while diminishing the risk of its slipping and lacerating the soft tissues of the mother or the operator.

The Smellie scissors consists of a heavy pair of sharp-pointed shears with a stop on the outer edge of each blade. Although it can also be used for other purposes, it was intended primarily as a skull perforator, to replace the complicated instruments previously used for this purpose.

Smellie's instruments are illustrated and their use described in his remarkable atlas, *A Sett of Anatomical Tables* [5] (Fig. 53–2), published in 1754, of which only 80 copies are believed to have been printed. The life-size obstetric drawings in it, far superior to any previously published and probably including some made by Smellie himself, show the normal anatomy of the genitalia, the pregnant uterus, the normal positions of the fetus during labor, twins, the use of forceps for vertex and face presentations and for the aftercoming head, molding, breech presentation, and the obstetric instru-

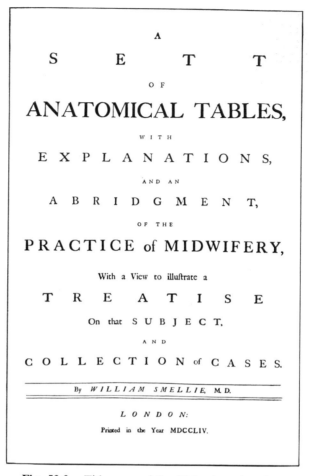

A

S   E   T   T

O F

ANATOMICAL TABLES,

W I T H

E X P L A N A T I O N S,

A N D   A N

A   B   R   I   D   G   M   E   N   T,

O F   T H E

PRACTICE of MIDWIFERY,

With a View to illuſtrate a

T   R   E   A   T   I   S   E

On that S U B J E C T,

A N D

C O L L E C T I O N of C A S E S.

By *WILLIAM SMELLIE*, M.D.

L O N D O N:

Printed in the Year MDCCLIV.

Fig. 53-2. Title page of Smellie's obstetric atlas.

ments. These last appear in the thirty-seventh to thirty-ninth tables, the first and last of which are here reproduced (Figs. 53-3, 53-4), with their respective annotations:

The Thirty-Seventh Table with the two following represents several kinds of Instruments useful in laborious and difficult Cases.

A The streight short Forceps, in the exact proportion as to the width between the Blades, and length from the points to the locking part: the first being two and the second six Inches, which with five Inches and a half (the length of the handles) makes in all eleven inches and a half. The length of the handles may be altered at pleasure. I find however in Practice that this standard is the most convenient, and with less difficulty introduced, than when longer, having also sufficient force to deliver in most cases, where their assistance is necessary. The handles and lowest part of the Blades may as here be covered with any durable leather, but

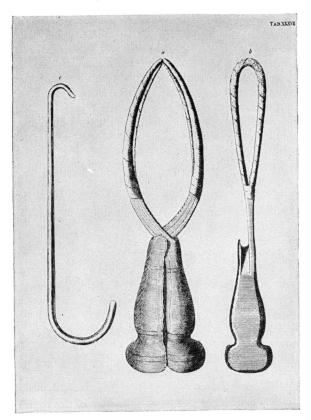

Fig. 53-3. Table XXXVII of Smellie's *Sett of Anatomical Tables,*[5] showing his short straight forceps and blunt hook.

the Blades ought to be wrapped round with something of a thinner kind, which may be easily renewed when there is the least suspicion of venereal Infection in a former Case: by being thus covered, the Forceps have a better hold, and mark less the Head of the Child. For their easier Introduction the Blades ought likewise to be greased with Hogs-lard.

B represents the posterier part of a single Blade in order to shew the width and length of the open part of the same, and the form and dimensions of the whole. The handles however as here represented are rather too large.

The Forceps were at first contrived to save the Foetus, and prevent, as much as possible, the use of sharp Instruments; but even to this salutary method recourse ought not to be had but in Cases where the degree of force requisite to extract will not endanger by it's consequences the life of the mother. For by the imprudent use of the Forceps much more harm may be done than good. . . .

C The Blunt Hook which is used for three purposes.

First, to assist the extraction of the Head after the *Cranium* is opened with the Scissars, by introducing the small end along the Ear on the outside of the Head to above the Under-jaw, where the point is to be fixed; the other extremity of the Hook being held with one hand, whilst two fingers of the other are to be introduced into the foresaid opening, by which holds the Head is to be gradually extracted.

Secondly, The small end is useful in abortions in any of the first four or five Months to hook down the *Secundines,* when lying loose in the *Uterus,* when the patient is much weakened by Floodings from the too long retention of the same, the pains also being unable to expel them, and when they cannot be extracted with the fingers. But if the *Placenta* still adheres it is dangerous to use this or any other Instrument to extract the same, as it ought to be left 'till it separates naturally. If a small part of the *Secundines* is protruded through the *Os Uteri* and pulled away from what still adheres in the Uterus, the mouth of the *Womb* contracts, and that irritation is thereby removed which would have continued the pains, and have separated and discharged the whole.

Thirdly, the large Hook at the other end is useful to assist the extraction of the Body when the Breech presents, but should be used with great caution, to avoid the dislocation or fracture of the Thigh. . . .

The Thirty-Ninth Table

a Represents a pair of curved Crotchets locked together in the same manner as the Forceps: It is very rare that the use of both is necessary, excepting when the Face presents with the Chin turned to the *Sacrum* and when it is impossible to move the Head to bring the Child footling or deliver with the Forceps. In that case if one Crotchet is not sufficient the other is to be introduced, and when joined together will act both as Crotchets, in opening the *Cranium,* and, as the Head advances, will likewise act as Forceps in moving and turning the Head more conveniently for the delivery of the same. They may also be useful to assist when the Head is left in the Uterus, and one Blade is not sufficient. There is seldom occasion however for the sharp Crotchet, when the Head presents, the blunt hook in Table XXVII [XXXVII] being commonly sufficient, or even the Forceps to extract the same, after it is opened with the Scissars. Great care ought to be taken when the sharp Crotchet is introduced, to keep the point towards the Foetus, especially in Cases where the fingers cannot be got up to guide the same. The dotted lines along the inside of one of the Blades represent a sheath that is contrived to guard the point 'till it is introduced high enough; the ligature at the handles, marked with the two dotted lines is then to be untied, the sheath withdrawn, and the point being uncovered is fixed as directed in Table XXXVI.

The point guarded with this Sheath may also be used instead of the blunt Hook.

b Gives a View of the back part of one of the Crotchets which is twelve Inches long.

c Gives a front View of the point to shew it's length and breadth, which ought to be rather longer and narrower than here represented.

d Represents the Scissars proper for perforating the *Cranium* in very narrow and distorted *Pelvis's.* They ought to be made very strong, and nine Inches at least in length with stops or rests in the middle of the Blades, by which a large dilatation is more easily made.

The above Instruments ought only to be used in the most extraordinary Cases, where it is not possible to save the Woman without their assistance.

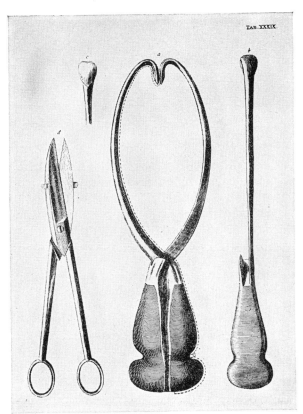

Fig. 53-4. Table XXXIX of Smellie's *Sett of Anatomical Tables,*[5] showing his double-curved crotchet and scissors.

In his *Treatise on the Theory and Practice of Midwifery,*[3] published in 1752, Smellie laid down a set of rules for using the forceps, these rules bearing a remarkable similarity to current teaching on the subject. He insisted on a precise determination of the position of the fetal head, to permit a cephalic application of the blades. Smellie was also the first to perform forceps rotation of the head from a persistent occiput posterior position and first to use forceps on the aftercoming head. The following paragraph from his *Treatise,* instructing the accoucheur in the niceties of forceps practice, provides an interesting glimpse of eighteenth-century obstetrics:

The woman being laid in a right position for the application of the forceps, the blades ought to be privately conveyed between the feather-bed and the cloaths, at a small distance from one another, or on each side of the patient: that this conveyance may be the more easily effected, the legs of the instrument ought to be kept in the operator's side-pockets. Thus provided, when he sits down to deliver, let him spread the sheet that hangs over the bed, upon his lap, and under that cover, take out and dispose the blades on each side of the patient; by which means he will often be able to deliver with the forceps, without their being perceived by the woman herself, or any other of the assistants. Some people pin a sheet to each shoulder, and throw the other end over the bed, that they may be the more effectually concealed from the view of those who are present: but this method is apt to confine and embarrass the operator. At any rate, as women are commonly frightened at the very name of an instrument, it is adviseable to conceal them as much as possible, until the character of the operator is fully established.

Before the development of his forceps Smellie's repertoire, when he was called as a consultant in cases of prolonged labor, was limited to version and destructive operations on the fetus. His conservative attitude toward multilating procedures is embodied in the following statement, taken from his *Collection of Cases and Observations in Midwifery* (Collection 20, Case 7):

During the first year of my practice, when I was called to lingering cases which were often occasioned by the imprudent methods used by unskilful midwives to hasten labour, such as directing the patient to walk about and bear down with all her strength at every trifling pain, until she was quite exhausted, and opening the parts prematurely so as to produce inflammations, and torture the woman unnecessarily; on such occasions, without knowing the steps that had been taken, I have been told that the patient had been in severe labour for many hours, and sometimes days, and that now I was called to prevent her from dying with the child in her belly. Thus sollicited, if the head was at the upper part of the *Pelvis*, I commonly turned the child, and brought it by the feet; and thus, if small, it was usually saved, provided it was not dead before my arrival: but, when the head was large, or the *Pelvis* narrow and distorted, the force necessary to extract it, was often the occasion of its death. On the other hand, when the head was so low in the *Pelvis*, that I could not raise it into the *Uterus*, in order to be turned, I was obliged to dilate the *Cranium* with the scissars, and extract with my fingers, assisted by the blunt hook. This method, however, I never practiced, except when the head was low down, and the patient so much exhausted that she could not be delivered by the pains. . . .

When circumstances required, however, Smellie did not hesitate to dismember a dead fetus to effect its delivery, as revealed in this account of a neglected transverse lie for which he was called in consultation (*Collection of Preternatural Cases,*[6] Collection 35, Case 7):

One of the arms had descended, and been so pulled by the midwife, that the shoulder was down to the *Os Externum*.

I tried to raise the shoulder by passing up along the arm which was excessively swelled and livid, it having been down in that position above four and twenty hours; but I could not introduce my hand. Considering that the child was probably dead from its being so long in that situation, and its not being felt to move by the mother for many hours, I thought it was most expedient to separate the arm from the shoulder. This last being low down, I guided the points of the scissars to it, and easily separated the arm; partly by cutting the skin and ligaments, and partly by pulling and twisting.

In pushing up the shoulder into the *Uterus,* I found that the *Pelvis* was small and the child large. I brought down only one of the legs, which was pulled off . . . then with great labour I brought down the other, which gave way also by the force of pulling.

I was afterwards obliged to tear down the body with the crotchet, and even to fix the same instrument on the head.

Being the straight kind, it slipped several times, and hurt the inside of my left hand in two places, while I guided the point from hurting the *Vagina* of the patient. At last, gaining a firmer hold above the ear, I fixed the fingers of my left hand over the shoulders, and pulled with great force, both at the body and crotchet. Finding it did not move, I wrapped a cloth round the shoulders, and pulled at them with so great force, as almost to separate the head. By these means, the head was brought a little lower; yet not daring to exert again such violence at the body, I pulled by the crotchet, which brought the head down to the *Os Externum;* and in raising the body and pulling it upwards, it at last separated.

The head however being brought low, I took hold of the under jaw, and pulling at that, while I exerted more force at the crotchet, the head was also delivered.

The woman behaved with great courage, although she had been much fatigued, and weakened by a flooding brought on by the great force that I was obliged to exert in turning the *Foetus.* This woman also recovered, contrary to every body's expectation.

Heroic obstetrics of this sort made great physical demands on the operator as well. As a concluding statement to another of his case reports Smellie wrote: "This case so fatigued me that I was obliged to . . . go to bed after I was carried home in a chair. My hands were so swelled that I could only use my fingers like a gouty person, for a day or two."

The use of the crotchet on the avulsed fetal head within the uterus is illustrated again in Collection 36, Case 4, of Smellie's *Collection of Preternatural Cases.* It is in this case report that the term "hour-glass" was first used in reference to the contracted lower uterine segment. The patient, aged 40, had a contracted pelvis, and the fetus presented by an arm. Smellie was called after the midwife and two consultants had performed a version and extracted the decapitated body and had become fatigued from their unsuccessful efforts to extract the head. Wrote Smellie:

After having placed her in a supine position, I introduced my left hand into the *Vagina,* then raised the head, so as to gain admission into the *Uterus.* In doing this, I found that the difficulty in the head's coming along proceeded from the *Pelvis* being distorted; and that the upper part of the *Os Sacrum,* and last *Vertebra* of the loins jetted considerably forwards.

Having found the mouth, I introduced a finger into it, and bringing it downwards, turned the forehead to the right side, at the brim of the *Pelvis*. . . . Between [the pubis] and the child's head, I slipped up the crotchet with my right hand, having the head grasped in the *Uterus* with my left, my fore and middle fingers being placed on the right parietal bone, near the *Vertex*. I fixed the point of my crotchet into this part, and after I found that I had tore open the skull, and that the crotchet had a firm hold, I withdrew my hand. Fixing again the fore and middle fingers into the mouth, and my thumb below the chin, I began to pull with both hands, *viz.* at the under jaw with my left, and at the crotchet with my right; but finding that it required a good deal of force, I pulled at first in a slow and cautious manner, that as the crotchet tore open the bones, I might allow time for the brain to evacuate, and the head to diminish its bulk. . . . By increasing the force at intervals, the head began to advance lower and lower. When I had brought it down into the *Pelvis* . . . I turned the forehead from the right *Ischium* backwards to the concave, and lower part of the *Sacrum;* and standing up, pulled the head upwards, in a semicircular manner, from below the *Pubis*. . . . Finding that the *Placenta* did not in a little time come down, I introduced my hand into the *Uterus,* and found the part where the head was lodged still pretty open. At the upper part of it I perceived the middle of the *Uterus,* contracted in the form of an hour-glass, below the *Placenta,* which adhered to the Fundus. I insinuated the fingers of my right hand gradually into this contracted part, while at the same time I pressed my left hand on the *Abdomen,* to keep down the *Uterus*. After it was fully stretched, so as to allow my hand to pass, I gradually separated and extracted the *Placenta,* which was adhering firmly to the *Uterus*.

SMELLIE'S LIFE

William Smellie, born in Lanark, Scotland in 1697, is commonly referred to as "the master of British midwifery." [1,2,7] Fasbender, in his history of obstetrics, has called him "one of the most important obstetricians of all times and countries." The details of Smellie's early life and education are unknown, but he probably entered the profession of medicine through apprenticeship to Dr. John Gordon of Glasgow, and began general practice in his native town in 1720, without a medical degree or license. It was not until considerably later that he enrolled for the study of medicine at Glasgow University, from which he received his M.D. in 1745. After 19 years' practice in Lanark, Smellie went to London in 1738 for further training in obstetrics and the following year took courses under Gregoire in Paris; but dissatisfied with the caliber of the obstetrics he witnessed, he returned to London, reestablished himself in practice, and began to give midwifery courses on his own.

Smellie's practice took him into the St. Giles and Holborn districts of London, where he encountered the worst possible living conditions and personal hygiene among his clientele and a staggering infant mortality, only one child out of every five born surviving to the age of six. Here he soon found obstetric patients in large number who were willing to serve as teaching subjects in return for his expert and kindly ministrations. His course of instruction was advertised in a brochure as follows:

I. The course is divided into Twelve Lectures, and no more than four Persons can attend at once, each paying Two Guineas at the First Lecture.

II. They who come on purpose from the Country, and cannot wait 'till the Number of Subscribers is complete, pay Three Guineas.

III. The Expence of being present at a real Labour, is One Guinea; but such as contract for Two Courses and Four Labours, pay only Five Guineas, and perform the last Delivery themselves.

IV. Pupils who engage for a Year pay Fifteen Guineas, and are entitled to attend all the Courses and Labours of that Time, whereby they will have the Opportunity of Seeing and Performing in several difficult Cases.

V. By paying Twenty Guineas they are admitted to this Course, with all the forementioned Advantages, for Two Years.

N.B. The Men and Women are taught at different hours.

The students were also required to pay six shillings toward a fund for the support of the poor patients. Smellie supplemented the clinical demonstrations on his patients with instructions on his "machine," an obstetric manikin of his own invention. He soon became well known as both a practitioner and teacher of midwifery and in ten years had given 280 courses of lectures and instructed 900 students on 1150 labor cases.

Smellie was the first to measure the diagonal conjugate of the pelvis. He showed that contracted pelves usually cause difficulty at the level of the superior strait. He called attention to the frequency with which a number of cases of eclampsia occur at about the same time and suggested the weather as a causal factor, an idea that even now is the subject of scientific investigation. His name is associated with the manual maneuver for assisting the aftercoming head in breech deliveries, described earlier by Guillemeau and Mauriceau. Smellie's most important contribution to obstetrics, however, is thought by many to be his description of the mechanism of labor, which comprises Section 5 in the first chapter of his *Treatise*.

Troubled by asthma, he retired from practice in 1759 and returned to Lanark, where he added to the property that he had retained, built a modest home, and created the small estate that became known as Smellom or Smyllom. Here he died, childless, March 5, 1763, after gathering together the material for *A Collection of Preternatural Cases*, which was published the following year. This, as well as the two earlier volumes published during his life, are generally assumed to have been carefully edited, if not actually written, by Tobias Smollett, the well-known poet and author, who was one of Smellie's few close friends; for these writings possess a literary style in striking contrast to the codicils to Smellie's will and the letters he wrote after leaving London.

Sadly lacking in the social graces, and a poor conversationalist, Smellie avoided London society and shunned public gatherings. His ascent to the foremost position in his profession, without the help of influential friends and without even the advantages of a hospital clinic, was achieved by dint of his own genius and sheer devotion to his work. He cultivated the arts as well, however, and is believed to have painted his own portrait (Fig. 53-1). His will, made jointly with his wife, mentions a violin cello, an organ, and a large collection of "English floots," now known as recorders. His excellent library was bequeathed to the town of Lanark.

REFERENCES

1. Findley, P.: *Priests of Lucina. The Story of Obstetrics.* Little, Brown & Co., Boston, 1939, pp. 169–77.

2. Johnstone, R. W.: *William Smellie. The Master of British Midwifery.* E. & S. Livingstone, Ltd., Edinburgh, 1952.

3. Smellie, W.: *A Treatise on the Theory and Practice of Midwifery.* D. Wilson & T. Durham, London, 1752.

4. Smellie, W.: *A Collection of Cases and Observations in Midwifery.* D. Wilson & T. Durham, London, 1754.

5. Smellie, W.: *A Sett of Anatomical Tables, with Explanations, and an Abridgment of the Practice of Midwifery.* London, 1754.

6. Smellie, W.: *A Collection of Preternatural Cases and Observations in Midwifery.* D. Wilson & T. Durham, London, 1764.

7. Spencer, H. R.: *The History of British Midwifery from 1650 to 1800.* John Bale, Sons & Danielson, London, 1927, pp. 43–60.

James Young Simpson and His Obstetric Forceps*

CHAPTER

54

The obstetric forceps has been modified and redesigned in new form probably more times than any of the other countless number of instruments and devices that man's mind has conjured up for the diagnosis and treatment of his ills. The Chamberlen family is often credited with invention of the first safe and effective forceps, in the late-sixteenth or early-seventeenth century; but archaeologic evidence (Fig. 54-1) shows the forceps to have been in use for the delivery of living infants much earlier, probably the second or third century A.D., in the days of the Roman Empire.[3] During the latter part of the nineteenth century almost every obstetrician of renown seems to have felt the need to add his own modification to the forceps; and even now, scarcely a year passes without the addition of at least one new instrument to our forceps arsenal. For fully a century, however, year in and year out, the vast majority of forceps deliveries has been carried out by means of an instrument popularized by Sir James Young Simpson and usually known as the Simpson forceps, although models embodying minor changes continue to bear the names of their new inventors.

SIMPSON'S DESCRIPTION OF HIS FORCEPS

Simpson demonstrated his forceps for the first time on May 10, 1848, at a meeting of the Edinburgh Obstetrical Society.[15] He explained:

* This chapter originally published in *J. Obst. & Gynaec. Brit. Emp.*, **64**:744–49, 1957; reprinted by permission.

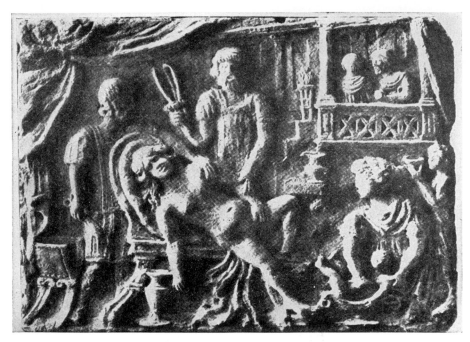

Fig. 54-1. Ancient marble bas-relief depicting a birth scene. The accoucheur, in the center, holds a pair of obstetric forceps aloft in his right hand. This marble tablet, measuring 74 x 55 cm, was discovered in the early-twentieth century in the vicinity of Rome. The attire and furnishings in the scene date it in the second or third century A.D. (Reproduced from *Fisiol. e Med.,* **8**:169–75, 1937.)

They differ from the short forceps in some points of construction, but more particularly in regard to their mode of application and working. They differ for example in their length; in the shanks being parallel for some distance beyond the lock, an indispensable point in order to prevent them injuring the outlet; in their blades being curved; and in the part intended to embrace the head being sufficiently long and large. . . . The blades are the same as Dr. F. Ramsbotham's, but scarcely so much curved. The lock is Smellie's, but with knees or projections above it of such size as to prevent the blades readily unlocking in the intervals between the pains, these giving it the fixed character of the locks of Levret and Bunninghausen's instruments, without their complexity. The joints are made so loose as to allow of their lateral motion and overlapping to a very considerable degree, thus facilitating their introduction and application. And, lastly, the handle is that used by Naegele and other German accoucheurs, viz. with transverse knees or rests below the lock for one or two of the first fingers of the right hand to drag by, the long forceps being only properly used as an instrument of traction, not of compression. In addition, the handles are grooved and marked on the anterior side, to distinguish that from the other side when the blades are within the pelvis. . . .

The forceps was used in the management of uterine inertia, hemorrhage during labor, and other complications, but Simpson regarded pelvic contraction as the chief indication:

. . . The common reason for employment of the long forceps is morbid contraction of the brim of the pelvis in its most general form, and from its most general cause, viz. in the conjugate or antero-posterior diameter, from projecting forward of the promontory of the sacrum. How are the long forceps applied when used in this, the case in which they are most generally had recourse to in practice? It is first requisite to state, that under this complication the child's head is found situated in the brim, with its long or fronto-occipital diameter lying in the transverse diameter of the brim, or with the forehead looking to one ilium, and the occiput looking to the other. In other words, the long diameter of the head is not placed, as usual, in the right diagonal diameter of the brim, and, consequently, the one in which the child's head comes to be placed by the uterine efforts . . . the lateral surfaces of the child's head come to be compressed between the protruding sacral promontory and the interior of the symphysis pubis. . . .

Modern obstetric teaching emphasizes the importance of symmetric, or cephalic, application of forceps to the sides of the fetal head. Simpson, by contrast, advised asymmetric, or pelvic, application of the blades. He said:

The blades of the long forceps should be placed obliquely upon the child's head,—one, the posterior, over the side of the occiput; and the other, or anterior, over the side of the brow or temple, and consequently should be situated in the oblique diameter of the brim. (See Woodcut [Fig. 54-2].)—The markings on the child's head after birth always show this mode of application of the instrument: when properly applied upon the mother, and when their situation relative to the pelvis is examined, they are found to have assumed this position; and in experiments with the instrument (when the head of a dead child is fixed in a pelvis with a contracted brim), this is the position and relation which the instrument will be seen to assume with relation to the infantile head and maternal pelvis. Besides, in thus placing the instrument, while we incur less danger of injuring the urethra and other important parts, we place the blades of the instrument in exactly those parts of the pelvic circle where there is least pressure and consequently most room for them. . . .

SIMPSON AND OBSTETRIC ANESTHESIA

Simpson is remembered eponymically for his forceps, but far greater to his credit was his introduction of anesthesia into obstetric practice. On January 19, 1847, for the first time, he administered ether to a patient in labor, reporting the case in the March issue of the *Monthly Journal of Medical Science.*[12] Wrote Simpson:

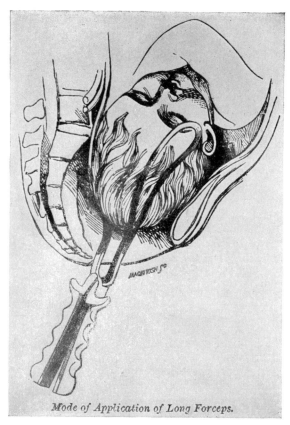

Mode of Application of Long Forceps.

Fig. 54-2.   Simpson's illustration,[15] showing application of his forceps.

The pelvis of the mother was greatly contracted in its conjugate diameter from the projection forwards and downwards of the promontory of the sacrum; the lumbar portion of the spine was distorted; and she walked very lamely. The present was her second confinement. Her first labour had been long and difficult . . . delivered by craniotomy. . . . Even after the cranium had been fully broken down, a considerable time and much traction had been required to drag the diminished and mutilated head of the infant through the contracted brim of the pelvis; and she was long in recovering. Contrary to the urgent advice of her medical attendant, Mr. Figg, he was not made aware of her present or second pregnancy till she had arrived at nearly the end of the ninth month. It was thus too late to have recourse to the induction of premature labour, which had been strongly pressed upon her as the only means of saving her child, should she again fall in the family way. The pains of her second labour commenced in the forenoon of the 19th. I saw her with Mr. Figg at five o'clock in the afternoon, and again at seven. The os uteri was pretty well dilated, the liquor amnii not evacuated, the presenting head very high, mobile, and difficult to touch; and a pulsating loop of the umbilical cord was felt floating below it in the unruptured bag of membranes. From five to nine o'clock the pains seemed only to push the circle of the os uteri further downwards, without increasing its dilatation or making the head in any degree enter into the pelvic brim. Assisted by Dr. Ziegler, Dr. Keith, and Mr. Figg, I shortly after nine o'clock made the patient inhale the ether vapour. As she afterwards informed us, she almost immediately came under the anodyne influence of the ether. But in consequence of doubts upon this point, its use was continued for nearly twenty minutes before I proceeded to turn the infant (as I had previously predetermined to do). A knee was easily seized, and the child's extremities and trunk readily drawn down; but extreme exertion was required in order to extract the head. At length it passed the contracted brim with the anterior part of its right parietal bone deeply indented by pressure against the projecting promontory of the sacrum, and the whole cranium flattened and compressed laterally. The infant gasped several times, but full respiration could not be established. . . .

On questioning the patient after her delivery, she declared that she was quite unconscious of pain during the whole period of the turning and extracting of the infant, or indeed from the first minute or two after she first commenced to breathe the ether. The inhalation was discontinued towards the latter part of the process, and her first recollections on awaking were "hearing," but not "feeling," the head of the infant "jerk" from her (to use her own expressions), and subsequently she became more roused by the noise caused by the preparation of a bath for the child. She quickly regained full consciousness, and talked with gratitude and wonderment of her delivery, and her insensibility to the pains of it. . . .

The ensuing controversy over the use of anesthesia in obstetrics has had few equals in the annals of medicine. Simpson's practices were violently opposed by many of the clergy as well as his medical peers, but to each attack the articulate Simpson replied with devastating logic, impeccable taste, albeit liberally salted at times with incisive sarcasm, and extensive biblical quotations in rebuttal of his critics' protestations against man's alleviation of the travail of childbirth.[17] The distinguished Meigs of Philadelphia referred to the pain of parturition as a "physiological pain," and the equally renowned Ashwell of London wrote in the *Lancet*[2] that to use anesthesia in obstetrics constitutes "unnecessary interference with the providentially arranged process of healthy labour . . . sooner or later, to be followed by injurious and fatal consequences."

Recalling the words of Galen: *Dolor dolentibus inutilis est* (Pain is useless to the pained), Simpson went further, demonstrating the mortal potentialities of pain. By widespread questionnaire study of the results of thigh amputation he showed that ether anesthesia had reduced the mortality from the operation by almost half. He wrote: [13]

Bodily pain, with all its concomitant fears and sickening horrors . . . is, with very few, if indeed any exceptions, morally and physically a mighty and unqualified evil. And, surely, any means by which its abolition could possibly be accomplished, with perfect security and safety, deserves to be joyfully and gratefully welcomed by medical science, as one of the most inestimable boons which man could confer upon his suffering fellow-mortals.

Arguing for the extension of anesthesia to obstetrics, Simpson made a forceful, impassioned plea: [12]

Now, if experience betimes goes fully to prove to us the safety with which ether may, under proper precautions and management, be employed in the course of parturition, then . . . instead of determining . . . whether we shall be "justi-fied" in using this agent . . . it will become, on the other hand, necessary to determine whether on any grounds, moral or medical, a professional man could deem himself "justified" in withholding, and *not* using any such safe means (as we at present pre-suppose this to be), provided he had the power by it of assuaging the agonies of the last stage of natural labour, and thus counteracting what Velpeau describes as "those piercing cries, that agitation so lively, those excessive efforts, those inexpressible agonies, and those pains apparently intoler-able," which accompany the termination of natural parturition in the human mother.

Simpson's entreaties were met at first by the reticence characteristic of his conservative colleagues, as evidenced by his address to the Medico-Chirurgical Society of Edinburgh on December 1, 1847. He lamented:

Probably at the date at which I write there is not one in twenty—perhaps not one in a hundred—of the physicians and surgeons of Great Britain who have, as yet, thought seriously upon the propriety of alleviating and annulling the tor-tures attendant on human parturition; or who have acknowledged to their own minds the propriety of bestirring themselves so as to be able, in the exercise of their profession, to secure for their patients an immunity from the throes and agonies of childbirth.

It soon became apparent to Simpson that ether suffered from certain shortcomings as an obstetric anesthetic, and in the autumn of 1847 he began his search for a better agent, in collaboration with Drs. Thomas Keith and J. Matthews Duncan. Their experiments were carried out at the conclusion of the day's work, in Simpson's dining room. A small quantity of the test liquid was placed in a cup or drinking glass, which was immersed in hot water, if necessary, to increase the volatility. The experimenters then pro-ceeded with their hazardous task of inhaling the vapors and noting the effects. It was in this manner that Simpson and his assistants came upon the anesthetic properties of chloroform on November 4, 1847.

Exhilarated by his new discovery, Simpson employed chloroform in the confinement of the wife of Dr. Carstairs of Edinburgh four days later, the child being named "Anaesthesia." Simpson reported the event to the Medico-

Chirurgical Society of Edinburgh on November 10, 1847,[14] in the following words:

> The lady to whom it was first exhibited during parturition had been previously delivered in the country by perforation of the head of the infant, after a labour of three days' duration. In this, her second confinement, pains supervened a fortnight before the full time. Three hours and a half after they commenced, and ere the first stage of the labour was completed, I placed her under the influence of the chloroform, by moistening, with half a teaspoonful of the liquid, a pocket handkerchief, rolled up into a funnel shape, and with the broad or open end of the funnel placed over her mouth and nostrils. In consequence of the evaporation of the fluid, it was once more renewed in about ten or twelve minutes. The child was expelled in about twenty-five minutes after the inhalation was begun. The mother subsequently remained longer soporose than commonly happens after ether. The squalling of the child did not, as usual, rouse her; and some minutes elapsed after the placenta was expelled, and after the child was removed by the nurse into another room, before the patient awoke. She then turned round and observed to me that she had "enjoyed a very comfortable sleep, and indeed required it, as she was so tired but would now be more able for the work before her." . . . In a little time she again remarked that she was afraid her "sleep had stopped the pains." Shortly afterwards, her infant was brought in by the nurse from the adjoining room, and it was a matter of no small difficulty to convince the astonished mother that the labour was entirely over, and that the child presented to her was really her "own living baby."

Three weeks later, at its meeting on December 1, 1847, Simpson employed his most impassioned oratory in an address to the same society. Singing again the praises of anesthesia for childbirth, and especially of the newly discovered merits of chloroform, he stated:

> I do not remember a single patient to have taken it who has not afterwards declared her sincere gratitude for its employment, and her indubitable determination to have recourse again to similar means under similar circumstances. All who happened to have formerly entertained any dread respecting the inhalation, or its effects, have afterwards looked back, both amazed at, and amused with, their previous absurd fears and groundless terrors. Most, indeed, have subsequently set out, like zealous missionaries, to persuade other friends to avail themselves of the same measure of relief, in their hour of trial and travail. . . . All of us, I most sincerely believe, are called upon to employ it by every principle of true humanity, as well as by every principle of true religion. Medical men may oppose for a time the superinduction of anaesthesia in parturition, but they will oppose it in vain; for certainly our patients themselves will force the use of it upon the profession. The whole question is, even now, one merely of time. It is not—Shall the practice come to be generally adopted? but, When shall it come to be generally adopted? Of course, it will meet from various quarters with all due and deter-

minate opposition. Medical men will, no doubt, ernestly argue that their established medical opinions and medical practices should not be harshly interfered with by any violent innovations of doctrine regarding the non-necessity and non-propriety of maternal suffering. They will insist on mothers continuing to endure, in all their primitive intensity, all the agonies of childbirth, as a proper sacrifice to the conservatism of the doctrine of the desirability of pain. They will perhaps attempt to frighten their patients into the medical propriety of this sacrifice of their feelings; and some may be found who will unscrupulously ascribe to the new agency any misadventures, from any causes whatever, that may happen to occur in practice. But husbands will scarcely permit the sufferings of their wives to be perpetuated, merely in order that the tranquillity of this or that medical dogma be not rudely disturbed. Women themselves will betimes rebel against enduring the usual tortures and miseries of childbirth, merely to subserve the caprice of their medical attendants. And I more than doubt if any physician is justified, on any grounds, medical or moral, in deliberately desiring and asking his patients to shriek and writhe on in their agonies for a few months or a few years longer—in order that, by doing so, they may defer to his professional apathy, or pander to his professional prejudices.

In 1853 John Snow, the first full-time physician anesthetist, administered chloroform to Queen Victoria during the birth of Prince Leopold, her eighth child; and Her Majesty was lavish in her thanks for the new agent and the pain relief it provided. This, probably more than any other single event, bowled over most of the remaining opposition to anesthesia in labor and led to the rapid and widespread acceptance of chloroform in obstetric practice. Not long thereafter Simpson was made a baronet, the inscription on his coat of arms reading "VICTO DOLORE" (pain conquered).

With his characteristic vision Simpson, after he introduced ether into obstetrics, foresaw the advantages of a special anesthesia room for surgical patients, for in September, 1847, he wrote: [13] "In our surgical hospitals, if a ward immediately adjoining the operating theatre were set aside for operation cases, it would in this way facilitate the process of etherization, and ensure more certain and perfect results from it."

SIMPSON'S LIFE

James Young Simpson was born June 7, 1811, in Bathgate, Scotland, the youngest of seven sons of the village baker.[1,4,5,6,7,8,9,10,11,18,19] At the age of 14 he enrolled in the University of Edinburgh, with the help of his family's combined resources, but withdrew from the arts course two years later to pursue the medical curriculum. After three years of medical study, when Simpson had completed all the required courses, he passed his final examination and received the diploma of the Royal College of Surgeons. Being only 18 years old, however, he had to wait two more years for his license to practice. During the interim he undertook further studies in midwifery, alternately assisted

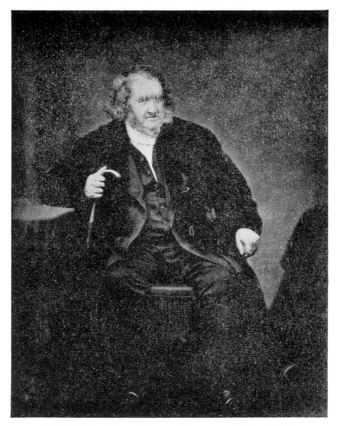

Fig. 54-3. James Young Simpson (1811–1870).

the professor of pathology at the university and Mr. Dawson, the family doctor in Bathgate, and visited the clinics of France and England. Simpson then returned to Edinburgh and entered general practice, but devoted his principal attention to obstetrics. He soon obtained an appointment at the Edinburgh Lying-in Hospital and in 1838 began giving courses of obstetric lectures on his own. When he was only 28 years old he became a candidate for the recently vacated chair of midwifery at the university, waging his campaign for this coveted position in a manner reminiscent of today's political contests. When his state of bachelorhood was mentioned in argument against his appointment, Simpson promptly took unto himself a wife. The Town Council finally elected him to the chair by a single vote's margin over his chief rival, Evory Kennedy, Master of the Rotunda in Dublin. Simpson's wife is said subsequently to have "poured out more tea than any woman in Scotland."

The lectures of the newly elected professor attained a new high in popularity, surpassing in attendance all the other medical courses in the university. In addition to his forceps and his introduction of anesthesia, Simpson made a number of other important contributions to obstetrics and gynecology. He invented a cranioclast for fracturing the base of the fetal skull, and contrived the uterine sound and the sponge tent for dilating the cervix, to provide access to the uterine cavity for the removal of endometrial polyps. Almost at the same time as Semmelweis he called attention to the contagiousness of puerperal fever, giving the most convincing exposition until then of the similarity between this scourge and surgical fever; but he failed to encourage Lister, working contemporarily at the University of Edinburgh, in the latter's experiments on antisepsis, and never accepted Lister's concept of the bacterial origin of infection. He wrote on hermaphroditism and on the freemartin, and dispelled the widely held, but erroneous, belief that among human twins the female was sterile if her cotwin was a male. Simpson was probably the first to stress the importance of bimanual examination of gynecologic patients. He wrote in 1850: [16]

In making this examination, as in making most other examinations of the uterus, a rule requires to be followed which is too often forgot, namely to use both hands for the purpose. For if we are examining the uterus internally with the forefinger, or fingers of the right hand, the facility and precision of this examination will be found to be immensely promoted by placing the left hand externally over the hypogastric region, so as to enable us by it to steady, or depress, or otherwise operate upon the fundus uteri. The external hand greatly assists the operations of that which is introduced internally; and farther we can generally measure, between them, the size, relation, & c., of the included uterus.

Simpson's interests ranged wide beyond the limits of his profession. He published extensively on archaeologic subjects; became an ardent and authoritative antiquarian; and remained constantly engrossed in literature, philanthropic enterprises, medical reforms, and civil and university politics. He served as president of the Edinburgh Obstetrical Society from 1841 to 1858. His nephew and successor to the chair of midwifery in the university, Sir Alexander Simpson, later recalled his uncle's house thus: [10]

[It was] a rendezvous for all sorts and conditions of men. The strangest streams of life were constantly flowing through it. Candidates for seats in Parliament or in the Council Chamber of the city, for vacant chairs in the University, for posts in the Infirmary, for lectureships in many schools of medicine, and for pulpits in town or country—all came to seek his advice and bespeak his influence. Antiquaries came with their latest finds; artists and architects sought his opinion of their designs; poets brought him their new poems, and novelists their stories; the Arctic voyager, the African explorer, the traveller from Mecca, missionaries from all parts of heathendom, came with news and gifts of every kind.

A companion who accompanied him to a reception in Madame Victor Hugo's salon in Paris reported that "the excitement was something tremendous, and for a time you could hear the sound of ss ss ss running through the room as there passed from mouth to mouth the exclamation 'C'est Simpson, C'est Simpson.' " [10]

Simpson died of coronary disease on May 6, 1870, at the age of 58, and was buried in Warriston Cemetery in Edinburgh, alongside the five of his nine children who had predeceased him. A day of public mourning was declared in Edinburgh, its shops and the university were closed, and it is said that 30,000 bereaved citizens attended the funeral. A bust of Simpson, erected in Westminster, bears the inscription, "To whose Genius and Benevolence the world owes the blessings derived from the use of Chloroform for the relief of suffering," a fitting but modest tribute to one of nature's true noblemen.

REFERENCES

1. Anderson, J.: Sir James Young Simpson's work in archaeology. *Edinburgh M. J.,* **6**(n.s.):516–22, 1911.

2. Ashwell, A.: Observations on the use of chloroform in natural labour. *Lancet,* **1**:291–92, 1848.

3. Baglioni, S.: Conoscevano gli antichi l'uso del forcipe ostetrico. *Fisiol. e. Med.,* **8**:169–75, 1937.

4. Ballantyne, J. W.: Sir James Y. Simpson's contributions to antenatal pathology. *Edinburgh M. J.,* **6**(n.s.):554–60, 1911.

5. Barbour, A. H. F.: Simpson as a gynecologist. *Edinburgh M. J.,* **6**(n.s.):534–42, 1911.

6. Croom, H.: Sir James Young Simpson's influence on the progress of obstetrics. *Edinburgh M. J.,* **6**(n.s.):523–33, 1911.

7. Findley, P.: *Priests of Lucina. The Story of Obstetrics.* Little, Brown & Co., Boston, 1939, pp. 234–44.

8. Hart, D. B.: James Young Simpson. An appreciation of his work in anaesthesia and of some of his outstanding papers. *Edinburgh M. J.,* **6**(n.s.):543–53, 1911.

9. Robinson, V.: *Victory over Pain.* Henry Schuman, Inc., New York, 1946, pp. 191–208.

10. Simpson, A. R.: Memories of Sir James Simpson. *Edinburgh, M. J.,* **6**(n.s.): 491–515, 1911. Oliver & Boyd, Ltd., Edinburgh.

11. Simpson, E. B.: Sir James Young Simpson. *Edinburgh M. J.,* **6**(n.s.):482–90, 1911.

12. Simpson, J. Y.: Notes on the employment of the inhalation of sulphuric ether in the practice of midwifery. *Month. J. M. Sc.,* **7**(2):721–28, 1847.

13. Simpson, J. Y.: Etherization in surgery: Part 1.—Its effects; objections to it, &c. *Month. J. M. Sc.,* **8**:144–66, 1847.

14. Simpson, J. Y.: *Account of a New Anaesthetic Agent, as a Substitute for Sulphuric Ether in Surgery and Midwifery. Communicated to the Medico-Chirurgical Society of Edinburgh at their Meeting on 10th November, 1847.* Edinburgh, 1847. (Reprinted in New York, 1848.)

15. Simpson, J. Y.: On the mode of application of the long forceps. *Month. J. M. Sc.,* **9**:193–96, 1848.

16. Simpson, J. Y.: On the detection and treatment of intra-uterine polypi. *Month. J. M. Sc.,* **10**:3–21, 1850.

17. Simpson, J. Y.: *The Obstetric Memoirs and Contributions of James Y. Simpson, M.D., F.R.S.E.* Ed. by W. O. Priestley and H. R. Storer. J. B. Lippincott Co., Philadelphia, 1856, Vol. 2, pp. 463–716.

18. Watson, B. P.: President's address. Sixty-first annual meeting of the American Gynecological Society. *Am J. Obst. & Gynec.,* **32**:547–59, 1936.

19. Watson, B. P.: Commemoration of the centennial of the introduction of anesthesia in obstetrics by Sir James Y. Simpson. *Am. J. Obst. & Gynec.,* **56**: 205–12, 1948.

Étienne Stéphane Tarnier and His Axis Traction Forceps

Since the invention of the obstetric forceps the number of really basic modifications of this instrument can be counted on the fingers of one hand. One of the fundamental changes was the addition of the traction apparatus of Tarnier. Paul Bar, in his lecture [1] at the Clinique d'Accouchement on the occasion of Tarnier's death, stated the need for axis traction in simple, if somewhat exaggerated, terms:

> The forceps had remained a pincer which, applied to the head, permitted its reduction and extraction. But by its very construction it could not attain this goal without considerable injury to the fetal head or maternal soft parts. The operators had tried to diminish these hazards by improving their technique and being more gentle and more precise in the site, method, and direction of application of traction, according to the position and station of the head. A few had made inadequate modifications of the forceps. One had used locks for traction. . . . Others had added a mechanical tractor. None answered the needs.

Tarnier was probably the nineteenth century's most astute student of the obstetric forceps and the mechanical principles underlying its use. His monograph of 1860 [6] revealed a long-standing interest in the subject. At that time the forceps of Levret was the standard instrument in France. Even then Tarnier had begun to feel dissatisfaction with this forceps, later expressed more forcefully with the introduction of his own invention. Wrote Tarnier: [7]

> All obstetricians know that in a proper application of the forceps, traction ought to be directed, as far as possible, in the axis of the pelvis; but all acknowledge that at the superior strait and above this strait it is impossible to pull far enough back,

481

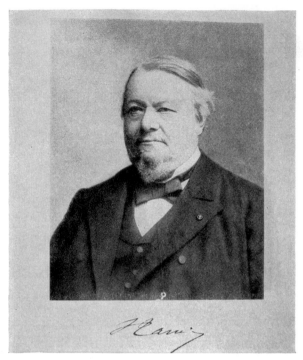

Fig. 55-1. Étienne Stéphane Tarnier (1828–1897). (Courtesy of American Gynecological Society.)

because the instrument is unavoidably maintained in the wrong direction by the resistance of the perineum. I will go farther and say that at the level of the inferior strait and of the vulval orifice, traction is always misdirected when one uses ordinary forceps, because of the very shape of the instrument, whether its blades be crossed or parallel. . . .

Obstetricians have so well understood the harmful effects of the wrong direction of traction made with the actual curved forceps that they try to carry the blades of the instrument as far back as possible; but they then run the risk of tearing the perineum by depressing it too forcefully. . . .

Advocates of the ordinary forceps will further maintain that at the inferior strait and at the vulval orifice they can place their hands in such a way that one of them exerts traction on the handles of the forceps while the other is applied to the articulation of the instrument's blades, exerting downward pressure at this point; that the direction of the resultant of the forces produced by both hands can parallel the axis of the birth canal. I do not deny the possible usefulness of this maneuver, but with it one proceeds empirically, acting haphazardly or by trial and error, and it is absolutely certain that the result obtained never has the exact direction of the axis of the pelvis; this I shall demonstrate experimentally upon request. With this maneuver, if the head progresses in line with the birth canal that it traverses, it is because it is guided by the resistance of the maternal parts despite the traction that pulls it in another direction and in spite of the fumbling of the operator. Finally, with this maneuver it is impossible to make traction as strong as when pulling directly on the handles of the forceps with both hands.

I will make the same objections in relation to another maneuver, which consists of steadying the handles of the forceps with one of the hands, while the other is applied at the level of the articulation, on which it applies pressure. Furthermore the forceps is thus transformed into a powerful lever, and if the head is not grasped firmly the blades may slip backward suddenly and tear the perineum.

Does one wish clinical proof of the ineffectiveness or the difficulties of all these maneuvers by which one attempts to bring traction back into the axis of the birth canal when the head is at the vulval orifice? To facilitate disengagement of the head the majority of obstetricians actually advise raising the instrument up in front of the pubic symphysis and resting it . . . on the patient's abdomen. It is obvious that in such a direction the forceps does not pull in the axis of the vulval orifice and it no longer acts as an instrument of traction. The forceps is now transformed into a lever with its fulcrum at the ischiopubic rami, while the force is applied at the end of the handles and the resistance at the center of the blades and of the head. This then is a convenient maneuver for the obstetrician but painful to the patient and hazardous to the perineum, which is depressed by the extremities of the blades when these are not as one with the fetal head. . . .

In natural deliveries the infant's head, in passing through the birth canal, from the superior strait to the vulval outlet, is constantly changing direction, and thanks to this mobility, describes a curve that follows the central line of the pelvis.

The head would describe the same curve if, the forceps being applied, the woman were to deliver spontaneously without the operator having to exert any traction, as one sees in some cases where the introduction of the blades of the instrument awakens the uterine contractions and stimulates them sufficiently so that they alone could bring about expulsion of the fetus. Indeed, in the foregoing hypothesis, the fetal head and the forceps are intimately united and form only a sort of single body; therefore all the movements of the head are infallibly transmitted to the forceps. . . . One could not deny, without committing a scientific heresy, that it is of the first order of importance to give the traction on the forceps the direction of the pelvic axis, which the fetal head has to traverse.

But what is this direction in the pelvis of the woman in labor? A skilled operator senses it approximately, but no one ever knows it exactly. The accoucheur is thus, so to speak, deprived of a compass and must orient the path of his forceps as best he can according to his anatomic knowledge. . . . The head of the fetus, in negotiating the birth canal, communicates to the forceps, it is true, an impulse that can be felt by the hand of the operator; but this sensation is a very inadequate guide for directing traction, for I have often seen the most experienced accoucheurs alternately raise and lower the forceps because they were not certain that they were pulling properly and they had to fumble a long time before finding the correct direction, if indeed they found it at all.

Having thus stated the problem, Tarnier proceeded to enumerate the following requisites of the ideal forceps:

1. To enable the operator to pull at all times in the axis of the pelvis, whatever the position of the head in the pelvic canal.

2. To allow the fetal head enough mobility to follow the curve of the pelvis freely.

3. To carry a needle indicator showing the obstetrician the direction that he should give his traction in order that it be absolutely correct.

During the winter of 1874–1875 an obstetrician named Pros, from Rochelle, visited Tarnier to show him a mechanical traction apparatus he had designed for attachment to the forceps. This visit freshly stimulated Tarnier to find an answer of his own to the problem he had posed himself, and for the next few years he worked at it, day and night. In this effort he enlisted the aid of two collaborators: Voilliard, a military ballistics expert; and Collin, an artisan. Together they made 30 different models before Tarnier was satisfied; and the resultant instrument (Fig. 55-3), or rather an early modification [2] of it (Fig. 55-4), was soon to replace that of Levret as "the French forceps."

TARNIER'S DESCRIPTION OF AXIS TRACTION FORCEPS

This instrument Tarnier described in a superb monograph published in 1877,[7] consisting of 55 pages of text and profusely illustrated with diagrams showing the mechanical disadvantages of the conventional forceps (Fig. 55-2) and the means by which his new invention could overcome them. The advantages of the new forceps he described as follows:

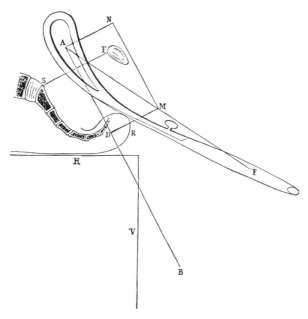

Fig. 55-2. An illustration from Tarnier's monograph,[7] showing the mechanical disadvantage of the conventional forceps in exerting traction at the superior strait.

1. Traction will not need to be as strong as with the ordinary forceps. Indeed, assuming that the head offers to extraction efforts made upon it a resistance of 17 kg above the superior strait or at the level of the vulval orifice, it will suffice to pull on the new forceps with a force of 17 kg, because all this force is used to overcome the resistance offered by the head. With the conventional forceps, on the

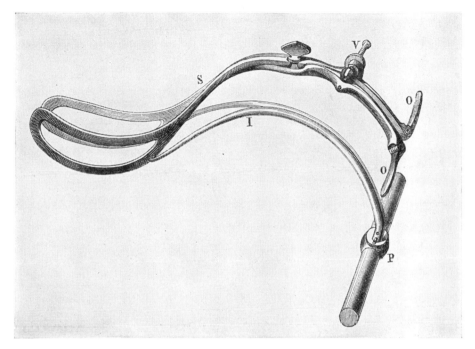

Fig. 55-3. Tarnier's original axis traction forceps.[1]

contrary, in order to obtain a similar result, it would be necessary to pull with a greater force, because the latter would distribute itself partly in useful force, partly in wasted force . . . the effect of which increases the resistance of the head. . . .

2. With the new forceps, all the applied force brings the head into the axis of the pelvis without producing any compression of the maternal tissues. With the conventional forceps, on the contrary, the tissues are compressed during the operation, because the traction is converted partly into wasted force. . . .

3. With the new forceps pulling in the axis of the pelvis, the fetal head has no tendency to slip out from between the blades, although this often occurs with the conventional forceps because, traction there being oblique in relation to the axis of the pelvis, the head, pressing against the pubis, slides between the blades and escapes posteriorly.

4. The handle of the new forceps, being directed transversely . . . gives the hands of the operator a much more convenient grip and a firmer one than that resulting from the application of his hands to the handles of the conventional forceps. Moreover, this handle, pivoting around the end of the traction bars . . .

can, at the last moment of the delivery, be directed in the line of the axis of the instrument. . . .

5. Once the blades of the new forceps are closed on the fetal head by means of the screw . . . the pressure does not increase with the strength of the traction made upon the transverse handle of the instrument; while the operator's hands produce on the handles of the conventional forceps . . . a pressure which, transmitted to the head, is proportional to the strength of the traction; and the head, thus compressed from side to side, elongates from front to back, thus increasing the difficulties of delivery when the pelvis is already too narrow in its anteroposterior diameter, as is commonly the case.

6. The blades of the new forceps, being short and raised in a sharp curve, grip the fetal head without extending below it. . . . Under these conditions the presenting part of the head is the first to touch the perineum, as is the case in natural delivery and one can always direct the traction in the actual axis of the pelvis without fear of tearing the posterior commissure of the vulva with the blades of the instrument. The opposite occurs . . . with the conventional forceps. . . . With the latter forceps one is therefore liable to tear the perineum if one persists

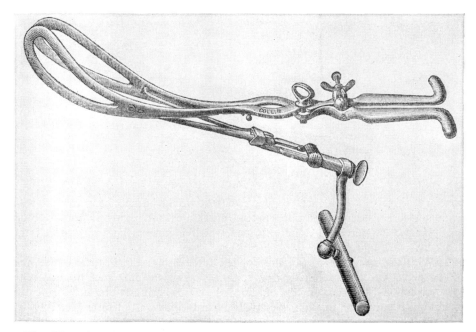

Fig. 55-4.   Tarnier's later modification of his forceps and the model now in use.[1]

in pulling in the axis of the pelvis; therefore one must promptly change the traction, bringing it too far anteriorly and thereby imparting to it an improper direction.

7. To the advantages of traction made in the axis of the pelvis there is added in the new forceps a feature that always leaves the head free to follow the curve of the birth canal. Thanks to the mobility of the articulation of the traction bars

with the prehensile blades, the head can still carry out its movement of rotation around the axis of the pelvis spontaneously and easily; but if one wishes to produce this rotation artificially, he must make sure to carry out this maneuver with the prehensile blades and the tractor joined together in his hand, for if one tried to make the head turn by means of the traction bars alone, one might bend them.

8. Finally, the new forceps is equipped with a needle indicator, which is completely lacking in all other forceps.

Tarnier's publication touched off a series of lively discussions concerning the merits of the new forceps and the rationale of axis traction in general, and brought Tarnier into public debate with Pajot, who regarded the new forceps as a challenge to his maneuver for bringing the head through the pelvis with the conventional instrument of Levret. The month of Tarnier's publication in 1877 is not recorded, but it must have been January or February, for in March of that year Pajot's criticism appeared in the *Annales de gynécologie*. Tarnier's rejoinder, in the very next issue of the same journal,[8] is a model of diplomacy, dispassionately discussing the disputed points in order and refuting the criticisms while maintaining an obviously sincere respect for his "master." Not content to let the matter rest with this, however, Pajot countered in the May issue of the *Annales* with a repetition of his earlier attack.

Glowing tribute was paid Tarnier's invention by Sir Alexander Simpson a few years later.[4] Wrote Simpson:

Let who will continue to use ordinary curved forceps, an obstetrician who has used the Tarnier forceps in a few test cases, will no more think of reverting to the other than a man who can afford to keep a carriage will continue to practice as a peripatetic. He may use the defective instrument occasionally to keep muscle and mind in exercise, or because the case is so easy that it can be finished with anything, as he may walk to some patient's house for the sake of his own health, or because she lives in the same street; but in the general run of his work, and in all his difficult cases, the axis-traction forceps becomes for him a valued necessity.

TARNIER'S LIFE

Étienne Stéphane Tarnier was born April 29, 1828, in Aiserey, a small village near Dijon, France, the son of a country doctor.[1,3,10] Very soon thereafter the family moved to Arc-sur-Tille, where Étienne grew up. He developed a deep attachment to the new family homestead and loved to return to it for his vacations in later life. After completing his secondary education at the Lycée of Dijon in 1848, he went to Paris to study medicine. His studies were soon interrupted, however, for he had to return home to help his father during the cholera epidemic that devastated the entire Dijon region in 1849. He then resumed his training in Paris. In 1856 Tarnier entered the

Maternité, not with the thought of going into obstetrics as a career, but merely to round out his internship with enough obstetric experience to equip him for general practice. Paul Dubois was then surgeon-in-chief but was absent most of the time and Tarnier had no real contact with him. Nevertheless, he soon developed a love of obstetrics, embarked on a series of clinical and pathologic investigations, and decided to devote himself to this specialty.

Puerperal fever was the most pressing problem of the day. From the period April 1 to May 10, 1856, Tarnier witnessed 64 maternal deaths in 347 deliveries at the Maternité, a ratio of more than 1 to 6. He immediately became engrossed in the study of this scourge and, despite violent opposition, was one of the first in Europe to insist on its contagiousness and to advocate the reforms necessary for its control. He showed that the maternal mortality was six to seven times greater in the hospitals of Paris than among the city as a whole. In his inaugural thesis in 1857 [5] he wrote: "We have not invented the facts, we have not let them be molded to a preconceived idea; we have discussed them without prejudice, in relying on the principles of pathology, and it is with sincerity and conviction that we maintain that puerperal fever is contagious."

Having to earn a living after his internship, Tarnier entered private practice, but the early days were so discouraging that he seriously considered giving up medicine. His clientele was both small and poor, and paid him little or nothing for his services.

Providentially for Tarnier, the Académie had just launched a four-month study of the nature of puerperal fever, during which his thesis was much quoted. To Paul Dubois, an important member of the study group, Tarnier furnished important data; and as a reward for this vital service he was later made chief of clinic at the Maternité. His promotions were rapid and in 1867 he became surgeon-in-chief, succeeding Trélat. During the 22 years of Tarnier's direction the maternal death rate declined dramatically. The Maternité eventually succeeded in confining 1000 consecutive women without the loss of a single mother. Tarnier developed a peritoneal exclusion technique for cesarean section, and was the first to use carbolic acid in obstetrics. He designed an isolation pavilion, erected in the garden of the Maternité. In 1889 he succeeded his erstwhile critic, Pajot, as professor of obstetrics in the University of Paris, and upon the latter's death became the leading figure in French obstetrics.

Tarnier made important contributions in several other spheres. Greatly interested in the problem of prematurity, he fostered the use of heated bassinets, and introduced gavage feedings in his clinic. Under his direction Budin, while an intern at the Maternité, carried out experiments, only recently revived and reported as new, showing the advantages of delayed ligation of the umbilical cord. Tarnier's milk diet in the treatment of pre-eclampsia remained in vogue until about two decades ago. He revised Cazeaux's textbook of obstetrics, collaborated with Sée in the revision of Lenoir's obstetric atlas, and later published under his own name, with the assistance of Budin and Chantreuil, his *Traité de l'Art des Accouchements*. In addition to his forceps he devised an intrauterine balloon for the induction of a labor; and, more important, his basiotribe,[9] still in use, to replace Baudelocque's cephalotribe and Simpson's cranioclast. Tarnier's basiotribe (Fig. 55-5) combined the force of action of the former with the surety of grasp of the latter.

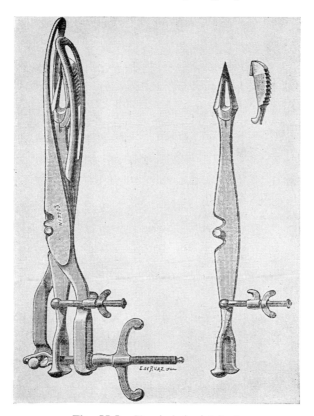

Fig. 55-5. Tarnier's basiotribe.[1]

Having taken ill once previously from the strain of overwork, Tarnier resolved to retire in 1897. On the very day of his scheduled farewell speech he suffered a stroke, from which he never recovered, and died on November 23. A monument in his honor (Fig. 55-6) has been erected in Paris at the corner of l'avenue de l'Observatoire and la rue d'Assas, in the wall of the very building where he carried on his teaching during his later years, now renamed "la Clinique Tarnier." *

* The birth date of 1820, shown on the plaque of the statue, is in error, and has recently been changed to the correct date, 1828.

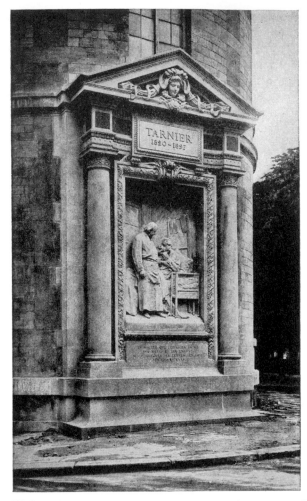

Fig. 55-6.   Monument to Tarnier in Paris. (See footnote, p. 489.)

REFERENCES

1. Bar, P.: *Le Professeur S. Tarnier, 1828–1897.* Carré et Naud, Paris.
2. Bulletin du Progrès Médical: Le forceps de M. Tarnier. *Progrès méd.,* **6**:517–19, 1878.
3. Pinard, A.: Tarnier. 1828–1897. Éloge prononcé a l'Académie de Médecine dans sa séance annuelle du 15 Décembre. *Ann. de gynéc. et d'obst.,* **6**(n.s.): 2–28, 1909.
4. Simpson, A.: Again on axis traction forceps. *Edinburgh M. J.,* **29**(1):289–303, 1883. Oliver & Boyd, Ltd., Edinburgh.
5. Tarnier, E. S.: Recherches sur l'état puerpérale et sur les maladies des femmes en couches. Inaug. diss., Paris, 1857.

6. Tarnier, E. S.: *Des Cas dans lesquels l'Extraction du Foetus est Nécessaire et des Procédés Operatoires relatif a cette Extraction*. Baillière, Paris, 1860.

7. Tarnier, E. S.: *Description de deux Nouveaux Forceps*. Martinet, Paris, 1877.

8. Tarnier, E. S.: Discussion relative au nouveau forceps. *Ann. de gynéc.,* **7**:241–64, 1877.

9. Tarnier, E. S.: Présentation d'instruments. *Bull. Acad. de méd., Paris,* **12**(n.s.): 1425–26, 1883.

10. Tarnier, E. S.: *American Gynecological Society Album of Fellows, 1876–1930*. Ed. by F. E. Keene. Dornan, Philadelphia, 1930.

Christian Kielland and the Kielland Forceps

The earliest models of the obstetric forceps were straight, having no pelvic curve. An intact perineum interfered with proper application and efficient traction, especially when the head lay high in the pelvis. Indeed, it was probably this difficulty that led to the development of the forceps' pelvic curve and the subsequent addition of the traction bar. Episiotomy was rarely carried out until this could de done painlessly and with the prospect of good healing of the perineum. Anesthesia and asepsis, which freed surgery from its fetters in the mid-nineteenth century, made this possible. With the popularization of episiotomy in the present century the pelvic curve of the forceps and the traction bar lost something of their crucial value, for forceps operations with a straight instrument now became mechanically simpler and clinically feasible. It has even been suggested [1,2] that Smellie and Tarnier might never have developed their forceps had the advantages of anesthesia and asepsis, and hence episiotomy, been available to them.

The straight forceps of Christian Kielland has achieved a position as one of the most valuable instruments in the modern obstetrician's armamentarium. It is particularly useful for midpelvic extractions and in cases of deep transverse arrest, asynclitism, and occiput posterior or face presentation; it has also been used for delivery of the aftercoming head in breech presentation, but is inferior to the Piper forceps for this purpose. Kielland first demonstrated his invention at the Copenhagen Rigshospitalet in 1910, but it received no recognition until five years later, when he again demonstrated it in the Univer-

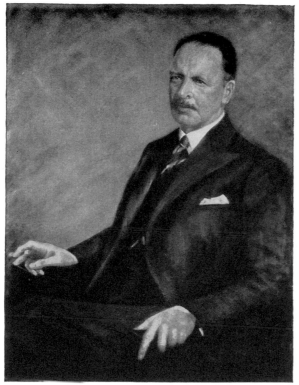

K. Teigen

Fig. 56-1. Christian Caspar Gabriel Kielland (1871–1941). (Courtesy of Dr. Erik J. Kielland.)

sity Clinic in Munich and at a meeting of the Munich Gynecological Society,[3] under the auspices of Professor Döderlein. Kielland's full description of the instrument and instructions for its use were published in 1916.[4] It found immediate favor with the profession, and in the ensuing quarter century fully 200 papers appeared, reporting the experience and attitude of as many obstetricians toward it. An excellent review of the literature on the Kielland forceps is to be found in Jones's monograph.[2]

KIELLAND'S DESCRIPTION OF STRAIGHT FORCEPS

Kielland's paper dealt first with the difficulties encountered in the use of the conventional forceps for extraction of an incompletely rotated head from the upper pelvis. He wrote:

[The position of the fetal head is such] that it cannot be grasped by the forceps blades in as ideal a manner as when the head is low and rotated. The forceps do not then grasp the lateral surfaces of the head, but rather the brow and occiput. . . . In most of such cases a greater force is required than can be accounted for by the resistance resulting from these factors alone.

In my search for an explanation for the extraordinary force necessary, I soon came to the conclusion that this lay principally in the misdirected traction resulting from the handles of the conventional forceps whose blades have a pelvic curve. When one attempts to exert traction in the direction of the pelvic axis, these forceps cannot be depressed so low against the perineum without running the risk of injuring it or losing the proper application to the fetal head. [This was, of course, the precise reason for Tarnier's invention of his axis traction forceps, as already discussed.]

In my opinion, most failed forceps operations are not caused by pelvic contraction. If actual cephalopelvic disproportion exists in such a degree that the head is held up at the inlet, then this is usually obvious to the obstetrician, who realizes how little can be accomplished with forceps in such a case. . . . Quite different, however, when the head is more or less engaged in the pelvic inlet. Then, of course, it may be difficult to recognize how much disproportion is present and to what extent pelvic contraction is responsible for the malposition. . . . Even when the pelvis is normal and the head is in the pelvic inlet, attempted forceps delivery is often unsatisfactory. . . .

Why then do the forceps often prove inadequate in normal pelves with the head at a more or less high station? . . . The cause is to be found less often in the high station of the head than in its position . . . that it lies in the transverse position, still incompletely rotated. In such cases attempts to apply the forceps in any way other than over the brow and occiput are usually unsuccessful. [A lengthy discussion of the maternal and fetal hazards of brow-mastoid applications follows.]

Kielland was apparently unaware that others * had previously inserted the anterior blade upside down. He wrote:

Stimulated by the fact that these injuries resulted from faulty application of the forceps, and by the advantages of . . . a symmetrical grip on the sides of the head, I devised a new method of application of the anterior blade of the forceps. For it should be emphasized that the difficulties were associated with the application of this blade.

A method was necessary by which the anterior blade could be placed in position against the anterior surface of the head with greater ease and safety than with the wandering method usually used.

A modification of the forceps was sought for this purpose. The procedure consists in inserting the anterior blade of the forceps behind the symphysis and directly into its position in the anterior part of the pelvis.

* "Andere, so z. B. Bökelmann, führten den Hebel so ein, dass die Concavität desselben nach den mütterlichen Theilen, die Convexität aber gegen den Kopf des Kindes gekehrt war, und drehten erst, sobald sie hinlänglich hoch gekommen waren, das Instrument auf die erforderliche Weise gegen den Kindestheil." (Kilian, H. F.: *Die operative Geburtshülfe,* 2nd ed. Weber, Bonn, 1849, Vol. 2, pp. 692–93.)

Since the forceps blade cannot be introduced directly in the position that it is to assume on the fetal head, that is, with the inner surface of the blade facing the head, except in cases where the head is very deeply engaged and the cervix dilated, it is introduced with the inner surface of the forceps blade *directed away* from the fetal head. After being introduced far enough in this position, it is turned 180° about its long axis, when it immediately assumes its correct position on the head. . . .

The other blade is inserted directly posteriorly into the pelvis, either in front of or alongside the promontory. The closed forceps now grasps the sides of the head symmetrically. . . .

To permit rotation of the blade, the part . . . where the shank joins the blade is made narrower than in other forceps, and has beveled edges.

I had already modified the forceps so that it had a bayonet-like shape from the side.

This was done in order to facilitate the application of the forceps around the oblique diameter of the head in the so-called wandering method. . . .

The bayonet-like shape permits the axis of the blade to lie parallel to the axis of the handle. . . . When applied symmetrically to the head at the pelvic inlet, with one blade behind the symphysis and the other in front of or alongside the promontory, the forceps grasps the head in the same ideal manner as does the conventional forceps when the head lies completely rotated at the pelvic outlet.

The tips of the blades lie against the cheeks, close to the corners of the mouth. The blades themselves, lying close against the head, extend along its lateral surfaces to the parietal bosses; the forceps thus completely enclose the head within the blades.

The tips of the blades, through which the greatest part of the traction force is transmitted to the head, encounter only the relatively hard parts of the face, parts that are also protected by a thick layer of soft tissue and can best withstand the pressure of the forceps. . . .

With the forceps blades in proper position on the fetal head the handles, because of their peculiar shape, point directly downward. Traction can therefore follow the direction of the handles. . . .

The most controversial aspect of the Kielland forceps has been the inventor's recommended method of application of the anterior blade. Kielland himself took full cognizance of the objections that were raised against this method from the very outset. He wrote:

The first thought that occurs to most people when confronted with this new method of application is that it must be dangerous. . . . It is easy to imagine that the forceps blade, in an inverted position and with the inner aspect of the blade facing anteriorly, could injure and even perforate the uterine wall while being led up along its inner surface. It can scarcely be denied that the forceps blade will impinge against the uterine wall and stretch it somewhat. But after brief consideration, one realizes that this is not necessarily any more dangerous than many other procedures in which the lower uterine segment is thinned out to the same extent, or indeed even more, without being injured.

More convincing than theoretic discussions is the fact that the introduction and rotation of the anterior blade usually proceed without any resistance. This surely disproves the assumption that the blade presses so strongly against the uterine wall as to distend it beyond the limit of its elasticity. And most significant of all, the procedure has caused no injuries despite the fact that it has been used several hundred times. . . .

. . . If the head approaches the oblique diameter . . . then the forceps blade can be pushed laterally along the anterior pelvic wall without resistance. This mobility of the forceps is especially advantageous in cases where the large fontanelle is turned more or less anteriorly [occiput posterior]. . . . The head can then be rotated surely and safely with the forceps, thus converting it from an occiput posterior presentation to an occiput anterior.

For a correct application of the forceps Kielland advised that the patient be placed "on a slanting couch, with her buttocks extending over the edge." Here are his precise instructions for use of the forceps on a head in the transverse position:

Before proceeding with the application of the forceps, the operator must have made an exact diagnosis of the position of the head, the direction of the sagittal suture, and the location of the large and small fontanelles.

The forceps are then held in front of the genitalia, in the position they are to occupy on the fetal head in the pelvis, with the concavity of the pelvic curve facing the occiput. The blade that now lies anteriorly and closer to the operator . . . is introduced between the symphysis and the fetal head. *This blade must always be introduced first.*

The index and middle fingers of one hand are placed inside the anterior lip of the cervix and against the fetal head. The other hand grasps the forceps blade with a full grip (like a sword, not a pen). The blade is held horizontally, with its inner surface, the concavity of the cephalic curve, facing upward. It is introduced along the two fingers in this position, until it encounters the fetal head (Fig. 1) [Fig. 56-2]. The handle is then depressed, the fingers having made certain that the tip of the blade is behind the anterior lip of the cervix and is sliding between it and the head.

. . . The blade is pushed up slowly and evenly, as long as it is felt to be sliding without resistance. When it has been introduced far enough, the shank of the forceps rests on the posterior vaginal wall. . . . Rotation can now be carried out, but in which direction? The blade should be rotated to the side faced by the pelvic curve of the forceps. After the first half of the rotation (about 90°) is completed, the blade thus comes to lie with the concave rim of its anterior edge against the convex surface of the head. On one side of the handle is an easily palpable, knob-shaped elevation, which makes it unnecessary to stop and consider the position of the blade within the pelvis in order to know in which direction the blade is to be rotated. *Rotation is carried out toward the side on which this knob is felt.* During the rotation the handle is held loosely, allowing the blade to adapt to the changing position imparted to it by the rotation. If not introduced deeply enough initially, the blade may sometimes be seen rising somewhat higher, like a corkscrew. After

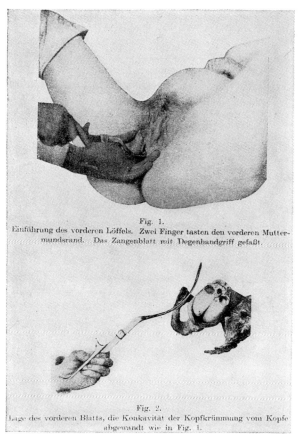

Fig. 1.
Einführung des vorderen Löffels. Zwei Finger tasten den vorderen Mutter-
mundsrand. Das Zangenblatt mit Degenhandgriff gefaßt.

Fig. 2.
Lage des vorderen Blatts, die Konkavität der Kopfkrümmung vom Kopfe
abgewandt wie in Fig. 1.

Fig. 56-2. Illustrations from Kielland's paper,[4] showing his method of applying the
anterior blade of his forceps. (Reproduced by permission of *Monatsschrift für Geburtshilfe und Gynäkologie.*)

the rotation the forceps lock comes to lie firmly against the perineum. The blade
is thus maintained in position; it does not need to be held manually while the other
blade is applied. . . . The handle should be made to lie in the midline, exactly
in the line of the vulval cleft. . . .

[For application of the posterior blade] one introduces two fingers of one hand
into the vagina again and seeks the posterior lip of the cervix. The forceps blade,
held in the other hand, is introduced into the vagina like the first, indeed on the
same side as the first, as indicated by the lock. Crossing of the handles is thus
obviated later when the blades are to be locked. The blade is now inserted behind
the head and in front of the posterior lip of the cervix, under control of the vaginal
fingers. It is then slowly pushed up in the pelvis, either posteriorly or alongside
the promontory, according to the available space. . . . *The posterior blade is the
only one whose insertion may present difficulties.* If the blade will not slide in,
it is either because its tip is striking the posterior pelvic wall (in which case the han-

dle is not depressed enough) or because it is impinging against the infant's head (in which case the handle is depressed too much). By elevating or depressing the handle one finds the correct position, in which the forceps blade can slide in without resistance. Under no circumstances should one try to overcome any resistance with force. The lock, especially constructed for this forceps, always permits meshing of the blades, even if they were not introduced to exactly the same level. Any small difference is equalized with the first pull. . . . *Subsequent traction is made exactly in the direction of the handles,* preferably somewhat more posteriorly than anteriorly. The symphysis should not be used as a fulcrum.

The head usually rotates spontaneously as it descends. If the head is in the pelvic cavity, rotation can be completed with the forceps, but this is actually unnecessary. . . . If much resistance . . . is anticipated, the head is rotated 90° from the transverse into the exact anteroposterior diameter before its extraction through the pelvic narrows is begun. In such a case rotation is carried out *without* simultaneous traction. The forceps, held tightly closed, are turned about the axis of the handles. Some pelvic forms do not allow the head to rotate spontaneously, nor will they permit artificial rotation, until the head is at the pelvic outlet. . . . When the head is brought down to the episiotomy, the handles should not be elevated any higher than would result from spontaneous extension of the head. One tends to do so when using the forceps for the first time, for the handles point lower than those of the conventional forceps. If the handles are elevated, then the tips of the blades are separated from their position on the cheeks and are forced onto the temporal regions. One should therefore exert traction only in the direction of the handles, following the change in direction imparted to them by the head.

Kielland's teachings have proven eminently sound, and their essentials remain unaltered in today's practice.

KIELLAND'S LIFE

Christian Caspar Gabriel Kielland was born November 10, 1871, in Zululand, South Africa, the son of a Norwegian vicar, whose forebears had lived near Stavanger, West Norway, since the seventeenth century. By 1800 the Kielland family of shipowners had achieved a position of wealth and prominence, but its fortunes were later decimated by wars. When young Kielland was three years old his parents left their African missionary station and returned with him to Norway. After preliminary education at his father's vicarage at Brönnöysund, North Norway, Kielland was sent to the Kathedralskole in Oslo. He then spent a year in the Officers' Training Corps before beginning the study of medicine in the Universitas Regia Fredrickiana, from which he graduated in 1899. After internships at the Gravdal Sykehus in Lofoten, Nordland, and the Rikshospitalet in Oslo, he devoted two years to special training in obstetrics at the Födselstiftelse, also in Olso, then entered private practice in that city in 1902. For the next seven years Kielland served as assistant to Professor Brandt, chief obstetrician at the university clinic, then spent three months in the gynecology department of the Rigshospitalet in Copenhagen. Kielland practiced during the ensuing five years in association with Dr. Egeberg, who held the position of Livemedicus (King's physician). From 1911 to 1914 Kielland also served as deputy medical officer at the Födselstiftelse and in 1915 received his appointment to the university clinic. In 1910 he made the first of a series of annual visits to various clinics in Germany, culminating in the demonstration of his forceps in 1915; and he visited the United States in 1931 and 1939. Kielland died in Oslo, March 8, 1941, survived by his wife, a daughter, and two sons, one of whom, Dr. Erik J. Kielland, owns the portrait shown in Figure 56–1.

REFERENCES

1. Jarcho, J.: The Kielland obstetrical forceps and its application. *Am. J. Obst. & Gynec.,* **10**:35–49, 1925.

2. Jones, E. P.: *Kielland's Forceps.* Butterworth & Co., Ltd., London, 1952.

3. Kielland, C.: Eine neue Form und Einführungsweise der Geburtszange, stets biparietal an den kindlichlen Schädel gelegt. *München. med. Wchnschr.,* **62**:923, 1915.

4. Kielland, C.: Über die Anlegung der Zange am nicht rotierten Kopf mit Beschreibung eines neuen Zangenmodelles und einer neuen Anlegungs- methode. *Monatschr. f. Geburtsh. u. Gynäk.,* **43**:48–78, 1916.

Edmund Brown Piper and His Forceps for the Aftercoming Head*

CHAPTER

57

Efforts to reduce the fetal mortality associated with breech delivery have been directed primarily toward improved methods for delivery of the aftercoming head. Evolution of the manual techniques began with the insertion of a finger in the infant's mouth, described by Guillemeau in 1621, with the subsequent addition of traction on the neck, as advocated by Mauriceau; suprapubic pressure on the fetal head, introduced by Wigand and Martin; and Smellie's method of allowing the infant's body to straddle the arm of the operator, designated by the Germans as *Reitenlassen des Rumpfes*.[3] Forceps for the aftercoming head have had a long and checkered career, a satisfactory instrument being a late and relatively recent development in the history of obstetrics.

The first use of forceps for the aftercoming head is illustrated in Table XXXV of Smellie's *Sett of Anatomical Tables*,[7] published in 1754: a "lateral view of pelvis showing method of assisting delivery of head of fetus with long curved Forceps in praeternatural cases, when it cannot be done with the hands" (Fig. 57–1). The "long curved Forceps," originally designed by Smellie for grasping a high head in cephalic presentations, was mentioned in the preface to his *Collection of Cases and Observations in Midwifery*[8] as also useful for delivery of the aftercoming head in breech presentations:

* This chapter originally published in *Surg., Gynec. & Obst.*, **103**:367–70, 1956; reprinted by permission. Copyright, 1956, by The Franklin H. Martin Memorial Foundation.

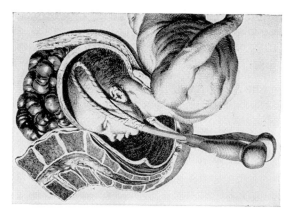

Fig. 57-1. Plate from Smellie's *Sett of Anatomical Tables,*[7] showing the first illustration of the use of forceps on the aftercoming head.

. . . Among the improvements and alterations that have been made in the forceps, I mentioned a long pair, curved to one side, which I contrived several years ago, for taking a firmer hold of the head in the *Pelvis* when high; but I did not then recommend the use of them, because I was afraid of encouraging young practitioners to exert too great force, and give their assistance too soon. Of late, however, I have found them very serviceable in helping along the child's head in preternatural cases, after the body and arms of the *Foetus* were brought down, and it could not be delivered without destroying the child, by overstraining the neck and jaw.

A Collection of Preternatural Cases and Observations in Midwifery,[9] published in 1764, after Smellie's death, contains three interesting reports of cases in which the use of forceps was attempted on the aftercoming head. The first (Collection 34, Case 5), in 1750, is a case of failed forceps following efforts at application to the unengaged head. Smellie's account reveals his awareness of at least one shortcoming of the instrument:

The head, in this case, was to the right side of the *Uterus:* the breech on the left, near the *Fundus,* with the arms and legs backwards, as in the former case; but as the *Uterus* was not so strongly contracted, some of the waters still remained. I grasped the body with my left hand, and raising the head and shoulder to the *Fundus Uteri,* by which the breech was brought to the lower part, the legs with great ease were grasped and brought through the *Os externum.*

In the mean time, the patient begged hard that I would do all in my power to save her child.

The midwife informing me, that the woman had lost one formerly which came in the wrong way, and I finding that the child was alive by the motion of its legs, and that although it was not uncommonly large, the *Pelvis* was narrow; resolved to proceed with great caution, and do all I could to save the *Foetus.*

The patient was in bed lying on her left side: but on this information I had her moved into the supine position. Having brought down the body and one arm of the child which lay before the face, I introduced two fingers of my left hand into the mouth . . . and the fingers of my other hand over the shoulders; then trying to deliver, I could not move the head down after several gentle efforts in this manner. I let go my hold of the under jaw, and tried *Daventer's* method by pressing down the shoulders to bring out the *Occiput* from below the *Os-Pubis;* but this failing also, and finding there was still a pulsation in the *Funis,* I resolved to try the Forceps.

I now desired the midwife to hold up the body of the child so as to give me more room for introducing that instrument: but it being too short, and the head above the brim of the *Pelvis,* I could not fix them properly so as to render them of any use to assist delivery.

Smellie's second case (Collection 34, Case 7) was in 1753. He was called to attend a patient with a compound or shoulder presentation, with an arm prolapsed in the vagina. After performing version and extracting the legs and trunk, he found:

. . . There was still a strong pulsation of the arteries in the *Funis Umbilicalis;* and . . . [I was] afraid of losing the child by overstraining the neck; although I had failed with the short straight Forceps . . . yet I resolved to try a longer pair that were curved to one side, to suit the curvature of the *Os Sacrum.* . . .

Being properly seated, I introduced my right hand up the left side of the child's face. Then with my left hand I insinuated a blade of the *Forceps* up to that part. As I withdrew my right hand to make more room, I slipped the blade farther, that the end of it might reach as high as the upper part of the child's head: then I moved it towards the left groin of the patient, that the blade might be over the left ear, which was at that part: the part of the blade that was bent to one side, was to the *Pubis;* and the convex part was backwards to suit the concavity of the *Sacrum.* . . .

My left hand was next introduced up the right side, betwixt the *Sacrum* and *Ischium,* and along on the inside of my hand the other blade in the same cautious manner, over the right ear: having locked them together, I introduced a finger of my left hand into the child's mouth, to keep the face from turning upwards; then pulling the handles of the instrument with my right, and increasing the force, I brought down the forehead past the narrow part of the *Pelvis;* and turning it backwards to the concavity of the *Sacrum,* brought the head through the *Os externum,* by pulling upwards over the *Pubis,* to prevent a laceration of the *Perinôeum.*

There was a small impression made by the Forceps on the scalp, which dispersed soon after: the child was strong and healthy; and although I used a good deal of force, the mother recovered without any uncommon complaints.

Two years later Smellie had another opportunity to use his long curved forceps on the aftercoming head, again with happy results. He wrote:

In the year 1755 I was called to a case [Collection 34, Case 2] in which . . .
after the body was delivered, the head of the child stuck at the brim of the *Pelvis*.
. . . I introduced a blade of the long *Forceps,* that were curved to one side, up
along each side of the Pelvis, while an assistant held up the body of the child
to give more room for their application; and having fixed them on the head, and
joined the blades of the instrument together, I introduced two fingers of my left
hand, and fixed them on each side of the child's nose, while my right pulled the
head with the instrument, and delivered it safely.

These two successful cases gave me great hope, that the above method would
be of great service to save the lives of many children, who are generally lost by
overstraining the neck in delivering the head; but a third in which I failed [Case 5],
shewed, that we ought never to trust too much, or be over sanguine, with respect
to any particular method of practice; but vary the same as we find it necessary. . . .

. . . The practice is advisable; especially when we are certain that the child
is alive from the pulsation of the *Funis,* or motion of the body, or would prevent
overstraining the neck, or avoid using the crochet. . . .

The use of forceps on the aftercoming head was soon taken up by others.
In Baudelocque's book, *L'Art des Accouchemens,*[1] published in 1781, 13
pages of text and two illustrations (Fig. 57–2) are devoted to this topic, and
the technique is described for using Levret's forceps for the aftercoming head
as well as in cephalic presentations.

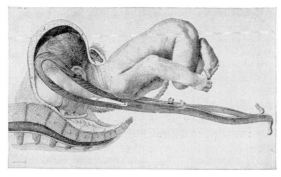

Fig. 57-2. Illustration from Baudelocque's *L'Art des Accouchemens,*[1] showing
Levret's forceps on the aftercoming head.

Forceps for breech deliveries later fell from grace and for a number of years
remained in disfavor as an instrument for the aftercoming head, especially in
Germany. The negative attitude that now prevailed among the profession
toward forceps extraction of the aftercoming head was attributable in part to
the lack of a truly satisfactory instrument for the purpose, but perhaps to a
greater extent to the hostility of certain authorities, notably Karl Schroeder.
In his textbook on obstetrics (1874) Schroeder [6] had written, referring to

the use of forceps on the aftercoming head: "In the not too difficult cases it is unnecessary and worsens the prognosis, at least for the child; and in very difficult cases it is of no value to the child but is far more dangerous to the mother than perforation of the aftercoming head."

Early in the twentieth century interest was renewed in forceps assistance in breech deliveries, largely through Döderlein's more sympathetic attitude toward the instrument's potential value for this purpose; and in 1922 a favorable report by Nürnberger on the results of forceps extraction of the aftercoming head appeared from the Universitäts-Frauenklinik in Hamburg.[4]

PIPER'S DESCRIPTION OF FORCEPS FOR AFTERCOMING HEAD

Piper's forceps for the aftercoming head (Fig. 57–3), described in 1929 after five years' use by the author, has now withstood the test of over a quarter century of clinical evaluation by the profession and remains the most satisfactory instrument of its type yet developed. In contrast to the vast array of obstetric forceps for cephalic presentations, the Piper instrument remains the principal forceps in current use for the aftercoming head, at least in the United States. Its characteristics, as described by Piper and Bachman,[5] are:

. . . (1) a blade having a somewhat flattened pelvic curve for high applications, as in the Tarnier forceps; (2) a lengthened shank, which permits an unusual degree of "spring" between the blades and thus prevents compression of the head; and (3) depressed handles for greater ease of application and manipulation in the presence of the delivered fetal body.

The technique of application was explained by Piper and Bachman as follows:

[It] requires aiming the blades directly at the intended positions on the sides of the head, without rotation, and from below. An assistant meanwhile holds the child's arms and legs . . . maintaining the trunk at not too great an angle of extension on the neck. Whether absolutely required for extraction of the head or applied as an elective maneuver, the chief function of the instrument is that of flexion and not traction; in addition, it serves to control the exit of the brow across the perineal edge, protecting the latter from the lacerations that sometimes occur as the head "jumps" out in this final act of the birth.

The recommended role of the Piper forceps in breech delivery was described thus:

Of the standard methods now available [for delivery of the aftercoming head] all are efficient in the average, uncomplicated case, but most of them, with the exception of those employing forceps, have disadvantages when one encounters

The advocacy of the routine use of forceps on the aftercoming head is not new,[4] and the plan has many points in its favor. To render the maneuver easier, however, the senior author has devised and used in the past five years a specially designed instrument (figs. 16 and 17) embodying the following features: (1) a blade having a somewhat flattened pelvic curve for high applications, as in the Tarnier forceps; (2) a lengthened shank, which permits an unusual degree of "spring" between the blades and thus prevents compression of the head, and (3) depressed handles, for greater ease of application and manipulation in the presence of the delivered fetal body. The technic of application (fig. 18) requires aiming the blades directly at their

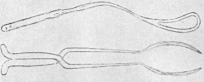

Fig. 17.—Piper's forceps for application to the aftercoming head.

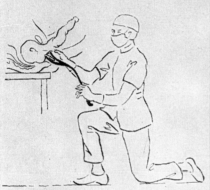

Fig. 18.—The introduction of the aftercoming head forceps requires their direct application, from below, to the sides of the fetal head.

intended positions on the sides of the head, without rotation, and from below. An assistant meanwhile holds the child's arms and legs as shown in figures 19, 20 and 21, maintaining the trunk at not too great an angle of extension on the neck. Whether absolutely required for extraction of the head or applied as an elective maneuver, the chief function of the instrument is that of flexion and not traction; in addition, it serves to control the exit of the brow across the perineal edge, protecting the latter from the lacerations that sometimes occur as the head "jumps" out in this final act of the birth.

SUMMARY

The factors of infant mortality in uncomplicated breech labor are reducible to compression of the cord, the occurrence of nuchal positions of the arm, and delay in delivery of the aftercoming head. The first

4. Nurnberger, L.: Die Zange am nachfolgenden Kopf. Monatschr. f. Geburtsh. u. Gynäk. 57: 305 (May) 1922.

accident is often inherent in the mechanism of breech labor. The other two are more often the result of poor obstetric judgment and technic. As a means of lowering this mortality, we believe, in hospital practice at least, in eliminating the late first stage of the labor, by early decomposition into the double footling attitude, and immediate extraction. For this, thorough dilation of the soft parts of the birth canal is essential, in the achievement of

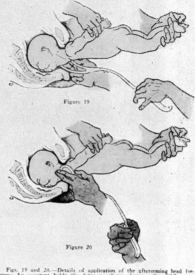

Figure 19

Figure 20

Figs. 19 and 20.—Details of application of the aftercoming head forceps: An assistant holds the fetus as shown, keeping the child's arms out of the way.

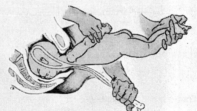

Fig. 21.—Forceps extraction of the aftercoming head: The forceps are used primarily to flex, and seldom to draw on, the head. See text.

which deep anesthesia is a necessary adjunct. The technic of extraction must be perfected, however, in order that nuchal positions of the arms may be avoided, and the aftercoming head guided into the pelvis with the face posterior. In the event of difficulty in delivery of the aftercoming head, the prompt use of forceps will save many infants heretofore lost by too long persistence in efforts to deliver by the standard manual methods.

Fig. 57-3. Pages from original paper by Piper and Bachman, illustrating the Piper forceps and its use. (Reproduced by permission of *The Journal of the American Medical Association*.)

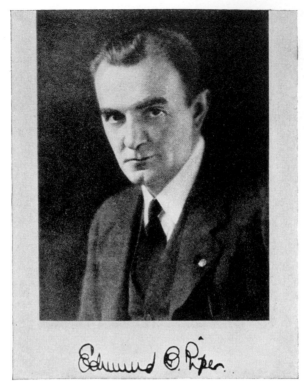

Fig. 57-4. Edmund Brown Piper (1881–1935). (Courtesy of American Gynecological Society.)

high arrests or failures of engagement. The least objectionable of the manual methods is the Wigand, as is any method which aims to avoid imposition of too great a degree of traction on the neck. Even in this, however, there is danger of inflicting tentorial lacerations from too vigorous suprapubic pressure, or of impacting the head in the anteroposterior diameter of the superior strait, in one's anxiety to effect rapid delivery. With this in mind we follow the plan of making only one gentle effort to deliver the head with the Wigand method and, in the event of failure, pass at once to the use of forceps.

PIPER'S LIFE

Edmund Brown Piper was born in Williamsport, Pennsylvania, April 20, 1881.[2] Although he was known to have organic heart disease from the age of 12, he managed to maintain his place among his contemporaries and was not seriously handicapped by it until his later years. He received his B.S. degree at Princeton in 1902 and then entered into the world of business, working for the Williamsport Water Company for five years before deciding to study medicine. He then entered the University of Pennsylvania Medical School, graduating in 1911. After internships at the Children's Seashore House in Atlantic City, the Mercy Hospital in Pittsburgh, and the University Hospital in Philadelphia, and a brief period in private practice, he enrolled with the University Unit of the Ambulance Service in France in 1915. In 1917, after the entry of the United States into World War I, he returned with the American Expeditionary Forces to France, where he commanded several camp hospitals. At the conclusion of the war, Piper returned to private practice in Philadelphia, specializing in obstetrics and gynecology. Here he held a number of important hospital and teaching positions, including the professorship of obstetrics and gynecology at the University of Pennsylvania, and headed the service at the Pennsylvania Hospital. In 1924 he served as president of the Philadelphia Obstetrical Society. He carried out some of the early experiments on the intravenous injection of mebromin (Mercurochrome), later adapted to human use in cases of bacteremia. Although Piper is best known for his forceps for the aftercoming head, he also devised other instruments, including an axis traction forceps. He died suddenly on January 14, 1935.

REFERENCES

1. Baudelocque, J. L.: *L'Art des Accouchemens.* Méquignon, Paris, 1781, Vol. 2, pp. 139–52.

2. Hirst, B. C.: Edmund Brown Piper—1881–1935. *Tr. Am. Gynec. Soc.,* **60**:331–34, 1936.

3. Klein, G.: Zur Geschichte der Extraktion und Expression des nachfolgenden Kopfes. *München. med. Wchnschr.,* **49**:1307–10, 1902.

4. Nürnberger, L.: Die Zange am nachfolgenden Kopf. *Monatschr. f. Geburtsh. u. Gynäk.,* **57**:305–40, 1922.

5. Piper, E. B., and Bachman, C.: The prevention of fetal injuries in breech delivery. *J.A.M.A.,* **92**:217–21, 1929.

6. Schroeder, K.: *Lehrbuch der Geburtshilfe.* Max Cohen & Sohn, Bonn, 1874, p. 274.

7. Smellie, W.: *A Sett of Anatomical Tables, with Explanations, and an Abridgment of the Practice of Midwifery.* London, 1754.

8. Smellie, W.: *A Collection of Cases and Observations in Midwifery,* 2nd ed. D. Wilson & T. Durham, London, 1758, Vol. 2, pp. v–vi.

9. Smellie, W.: *A Collection of Preternatural Cases and Observations in Midwifery.* D. Wilson & T. Durham, London, 1764, Vol. 3, pp. 193–95, 199–201, 205–8.

David Hillis, Joseph Bolivar DeLee, and the Hillis-DeLee Stethoscope

The pulse of the fetus provides the principal clinical criterion of its functional status in utero. The heart tones give assurance of fetal life during pregnancy; alterations of rate and rhythm serve as the most reliable index of fetal distress during labor. Contractions of the embryonic heart muscle begin as early as the fourth week of development; but auscultation of the cardiac beat, transmitted through the uterine and abdominal walls of the mother, is difficult at best before the fifth month. Even later in pregnancy the fetal heart sounds may be dampened to the point of inaudibility by maternal obesity or hydramnios if the observer relies on the conventional type of binaural stethoscope. During the final minutes of labor not only must the obstetrician give special attention to the fetal heart rate, but after all preparations have been made for delivery he must maintain the sterility of his garb while keeping his hands free for intervention if dictated by a faltering fetal circulation. In answer to these special requirements of obstetric practice an instrument, known as the Hillis-DeLee stethoscope, has come into use. Affixed to the head of the obstetrician, it facilitates auscultation through the medium of bone as well as air conduction, while its bell requires no manual control for its application against the maternal abdomen. This instrument is well adapted, therefore, for augmentation of questionably audible heart sounds of the fetus and is ideally suited to the obstetrician who must conduct the second stage of labor without a trained assistant to count the fetal heart rate at frequent intervals.

508

The audibility of the fetal heart in utero was announced as early as 1650 by Marsac, a poet and physician of Limousin, one of the provinces of seventeenth-century France. Philippe Le Goust,[11] one of Marsac's colleagues, told of this discovery in an ode, written in the now obsolete Limousine tongue:

> Ma quand eu voglio qu'eu fautesso
> Qu'eu se viress' et se tournesso
> Et qu'en fuss' en sa libertat
> De changea souuen de posturo,
> L'aguet vougut que sa senturo
> Et sou langeou fussan mai eycartat.

[But when he insisted that it (the fetus) jumps, turns, whirls, moves about freely, and is able to change its position frequently, she (Nature) wished that its waistband and its waddling reins were looser.]

> Et aleydon qu'en hauto noto
> Eu chantauo que lou cor troto
> Comm' un traquet, et forgeo sou esprits
> Sey materio de sang et d'airé
> Ell' enuoyet Galien brairé
> D'aucy dit autromen din sou eycrits.

[And when he sang in a loud voice that the heart beats like a millclapper and forges its spirits without blood or air, She scolded Galen for having said otherwise in his writings.]

For many years Marsac's priority lay overlooked, François Mayor (1779–1854), a Swiss surgeon, commonly being credited[10] as the first to resort to auscultation for determining fetal life by applying his ear to the abdominal wall of the mother in 1818.[12] Lejumeau de Kergaradec,[5,6,9] a Frenchman, reported his rediscovery of this phenomenon four years later, but his acknowledgment of Mayor's earlier experience failed to prevent a heated dispute over priority, stirred by regional rivalry. However, not until the publication of Kennedy's monograph,[8] two decades later, was attention forcefully directed to the value of stethoscopic auscultation in obstetrics. Wrote Kennedy:

It is a matter of regret to us that auscultation in midwifery has not met with more opposition, as the more it meets with, the more it will attract the attention of the profession, which is all that is required to establish its utility. . . . In exploring with the stethoscope the abdomen of a woman at the full period of pregnancy, whose child is alive, we shall detect over a surface, more or less extensive according to the position of the child, and disposition of the foetal and maternal organs, a pulsatory sound generally much more rapid than the pulse of the mother, and exhibiting the characteristic marks of a distinct and independent circulation. . . . On the score of delicacy, as well as accuracy, it may be looked upon as a vast acquisition to the accoucheur, inasmuch as he may arrive at often much more accurate conclusions, by merely applying the stethoscope, and detecting the foetal

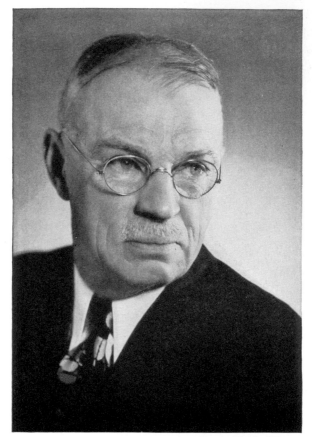

Austen Field, Chicago

Fig. 58-1. David Sweeney Hillis (1873–1942).

heart, than he could possibly expect to do by the assistance of a vaginal examination, which is, to many females, particularly those who are unmarried, not only objectionable, but often so revolting as not to be submitted to. Again, in concealed pregnancy, we may by this means often acquire a knowledge of the true nature of the case, before the female is even aware of our suspecting her. . . . Although we have in a few cases detected this sound even before the expiration of the fourth month, it will not, in the majority, be possible, until a later period; and in those cases where it can be detected about this time, it is sometimes so delicate and feeble as to render it necessary for the individual exploring, to have an ear well trained to stethoscopic sounds.

THE HILLIS STETHOSCOPE

An obstetric head stethoscope, sometimes designated as a fetoscope, was first developed at the Chicago Lying-in Hospital and described by David Hillis in 1917.[7] Hillis' report, showing the instrument in use, is reproduced in its entirety in Figure 58–2.

HILLIS' LIFE

David Sweeney Hillis was born in Chicago, July 19, 1873. He graduated from Northwestern University Medical School in 1898 and subsequently became professor of obstetrics in his alma mater. He also served, at various times, on the staffs of the Chicago Lying-in, Provident, and Passavant Memorial Hospitals, as chairman of Cook County Hospital's Department of Obstetrics, and as president of the Chicago Gynecological Society. During World War I he held the rank of lieutenant commander in the Medical Corps of the U.S. Navy. Hillis died of lung cancer on November 9, 1942.[2] He is also remembered eponymically in association with the Müller-Hillis maneuver for evaluating the cephalopelvic relationship.

THE DeLEE STETHOSCOPE

Not until 1922, five years after Hillis' report on the head stethoscope, did DeLee publish [3] a description of an almost identical instrument (Fig. 58–4) under his own name; but bitter dispute raged between the two principals over the question of priority. The proper division of credit for the invention is still a matter of uncertainty. Thus was precipitated but one of a long succession of quarrels, which led to a constant state of feuding and bickering between these two talented, ambitious, and sensitive men, whose personalities were too much alike to permit them to work together in harmony. The running battle between Hillis and DeLee, which continued throughout most of their professional lives, is given further documentation in Fishbein's biography of the latter.[4]

An example of the relations between the two men is well revealed in one of DeLee's letters to Hillis, when they were both working in the Chicago Lying-in Hospital. DeLee, then chief of staff, had just invented his obstetric forceps, which he requested Hillis to demonstrate before a group of observing doctors and nurses in the delivery room. Hillis, however, ignored the DeLee forceps that had been placed on the instrument table and selected the other, older pair instead. Stung by this rebuff, DeLee promptly wrote his colleague:

> I thought I would let you know that I am duly sensible of the intention of your action yesterday when I politely requested you to try my forceps and make suggestions for their improvement. This action has been registered in my memory together with the numerous other ones. Had you heard the comment on the incident by one who was present you might have realized its futility and the harm it has done you.
>
> I would like to contrast your attitude with my own in a similar case. For many

Jour. A. M. A.
March 24, 1917

Thomas or extension splint in the groin may be relieved by elevating the foot of the bed and attaching to the end of the splint an additional rope which runs through a pulley on this crossarm and is balanced by a weight. In this way extension is secured and the patient can also move on the bed.

The cost of this apparatus is very slight, and any carpenter can make it, from the diagram (Fig. 4), which gives the various measurements.

923 North Broadway.

ATTACHMENT FOR THE STETHOSCOPE

DAVID S. HILLIS, M.D., CHICAGO

Attending Obstetrician, Cook County and Provident Hospitals; Assistant Obstetrician, Chicago Lying-In Hospital; Instructor in Obstetrics, Northwestern University Medical School

Frequent observation of the fetal heart tones during the last part of the second stage of labor presents certain technical difficulties after the attendant is surgically prepared for the delivery. In breech labors in which the heart tones must be watched very carefully, it is always desirable and often

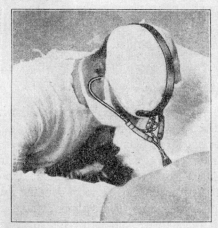

Attachment for the stethoscope facilitating the observation of heart tones.

necessary for the operator to observe the heart tones himself.

In order to make this easily possible, an attachment for the stethoscope was devised which consists of a metal band such as is used on a head mirror, passing from front to back over the top of the head. The Y of the binaural stethoscope is fastened to the front plate of this band by means of a short spiral spring and a universal joint which is capable of being made rigid by a thumb screw. This permits proper adjustment of the ear pieces and holds the stethoscope in a position above the line of sight at right angles to the forehead. The spiral spring gives enough flexibility to the bell of the instrument to make it easily adaptable to the surface.

An experience of several months with its use at the Chicago Lying-In Hospital indicates that it has the following advantages:

It gives easy and accurate control of heart tones.

After adjustment, no handling is required.

Heart tones are heard better, since there is bone conduction through the metal parts of the instrument, in addition to the air conduction of the ordinary stethoscope.

The bell may be pressed firmly against the abdominal wall without interference from muscle sounds.

Fig. 58-2. Hillis' report of his head stethoscope. (Reproduced by permission of *The Journal of the American Medical Association.*)

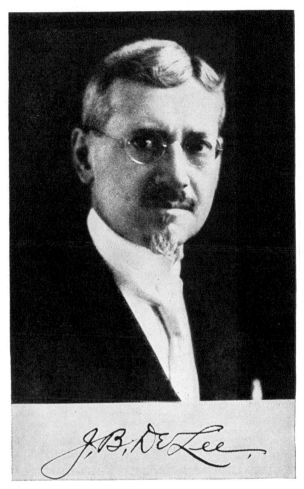

Fig. 58-3. Joseph Bolivar DeLee (1869–1942). (Courtesy of American Gynecological Society.)

years I have been using your membrane perforator and have always called it by its proper name. . . . I have had, and kept at home for more than fifteen years, a membrane perforator infinitely superior to yours. Recently I found your instrument totally inefficient and felt it was time to bring over one that would do the work. . . . It was invented by Dr. Fried in 1840. I kept it hidden because I did not want it to supersede yours.

Yesterday morning I gave you four different psychological tests. I wanted to know if you had undergone a change of heart. In all four tests, however, much to my regret, it was apparent that you were traveling true to your old form.[4]

DeLee's version of the stethoscope controversy is far from clear. In a note dated March 10, 1926, he wrote:

1688   Zentralblatt für Gynäkologie 1922. Nr. 42.

sie mir lachend, sie habe eine ganze Reihe Kinder. Bei mehreren sei sie während
der letzten Schwangerschaftsmonate heiser gewesen. Sie habe deswegen auch
schon vor einigen Jahren den inzwischen verstorbenen Chirurgen Roser (Marburg)
konsultiert, und der habe ihr beinahe wörtlich dasselbe gesagt, wie ich. Sie wisse
das aber besser: das Halsleiden ginge mit Beendigung der Schwangerschaft allein
vorüber. Daraufhin bat ich natürlich, sie möchte sich nach der Entbindung noch
einmal vorstellen. 6 Wochen später konnte ich einen gesunden Kehlkopf mit
klarer Stimme feststellen. Über das weitere Ergehen der Frau vermag ich nichts
mitzuteilen.

II.

Northwestern University Chicago, U.S.A.

Ein neues Stethoskop,
für die Geburtshilfe besonders geeignet.

Von

Prof. der Geburtshilfe M. D. Jos. B. De Lee.

Den deutschen Ärzten möchte ich ein Instrument vorlegen, dessen Gebrauch,
ich bin überzeugt, vielen Kindern das Leben retten wird.

Man weiß, wie umständlich es ist, in der Austreibungsperiode der Geburt die
kindlichen Herztöne beständig zu überwachen.

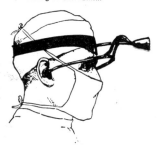

Fig. 1.

Kopfstethoskop nach Prof. Dr. Lee, Chicago.

Bei meinen Assistenten hat sich öfters das Bedürfnis geäußert für ein elek-
trisch-akustisches Instrument, das man am Abdomen einer Kreißenden zu fixieren
vermag, und das an einer entfernten Tafel (Dial) die Herzbewegungen des Kindes
abzulesen, oder am Kopfe getragen, die Herztöne fortwährend zu hören gestatte.
Dozent Dr. Hillis schlug vor, man soll das gewöhnliche Stethoskop einfach am
Kopfe fixieren.

Fig. 58-4.   First page of DeLee's report of his head stethoscope. (Reproduced by permission of *Zentralblatt für Gynäkologie*.)

For several years Dr. Hillis has claimed that I stole the idea of the Head
Stethoscope from him. The facts are that for years before he began the study of
medicine [Hillis received his M.D. in 1898, when DeLee was not quite 29 years
old] I spoke of such an instrument. The idea of fastening a listening device to
the head for [listening to] the fetal heart tones is mine.[4]

Years later, in 1941, DeLee dated his conception of the idea as 1898, when
he experimented with a number of mechanical and electrical models, none
of which proved satisfactory. Then in 1915, according to DeLee's letter,
Hillis either suggested or agreed (the choice of words here is crucial) that
the conventional-type stethoscope might be worn on the head. It was at this
time, DeLee recalled, that "I immediately designed the instrument now used
under the name DeLee-Hillis Head Stethoscope."

A totally different version was recounted by Hillis. The original idea of a stethoscope that would not require manual control by the obstetrician emanated from DeLee, Hillis admitted, but after joint discussion, he (Hillis) actually designed the instrument. DeLee then expressed his dissatisfaction with the Hillis model, according to this account, made a few insignificant changes, and called the invention his own.

The early models of the instrument, Fishbein states,[4] were advertised by the manufacturer as the DeLee Stethoscope, Hillis' name being added later at DeLee's request.

DeLEE'S LIFE

Joseph Bolivar DeLee was born October 28, 1869, the son of a dry-goods merchant and the ninth of ten children, in the small community of Cold Spring, New York, just across the Hudson from West Point.[1,4] After attending the public schools of New York City he worked for a while at odd jobs, including drugstore clerk and electrician's helper. Over the objections of his father, who wanted him to be a rabbi, young DeLee then enrolled in the Chicago Medical College, later to become the medical school of Northwestern University, helping finance his education by working during his spare time as medical attendant in a farm for illegitimate and unwanted babies. "The mortality was fearful," DeLee later recalled, but this provided abundant opportunity for postmortem examinations, which impressed him with the frequency of cerebral hemorrhage as a cause of neonatal death, a problem that engaged much of his attention in later years.

Medical education in America was in a sorry state at that time. The school of DeLee's choice had only two full-time employees: the professor of chemistry and the janitor. DeLee made the most of his opportunities, however, and graduated with honors in 1891. Inspired by his professor of obstetrics and disturbed by the plight of Chicago's unwed mothers, he decided on a career in obstetrics. After an internship at Cook County Hospital, a year of teaching anatomy and physiology, and a period of postgraduate study in Paris, Berlin, and Vienna, he opened a free maternity clinic in the slums of Chicago under the auspices of the medical school, in addition to his own office for private practice. The clinic proved a fiasco, however, failing to attract any patients. Undaunted, DeLee enlisted organized philanthropic aid and established the Chicago Lying-in Dispensary in 1895. This took hold from the start, and by the end of the following year he had supervised the confinement of 204 patients and had given practical obstetric instruction to 12 physicians and 52 students. Flushed with success, he soon began to plan for expansion of the dispensary's services, a frequently recurring project that culminated in the present Chicago Lying-in Hospital. The main building of this institution was subsequently named for him.

For nearly 40 years DeLee held the rank of professor of obstetrics in Northwestern University; but when the Chicago Lying-in Hospital was merged with the University of Chicago, DeLee, as the hospital's chief of staff, was made chairman of the Department of Obstetrics and Gynecology in the latter university. He held this position until 1932, when he founded the Chicago Maternity Center. Ten years later, on April 2, 1942, he died of coronary thrombosis, still a bachelor at the age of 72. Long before his death he had won for himself the reputation as one of America's most distinguished obstetricians. In addition to his stethoscope and forceps, he designed approximately 40 other instruments, as well as a delivery bed and an incubator for premature infants. A prolific writer throughout his professional life, his *Obstetrics for Nurses* went into 12 editions, and the *Yearbook of Obstetrics* enjoyed his editorship from 1904 until his death. His greatest literary monument was *The Principles and Practice of Obstetrics,* first published in 1913, which enjoyed seven editions during his lifetime and which has been carried on subsequently by Greenhill, one of his disciples. DeLee pioneered in the use of motion pictures for medical teaching, and a number of his obstetric films are still in use. He was also instrumental in popularizing the low cervical cesarean section in America. Greatly in demand as a consultant, his practice was highly lucrative, but most of the proceeds from it and from his books were donated to the institutions to which he had dedicated himself. Despite his wide professional acclaim, DeLee remained fundamentally a lonely, unhappy man, constantly plagued by his excessive sensitivity and the compulsive tendencies of the perfectionist he was.

REFERENCES

1. Deaths: Joseph Bolivar DeLee. *J.A.M.A.*, **118**:1314, 1942.

2. Deaths: David Sweeney Hillis. *J.A.M.A.*, **120**:1055, 1942.

3. DeLee, J. B.: Ein neues Stethoskop, für die Geburtshilfe besonders geeignet. *Zentralbl. f. Gynäk.*, **46**:1688–89, 1922.

4. Fishbein, M., and DeLee, S. T.: *Joseph Bolivar DeLee, Crusading Obstetrician.* E. P. Dutton & Co., Inc., New York, 1949.

5. Fodera, D. M.: Mémoire sur l'auscultation appliquée à l'étude de la grossesse, ou recherches sur deux nouveaux signes propres à faire reconnaitre plusieurs circonstances de l'état de gestation; par Lejumeau de Kergaradec, M. J. A., *J. de physiol.*, **2**:112–17, 1822.

6. Glück, E.: *La Découverte de Lejumeau de Kergaradec. L'Auscultation appliquée à l'Art des Accouchements. Étude Historique.* Thesis, Paris, 1939.

7. Hillis, D. S.: Attachment for the stethoscope. *J.A.M.A.*, **68**:910, 1917.

8. Kennedy, E.: *Observations on Obstetric Auscultation, with an Analysis of the Evidences of Pregnancy and an Inquiry into the Proofs of the Life and Death of the Foetus in Utero.* J. & H. G. Langley, New York, 1843.

9. Lejumeau de Kergaradec, J. A.: Mémoire sur l'auscultation appliquée à

l'étude de la grossesse, ou recherches sur deux nouveaux signes propres à faire reconnaitre plusieurs circonstances de l'état de gestation, lu à l'Académie royale de Médecine, dans la séance générale du 26 décembre 1821. *Ann de méd. physiol.,* **1**:344–47, 1822.

10. Moulinié: Notice nécrologique sur feu le docteur Mayor père, ancien président de la Section des Sciences naturelle et mathématiques. *Bull. Inst. Nat. Geneva,* **5**:328–39, 1854.

11. Phélippeaux: Notice biographique et bibliographique sur Philippe Le Goust, médecin du XVIIe siècle, lue à la séance générale de la Société des archives historiques de la Saintonge et de l'Aunis, le 12 mars 1879, par le Dr. Phélippeaux (de Saint-Savinien). *Arch. de tocol.,* **6**:304–20, 1879.

12. Pictet: *Footnote to* Notice des séances de l'Académie Royale des Sciences de Paris, pendant le mois de juin. *Bibliothéque Universelle des Sciences, Belles-Lettres, et Arts.* Geneva, 1818, Vol. 9 (*Sciences et Arts*), pp. 249–50.

Champetier de Ribes, James Voorhees, and Their Metreurynters*

For over a century, bags, balloons, and animal bladders [4] have been inserted into the pregnant and puerperal uterus for a variety of purposes, including tamponade in cases of postabortal and postpartum uterine hemorrhage and placenta previa, induction of labor, treatment of uterine inertia, management of fetal malpresentations, and promotion of adequate cervical dilatation for passage of the aftercoming head in premature births. These metreurynters still linger on the horizon of modern obstetric practice, having been almost, but not quite, replaced by other methods of treatment. In many delivery rooms they are still called into use occasionally.

Two models of the intrauterine bladder have survived the test of professional acceptance: the Champetier de Ribes balloon and the Voorhees bag. Neither, however, quite qualifies as an original invention, each representing but a modification of a pre-existing instrument of the same general type.

Until the latter part of the nineteenth century the danger of abdominal operation limited the methods of treating pelvic dystocia largely to forceps extraction, version, embryotomy, and induction of premature labor. The principal devices for inducing labor consisted of artificial rupture of the membranes, bougies, and intrauterine balloons. Champetier de Ribes, while an intern under Tarnier at the Maternité in Paris in 1878, learned the use of his master's *ballon excitateur,* a soft rubber bag, hen's egg size, which was inserted through the cervix on the end of a male catheter for dilatation of the

* This chapter originally published in *Bull. Sloane Hosp. for Women,* **2**:13–20, 1956; reprinted by permission. Copyright © 1956, by The Sloane Hospital.

canal. Tarnier's intracervical balloon, introduced in 1862, at about the same time as Barnes's fiddle-shaped bag, had already been anticipated during the preceding two decades by Hüter and Busch, who had used the urinary bladder of the pig and dog to stanch the hemorrhage from placenta previa, and by Slyman, who had employed a rubber intrauterine bag for the control of post-abortal bleeding.

THE DE RIBES BALLOON

Finding Tarnier's round balloon too small and not well shaped for his purpose, de Ribes experimented with a number of models and sizes of his own design, the largest being a conical, rubber-covered, silk balloon, 21 cm in circumference. This he used for the first time on August 25, 1887; and the following year he published a report on 18 patients treated with his new balloon.[2] Contracted pelvis was the indication for induction of labor in 14 cases, heart disease in one. Two additional patients suffered from uterine inertia plus a contracted pelvis; and in the final case the balloon was used in a primigravida with a dead fetus presenting by the shoulder. Wrote de Ribes:

I have sought a method to induce labor surely and rapidly, and at the same time to dilate the whole birth canal in order to remove the obstacles presented by the soft parts at the time of delivery, whether left to nature or terminated by operation.

I believe I have attained this objective by a simple, harmless procedure, easy to use.

In order to accomplish this result I insert an impermeable empty balloon, made of nondistensible material, above the internal os; I inject it with fluid: then its largest circumference becomes equal to or a little larger than that of the fetal head; then I let the maternal organism expel the foreign body spontaneously.

. . . When the dilating balloon has passed the vulva the road is clear, and the fetus in its passage will then encounter no further difficulties from the maternal soft parts.

Additional situations in which de Ribes suggested insertion of the balloon he listed as follows:

1. In some cases of hydramnios, in which I would advise rupture of the membranes at the time of insertion of the balloon. . . .

3. In cases of severe albuminuria necessitating interruption of pregnancy.

4. At the onset of labor in cases of unengaged shoulder presentation, the membranes being ruptured and internal version being impossible because of retraction of the uterus; in order to hasten [cervical] dilatation and at the same time descent of the shoulder. . . .

6. In cases of retained placenta, in order to reopen the uterus if manifestations of serious infection are present.

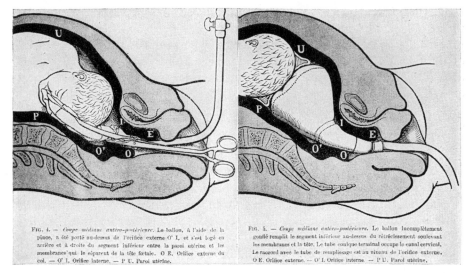

Fig. 59-1. Illustrations from de Ribes' paper,[2] showing insertion of the balloon, and the inflated balloon in position in the uterus. (Reproduced by permission of Masson & Cie, Paris.)

7. Finally, in cases of severe hemorrhage resulting from abnormal attachment of the placenta, I would be very much inclined to rupture the membranes even before the onset of labor, if I could reach them, and to insert a balloon into the amniotic sac. I am convinced that the balloon will act as an excellent tampon while bringing on labor rapidly, thus fulfilling all the conditions for producing the best possible results for both mother and child in these serious cases.

The effect of the balloon on the uterus and the character of the labor it produced were carefully recorded by de Ribes. He wrote:

For a variable time after the insertion of the balloon one sees nothing special; some women complain of a sensation of tightness in the hypogastric region; sometimes dull pains appear immediately.

Most often true labor sets in after three or four hours, and it is usually very painful and progresses rapidly. As a result of the contractions one soon feels the lower segment, which bulges gradually while the cervix effaces and the balloon begins to descend. One can determine, by actual palpation, that the apparatus lies in the midline during its descent.

As the contractions increase and the margins of the external os thin out, an increasingly larger part of the balloon is palpable to the examining finger around the insertion of the tube. From the moment when the os reaches the size of a 5-franc piece during a contraction, dilatation proceeds very rapidly; suddenly, under the influence of a contraction, the largest circumference of the balloon clears the os and the balloon drops into the vagina.

When the balloon has passed through the external os the period of expulsion [second stage of labor] begins. It is always very rapid, even in primigravidas. It is very advantageous to have as much dilatation as possible of the vagina and vulva; I therefore advise leaving the balloon full during this entire period, to ensure its largest dimensions.

The balloon's action, according to de Ribes, is twofold: (1) direct mechanical distention of the lower uterine segment and internal cervical os; and, more important, (2) reflex stimulation of the expulsive powers of the uterine fundus and abdominal musculature.

The balloon acts like the bag of waters: in addition to the increase in tension produced by its volume, which, contrary to what I had reasoned theoretically, is rather small, its whole value in bringing about expulsion is due to the contraction of the uterine and abdominal muscles. The force that it exerts against the walls that it dilates is thus borrowed almost entirely from the maternal organism, which reacts to it as it would to a whole small fetus presenting itself in front of a second well-developed fetus in a twin delivery, the first fetus being dead and macerated.

The management counseled by de Ribes following the balloon's expulsion was governed by the circumstances:

Palpation immediately after exit of the balloon gives precise information concerning the condition of the cervix, lower uterine segment, and the presenting part of the fetus. If the flexed head is only at the level of the superior strait and has not descended, one can allow labor to follow its course for an hour or two; the membranes should be ruptured if intact.

If the uterus contracts vigorously and if the pelvis is not too small or the fetal head too big, the latter descends into the pelvis and spontaneous delivery occurs.

If after a limited time the head fails to descend and the cervix begins to close again, delivery should be accomplished by forceps or embryotomy; there is no advantage in waiting.

When the breech presents, it always descends behind the balloon, if pelvic contraction is not too great, and one only has to intervene for the shoulders and head.

If a complication occurs, such as prolapse of the cord, one is in an excellent position to perform a version.

My final advice is that one ought to complete the delivery after expulsion of the balloon, unless spontaneous delivery appears imminent. In other words, *one ought to act as one would for the delivery of a second twin.*

CHAMPETIER DE RIBES' LIFE

Camille Louis Antoine Champetier de Ribes was born in Draveil, France, June 3, 1848.[1,3,6] He studied medicine in Paris and in 1879, under Tarnier's direction, published his thesis, *Le passage de la tête foetale dernière à travers les bassins retrecis,* a timely topic, for the principal subject of obstetric study at that time was the mechanics of labor and delivery. In this thesis de Ribes described the passage of the aftercoming head through the flat rachitic pelvis and called attention to the importance of flexion and posterior asynclitism. He also described a maneuver, sometimes called by his name, for directing the head into the pelvis with the bitemporal diameter substituted for the larger biparietal. He became best known for his intrauterine balloon, which soon attained great popularity, not only for induction of labor, but also for arresting hemorrhage in placenta previa; and for several years it remained the principal means of treatment for this condition. De Ribes was made accoucheur of the maternity hospital of Tenon in 1889 and in 1897 became director of obstetrics at the Hôtel-Dieu as well. Here he remained until 1911, when he retired to the family homestead at Bearn in Argagnon. He died on April 1, 1935, at the age of 86.

THE VOORHEES BAG

The de Ribes balloon was tried out in New York in the fall of 1897 by Dr. James W. McLane, first director of the Sloane Maternity Hospital, but was found unsatisfactory. It was not strong and durable enough, it held insufficient fluid, it ruptured easily at the seams, and its tube withstood but little traction. In addition, the balloons were expensive, costing $1.50 each, or $9.00 per set, and had to be ordered from Paris. Dr. James Voorhees, then resident obstetrician, therefore set out to improve on the de Ribes balloon, and succeeded in having a canvas bag, covered with heavy rubber, manufactured in New York. Its retail price was $1.00 for a set of four.

By September 1, 1899, Voorhees' bag had been used in 72 out of 2113 obstetric cases at the Sloane Hospital. Voorhees' report,[7] which received the Stevens Triennial Prize from Columbia University, was published in the *Medical Record* for September 8, 1900. Complete instructions were given for use of the bag, and the indications listed as follows:

(1) To start pains, when the membranes have been long ruptured, especially in breech cases; (2) in dry labors when the child is in bad condition—there is an umbilical souffle, or it is passing meconium, or the heart is slow or irregular; (3) in prolonged and protracted labors, oxytocics and chloral failing; (4) in rigid cervices of all kinds; (5) in hydramnion, when it is necessary to rupture the membranes; (6) in cases of twins, when it is necessary to rupture the membranes; (7) in shoulder presentations, when a Braxton Hicks version cannot be easily done; (8) to induce labor: (a) in cases in which a bougie fails or when the membranes are ruptured in its introduction; (b) in albuminuria; (c) in contracted pelves—to let the head down against the brim to engage; or preparatory to forceps or version; (d) in case of a dead fetus; (e) in chronic endocarditis;

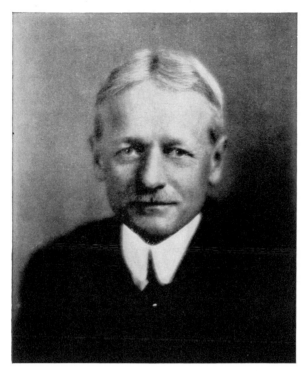

Fig. 59-2. James Ditmars Voorhees (1869–1929). (Courtesy of New York Academy of Medicine.)

(9) in placenta previa, especially those cases in which the cervix is tough, or in which the placenta is over the os and one cannot turn easily, preparatory to version.

The Voorhees bag rapidly replaced Champetier de Ribes' model, and for more than a quarter of a century occupied a prominent place in the armamentarium of the American obstetrician.

VOORHEES' LIFE

James Ditmars Voorhees was born in Morristown, New Jersey, May 21, 1869, a descendant of Albert Coerte Van Voor Hees, who emigrated from Holland and was one of the first settlers on Long Island in 1620.[5] After his preliminary education in Morristown, Voorhees attended Princeton University, where he received his B.A. in 1890. In 1893 he graduated from the College of Physicians and Surgeons of Columbia University, being awarded the second Harsen prize. His postgraduate training consisted of two years as assistant resident in the Presbyterian Hospital in New York and a year at the New

York Foundling Hospital, following which he spent three and one-half years as resident physician in the Sloane Maternity Hospital, beginning in 1897, and was made instructor in obstetrics in the College of Physicians and Surgeons. At the completion of his residency he entered private practice in New York, and in 1901 was made secretary to the medical faculty. One of New York's most prominent obstetricians, Voorhees confined most of his patients in private nursing establishments throughout the city during the latter years of his practice and delivered many in their own homes. He died in Santa Barbara, California, July 30, 1929, while vacationing there a few years after his retirement.

REFERENCES

1. Brindau: Notice nécrologique sur M. Champetier de Ribes (1848–1935). *Bull. Acad. de méd., Paris,* **113**:435–36, 1935.

2. Champetier de Ribes: De l'accouchement provoqué. Dilatation du canal génital (col de l'utérus, vagin et vulve) a l'aide de ballons introduit dans la cavité utérine pendant la grossesse. *Ann. de gynéc.,* **30**:401–38, 1888.

3. *Index Biographique des Membres, des Associés et des Correspondants de l'Académie de Médecine. Décembre 1820 a Juillet 1939.* Masson & Cie, Paris, 1939, p. 24.

4. Ricci, J. V.: *One Hundred Years of Gynaecology, 1800–1900.* Blakiston Co., Philadelphia, 1945, pp. 502–3.

5. Shrady, J.: *The College of Physicians and Surgeons, New York and Its Founders, Officers, Instructors, Benefactors and Alumni. A History.* Lewis Publishing Co., New York.

6. Siredey, A.: Champetier de Ribes (1848–1935). *J. de méd. et chir. prat.,* **106**: 297–98, 1935.

7. Voorhees, J. D.: Dilatation of the cervix by means of a modified Champetier de Ribes balloon. *M. Rec.,* **58**:361–66, 1900.

Leonardo Gigli and the Gigli Saw | CHAPTER 60

One of the gravest errors in the history of obstetrics was the belief that the innominate bones separate during labor to facilitate passage of the fetus through the pelvic canal. This teaching, which probably originated with Hippocrates, was persistently cherished by his followers for many generations, even after the anatomic demonstration of its untenability by Vesalius in the sixteenth century.[4] Progress in labor was thought of in relation to pubic separation, and Soranus actually listed too firm a union at the symphysis as a cause of dystocia. Based on this concept, although faulty, there arose a method of therapy consisting of surgical division of the pelvic brim, which was practiced intermittently by obstetricians for two and one-half centuries, its rationale unimpaired by the ultimate understanding of the unyielding character of the bony girdle.

Artificial spreading of the pubes to expedite delivery of the infant was first suggested in 1592 by Pineau [12] but was not actually carried out until 1655, when de la Courvée [3] performed the operation on a patient who had died in labor. Postmortem division of the symphysis, le Roy showed, permitted the pubic bones to be separated up to 2½ in. The same author later assisted in the first symphysiotomy on a live subject, and the following account is based on his subsequent report.[14]

The patient, Mme. Souchot, was a 30-year-old rachitic dwarf, 3 ft 8 in. tall. Each of her four previous pregnancies had ended in the birth of a dead child following a difficult and traumatic delivery. The diagonal conjugate of her pelvis had been measured at 2½ in. by the distinguished Levret, who saw the patient in consultation during her fourth confinement. Sigault, her obstetrician, in collaboration with le Roy, had decided in advance to deliver Mme. Souchot of her fifth pregnancy with the aid of symphysiotomy, the only alternative to cesarean section if a living child were to be obtained. When labor began, on the afternoon of September 30, 1777, the plan of management had already been carefully formulated. The operation was carried out shortly after midnight, by the light of a candle, and, of course, without anesthesia. The incision over the symphysis deviated somewhat to the left of the midline and went through the crus of the clitoris, part of the labium minus, and into the urethra. After cutting through the soft parts Sigault inserted the index finger of his left hand behind the symphysis and divided the cartilage and ligament from above down. He then separated the pubes 2½ in. and ruptured the membranes, whereupon le Roy carried out breech extraction of a living male child whose biparietal diameter measured 3½ in.

The patient became incontinent of urine immediately after the operation. By the sixteenth postoperative day the upper surface of the symphysis had closed and the lower edge had begun to heal. Mme. Souchot made her first attempt to walk on the forty-sixth day. Two weeks later a special committee that had been appointed by the medical faculty of Paris to report on the case announced that the patient was able to walk with the aid of a cane, sometimes even without one, but her involuntary loss of urine continued. On December 3, 1777, Sigault triumphantly presented Mme. Souchot before the medical faculty, which awarded him and le Roy a special silver medal in recognition of their achievement. Eight years later the patient, still incontinent, could not yet walk without support, her pubic bones remained ununited, her prolapsed uterus and inverted vagina hung out of the pelvis, and a fistulous ulcer persisted on the left side of the vulva.

As a result of the successful confinement of Mme. Souchot, with survival of both mother and child, symphysiotomy soon rose to great favor among Parisian obstetricians; but as increasing experience accentuated its hazards, the operation's popularity began to wane. Infections, hematomas, prolapse of the bladder, and injuries to the urethra, external genitalia, cervix, and sacroiliac joints occurred so frequently that most abandoned it.

Baudelocque was particularly vocal in his condemnation of the procedure, for of the 33 patients on whom it was performed 12 mothers succumbed and only 13 infants survived. In the English abridgment [2] of Baudelocque's textbook, Dewees even deleted symphysiotomy from the author's list of seven methods for dealing with pelvic contraction, dismissing it with the following editorial footnote:

This operation is now so entirely laid aside, that it is not any longer by judicious practitioners considered as a resource of the art. It is but justice to add, that our author has, by demonstrating most satisfactorily its insufficiency for the end proposed, contributed much to the cause of humanity, by bringing this horrible operation into complete disgrace.

Only in Italy did symphysiotomy continue to enjoy any favor. John Whitridge Williams, in the first edition of his *Obstetrics*,[15] published in 1903, expressed the attitude of American obstetricians toward the operation when he wrote: "Personally, at the present time, I do not expect to perform symphyseotomy under any circumstances, and consider that the present enthusiasm for it will eventually disappear."

To obviate the hazards of symphysiotomy Aitken of Edinburgh suggested a modified procedure for enlarging the pelvic brim by dividing the superior ramus of the pubis itself. In the third edition of his *Principles of Midwifery*,[1] published in 1786, he wrote, referring to cesarean section:

In Britain it has never had the desired effect, for all the mothers have died. May not this and embryotomy be superseded by a pelvitomia nova? viz. Two incisions, one on each side, reaching to the ossa pubis, as near the crural vessels as safely may be, so that one may be distant from the other about four inches; and two corresponding to and touching the joinings of the rami pubis and ischiorum. The bones are then divided by the flexible saw, without wounding the peritonaeum, bladder, urethra, or vagina. Thus the segment of the pelvis becomes moveable, and yields to the pressure of the child, so as to allow delivery. If due attention be paid to the wound, may not the healing take place in such sort, that in future sufficient capacity of the pelvis may be preserved?

It is clear that Aitken had not yet resorted to this procedure himself, for in a footnote he added: "I am just now employed in trying the effect of this operation on brutes."

This operation, commonly known as pubiotomy but more properly as hebotomy or hebosteotomy, was taken up later by Champion of Bar le Duc, France, and by Stoltz in Strasbourg, who used a chain saw for the purpose. The chain saw proved generally unsatisfactory, however, for it was cumbersome, hard to sterilize, and broke easily. From Stoltz the idea of a filiform wire saw was imparted to Leonardo Gigli, who proceeded to develop such an instrument for dividing the pubis. The Gigli saw, as it soon came to be known, has long since been abandoned for the original purpose for which it was intended, but remains in use to this day as a standard item of equipment in orthopedic and neurologic surgery.

GIGLI'S DESCRIPTION OF STRING SAW

With the collaboration of Härtel, an instrument maker in Breslau, Gigli embarked on a series of experiments on cadavers, sawing through ribs and mandibles with serrated wires ranging from 0.45 mm to 1 mm in diameter.

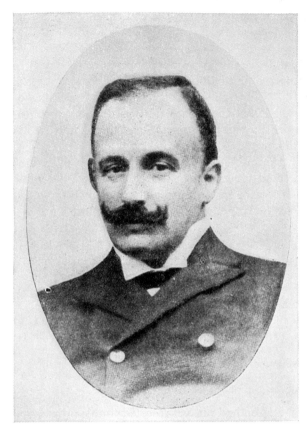

Fig. 60-1. Leonardo Gigli (1863–1908).

His perfected string saw and his recommended technique for the newly revived operation of hebosteotomy were reported in a series of papers [5,6,7] published in 1893 and 1894. Wrote Gigli: [6]

> I thought I could simplify symphysiotomy by means of these wires and make its technique more reliable. An oblique cut through the os pubis, to the right or left of where the head lies . . . is much easier and much more certain than the median incision, because all the dangers of the latter are thereby avoided and its advantages preserved.

The saw finally adopted by Gigli and Härtel was described as follows: [7]

> [It consists of] a single steel wire with a rough surface, its ends attached to two small handles with which the to-and-fro movements are carried out. . . . The wire saw, made in a diameter of 0.65 mm, has smooth end pieces, which have been heated and bent into a curve to correspond with the bone around which they are to be led.

The operation was carried out thus:

The patient is scrupulously cleansed, and the previously shaven mons veneris, the external genitalia, and the vagina disinfected. . . . The patient is placed in the obstetric position, her legs spread apart and held by assistants. The operator, sitting between the patient's legs, incises the soft parts above the pubis, the incision following a slightly curved line, its concavity facing him, and terminating above the subpubic tubercle, at the insertion of the triangular ligament.

The incision may be made through all the tissue layers or we may reflect the skin back first, for by the latter method the lower angle of the wound will be found farther away from the vaginal introitus. Hemostasis is imperative once the soft parts are incised. After introducing two fingers of the left hand into the vagina, laterally and well up behind the pubis, the operator directs a special large needle, mounted on a stout needle holder, behind the middle of the bone, the vaginal hand guiding the needle around its posterior surface. I try, if possible, to pass the needle lateral to the bladder attachment of the pubovesical ligament at the symphysis. In order to accomplish this I direct the needle straight down and try to bring it out at the subpubic tubercle, between the bone and the corpus cavernosus of that side.

We now pass a silk suture along a line . . . parallel to the symphysis and ending below at the subpubic tubercle. Taking hold of the upper end of the suture, we then bring it to the midline by passing it transversely behind the rectus muscle. The suture is now in an oblique position, according to the direction in which the bone is to be sawed, for severing or detaching the intervening soft parts. We are thus sure not to destroy the bladder fibers attached to the symphysis. With the silk suture in position, one end of the metal thread is tied to it and thus drawn into the place of the former. . . . In order to make the operation as similar as possible to the classic method, I incise the upper third of the symphysis exactly in the midline, with scissors or a knife, and draw one end of the string saw into this incision. By dividing the pelvic inlet in this manner, in a broken line, with the objective of opening the superior strait in the midline, the descent of the fetal head is facilitated, for the parietal boss can then impinge between the two separated ends of the pubic bone.

Having thus applied the string saw, we can accomplish the division of the bone with a few strokes, easily and with great safety, as though the bone were not being sawed but cut with a knife. I have done this very rapidly with the string saw many times. . . .

The bones divided in this manner separate promptly. Any remaining ligamentous tissue that inhibits adequate separation can be divided with scissors during a contraction, when the two bones are most widely separated.

Gigli recommended that spontaneous delivery of the infant then be allowed, if possible, with minimal interference. Repair of the soft parts was carried out postpartum. In a separate paper describing his new saw Gigli cautioned: [6]

Although the instrument has now been brought to a stage of complete development, it is still the operator's responsibility to exercise special skill at all stages of the operation and to develop the dexterity necessary for manipulation of the saw. For example, the angle into which the saw is bent must not be smaller than 45° and must be enlarged gradually but as much as possible, especially just before the complete transection of the bone. Also, too vigorous a pull on the saw . . . must be avoided, for it serves no purpose, and the application of too much force may cause the wire to break. Irrigation while sawing is likewise contraindicated, because the saw, having become hot and then being cooled unevenly by the stream of water, can break more easily.

By 1905 Gigli was able to report a series of 100 pubiotomies at the Eleventh Congress of Italian Obstetricians and Gynecologists in Rome. Following a simplification in its technique by Döderlein, the operation enjoyed a wave of increased popularity in Europe and parts of South America. Jellett,[9] Master of the Rotunda in Dublin, even proposed in 1919 that prophylactic pubiotomy be performed in nonpregnant women, for the radical cure of pelvic contraction. "It should never be postponed willingly," he wrote, "to the end of the second stage, but should ideally be carried out independently of pregnancy when its effects are likely to be required."

In the United States, by contrast, pubiotomy never attained a position of great favor. Williams, its staunchest supporter, reported 43 of these operations on 40 women, carried out in his clinic in the Johns Hopkins Hospital up to April, 1915, without a maternal death; but the procedure was abandoned shortly thereafter in favor of cesarean section.

The changing attitude to pubiotomy in the twentieth century is well illustrated by statements in the various editions of Williams' textbook.[15] Mentioning the operation for the first time in the second edition, published in 1909, Williams predicted:

I feel that one may look forward to pubiotomy practically displacing Caesarean section in the so-called "borderline" cases, as it enables one to subject the patient to the test of labour and to operate after several hours of second-stage pains have demonstrated that the head cannot pass through the superior strait.*

In the fourth edition, published in 1922, Williams' enthusiasm for pubiotomy was tempered somewhat and the indications defined more precisely. He now wrote:

In my experience the chief indication for the operation is presented by patients in whom the disproportion appears to be so slight that one feels that spontaneous delivery will probably occur, but in whom the test of several hours of second stage pains has demonstrated that the head cannot be forced through the superior strait. . . . I consider that the ideal indication for pubiotomy is afforded by pronounced grades of funnel pelvis; as in them the operation will not only permit the

* From J. W. Williams, *Obstetrics. A Text-Book for the Use of Students and Practitioners,* 2nd Edition, 1909. Courtesy of Appleton-Century-Crofts, Inc.

delivery of the child, but in all probability will lead to such permanent enlargement of the outlet that spontaneous labor will be possible in the future.*

The death knell for pubiotomy in the United States was finally sounded by Stander in the seventh edition of Williams' book, published in 1936: "With the introduction and development of low cervical cesarean section the operation of hebosteotomy has fallen into disuse in this country. . . . We doubt whether at the present time there is any sound indication for this operation." †
Harper's prediction, published only a few years earlier in his *Clinical Obstetrics*,[8] that pubiotomy "will re-assert itself and its position among valuable operative procedures will be restored," has failed to come true. The obstetrician has bequeathed his Gigli saw to the orthopedist and the neurosurgeon.

GIGLI'S LIFE

Leonardo Gigli was born in Sesto Fiorentino, Italy, April 30, 1863.‡ [10,11,13] He received his medical degree from the University of Florence in 1889; and after a brief apprenticeship in pediatrics under Professor Bajardi he was made assistant to Domenico Chiara in the obstetric and gynecologic clinic. In 1891, following Chiara's death, Gigli went to Paris for further training in the clinics of Tarnier, Pinard, and Budin, and then on to London and finally Breslau, where he studied under Fritsch from 1892 to 1893 and where he developed the idea for his pubiotomy saw. He then returned to Florence, obtaining an appointment on the staff of the Hospital of S. Maria Nuova, of which he was made director in 1899. He never succeeded, however, in his ambition to obtain a teaching position in the University of Florence. Opposed by his Florentine contemporaries, very sensitive to their criticism, and embittered over his failure to win an academic appointment, he resigned from the hospital in 1901 to devote himself exclusively to his private obstetric practice and research. In this same year he was made secretary of the Tuscan Obstetrical and Gynecological Society, a position he held until his death seven years later. Gigli achieved very little recognition during his lifetime among Italian obstetricians, in contrast to the reputation he enjoyed elsewhere, especially in Germany after his triumphant appearance before the 1907 gynecologic congress in Dresden. He died of pneumonia on April 4, 1908. A bibliography of Gigli's writings is appended to Resinelli's obituary of him.[13]

REFERENCES

1. Aitken, J.: *Principles of Midwifery, or Puerperal Medicine,* 3rd ed. J. Murray, London, 1786, p. 83.

* *Ibid.,* 4th Edition, 1922. Courtesy of Appleton-Century-Crofts, Inc.
† *Ibid.,* 7th Edition, 1936. Courtesy of Appleton-Century-Crofts, Inc.
‡ La Torre [11] gives 1866 as Gigli's year of birth.

2. Baudelocque, J. L.: *An Abridgement of Mr. Heath's Translation of Baude-locque's Midwifery. With Notes, by William P. Dewees, M.D.*, 3rd ed. Thomas Desilver, Philadelphia, 1823, p. 516.

3. Courvée, J. C. de la.: *De Nutritione Foetus in Utero Paradoxa.* Förster, Danzig, 1655.

4. Fasbender, H. F.: *Geschichte der Geburtshilfe.* Gustav Fischer, Jena, 1906, pp. 864–73.

5. Gigli, L.: Della sezione della sinfisi con la sega in filo metallico (Drahtsäger). *Ann. ostet. e ginec.,* **15**:557–60, 1893.

6. Gigli, L.: Über ein neues Instrument zum Durchtrennen der Knochen, die Drahtsäge. *Centralbl. f. Chir.,* **21**:409–11, 1894.

7. Gigli, L.: Taglio lateralizzato del pube. Suoi vantaggi—sua tecnica. *Ann. ostet. e ginec.,* **16**:649–67, 1894.

8. Harper, P. T.: *Clinical Obstetrics.* F. A. Davis, Philadelphia, 1930, p. 606.

9. Jellett, H.: The radical cure of pelvic deformity. *Surg., Gynec. & Obst.,* **29**:117–25, 1919.

10. La Torre, F.: Leonardo Gigli. *Clin. ostet.,* **10**:178–83, 1908.

11. La Torre, F.: Nel giorno dell' apoteosi di Leonardo Gigli. *Clin. ostet.,* **14**:121–35, 1912.

12. Pineau, S.: *Oposculum Physiologum, Anatomicum . . . libris duobus distinctum.* Z. Palthenius, Frankfurt, 1599 (first edition: Paris, 1592).

13. Resinelli, G.: Leonardo Gigli. *Ginecologia,* **5**:193–98, 1908.

14. Roy, A. le: *Recherches Historiques et Pratiques sur la Section de la Symphyse du Pubis, Pratiquée, pour Suppléer, à l'Opération Césarienne, le 2 Octobre 1777, sur la Femme Souchot.* Le Clerc, Paris, 1778.

15. Williams, J. W.: *Obstetrics. A Text-Book for the Use of Students and Practitioners.* D. Appleton & Co., New York & London, 1903, pp. 410–15; 2nd ed., 1909, pp. 456–60; 3rd ed., 1916, pp. 464–68; 4th ed., 1922, pp. 493–98; 5th ed., 1927, pp. 518–23; 6th ed., 1930, p. 559; 7th ed. (ed. by H. J. Stander), 1936, pp. 624–27.

Man is sometimes most emphatic about that which he is least able to prove. For more than 100 years obstetricians have been sharply divided in their attitude toward the intrauterine tampon for the arrest of postpartum hemorrhage from the atonic uterus. It is the exceptional practitioner who hesitates either to stoutly uphold the intrauterine pack and testify of its life-saving value, or to denounce it as an ineffective and even dangerous device. Of no other therapeutic measure do obstetricians speak with greater conviction or feeling. Yet no convincing clinical data have been collected to justify either endorsement or rejection of tamponade of the atonic postpartum uterus.

British obstetricians, as a group, have roundly condemned the uterine pack for the control of bleeding. William Smellie,[11] in the mid-eighteenth century, and others even before him, spoke occasionally of the use of vaginal pluggings, made of "dossils of lint" or "fine tow" impregnated with various styptic solutions, in the treatment of hemorrhage associated with abortion; but to combat flooding from the postpartum uterus the British accoucheur has always regarded manual compression of the organ as the more rational, effective, and safer procedure.

In America, by sharp contrast, the pack, in the form of plain gauze, iodoform gauze, or oxidized cellulose, continues to enjoy favor among the profession, and is commonly resorted to when massage and oxytocic drugs fail to stanch the flow of blood from the relaxed postpartum uterus. In a recent questionnaire study [8] of the 50 largest obstetric training centers in the United States, 95 per cent of the 37 responding institutions reported their current use of the intrauterine pack for postpartum hemorrhage; in only two was the pack never employed. For over a century it has successfully withstood the deprecation of some of the most eminent and articulate teachers of the specialty. Charles D. Meigs, for example, wrote in his *Obstetrics,*[10] published in 1849:

Tampon Never.—I repeat the opinion already expressed, that the blood that issues from the placental surface of the womb after delivery at Term, ought to be permitted to flow freely out from the vagina. . . . A very firm clot, shutting the mouth of the womb, may serve as a tampon which shall wholly prevent the escape of blood from the cavity, which expands as it continues to receive the effusion, until the womb becomes fully as large as at the sixth month. Such clots are as dangerous as, but not more so than the artificial tampon, when used after delivery at term. I have never used a tampon after delivery at term; but I have seen them used, which came very near causing the patient to sink, by detaining the effusion within the cavity. The principle is false, and the practice dangerous, which resorts to such a mode of arresting uterine hemorrhage, at term; he who resorts to it, does so under the ignorant presumption that uterine-like chirurgical hemorrhage is to be arrested by coagulation of the outflowing blood.

A few years later Bedford [2] lectured, with even greater ardor, against the evils of the uterine pack:

There is an unfortunate and far too common belief that the great remedy for hemorrhage is the *tampon;* with this conviction, many physicians have recourse to it the moment they are aware that flooding exists. The vagina is immediately plugged up, and in order to make matters doubly sure, a T bandage is employed for the purpose of retaining the tampon *in situ.* With the slightest possible reflection, the absurdity of this practice as a remedial means . . . must be too apparent to need comment, for do you not at once perceive that it can have no effect whatever in producing the only thing that will arrest the bleeding—contraction of the uterus? But, gentlemen, there is something more than absurdity in the application of the tampon in these cases; there is positive danger, which almost always results fatally to the unhappy patient. . . . When the child is delivered, and the tampon resorted to for the purpose of relieving the hemorrhage, the only effect is, by occluding the mouth of the womb, to convert an external into an internal flooding. It is true, the blood ceases to flow through the vagina, and this may afford you momentary consolation, under the erroneous impression that, because there is no longer any external sign of bleeding, therefore, all danger is at an end. Delusive and fatal hope! It will not, however, be long that you will be permitted to indulge in this fiction, for the evidences of exhaustion will be fast accumulating; the strength of the patient becomes more and more dilapidated, and you will soon be brought to a full, but melancholy appreciation of your folly, by seeing her sink at the very time you imagined you were rendering a most essential service! My advice to you is—*never resort to the tampon as a means of checking hemorrhage*

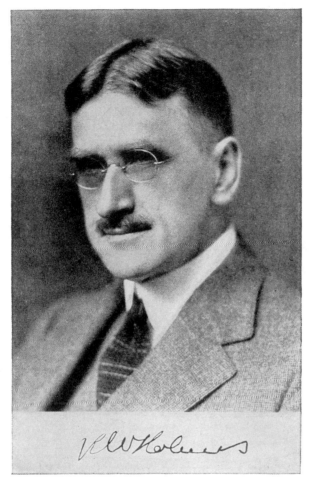

Fig. 61-1. Rudolph Wieser Holmes (1870–1953).

after the birth of the child, for the reason that it exercises no possible good in accomplishing the important object in view—the contraction of the uterus—but, on the contrary, its direct and necessary tendency is to convert an external into an internal hemorrhage, thus lulling the practitioner into false hope, and insidiously, but most certainly, destroying the patient; for . . . whether the flooding be internal or external, if it be not checked, the tendency is the same—death.

Leroux, generally credited with introducing the tampon into obstetric practice in France in 1776, filled the vagina with linen or tow previously saturated with vinegar, in order to make the blood coagulate more quickly. He subsequently reported a number of cases of severe hemorrhage resulting from uterine atony, in which his tampon allegedly saved the patient from almost certain death. Tarnier,[3] commenting years later on the claims of his country-man, remarked: "It often happens that men, even those who are otherwise worthy of credence, are often more successful with remedies of their own invention than any one else. In fact, the only effect of the tampon in many cases is to convert an external into an internal discharge."

Packing for the control of postpartum hemorrhage received great impetus in 1887, as a result of a paper by Dührssen.[7] Previously employed techniques had been rather haphazard, with little attention to methodical tamponade of the fundus. Dührssen grasped the cervical lips with tenaculum forceps, and with his left hand in the lower uterine segment as a guide, fed iodoform gauze into place with a dressing forceps in his right hand. Dührssen's method and its subsequent modifications suffered, however, from three major disadvantages: (1) the gauze, rubbing against the vulva and vagina, carried bacteria into the uterine cavity; (2) the repeated introduction of the dressing forceps was traumatic, frequently producing lacerations of the vagina and occasionally even perforation of the uterus; (3) insertion of the packing was difficult and dangerous when the cervix was contracted.

HOLMES'S DESCRIPTION OF UTERINE PACKER

To circumvent these difficulties, Rudolph Holmes [9] introduced a tamponade instrument (Fig. 61-2) in 1902, which further enhanced the popularity of the

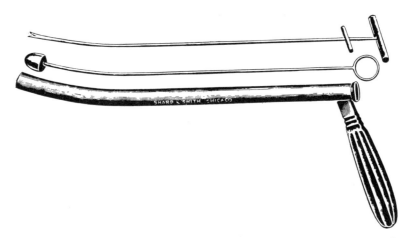

Fig. 61-2. Holmes's uterine packer, as illustrated in his paper of 1902.[9]

uterine pack in the United States. Wrote Holmes:

The Instrument comes in three parts—the tube, the obturator, and the introducer. The tube has a length of twenty-eight centimetres and a calibre of eighteen millimetres. On the proximal end is a handle similar to that on Kelly's graduated urethral speculum. There is a pelvic curve of five centimetres; this curve is in the distal half of the tube, and its measure is taken from the centre of the lumen at the distal end to the prolongation of the line coincident to the external lower surface of the straight portion of the tube; a greater curve than this prevents a proper working of the introducer. The obturator has a conical shape and accurately fits the distal opening; its use is merely to facilitate the introduction of the tube. The introducer is a strong, highly tempered steel rod with three sharp prongs on its distal end (the clefts between the prongs must be so rounded that by no chance may the gauze be caught); near the proximal end is a small cross-bar at such a distance from the prongs as to prevent their appearance beyond the distal end of the tube; some six centimetres further is the handle; the rod should be at least No. 12 French scale.

Holmes explained the use of the instrument:

The tube, with obturator in place, is pushed up to the fundus uteri, guided by the left hand introduced into the lower uterine segment. The obturator is removed without withdrawing the hand from the vagina. An assistant brings the jar of properly prepared gauze within an inch or two of the proximal end of the tube; the end of the gauze is picked up with a forceps and pushed into the tube a short distance—i.e. two inches; then the introducer is pushed home, carrying the gauze with it; rapidly withdrawing the introducer an inch, or at most two inches, again it is pushed home, repeating the maneuvre until the uterus and vagina are full. It is a useful expedient while packing to gently oscillate the distal end of the tube from side to side to throw the gauze in folds across the cavity. Two facts must be kept in mind: one, that if the introducer is withdrawn too much the gauze will be packed into the tube, thus preventing further working of the instrument, or at least hindering the progress of the gauze; second, the gauze must be of proper size, and so "felted" in the container that it feeds out easily—under no circumstances must the gauze be rolled in the jar. . . . The most convenient gauze for tamponing by the introducer . . . is a strip one-half yard wide and nearly twelve yards long; this gauze is folded into a strip about two inches wide. In cases of extreme atony full twelve yards may be introduced into the utero-vaginal tract; in other cases the amount will depend on the laxity of the uterus and roominess of the vagina.

HOLMES'S LIFE

Rudolph Wieser Holmes was born in Chicago, Illinois, June 27, 1870.[1,5] He attended Harvard College from 1888 to 1890, and then Rush Medical College, from which he graduated in 1893. After an internship in the Presbyterian Hospital of Chicago, he joined the faculty of his alma mater, where he rose from instructor to professor emeritus of obstetrics and gynecology. He also served on the medical faculties of the University of Illinois and Northwestern University. In 1924 he was elected chairman of the Section on Obstetrics, Gynecology, and Abdominal Surgery of the American Medical Association, and the following year was made a member of the Advisory Committee of the U.S. Department of Labor's Bureau of Child Welfare. A fellow of the American Gynecological Society, he also served at various times as president of the Chicago Gynecological Society and of the Central Association of Obstetricians and Gynecologists, and as a director of the American Committee on Maternal Welfare. Holmes died in Charlottesville, Virginia, April 25, 1953, at the age of 82.

MODERN ATTITUDE TOWARD UTERINE TAMPONADE

John Whitridge Williams, the principal standard-bearer of American obstetrics during the first three decades of the twentieth century, endorsed uterine tamponade in every edition of his textbook [12] whose publication he oversaw. He wrote:

Whenever there is persistent loss of blood following the third stage of labour, which does not yield to the ordinary methods of treatment, this procedure offers a most efficient method of controlling it, as the pack not only exerts pressure upon the bleeding vessels but mechanically stimulates the uterus to renewed contraction.*

In the fifth edition of his *Obstetrics,* published in 1927, Williams took note of the Holmes packer; and the sixth (1930), seventh (1936), eighth (1941), and ninth (1945) editions, the last three edited by H. J. Stander, warmly endorsed it: "We have employed this instrument . . . with great satisfaction and believe that it should always form part of the equipment of an obstetrical operating room." †

The rumblings of dissent are now being heard again, however. In an editorial entitled "The Passing of the Pack," published in 1955, Douglass [6] stated:

Times change and medicine moves ahead. And as advances occur it is inevitable that drugs, operations and procedures which at one time were accepted as being highly efficacious should be found wanting and should be discarded. . . . The intrauterine pack for the control of postpartum hemorrhage . . . was a method much in use until 10 or 15 years ago simply because there was no better way known to combat the condition. Today the situation is quite different. No longer do we have to depend upon the uncertain fluid extract of ergot, which constantly varied in its oxytocic property, and could only be given by mouth. In its place we have the active oxytocic principle of ergot, ergonovine, and the oxytocic factor of the posterior pituitary gland. . . . The action of these 2 drugs upon the uterus is so constant that we can almost say they "never" fail to cause uterine contraction.

* From J. W. Williams, *Obstetrics. A Text-Book for the Use of Students and Practitioners,* 1st Edition, 1909. Courtesy of Appleton-Century-Crofts, Inc.

† *Ibid.,* 6th–9th Editions, 1930, 1936, 1941, 1945. Courtesy of Appleton-Century-Crofts, Inc.

Douglass also noted that the intrauterine pack had been used unsuccessfully in each of the ten fatal cases of postpartum hemorrhage in Maryland during a recent two-year period; whereas no deaths occurred from this cause during the same two years in three of Baltimore's largest obstetric clinics, where the pack is practically never used.

Among the most outspoken of the modern American critics of uterine tamponade is Samuel Cosgrove,[4] who wrote in 1936:

It seems to me entirely unphysiological. Up to this time all effort has been made completely to empty the uterus in order to permit it to contract down, and by its contraction to squeeze shut the bleeding sinuses and permit their occlusion by clots formed in the mouths thereof. Now, to reverse this physiological effort to empty the uterus, and proceed to introduce a large mass of foreign material with the avowed purpose of stimulating the uterus to contract and of controlling bleeding by direct pressure of the foreign mass against the sinuses, necessarily mechanically held wide open by the pressure of that mass, does not seem to me good sense. . . . If the uterus is so truly atonic as not to be capable of response to the mechanical stimulation of manual control . . . and powerfully acting oxytocics, one can hardly expect that it will be capable of responding to the less efficient irritation of a wad of gauze pushed into it. If it does not so contract, it will merely balloon more and more as blood accumulates above the pack, and the supposed function of direct pressure of the packing against the whole surface of the uterus will be nullified. In this way the packing may do little more than stop the obvious flow of blood escaping from the uterus and lull the operator into a false sense of security.

How reminiscent are the words of Cosgrove and Douglass of those written by Meigs and Bedford a century earlier! Condemnation of uterine tamponade has come full circle, but the operation remains in use nonetheless, and the Holmes packer still sees occasional service.

REFERENCES

1. *American Gynecological Society Album of Fellows, 1876–1930.* Ed. by F. E. Keene. Dornan, Philadelphia, 1930, pp. 292–93.
2. Bedford, G. S.: *The Principles and Practice of Obstetrics,* 5th ed. William Wood & Co., New York, 1871, p. 393.
3. Cazeaux, P.: *A Theoretical and Practical Treatise on Midwifery, Including the Diseases of Pregnancy and Parturition.* Revised and annotated by S. Tarnier. 5th American ed. from 7th French ed. (ed. by W. R. Bullock). Lindsay & Blakiston, Philadelphia, 1873, p. 891.
4. Cosgrove, S. A.: Obstetrical hemorrhage and its management. *South. M.J.,* **29**:1219–25, 1936.
5. Deaths. Holmes, Rudolph Wieser. *J.A.M.A.,* **152**:255, 1953.
6. Douglass, L. H.: The passing of the pack. *Bull. School Med. Univ. Maryland,* **40**:38–39, 1955.

7. Dührssen, A.: Die Uterustamponade mit Jodoformgaze bei Atonie des Uterus nach normaler Geburt. *Centralbl. f. Gynäk.* **11**:553–59, 1887.

8. Fisher, J. J.: Present status of the intrauterine pack in postpartum hemorrhage. *J. Florida M. A.,* **41**:634–36, 1955.

9. Holmes, R. W.: A new method of tamponing the uterus post partum. *Am. J. Obst. & Gynec.,* **45**:245–50, 1902.

10. Meigs, C. D.: *Obstetrics: The Science and the Art.* Lea & Blanchard, Philadelphia, 1849, pp. 309–10.

11. Smellie, W.: *Smellie's Treatise on the Theory and Practice of Midwifery.* Ed. by A. H. McClintock. New Sydenham Society, London, 1876, Vol. I, p. 168.

12. Williams, J. W.: *Obstetrics. A Text-Book for the Use of Students and Practitioners.* D. Appleton & Co., New York & London, 1903, p. 432; 5th ed., 1927, p. 542; 6th ed., 1930, p. 581; 7th ed. (ed. by H. J. Stander), 1936, pp. 642–43; 8th ed., 1941, pp. 1245–46; 9th ed., 1945, p. 1126.

Hugh Lenox Hodge and His Vaginal Pessary

"The hysterical passion is of so ill fame among the Diseases belonging to Women, that like one half damn'd, it bears the faults of many other Distempers: For when at any time a sickness happens in a Womans Body, of an unusual manner, or more occult original, so that its cause lies hid, and the Curatory indication is altogether uncertain, presently we accuse the evil influence of the Womb (which for the most part is innocent) and in every unusual symptom, we declare it to be something Hysterical, and so to this scope, which oftentimes is only the subterfuge of ignorance, the medical intentions and use of Remedies are directed." Thus wrote Thomas Willis [10] in the seventeenth century, more than 200 years ahead of his time.

Gynecologic faddism enjoyed its heyday throughout most of the nineteenth century. During its early decades most of the ills of womankind were attributed to inflammation of the uterus, but toward the middle years these views were supplanted by the Galenic doctrine that displacements of that organ are the principal source of female complaints. Illnesses of all sorts were interpreted as "uterine sympathies," to be treated gynecologically; but therapy, fortunately, was usually limited to nonsurgical measures. From 1848 to 1851, for example, not a single gynecologic operation was performed at the New York Hospital. The pessary school of gynecology began to flourish. Indeed, it has been said that fortunes were to be made by two groups of gynecologists of that day: those who inserted pessaries, and those who removed them.

541

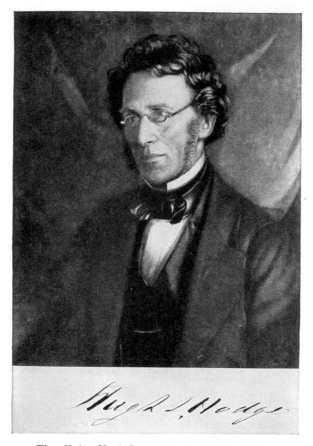

Fig. 62-1. Hugh Lenox Hodge (1796–1873).

HODGE'S DEVELOPMENT OF A VAGINAL PESSARY

Hugh Hodge spoke for a large segment of the profession when he stated in 1860: [4]

. . . The mechanical treatment of uterine displacements by intra-vaginal supports is essential, a "sine qua non," for their perfect relief; that by pessaries, of suitable material, size, and form, the uterus may very generally be replaced and be maintained in situ; that the local symptoms of weight, pain, etc., the leucorrhoea, the menorrhagia, the dysmenorrhoea, and all the innumerable direct and indirect symptoms of spinal and cerebral irritation, including neuralgia, nervous headache, nervous affections of the larynx, lungs, heart, stomach, bowels, etc., as also spasms, cramps, and convulsions, may often thus be dissipated; that the intellectual and spiritual being may be elevated from the lowest states of depression, bordering on melancholy, or be delivered from the highest degree of maniacal excitement; and that the whole economy may thus be revolutionized.

Patients often are amazed at their own altered sensations; they can hardly realize their identity—feeling as if they were either renovated, or that they had been transported to a "new world." . . .

The important declaration may be safely made that pessaries can be worn for many months, not merely with impunity, but with great advantage, keeping the organ in its natural position, relieving the symptoms of displaced and irritable uterus, the terrible irritations of the cerebro-spinal system, and allowing the bedridden and nervous patient to exert again her powers of locomotion and resume the duties of her social position, without any local disturbance or uneasiness. She finds herself relieved without being conscious of the presence of the agent by which she is benefited. A vaginal injection of pure water every day is almost the only attention required. I am abundantly satisfied that these bright hopes may be realized by the scientific employment of suitable pessaries. The difficulties may be great, and the means of success perhaps imperfect; but there is no doubt in the author's mind that proper indications can be established, and that human ingenuity, in unison with skill and patient perseverance, will insure a success which, to the minds of many, may now be deemed Utopian.

The vaginal pessary is among the oldest of all medical instruments; no one knows precisely when the first models were invented.[6] Indeed, what could have been more natural to the ancient midwife than that she shove something into the patient's vagina in an attempt to support a prolapsing womb? Over the years countless pessaries had been designed, fabricated in many shapes and sizes and of a variety of materials, including wood, leather, glass, and metal. None proved entirely satisfactory. Hodge listed the following requirements:

A pessary should be made of incorruptible materials. It should restore and maintain the uterus in its normal position at all times, under the ever-varying pressure from above. It should be movable with the uterus, allowing the natural motions of this organ, yet effectually preventing any displacement. It should be one with the uterus. It should be worn without pain, uneasiness, or discomfort, indeed, without any consciousness on the part of the patient. It should relieve, and not increase, nervous irritations. It should excite no organic or vascular disturbance, no engorgement, no inflammation; and therefore, it should be influential, not in increasing leucorrhoeal and menorrhagic discharges, but . . . in contributing to the resolution of chronic inflammations of the os and cervix uteri.

Vulcanization of rubber proved an ineffable boon to the purveyors and wearers of pessaries, greatly enhancing their popularity. Hodge enthused over the "new preparation of caoutchouc, brought into use and patented by Goodyear." He wrote:

It is commonly termed *"hard India-rubber"* or "hard vulcanite," and . . . is represented as being incapable of decomposition, and able to resist the action of

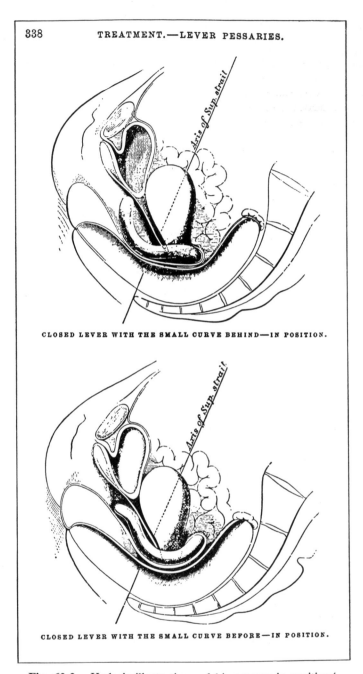

CLOSED LEVER WITH THE SMALL CURVE BEHIND—IN POSITION.

CLOSED LEVER WITH THE SMALL CURVE BEFORE—IN POSITION.

Fig. 62-2. Hodge's illustrations of his pessary in position.[4]

concentrated acids and the most powerful chemical reagents. The experiments that I have made with this article for pessaries have been very favorable; no perceptible change has been manifested in the integrity of the ring after being worn for twelve to fifteen months, even in cases where leucorrhoea existed. The smooth, polished surface has not been disturbed by any deposits, which not infrequently are observed even on gold pessaries. It promises, therefore, to be a cheap and excellent material for such agents.

But Hodge remained dissatisfied with the shapes of the existing pessaries and set out to design a new one. Countless hours of contemplation and many experiments had proved fruitless, when he came upon the idea for his lever model, soon referred to as the consummate in vaginal pessaries. The inspiration for Hodge's invention was later recounted by Richard Penrose,[7] who had been quizmaster under Hodge at the University of Pennsylvania. Recalled Penrose:

One evening while sitting alone in the room where the meetings of the medical faculty of the University were held, his eyes rested on the upright steel support by the fireplace, designed to hold the shovel and tongs; the shovel and tongs were kept in position by a steel hook, and, as he surveyed the supporting curve of this hook, the long-looked for illumination came; the shape, apparently so paradoxical, revealed itself in the glowing light and flickering flame of the burning grate, and the Hodge lever pessary was the result.

The lever pessary was designed especially for cases of uterine retroversion. As Hodge saw it: [4]

The important modification consists in making a ring oblong, instead of circular, and curved so as to correspond to the curvature of the vagina. Great advantages result from this form; the convexity of the curve being in contact with the posterior wall of the vagina, corresponds, with more or less accuracy, to the curve of the rectum, perineum, and sacrum. Hence, when properly arranged, there is no pressure against the rectum; and the higher the instrument rises, the superior extremity, instead of impinging against the rectum, passes upwards and behind the uterus—between this organ and the intestine—giving . . . a proper position to the womb, and yet allowing its natural pendulum-like motion to remain unrestrained.

Hodge soon added an additional curve to his new pessary:

The *double-curved closed lever* [as he referred to it] is equally advantageous, and is preferable, as being less liable to press injuriously on the bladder or urethra. . . . Its curves may be named the greater and the less; the former may be regarded as perfectly similar to that of the open pessary, but the other extremity is slightly bent in the opposite direction, so that when the instrument is viewed laterally its curves resemble somewhat those of the letter S. . . .

In most cases at the commencement of the treatment, especially when there is a rigid and short vagina, and the uterus not very movable, *the extremity with the small curve* should be placed under the uterus, with its convexity towards the posterior surface of the retroverted uterus, and its concavity towards the rectum; the concavity of the greater curvature will be in front towards the uterus, and the convexity towards the perineum. Then the index-finger, pressing on the lower portion of the pessary, should cause the instrument to glide slowly between the rectum and the uterus; and afterwards, by depressing the lower extremity towards the perineum and rectum, the fundus and body will be raised. . . . The advantage in this case is, that the convexity of the small curve presents a broader surface towards the irritable tissue of the uterus, and is therefore less likely to give pain; on the contrary, however, rather more pressure is made towards the sacrum, which may occasionally be an inconvenience.

After some days or weeks, when the uterus has yielded to this pressure, the pessary may be turned around in the vagina, so that the *concavity of the large curve* shall be towards the uterus behind, and the convexity of the small curve in front of the uterus and under the bladder. It now acts much more powerfully as a lever, and care must be taken that it does not press too firmly against the uterus behind.

Hodge's instructions for inserting the instrument were detailed and clear:

The pessary is to be held obliquely, say with the small curve to the orifice of the vagina, its convexity towards the pubis and concavity towards the perineum. It should be passed with one edge to the left of the urethra, the opposite edge being to the right of the perineal raphé. The whole instrument must be held so that the extremity may enter perpendicularly to the opening of the vagina. By firm pressure downwards against the perineum, the pessary enters the vagina; but the upper extremity, instead of passing under the uterus, necessarily, owing to the large curve, rises up in front of the organ and against the bladder. Pressure, often quite painful, is for the time made on the neck of the uterus; the practitioner, therefore, hastens to introduce his finger through the opening of the pessary, and to press down the upper extremity under the uterus as soon as possible, thus affording immediate relief to the pain. When the large curve is to be introduced first, the whole operation should be conducted in a similar manner.

Comparing his invention with intrauterine pessaries, Hodge concluded:

The lever pessary will more slowly accomplish the restoration of the displaced organ, but eventually, with equal certainty. It does not necessarily produce any irritation, organic or nervous, or any leucorrhoea, menorrhagia, inflammation, &c. It can be worn at all times, night and day; it interferes with no motion, and no function; the patient has no attentions to pay to it, excepting a daily vaginal wash; she may, and often does forget its presence, can enjoy her connubial pleasures, can move about in society without anxiety, is free from local and general nervous irritations, from corporeal, intellectual, and spiritual disturbance; and her physician may hope, that the uterus being perfectly sustained, the ligaments, now free from every counteracting influence, will continue to contract to their normal length, and acquire their original tonicity, so that a permanent cure may be effected, or that pregnancy ensuing, the continued use of the pessary will preserve his patient from those irritations so frequently excited by displacements, and so apt to result in abortions.

Albert Smith of Philadelphia later narrowed the front end of the Hodge pessary and widened the posterior limb; and T. Gaillard Thomas and Paul F. Mundé of New York subsequently added minor modifications of their own. Indeed, it has been said that in the spate of enthusiasm for pessaries that followed Hodge's invention every gynecologist felt himself called upon to devise a pessary of his own or to modify someone's else. However, this new fashion in gynecology was not without its critics, exemplified by W. D. Buck, president of the New Hampshire State Medical Society, who commented in 1866:[1]

When Dupuytren's operation for relaxation of the *sphincter ani* was in vogue, every young man who came from Paris found every other individual's anus too large, and proceeded to pucker it up. The result was that New York anuses looked like gimlet-holes in a piece of pork. It seems to me that just such a raid is being made upon the uterus at this time. . . . Had Dame Nature foreseen this, she would have made it iron-clad. . . . The *Transactions* of the National Medical Association for 1864 has figured one hundred and twenty-three different kinds of pessaries, embracing every variety, from a simple plug to a patent threshing machine, which can only be worn with the largest hoops. They look like the drawings of turbine water-wheels, or a leaf from a work on entomology. Pessaries, I suppose, are sometimes useful, but there are more than there is any necessity for. I do think that this filling the vagina with such traps, making a Chinese toy-shop of it, is outrageous.

HODGE'S LIFE

Hugh Lenox Hodge was born in Philadelphia, June 27, 1796.[2, 5, 7, 8] His father, who had been an army surgeon during the Revolution and one of the first teachers of anatomy in America, died in the yellow fever epidemic the year after Hugh's birth. After a preliminary education in Philadelphia and in boarding schools in Summerville, Pennsylvania, and New Brunswick, New Jersey, young Hodge entered the College of New Jersey, now known as Princeton University, graduating in 1814; four years later, at the age of 22, he received his medical degree from the University of Pennsylvania. A voyage to India followed, Hodge sailing aboard the "Julius Caesar" in the capacity of ship's surgeon. He entered private practice after returning to Philadelphia, and was promptly appointed to the staffs of the Southern Dispensary and the Philadelphia Dispensary. In 1823 he was named a lecturer in surgery in Nathaniel Chapman's summer school. Hodge's clientele grew very slowly, and it is said that 15 years passed before he could afford a horse and carriage. But when his practice did at last begin to flourish he became plagued by failing vision, which ultimately required the abandonment of his surgical work. It was only at this stage of his career that he began to concentrate on obstetrics. Recognition came fast in his newly chosen specialty. In 1832 he was put in charge of obstetrics at the ill-fated Pennsylvania Hospital, whose doors were later closed because of an outbreak of puerperal fever; and in 1835, victor in his contest with Charles D. Meigs, he returned to the University of Pennsylvania as professor of obstetrics and diseases of women and children, succeeding Dewees. In the role of professor, Hodge was most impressive, with his spare physique, sepulchral voice, and gold spectacles perched on his long nose. One of his students said that when Hodge entered the lecture hall one might have expected him to begin with the words: "Let us pray."

Hodge's first major literary effort, his *Diseases Peculiar to Women,*[4] published in 1860, dealt at great length with displacements of the uterus and their correction by means of pessaries. Far surpassing this work in value was his *Principles and Practice of Obstetrics,* published in 1864. All the more amazing because it was written from memory, John Whitridge Williams,[9] as late as 1903, referred to it as "a model of scrupulous observation . . . the most original work that had appeared in America and, with few modifications, still retaining its value." In it Hodge clearly described the pelvic types and the mechanism of labor, directed attention to the inadequacy of external pelvimetry, urged more frequent resort to the forceps in cases of dystocia, and introduced a placental forceps for the completion of incomplete abortion. This volume, one of the classics of American obstetrics, has become quite scarce through the attrition of use, attested by the worn pages of the present writer's treasured copy.

Like his Philadelphia contemporary, Charles D. Meigs, Hodge opposed the use of anesthesia in obstetrics and was critical of Oliver Wendell Holmes's views of the contagious character of puerperal fever. In contrast to Meigs, however, Hodge voiced his disagreement with greater restraint and dignity. Concerning the newly expressed doctrine of Holmes, Hodge wrote in 1852:[3]

It has been asserted, not only by unprofessional individuals, but even by medical men, that the obstetrician may become the minister of evil rather than of good: that he may actually, in the practice of his self-denying and anxious vocation, occasionally convey from one patient to another a terrible poison—by which disease, too often fatal in its tendencies, may be excited. That this is especially true, as regards puerperal, or childbed fever, the terror of the parturient female, and of her friends and physician. The mere announcement of such an opinion must strike every one of you with horror, and might induce you, at once to abandon a pursuit fraught with such danger and involving such terrible responsibilities; for what rewards can possibly compensate the obstetrician, who has reason to believe that he has actually poisoned even one of those valued and lovely beings who rested confidently and implicitly on him for safety and deliverance?

By 1850 Hodge's vision had deteriorated to such a degree that he could scarcely read. His lectures had to be given from memory, and he began to dictate rather than write his material for publication. Finally, in 1863, he resigned his professorship and, with the assistance of one of his seven sons, devoted himself to the completion of his textbook of obstetrics. Ten years later, on February 23, 1873, he died suddenly of a heart attack, at the age of 76.

REFERENCES

1. Buck, W. D.: A raid on the uterus. (Extract from an address by the president of the New Hampshire State Medical Society.) *New York M. J.,* **5**:464–65, 1867.

2. Cato: Sketches of eminent living physicians. Hugh L. Hodge, M.D., Prof. of Obstetrics and Diseases of Women and Children in the University of Pennsylvania. *Boston M. & S. J.,* **40**:518–20, 1849.

3. Hodge, H. L.: *On the Non-contagious Character of Puerperal Fever: An Introductory Lecture.* T. K. & P. G. Collins, Philadelphia, 1852.

4. Hodge, H. L.: *On Diseases Peculiar to Women, Including Displacements of the Uterus.* Blanchard & Lea, Philadelphia, 1860, pp. 302–50.

5. Kelly, H. A., and Burrage, W. L.: *American Medical Biographies.* Norman, Remington Co., Baltimore, 1920, p. 535.

6. Kelly, H. A., and Fricke, R. E.: The use of pessaries. *Therap. Gaz.,* **45**:5–9, 1921.

7. Penrose, R. A. F.: *A Discourse Commemorative of the Life and Character of Hugh L. Hodge, M.D., LL.D.* Collins, Philadelphia, 1873.

8. Thoms, H.: Hugh Lenox Hodge. A master mind in obstetrical science. *Am. J. Obst. & Gynec.,* **33**:886–92, 1937.

9. Williams, J. W.: Die Geburtshülfe in Amerika. In Dohrn, R.: *Geschichte der Geburtshülfe der Neuzeit.* Part 1 (1840–1860). Franz Pietzcker, Tübingen, 1903, pp. 193–267.

10. Willis, T.: *An Essay of the Pathology of the Brain and Nervous Shock: In which Convulsive Diseases are Treated of.* Translated from Latin into English by S. P. T. Dring, J. Leigh, & C. Harper, London, 1684, p. 69.

Operations and Therapeutic Procedures

PART IX

·

One of the cardinal requirements for the vaginal delivery of a viable infant is complete dilatation of the cervix. Attempts at delivery through an incompletely dilated os are hazardous to both mother and child and absolutely contraindicated in modern obstetric practice. When, for whatever reason, delivery of the infant becomes urgent before the stage of full cervical dilatation is reached, recourse must be had to either cesarean section or dilatation of the cervix by artificial means. Surgical incisions of the cervical rim for the latter purpose, or hysterostomatomy, are referred to more often by their eponymic designation, Dührssen's incisions. This procedure, like a number of other obstetric operations, has waned in popularity as the indications for and safety of cesarean section have increased. In modern practice Dührssen's incisions are seldom performed; yet many obstetricians still regard them occasionally as the method of choice, and nearly every large obstetric service lists several such operations every year.

The first reference to hysterostomatomy in the management of dystocia was in 1755 by Andreas Lindemann,[4] who recommended this operation to overcome a rigid, unyielding cervix, in preference to the more formidable operation of cesarean section with its then prohibitive maternal mortality. The value of cervical incisions remained overlooked, however, for more than a hundred years. In 1883 the procedure was employed again by A. Martin and reported by von Rabenau.[5] The patient had suffered earlier from typhus, as a result of which gangrene of the cervix developed and the portio sloughed away. When the healed external os failed to dilate in labor von Rabenau

553

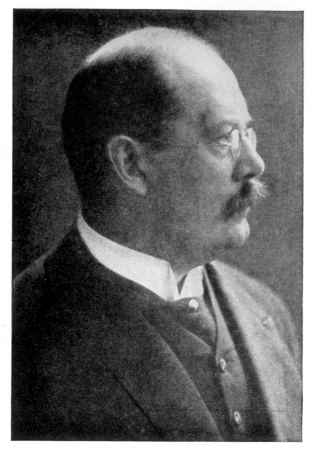

Fig. 63-1. Alfred Dührssen (1862–1933). (Reproduced from *Zentralbl. f. Gynäk.,* 58:145, 1934.)

summoned Martin, who had attended the patient previously. Martin incised the cervix and completed the delivery, but with great loss of blood.

Cervical incision during labor was soon adopted by others, and within the next few years communications on the subject were made by Skutsch,[6] Knoch,[3] and Wulsten,[8] culminating in 1890 in Dührssen's papers.[1,2] The last gained for hysterostomatomy an established place among the standard operations of obstetrics, and for their author the reward of eponymy.

DÜHRSSEN'S TECHNIQUE OF CERVICAL INCISION

Dührssen distinguished sharply between primigravidas and multiparas in their suitability for hysterostomatomy. He wrote: [1]

Enlargement of the external os by incision is indicated only in cases where the entire supravaginal part of the cervix is already dilated, as well as the internal os. For if this upper part of the uterus is not yet completely dilated, the obstruction to the progress of labor lies at this level and the external os does not even come into consideration. It therefore follows that the incisions are indicated almost exclusively in primigravidas, for in them the supravaginal part of the cervix is often dilated already as a result of the Braxton Hicks contractions, indeed always so from the first labor pains. . . . Thus while in primigravidas the lacking or deficient dilatation is limited to the portio vaginalis, faulty dilatation in multiparas always involves the supravaginal part more. As soon as this is fully dilated the external os and surrounding tissues offer no more resistance. To achieve sufficient dilatation for the passage of the head, one would have to carry out incisions into the supravaginal part of the cervix, not only through the internal os but through the lower uterine segment and surrounding pelvic tissues also. Such incisions are not possible. Therefore, the incisions are usually contraindicated in multiparas.

Modern obstetricians still insist on complete effacement of the cervix as a prerequisite for Dührssen's incisions, but no longer draw this sharp distinction based on the patient's parity.

Today's practice continues to follow Dührssen's advice with respect to the extent of the cervical incisions, but their number and placement have undergone gradual change. Standard procedure now calls for three incisions, corresponding in position to the numbers 10, 2, and 6 on the face of a clock. Counseled Dührssen: [1]

If one wishes to undertake delivery in a case of incomplete dilatation of the external os and to save the infant also, then all resistance must be made to disappear from the sides of the cervical rim. This can only result from incisions that extend to the vaginal attachment, and indeed four of them: two laterally, one anteriorly, and one posteriorly. The cervical rim is thus divided into four triangles, which merge with the vaginal wall as the presenting part descends. Only in this way is the barrier separating the uterus from the vagina removed and the lower uterine segment and vagina converted into a "passageway."

Dührssen's reports were based on his experience in 12 cases. He himself did not employ four incisions in every case, however; he sometimes used only two or three, while in one case, of a patient with eclampsia, he made six. Some of his indications, such as contracted pelvis and placenta previa, would now be considered absolute contraindications to hysterostomatomy.

In describing his technique Dührssen wrote: [1]

I never used a speculum. I cut while holding the cervical rim between the index and middle fingers of my left hand, using the ordinary Siebold scissors. The objective can be achieved in this manner if the rim is very firm, unyielding, and therefore not easily displaced. If the rim is flexible and soft, on the other hand, it is impossible to extend the incision to the vaginal attachment. It is then pushed back upward; it is impossible to grasp it with the fingers, for the cervix seems to have slipped away. In one of such cases I applied the forceps without making any incisions. Extraction, however, proved impossible, for the rim that had seemed flexible at first now encircled the head like an iron ring. I therefore fixed the rim by means of two bullet-forceps at the place of the appropriate incision, first on the left; and after introducing two fingers I was able to cut through the taut rim to the vaginal attachment with ease. I generally prefer this procedure as the one of choice, for it facilitates the incision in every case.

Obstetricians today would take issue with Dührssen's view that "repair of the incisions in the cervix is unnecessary for the control of bleeding, and I doubt whether healing occurs more often with suturing than without. . . ." Careful coaptation of the wound edges postpartum is now regarded as a cardinal part of the operation.

Although hysterostomatomy was performed almost a century and a half before Dührssen, and although the indications for and technique of the operation have undergone marked changes since his description of it, the procedure continues to be associated with the name of Dührssen because of the impetus he gave to its popularization and incorporation into obstetric practice.

DÜHRSSEN'S LIFE

Alfred Dührssen was born on March 23, 1862, in Heide, Germany, the eldest of six children.[7] His father and grandfather had been physicians before him; but the former suffered poor health, and Alfred, therefore, spent his early years accompanying him on trips to country resorts and spas. After completing his education in Marburg and Berlin, Dührssen embarked on his medical career in Königsberg under his uncle, Professor Dohrn. In 1886 he was appointed assistant to Gusserow at the Charité-Frauenklinik, and shortly thereafter was put in charge of a large school for midwives, receiving the title of professor in 1895. He later established a Frauenklinik of his own in Berlin. Dührssen's earliest scientific work was on the use of iodoform gauze for packing the uterus in the treatment of postpartum hemorrhage, a procedure still employed by many obstetricians. Prior to his papers on hysterostomatomy in 1890, faulty dilatation of the cervix in labor had been treated by a variety of ineffective or hazardous methods, including hot enemas, electrical stimulation of the nipples, bags, bougies, manual dilatation, and special instruments for stretching the os. Dührssen's incisions comprised a significant addition to existing techniques.

Dührssen became one of the leading advocates of the vaginal approach for all varieties of obstetric and gynecologic surgery. He introduced vaginal cesarean section and published a monograph on the subject, *Der vaginale Kaiserschnitt,* in 1896, but this operation failed to achieve widespread acceptance. The following year he presented a report, together with A. Martin, on 200 pelvic operations for adnexal disease, all by the vaginal route. His monograph, *Die Einschränkung des Bauchschnitts durch die vaginale Laparotomie (Kolpocoeliotomia anterior),* published in 1899, described his vaginal operations for multiple myomectomy, plastic reconstruction of the double uterus, salpingectomy for tubal pregnancy, and tubal sterilization. He also wrote an obstetric manual that went into 15 editions, and a gynecologic manual that went into 16.

In 1906 Dührssen visited the United States and Argentina, repeating the latter visit in 1921. He retired from academic life in 1913 to allow more time for the outdoor sports he loved so, including riding, sailing, hunting, and mountain climbing. The last four years of his life were marred by Parkinson's disease. He died October 11, 1933, at the age of 71.

REFERENCES

1. Dührssen, A.: Ueber den Werth der tiefen Cervix-und Scheiden-Damm-Einschnitte in der Geburtshülfe. *Arch. f. Gynäk.,* 37:27–66, 1890. (Abstracted in *Centralbl. f. Gynäk.,* 14:548–49, 1890.)

2. Dührssen, A.: Über einige weitere Fälle van tiefen Cervix-und Scheidendammincisionen in der Geburtshilfe. *Centralbl. f. Gynäk.,* 14:245–46, 1890.

3. Knoch, W.: Über die Berechtigung der seitlichen Incisionen der Cervix bei unvolkommen eröffnetem Muttermunde. Inaug.-Diss. Friedrich-Wilhelms-Universität, Berlin, 1888.

4. Lindemann, A.: *De Partu Praeternaturali, quem sine Matris aut Foetus Sectione Absolvere non Liceat Operatori.* E. Luzac, Göttingen, 1755.

5. Rabenau, von: Verschluss des Orificium externum als Geburtshindernis. *Centralbl. f. Gynäk,* 7:108–9, 1883.

6. Skutsch: Ueber Incisionen und Blutungen der Cervix uteri bei Geburten (Selbstbericht). *Arch. f. Gynäk,* 31:460–64, 1887.

7. Strassmann, P.: Zum Andenken an Alfred Dührssen. *Zentralbl. f. Gynäk,* 58:146–52, 1934.

8. Wulsten, M.: Zur Indicationsstellung des hohen Forceps. Inaug.-Diss. Friedrich-Wilhelms-Universität, Berlin, 1889.

François Mauriceau and
the Mauriceau Maneuver*

Until the popularization of the obstetric forceps and before cesarean section on the living woman became an acceptable operation, version and extraction was the accoucheur's sole device for delivery of a living child in labors complicated by mechanical difficulties, as well as the principal method of dealing with a variety of other obstetric complications. Operative obstetrics consisted in large part, therefore, of breech delivery, and then, as now, its bête noire was the aftercoming head.

Version and extraction on a dead infant was first described by Celsus, about 13 A.D., but it was not until almost a hundred years later that Soranus performed this operation on a living fetus. Version then fell into disuse until its revival by Ambroise Paré in the sixteenth century, remaining an important part of the obstetrician's repertoire from that time until the most recent years.

An important manual technique for delivery of the aftercoming head, whether the infant was turned in utero or presented initially by the breech, is identified with the name of François Mauriceau. This procedure, the *Mauriceau maneuver,* was subsequently modified by a number of later obstetricians, including Smellie, Levret, Gifford, Lachapelle, Veit, Wigand, Martin, and von Winckel, whose names have also been associated with the technique for extraction of the aftercoming head. Its principal features consist in turning the

* This chapter originally published under the title "François Mauriceau and His Maneuver in Breech Delivery" in *Obst. & Gynec.,* **9**:371–76, 1957; reprinted by permission. Copyright © 1957, by the American College of Obstetricians and Gynecologists.

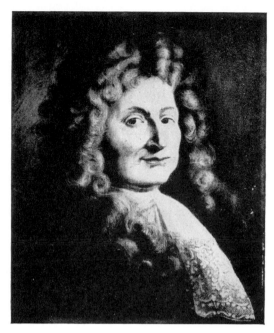

Fig. 64-1. François Mauriceau (1637–1709).

infant so that it faces posteriorly (away from the pubic symphysis) and inserting one or two fingers into its mouth, to aid flexion of the head and provide gentle traction for its delivery.

Long overlooked by obstetric historians as the probable originator of what is now called the Mauriceau maneuver, but antedating Mauriceau, was Jacques Guillemeau. This distinguished French obstetrician was born in Orléans in 1550 and died in Paris, in 1609 according to some authorities, and in 1612 according to others.[2,4] Guillemeau, a pupil of Paré, from whom he had learned the technique of podalic version, was probably the first to advocate it in the treatment of placenta previa. Unlike his master, Guillemeau had also studied the humanities and, being well versed in the classics, was able to read the writings of Hippocrates. In the latter's *De Superfoetatione,* dating back to about 400 B.C., Guillemeau had read the recommendation to insert a finger into the mouth of a dead fetus to assist in its delivery in cephalic presentations. Applying this principle to the aftercoming head, Guillemeau wrote in his textbook, *De la Grossesse et Accouchement des Femmes:*[3]

One would have to turn the body of the infant upside down gently, placing it face downward. . . . Working the head loose by moving it up and down in this situation, and holding the infant with one hand, and with the index finger of the other hand placed in the infant's mouth, it will be easy to extract [the head] with the body.

These lines were probably written, as a matter of fact, by Charles Guillemeau, son of Jacques, after the latter's death. The first edition of the book, which appeared in 1609, the probable year of Jacques's death, contains a chapter on breech delivery, but in a very rare copy of the 1612 English translation that I was able to examine, the above passage does not appear, the author merely mentioning the importance of having the infant's back toward the symphysis to prevent impaction of the chin. It is in the second edition, "corrected and enlarged by Charles Guillemeau," and published in 1621, after Jacques's death, that this technique for delivery of the aftercoming head is first described.

It is obvious that Mauriceau was familiar with the writings of the Guillemeaus, for although no acknowledgment of their priority in this technique is made, striking similarities are to be found in their respective chapters on breech delivery.

MAURICEAU'S INSTRUCTIONS FOR BREECH EXTRACTION

Mauriceau's celebrated text, *Traité des Maladies des Femmes Grosses,*[6] was published initially in 1668, but the early editions and their English translations by Hugh Chamberlen did not contain the famous chapter on breech delivery. The earliest edition of Mauriceau's book in which I have succeeded in finding his instructions for breech delivery is the third (Figs. 64-2, 64-3) published in 1681, from which the following excerpt is taken (Chap. XIII, pp. 271–76):

Now as soon as the Surgeon will have recognized that the infant is presenting in this position, and that the uterus is sufficiently dilated to allow the passage of his hand (otherwise he brings about gradual dilatation, lubricating its entire passage with oil or fresh butter, also using his fingers for this purpose, spreading them apart after having introduced his hand with the fingers together, and continuing to do so until it [the cervix] is sufficiently dilated) and having his nails cut short, his fingers without any rings and his whole hand anointed with oil or fresh butter, he will introduce it gently into the entrance of the uterus where, finding the feet of the infant, he will extract it in this position, in the manner that we are about to describe. But if only one of the feet presents itself, he must determine which it is, whether right or left, and in which position it is presenting; for these points will help him determine on which side the other foot lies. Having noted this, he will go after it and having found it, he will extract it very gently together with the first foot. Before doing this, he must be very careful that the second foot is not that of another child; because if it were so, he would burst the mother and infants before extracting them thus. This he will recognize easily if, having slid his hand along the leg and thigh of the first infant up to the groin, he finds that the two thighs are part of one and the same body. This is also an easy means of finding the other foot, when only one presents at first.

Several authors recommend that for fear of losing hold of the first foot, one

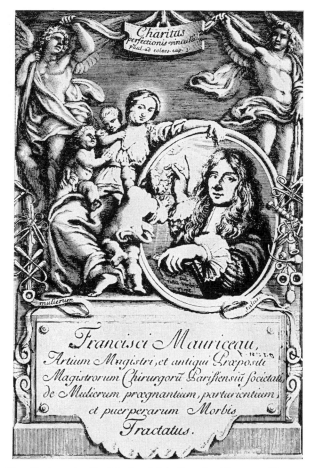

Fig. 64-2. Frontispiece in *Traité des Maladies des Femmes Grosses.* (Courtesy of New York Academy of Medicine.)

tie it with a ribbon with a slip knot, in order not to have to search for it again after having found the other foot; but this is not often necessary; for ordinarily when one has hold of one foot the other is not very hard to find. Nevertheless let him who wishes take this precaution, which does no harm except that it prolongs the time of the operation. Now as soon as the Surgeon will have found both of the infant's feet, he will extract them. Then taking them by both hands, above the malleoli, and holding them close together, he will pull evenly in this manner, until the thighs and hips of the infant are extracted. For this purpose he will grasp the thighs firmly above the knees as soon as he is able to, being careful to wrap these parts in an ordinary cloth, which should be dry, so that his hands, which are already greasy, will not slide on the body of the infant, which is very slippery because of the mucoid material with which it is covered and which would prevent him from being able to hold firmly. This done, and always holding the infant by

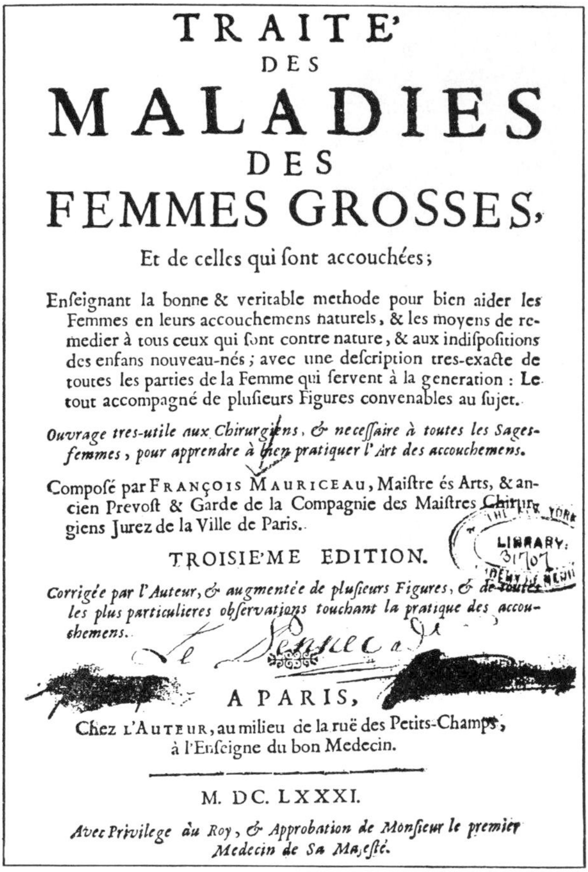

TRAITE'
DES
MALADIES
DES
FEMMES GROSSES,

Et de celles qui ſont accouchées;

Enſeignant la bonne & veritable methode pour bien aider les Femmes en leurs accouchemens naturels, & les moyens de remedier à tous ceux qui ſont contre nature, & aux indiſpoſitions des enfans nouveau-nés; avec une deſcription tres-exacte de toutes les parties de la Femme qui ſervent à la generation: Le tout accompagné de pluſieurs Figures convenables au ſujet.

Ouvrage tres-utile aux Chirurgiens, & neceſſaire à toutes les Sages-femmes, pour apprendre à bien pratiquer l'Art des accouchemens.

Composé par FRANÇOIS MAURICEAU, Maiſtre és Arts, & ancien Prevoſt & Garde de la Compagnie des Maiſtres Chirurgiens Jurez de la Ville de Paris.

TROISIE'ME EDITION.

Corrigée par l'Auteur, & augmentée de pluſieurs Figures, & de toutes les plus particulieres obſervations touchant la pratique des accouchemens.

A PARIS,
Chez L'AUTEUR, au milieu de la ruë des Petits-Champs, à l'Enſeigne du bon Medecin.

M. DC. LXXXI.

Avec Privilege du Roy, & Approbation de Monſieur le premier Medecin de Sa Majeſté.

Fig. 64-3. Title page of *Traité des Maladies des Femmes Grosses.* (Courtesy of New York Academy of Medicine.)

both feet, or above the knees, he will extract it to the top of the chest in this manner, after which he will with his hand bring down both arms of the infant alongside its body. The arms he will then find easily, being careful to hold them near the wrists rather than at any other point, and to disengage them skillfully one at a time, without using too much force, for fear of breaking them, as those who operate unmethodically often do; and being very careful then to hold the abdomen and face directly downward, to prevent the head, if facing upward, from getting caught by the chin on the os pubis. This is why, if it were not so turned, one would have to put it in this position, which one can easily do if, as soon as one starts to pull the infant by the feet, one lowers them while turning them gradually, proportionately to the amount of extraction, until the heels directly face the mother's abdomen. And if they are not in exactly this position when one has extracted the infant to the upper part of its thighs, before extracting it any farther the Surgeon must slide one of his flattened hands up to the infant's pubis and hold both its feet with the other hand, in order to turn its body at the same time to the side more favorable to a good position, until it is as it should be, that is to say, with the chest and face downward. Having thus guided it to the top of the shoulders, it is then necessary to take one's time (urging the patient to bear down now) in order to make sure that by pulling on it, the head can take the shoulders' place at the same time, and by so doing, will not be arrested in the birth canal. Several authors recommend, in order to prevent this mishap, bringing down only one of the infant's arms, and leaving the other up [in the uterus]; so that the other may serve as a splint for its neck, the uterus not being able to close before the infant's head is completely delivered. But if the Surgeon is able to take his time without losing his head, he will not need this precaution to prevent this accident, which would be more likely to occur if he left one arm of the child up [in the uterus]; for besides occupying by its size a part of the birth passage which is not too large anyway, by inclining the head more to one side than to the other, it would result in its surely being arrested where the infant's neck is not thus splinted. When I have sometimes wished to try to leave one arm up [in the uterus] in this manner while extracting infants by the feet, I have always been obliged to bring both arms down, after which I have completed my operation much more easily.

There are nevertheless some infants with a head so large that it remains caught in the passage after the body is completely out, in spite of all the precautions one can take to prevent this. In this case one must not fool around simply pulling the infant by the shoulders; for sometimes one would do better to quit and separate the neck than to continue thusly. But while some other person will pull unskillfully on the infant's body, holding it by both feet or above the knees, the Surgeon will disengage the head gradually from the bones of the pelvis. This he will do by gently sliding one or two fingers of his left hand into the infant's mouth, in order to release the chin first, and with his right hand he will grasp the back of the infant's neck, above the shoulders, with the help of one of the fingers of his left hand placed in the infant's mouth, as I have just said, to disengage the chin; for it is chiefly this part that causes the head to be held up in the pelvis, out of which one cannot extract it until the chin is completely disengaged. One must take care to do this as promptly as possible, for fear that the infant may suffocate, as would doubtlessly occur if it were to remain thus caught and arrested for a long time. This is because the umbilical cord that is outside, being cold and tightly compressed by the body or by the infant's head which remains too long in the birth canal, can then no longer keep the infant alive by the mother's blood, the movement of which is arrested in the cord, as much by its cooling, which makes it clot in it, as by its compression, which prevents its circulation, in the absence of which the child should breathe immediately. This it cannot do until its head is completely out of the uterus. This is the reason why after one has begun to extract the infant, he must try to deliver it completely as soon as he can; this being properly done, one will immediately deliver the woman of the afterbirth, in the manner that we have already described.

The next (fourth) edition of Mauriceau's *Traité* was published in 1694 together with a companion work, *Observations sur la Grossesse et l'Accouchement des Femmes*,[7] which consisted of illustrative case reports to document his teachings. Three of these case reports relate his use of the Mauriceau maneuver for the aftercoming head, the following one serving also to air his attitude toward the Hippocratic belief, then still popular, that an infant born after seven months' gestation has a better chance for survival than one born after eight months:

On the second of October, 1672, I delivered a young woman who, being seven months pregnant with her first child, was injured the day before while taking a rough carriage ride to Versailles. When I was called to help her I found that the midwife, having attempted to deliver her of the child, which was presenting by the feet, had extracted the body well, but the head was still in the birth passage, the midwife being unable to deliver it. This I did the very moment I arrived, after disengaging the chin from the passage with the help of my finger introduced into the mouth of the little infant, whose heart was still beating after I had extracted it. After I had thus completed the delivery of this woman, she told me that when she felt the first pains of labor she consoled herself with the common belief that, being pregnant seven months, her child could survive. But she was quite disillusioned of this common opinion by her own experience, for her child was so small, as are all children at this stage, that it could never have survived even if she had delivered it without any accident at this stage of seven months, when the deliveries, which are always premature, ought to be called abortions rather than true deliveries, as they are mistakenly called.

MAURICEAU'S LIFE

François Mauriceau was born in Paris in 1637.[1,5,8] Although not a doctor of medicine but rather an "ordinary surgeon," belonging to the community of surgeons of Saint-Côme, he became the most accomplished obstetrician of his day in France and the dominant figure in obstetrics of the seventeenth century. He acquired his early obstetric experience at the Hôtel-Dieu before entering private practice in Paris, but the record of this stage of his career is not entirely clear. According to the books of the Hôtel-Dieu, a young surgeon named François Mauriot on November 19, 1660, applied for permission, which was subsequently granted, to perform obstetric deliveries in that institution. He was expelled from the obstetric service on January 28, 1661, following a maternal death for which he was held responsible, and also because the allotted time of his appointment had expired. One of Mauriceau's biographers [5] concluded that François Mauriot and François Mauriceau were the same person, because (1) Mauriot and Mauriceau would both have been young men in 1660, (2) there are records indicating that Mauriceau was working in the maternity division of the Hôtel-Dieu at the end of 1660, and (3) no other record can be found of a seventeenth-century surgeon named Mauriot.

The publication of Mauriceau's text in 1668 was a milestone in the history of obstetrics, providing a tremendous impetus toward its establishment and recognition as a specialty. This book was soon translated into English, German, Dutch, Italian, Latin, and Flemish, and enjoyed the popularity of many editions. Much in the treatise, as in practically all textbooks, parroted the erroneous teachings of previous generations, but it also contained much that was original and important. In the former category was Mauriceau's perpetuation of the glaring anatomic error that regarded the ovarian ligaments as ejaculatory vessels leading from the ovaries to the uterus for the transmission of the female semen. Consistent with this view was his steadfast refusal to accept the concept of tubal pregnancy, and his rigid adherence to the Galenic doctrine that impregnation occurs in the uterine cavity by mixture of the male and female semens. Mauriceau attributed hydatidiform moles to excessive frequency of intercourse.

Among the significant new features of Mauriceau's work was his detailed analysis of the mechanism of labor and his description, probably the first, of brow presentation. He drew sharp distinction between the uterine forces during labor and the passive role of the fetus. Earlier generations of accoucheurs had delivered their patients in the squatting position or on the birth-stool; it was Mauriceau who introduced the practice of delivering women in bed. His book contains the earliest account of the prevention of congenital syphilis by antisyphilitic treatment during pregnancy. Rupture of the membranes had been employed for about 75 years for the induction of labor, but Mauriceau was the first to treat placenta previa by this method. In cases of ruptured perineum associated with childbirth he pioneered in advocating primary repair, recommending "cleansing the womb from such excrements as may be there, with red wine, then applying three or four stitches." He remained immovable in his opposition to cesarean section, which was almost invariably fatal to the mother, and stated that the few cases of reported success existed only in the imagination of the authors.

Mauriceau described the main differences between the male and female pelvis, but discredited Paré's observation of pubic separation in a woman who had been hanged two weeks after giving birth:

I will not in this case accuse him of imposture, for I have too much respect for him, and esteem him too sincere for it; but I indeed believe that he was mistaken in this separation; for there is no likelihood that, being so at the time of her labor, it would remain so a fortnight at the breadth of half a finger, for then they should have been obliged to carry this woman to her execution; for she would not have been able to have supported herself to climb the ladder of the gibbet and to keep herself on her legs . . . because the body is only supported by the stability of these bones: Wherefore we must rather believe . . . that such a disjunction and separation was caused either by the falling of this woman's corpse from the high gibbet to the ground after execution, or rather by some impetuous blow on that place received from some hard or solid thing.

In further support of his argument, Mauriceau informed his readers of his practice of having his hospital patients walk from the birthroom back to their bedroom immediately after delivery, perhaps the first record of early ambulation in organized obstetrics.

In 1694 Mauriceau published his *Aphorismes Touchant la Grossesse, l'Accouchement, les Maladies et les autres Indispositions des Femmes,* in which he demonstrated a familiarity with gynecologic problems as well. Among his numerous observations he gave the first clear reference to membranous dysmenorrhea and called attention to the significance of postmenopausal bleeding as a probable sign of genital cancer.

With Mauriceau's constantly growing fame came an ever-increasing demand for his services as a consultant, leading him finally to the decision to abandon his lucrative practice and retire to the country. Here he enjoyed several years of leisure before his death, October 17, 1709.

REFERENCES

1. Bayle and Thillaye: *Biographie Médicale.* Adolphe Delahays, Paris, 1855, p. 523.
2. Fasbender, H.: *Geschichte der Geburtshülfe.* Fischer, Jena, 1906, pp. 129–35.
3. Guillemeau, J.: *De la Grossesse et Accouchement des Femmes,* Abraham Pacard, Paris, 1609 (1621). Translated by A. Hatfield: *Childbirth, or the Happy Deliverie of Women.* A. Hatfield, London, 1612.
4. Klein, G.: Zur Geschichte der Extraktion und Expression des nachfolgenden Kopfes. *München. med. Wchnschr., 49:*1307–10, 1902.
5. Le Prieur, E.: *Étude sur l'Oeuvre de François Mauriceau.* Thesis, Paris, 1902.
6. Mauriceau, F.: *Traité des Maladies des Femmes Grosses, et de Celles Qui Sont Accouchées.* Paris, 1668. Translated by H. Chamberlen: *The Diseases of Women with Child and in Child-bed.* B. Billingsley, London, 1673.
7. Mauriceau, F.: *Observations sur la Grossesse et l'Accouchement des Femmes.* Paris, 1694.
8. Robb, H.: The writings of Mauriceau. *Bull. Johns Hopkins Hosp., 6:*51–57, 1895.

Erich Bracht and His Maneuver for Breech Delivery

CHAPTER

65

Obstetrics of the mid-twentieth century has been characterized by two divergent trends: increased radicalism, manifested by the broadened application of cesarean section to the manifold problems of parturition; and a growing swell of conservatism, augmented by the popular demand for "natural childbirth." Breech presentation exemplifies nicely this therapeutic dichotomy. Unless the prognosis is unreservedly good for unobstructed vaginal delivery, a breech is best managed by abdominal section. In all normal cases minimal intervention is advocated.

The "assisted breech" has long been taught as the properly conservative method of managing most breech births. This technique allows spontaneous expulsion of the infant to the umbilicus, followed by downward traction and rotation by the obstetrician for delivery of the trunk and arms, with birth of the head being assisted by forceps or suprapubic pressure. Yet the infant mortality resulting from breech delivery remains around 5 per cent. It has been estimated that 13,000 babies are lost from this cause in the United States each year.[5]

BRACHT'S TECHNIQUE

In 1935 Erich Bracht pointed out that the conventional method of "assisting" breech delivery interferes with the normal mechanism of labor, and proposed a new technique permitting spontaneous delivery of the infant. In

567

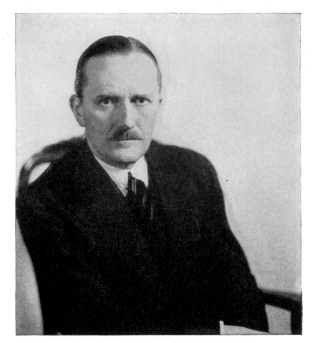

Fig. 65-1. Erich Franz Eugen Bracht (1882–　).

this method, which has come to be known as the Bracht maneuver, the principal function of the obstetrician is to support the infant's body against the force of gravity during birth, without traction, expulsion being accomplished by the force of the contracting uterus, augmented if necessary by suprafundic pressure. As described by Plentl and Stone: [4]

> The breech presents in transverse position or rotates to a transverse position as it passes through the outlet. With each succeeding contraction the posterior hip rolls over the perineum and when delivered, the baby's pelvis begins to rotate upwardly and anteriorly. The corkscrew motion of this compact form continues upward and forward until the baby's back lies directly against the mother's symphysis. At this point the feet pass over the perineum, and their release allows a further lordotic curvature around the mother's symphysis. This, in turn, is followed by spontaneous and simultaneous delivery of the elbows, succeeded by arms and shoulders in the transverse position. The expulsive force transmitted, but not exerted, by the aftercoming head, will invariably produce this effect if arms and head compete for room in the midpelvis. An attitude of extreme extension is now produced by the curvature of the baby's back allowing the head to pass through the outlet in its most favorable diameter. . . . The breech is allowed to deliver spontaneously up to the umbilicus without pull or push, the body and extended legs are held together with both hands maintaining the upward and anterior rotation of the body. When the anterior rotation is nearly complete the

baby's body is held, not pressed, against the mother's symphysis. The force applied in this procedure should be equivalent to the force of gravity; that is, equivalent to the weight of that portion of the baby which has already been born. The mere maintenance of this position added to the effects of uterine contractions and moderate suprapubic pressure by an assistant, suffices to complete the delivery by the spontaneous mechanism. . . .

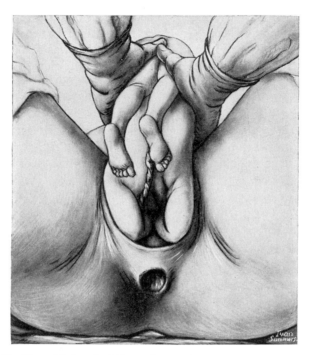

Fig. 65-2. Position of infant in delivery by Bracht maneuver. Note simultaneous birth of arms. (Reproduced from Plentl, A. A., and Stone, R. E.: The Bracht maneuver. *Obst. & Gynec. Surv.,* **8:**317, 1953.)

Bracht demonstrated his maneuver for the first time at a meeting of the Berlin Obstetrical and Gynecological Society on October 4, 1935,[1] but made no effort to publicize the method further until the International Congress for Obstetrics and Gynecology in Amsterdam in May, 1938,[2,3] when he showed his motion-picture film of the procedure and reported his experience with 206 cases with no mortality.

The Bracht maneuver was promptly adopted and subjected to extensive trial in Germany, France, Holland, and South America, with published fetal mortality figures [4] suggesting its superiority to the methods of breech delivery based on active intervention by the accoucheur. In the United States, however, the Bracht maneuver still awaits clinical evaluation.

BRACHT'S LIFE

Erich Franz Eugen Bracht was born in Berlin, Germany, July 5, 1882, the son of a physician.[6] After completing his formal medical education, he worked in the pathology laboratory of Aschoff in Freiburg, where he made an important contribution to the etiology and pathologic anatomy of rheumatic myocarditis. Having decided on a career in obstetrics and gynecology, he served as assistant to Menge in Heidelberg, then Pfannenstiel and Stöckel in Kiel, and finally Franz in Berlin. In 1922 Bracht was made extraordinary professor in the University of Berlin, and after Franz's death served for two years as acting director of the Charité Frauenklinik. Since 1945 he has been in charge of the Provincial Frauenklinik at Berlin-Neukölln, which was rebuilt after World War II into the city's largest hospital for women. He served also as consultant in obstetrics and gynecology to the U.S. Occupation Forces in Berlin. In addition to his professional activities, he is known as a collector of antique paintings and old Chinese and Japanese prints.

REFERENCES

1. Bracht, E.: Zur Manualhilfe bei Beckenendlage, *Ztschr. f. Geburtsh. u. Gynäk.*, **112**:271, 1936.
2. Bracht, E.: Zur Behandlung der Steisslage. *Handl. Int. Cong. v. Verloskunde en Gynaecologie.* Amsterdam, 1938, Vol. 2, pp. 93–94.
3. Bracht, E.: Zur Behandlung der Steisslage. *Zentralbl. f. Gynäk.*, **62**:1735, 1938.
4. Plentl, A. A., and Stone, R. E.: The Bracht maneuver. *Obst. & Gynec. Surv.*, **8**:313–25, 1953.
5. Ward, S. V., and Sellers, T. B.: Controversial issues in breech presentations. *South. M. J.*, **43**:879–86, 1950.
6. *Wer ist's*, 10th ed. Ed. by H. A. L. Degener. Berlin, 1935, p. 176.

Friedrich Wilhelm Scanzoni and the Scanzoni Maneuver

Failure of the occiput to rotate anteriorly from a posterior position in labor usually calls for obstetric assistance. Spontaneous delivery of the head with the occiput posterior almost always requires an unduly prolonged second stage. Forceps extraction of the head in this position is difficult, entailing excessive traction. The head delivering from the posterior position fails to present its smallest diameters to the vaginal outlet, often resulting thereby in a deep tear of the perineum or extension of the episiotomy. Delivery as an occiput posterior is mechanically inexpedient and hence aesthetically offensive to the obstetrician. He therefore treats arrested labor with the occiput posterior by rotating it first to an anterior position.

William Smellie [6,8] was the first to show an understanding of the mechanics of this problem and to provide a method for its solution in cases "when the forehead, instead of being towards the *Sacrum,* is turned forwards to the *Os pubis.*" He wrote:

The blades of the forceps, being introduced along the ears, or as near them as possible . . . the head must be pushed up a little, and the forehead turned to one side of the *Pelvis;* thus let it be brought along, until the hindhead arrives at the lower part of the *Ischium:* then the forehead must be turned backward, into the hollow of the *Sacrum,* and even a quarter or more to the contrary side, in order to prevent the shoulders from hitching on the upper part of the *Os pubis* or *Sacrum,* so that they may be still towards the sides of the *Pelvis;* then let the quarter turn be

571

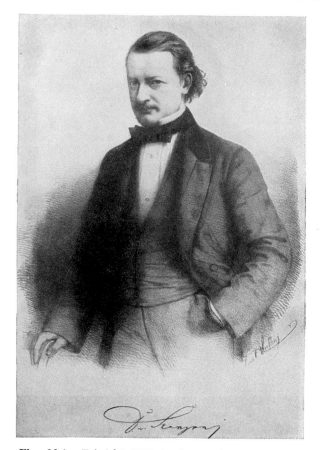

Fig. 66-1.   Friedrich Wilhelm Scanzoni (1821–1891).

reversed, and the forehead being re-placed in the hollow of the *Sacrum,* the head may be extracted. . . . In performing these different turns, let the head be pushed up or pulled down occasionally, as it meets with least resistance.

Smellie, it will be noted, carried out both rotation and extraction of the head with a single application of his forceps, as indicated in the above description and as illustrated further in Table XXI of his *Sett of Anatomical Tables;* [7] this was possible because the instrument pictured was short and possessed only a mild pelvic curvature.

SCANZONI'S TECHNIQUE

Rotation from the posterior and subsequent extraction cannot be carried out in the same operation with the conventional forceps, however, because of its pronounced pelvic curve. One solution to this problem was provided by Friedrich Scanzoni, who advocated that the procedure be carried out in two steps, with reapplication of the blades after rotation of the head. His operation continues to be used, in modified form, still known as the Scanzoni maneuver. Its rationale and technique were outlined at a meeting of the Physikalisch-medicinische Gesellschaft in Würzburg on April 26, 1851.[4] Explained Scanzoni:

If one considers the construction of the forceps, on the one hand, and the shape of the fetal head and of the maternal pelvis, on the other, one sees at a glance that the instrument will function most effectively and least traumatically when it is applied to both temporal regions and is so situated in the pelvis that its pelvic curve corresponds exactly with the direction of the pelvic axis. This is possible, however, only when the anteroposterior diameter of the head lies parallel to the anteroposterior of the pelvis, in which case the blades, applied along both side walls of the pelvis, grasp the head at its two lateral surfaces. . . .

If the forceps are applied to the sides of the head, however, when the anteroposterior diameter of the latter lies parallel to the transverse or an oblique diameter of the pelvis, then the tips of the instrument have to be turned more or less toward one of the pelvic side walls in order to bring the instrument into the relation to the pelvic axis necessary for extraction. Extraction may be very dangerous, often quite impossible, when attempted with improperly applied forceps.

[Turning now to the case in which] one has to deal with the position of the skull wherein the brow of the engaged head lies anterior [occiput posterior]: if natural rotation of the head and forceps occurs in such a case, the brow is brought directly anterior. It is obvious that in this position forceps extraction of the head is extremely difficult, as a rule, requiring considerable force and time, which could have been avoided if the brow had been rotated toward the posterior pelvic wall before the extraction.

In the application of the forceps one must abide by the general rule, that the blades be so placed that after being locked they lie against the head with their tips and concave edges facing the part that one proposes to rotate toward the anterior pelvic wall. An exception to this rule is permissible only in cases . . . that require a second, different application of the instrument for the complete achievement of rotation. In such cases the forceps are first applied with their tips pointing toward the part of the head to be rotated away from the anterior pelvic wall; and only after this is accomplished is the instrument reapplied with its tips pointing toward the part of the head that is now to be brought under the pubis by the second rotation. When this too is accomplished, the pelvic curve of the instrument corresponds to the pelvic axis. . . .

If the sagittal suture lies parallel to an oblique diameter but the brow faces the anterior pelvic wall, then a single application of the instrument does not suffice to turn anteriorly the occiput, which is in contact with the posterior pelvic wall. If we visualize the sagittal suture in the left oblique diameter, for example, with the brow near the right obturator foramen, it is then impossible to apply the forceps, because of its pelvic curve, in such a way that the blades grasp the head at its lateral surfaces and with their tips and concave edges at the same time facing the occiput, which lies at the left sacroiliac synchondrosis.

After roundly condemning brow-mastoid, or pelvic, application of the forceps, as advocated by Lange and others, and reaffirming the importance of an accurate cephalic application, Scanzoni continued:

> We therefore regard it as essential in such cases that the instrument be applied twice in order to bring about the necessary correction of the head's position, but always to the lateral surfaces of the head insofar as possible.
>
> Our procedure is as follows: If the head lies with the brow facing anteriorly and to the left [R O P], so that the sagittal suture runs in the right oblique diameter, then the left blade is applied in front of the left sacroiliac articulation, the right behind the right obturator foramen. The transverse diameter of the forceps thus lies in the left oblique of the pelvis, the concave edges and tips facing the anterior border of the left lateral half of the pelvis, and therefore the brow also, which lies there. Rotation of the instrument is now carried out, from right to left [clockwise], describing an eighth of a circle, as a result of which the right blade comes to lie almost behind the pubic symphysis, the left in front of the concavity of the sacrum. The head is thus rotated so that the brow, which previously lay anteriorly and on the left, moves to the middle of the left side wall of the pelvis, the occiput to the middle of the right side wall, and the sagittal suture lies parallel to the transverse diameter of the pelvis.
>
> Both blades of the forceps are now removed and reapplied in such a way that the left blade comes to lie behind the left obturator foramen, the right in front of the right sacroiliac articulation; whereupon renewed rotation of the instrument brings the occiput directly under the pubic arch.

Scanzoni anticipated, correctly but only in part, the criticism to be raised against his rediscovered technique of forceps rotation. He wrote:

> We believe we can parry any possible objection that this operation cannot be carried out on a head high in the pelvis because of the obstacle presented to the movement of the posterior blade by the anterior protrusion of the promontory, by simply stating that we do not regard as permissible any attempt at rotation of a high head. Even our method is not intended for such cases. It is just as safe as it is easy, however, when the head is deeply engaged.

Despite Scanzoni's satisfactory personal experience with his method at the time of his report, he would surely have wished to modify this statement, could he have anticipated the countless vaginal and cervical lacerations that were to result from the use of the "Scanzoni maneuver" by others.

SCANZONI'S LIFE

Friedrich Wilhelm Scanzoni was born in the village of Lichtenfels, near Prague, December 21, 1821.[1,2,3] He studied in Prague, graduating from the medical school in 1844. Soon after obtaining a small position in the gynecologic division of the general hospital in Prague he was appointed to the gynecologic staff in the university, under Professor Jungmann, who allowed his young assistant abundant opportunity for development of his gynecologic interests. He also served as assistant to Kiwisch in the obstetric clinic, until the latter went to Würzburg as professor of obstetrics. After Jungmann's death, when Kiwisch was recalled to Prague, Scanzoni was chosen to succeed Kiwisch as ordinary professor of obstetrics and gynecology at the Würzburger Hochschule, in 1850. His three-volume *Lehrbuch der Geburtshilfe,* the first volume of which had just been published (1849), was warmly received and soon became recognized as the leading textbook in the field, a position it enjoyed for several years. Scanzoni's move to Würzburg marked the beginning of his meteoric rise to the unchallenged position as the outstanding obstetrician and gynecologist on the Continent, the accumulation of many honors, the development of a very extensive private practice, and a phenomenal pecuniary reward. His fame was climaxed by a call to St. Petersburg to attend the Empress of Russia in her confinement, for which service he is said to have received 100,000 rubles and a fine house in Würzburg. For several years thereafter the aristocracy of Russia flocked to him in such numbers as to provide the principal support for several of the hotels of Würzburg. Students and practitioners likewise came from near and far for training under the great Scanzoni. From 1850 to 1870 none in Europe could match his reputation. When he was about to resign his chair in 1863, the citizens of Würzburg petitioned King Max of Bavaria, begging that means be found to induce Scanzoni to remain. Scanzoni, in deference to a personal letter and a baronetcy from the King, stayed on for a few more years, then withdrew completely from his active professional life, resigned his professorship, and retired to his estate at Arco-Zinneberg in the Bavarian Alps. Here he lived a life of leisure for the next 20 years, completely isolated from the medical world. When he died, June 12, 1891, from general paresis it is believed, little attention was paid to his passing, for his contributions had been missing from the medical literature for such a time that many had thought him long dead.

In addition to his textbook of obstetrics, Scanzoni was the author of a volume on gynecology, *Lehrbuch der Krankheiten der Weiblichen Sexualorgane;* a monograph on "chronic metritis"; an annual series of contributions, *Beiträge zur Geburtskunde und Gynäkologie* (popularly known as *Scanzoni's Beiträge*), published in seven volumes; and several other works.

Scanzoni is remembered primarily as an obstetrician, both for his positive contributions and for his bitter opposition to Semmelweis' doctrine of contagion in puerperal sepsis. His gynecologic interests were almost exclusively of a medical character. Surgical gynecology was in its infancy, and after his initial efforts in the field produced unsatisfactory results, he treated the "newer gynecology" with a full measure of disdain. Even the curette of Récamier was denounced by Scanzoni as "an instrument based upon an entirely erroneous thought, which takes from it all practical utility." His use of leeches in the treatment of cervical inflammations, acute metritis, and uterine prolapse exemplifies Scanzoni's gynecology. Concerning uterine cancer, he wrote:[5]

The most important causes are assuredly emotions of grief, fretfulness, the cares of life, affliction after some bereavement, etc. . . . We have been able to convince ourselves that eighty-four of our patients have for a long time undergone the pernicious influence of such causes, and almost always the first symptoms of the disease appeared a little after the fatal emotion.

We are further persuaded that immoderate coitus and excessive sexual excitation are not without importance in the etiology of cancer. In fact, we have been able, in fifteen of our patients, to recognize an insatiable desire, sometimes from the avowal of the patients themselves, sometimes from the complaints of their husbands, who accused their wives of having tormented them when the disease had already made considerable progress. The rarity of carcinoma of the uterus among public women (three of our patients had formerly belonged to this class) does not appear to be in contradiction to what we have affirmed, for in general they are not in coitus affected with the same intensity as a woman who yields herself to a husband she loves. It is not the frequency of the coitus, but the moral excitation which accompanies it, which seems here to be the important point.

No less fanciful, perhaps, are current concepts of the etiology of cervical cancer, a century later!

REFERENCES

1. *American Gynecological Society Album of Fellows, 1876–1930*. Ed. by F. E. Keene. Dornan, Philadelphia, 1930, p. 516.
2. Dohrn, R.: *Geschichte der Geburtshülfe der Neuzeit*. Part 1 (1840–1860). Franz Pietzcker, Tübingen, 1903, pp. 29–32.
3. Mundé, P. F.: In memoriam. Friedrich Wilhelm von Scanzoni. Born 1821; died June 12th, 1891. *Am. J. Obst.*, 24:935–38, 1891.
4. Scanzoni, F. W.: Die Anwendung der Geburtszange als Mittel zur Verbesserung der Stellung des vorliegenden Kindeskopfes. *Verhandl. d. phys.-med. Gesellsch. in Würzburg*, 2:184–201, 1851.
5. Scanzoni, F. W.: *A Practical Treatise on the Diseases of the Sexual Organs of Women*, 4th American ed. English translation by A. K. Gardner from the French of H. Dor and A. Socin. De Witt, New York, 861, pp. 58–60, 153, 179, 206, 300.
6. Smellie, W.: *A Treatise on the Theory and Practice of Midwifery*, 2nd ed. D. Wilson & T. Durham, London, 1752, Book III, Chap. III, Sect. IV, Numb. III, pp. 273–74.
7. Smellie, W.: *A Sett of Anatomical Tables, with Explanations, and an Abridgment, of the Practice of Midwifery*. London, 1754.
8. Smellie, W.: Laborious cases, in which, the vertex presenting with the forehead to the pubes or groin, the patient was delivered with the forceps. *A Collection of Cases and Observations in Midwifery*, 3rd ed. D. Wilson & T. Durham, London, 1764, Collection XXVIII, pp. 471–82.

A time-honored criterion of the accoucheur's handiwork is the integrity of the patient's perineum. The curve of the pelvis directs the presenting part of the fetus against this barrier, resulting in its distention and frequent rupture from the expulsive forces of the birth act. In modern obstetrics this tendency toward perineal laceration is circumvented by the frequent resort to prophylactic episiotomy, especially in primigravidas. But deliberate incision and reconstruction of the perineum is a relatively recent addition to obstetric practice. Before the twentieth century, physicians showed great aversion to episiotomy, their surgical efforts at enlarging the vaginal outlet being limited to multiple short and superficial nicks in the membrane of the dilated introitus. From the time of Soranus, early in the second century, manual support of the perineum was advocated as the expedient best suited for maintaining the entirety of this structure during birth of the infant's head.

Although now known as the Ritgen maneuver, the procedure was thus actually employed long before the time of this celebrated German obstetrician. Case reports from Giffard's *Cases in Midwifry*,[3] published posthumously in 1734 by his friend, Edward Hody, make clear reference to it. In Case 164 Giffard described his delivery of a stillborn infant on December 4, 1730. He wrote:

A Man came to me out of *Butcher-Row* about five o'Clock in the morning, desiring me to go to his Wife, who had been in Labour about thirty hours: The Membranes were broke, and the Waters pass'd off some hours before I came; the upper and back part of the Child's Head was advanced forwards into the

Vagina, and the upper and fore part was press'd against the *Os Sacrum;* it had lain in this condition at least two hours, and had not made the least advance, notwithstanding her Pains were quick and forcing. . . . As the head seem'd to be lock'd above between the bones, I therefore thought it advisable to pass up one Side of my *Extractor* between the upper edge of the *Os Pubis* of the Mother, and the back part of the Child's Head, and fixed it about the lower part of the *Occiput,* and then, by lifting it from off the said Bone, and drawing it downwards, I soon brought it lower, till it appeared between the *Labia Pudendi,* nevertheless the fore part made no advance: I therefore was obliged to pass up the other Side of my *Extractor* between the *Rectum* and the Head of the Child, and endeavoured to fix it against some part of the Head, in hopes that by pulling, I might bring the middle part of the Crown more opposite to the Passage, and thereby prevent it's being press'd so much backwards: by which means I, in some measure, obtain'd the end I desired; but as there was danger of tearing the *Perinaeum,* should I have proceeded further in that manner, I therefore withdrew my Instrument, and afterward clapp'd my Hand flat to her Back, near to the *Anus,* and whenever her Pains seiz'd her, I press'd my Hand against that part, and by pressing and drawing it downwards at the same time, I forced the Crown more forward and lower into the Passage, so that in a few Pains I disengaged the whole Head, and brought it out, and the Shoulders and other parts readily followed. . . .

A month later, on January 12, 1731, Giffard again found occasion to employ this maneuver of supporting the perineum. The circumstances are described in Case 173 of his book:

About eight o'Clock in the evening . . . a Carpenter in *Orchard-Street, Westminster,* came to desire me to go to his Wife. The Midwife upon my coming there told me, that the Child presented right, with the upper part of the Head foremost, and that it was sunk low into the *Vagina,* and that there it stuck, and for several hours had not advanced in the least, notwithstanding her Throws were both strong and forcing: from hence I concluded, as the Head was large, and the Woman not young, and this being the first time of her being in Labour, that the Head was lock'd between the Bones, so that there might be occasion for some help to bring it forwards: Whereupon I examined and found it as before represented, and therefore pass'd up one side of my *Extractor* between the *Os Pubis* of the Mother and the Head of the Child; and endeavour'd to fix it at the lower part of the *Occiput,* near to the first *Vertebra;* this done, I attempted to lift the Head from off the said Bone, and to draw it more downwards towards the *Labia Pudendi*: But as my Instrument slipp'd several times, I was as often forced to repass it, and, at last, with no small difficulty, I brought out the upper and hinder part of the Head beyond the *Labia,* and as the Fore-part press'd very much backwards against the *Rectum,* I press'd outwardly with the Flat of my Hand against that part, by which means I forced the Head more forewards, and more towards the *Labia,* and at length brought out the whole Head. . . .

In 1767 a pamphlet was published by John Harvie entitled *Practical Directions, Shewing a Method of Preserving the Perinaeum in Birth, and Delivering the Placenta Without Violence.*[4] In it more detailed instructions were given for manually protecting the perineum from laceration during birth of the infant. Explained Harvie:

From the natural formation of the *os externum* of women, and the largeness of the heads of children at their birth, were the delivery left to nature, the perinaeum would generally be torn at the time when the head of the child protrudes through the *os externum,* particularly at the birth of a first, or second child. The preservation of the *perinaeum* being of the greatest consequence ought to be principally attended to by midwives; and this I think may be best done by observing the following rules, the importance of which experience has taught me, and therefore I wish to recommend them to the consideration of all practitioners.

So soon as the *vertex* of the child's head begins to push into the *os externum,* it must only be allowed to advance in a slow and gradual manner, by the action of the labour pains.

To do this properly, the accoucheur having directed his patient to lie down upon the bed in the usual position, every pain must be attended to; and as soon as a pain has acted long enough to render the *froenum* of the *perinaeum* tight, the farther action of that pain must be totally prevented, by the palm of the left hand applied against the *perinaeum* with a proper force.

By observing this method in every following pain, a safe dilatation will be gradually produced. During the interval of pain, fresh hogs lard, the best ointment for that purpose, is to be insinuated upon the inside of the *perinaeum* and into all the *os externum.*

When the parts are greatly dilated in this gradual manner, the accoucheur, with the palm of his hand applied as already directed, is to prevent the forehead of the child making its rise from under the *perinaeum,* till he feels by the nape of the neck, that the *vertex* is entirely out from below the *ossa pubis.* Thus the external parts will not be put upon the stretch so much by one inch and a half, as they would be were the forehead allowed to rise at the time that the *vertex* is under the pubes.

To explain this rule, I must observe that the distance in a streight line between a child's forehead and *vertex* (when the head is not altered from its natural figure) is one inch and a half more than it is between the forehead and the nape of a child's neck. And frequently a much greater difference is observed in laborious cases, as in these the head is commonly lengthened in proportion to the difficulty.

In a later paragraph Harvie continued:

We must be careful to prevent the lengthening of the *perinaeum* from the time that the head first makes any pressure, to its full delivery. To accomplish this, the *perinaeum* is by the palm of the left hand to be pretty strongly carried back towards the *anus,* and kept so all the time of every pain.

Thus it will be preserved in its natural state, without being rendered thinner, or having it's fibres internally torn, the miserable consequence of these parts being too much extended.

The accoucheur ought to have a single fold of a warm and clean cloth between the palm of his left hand and the *perinaeum;* without which he could not have a commanding hold, and consequently could not attend to the rules here laid down.

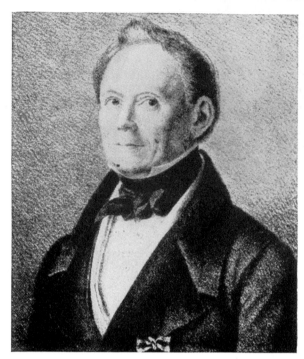

Fig. 67-1. Ferdinand August Maria Franz von Ritgen (1787–1867). (Reproduced from Tilanus, C. B.; Deelman, H. B.; and Bles, J.: *Surgery A Hundred Years Ago.* Geoffrey Bles, Ltd., London, 1925.)

VON RITGEN'S TECHNIQUE

Not until 1828, 61 years after the publication of Harvie's pamphlet and almost a century after Giffard's book, did Ferdinand von Ritgen first describe a manual method of perineal protection.[5] The early technique of von Ritgen differed in two essentials from that of his predecessors: his manual intervention was aimed at flexion rather than extension of the head, and his prophylactic efforts were made between, rather than during, the uterine contractions. Wrote von Ritgen:

[I employed the procedure] when the greatest diameter of the head was not quite ready to be born, the presenting part being near the midportion of the skull rather than the occiput. When a considerable part of the head was visible I then often succeeded in bringing the occiput to the front. Sitting behind the parturient, who lay on her side, I first placed the flat of my hand under the coccyx and applied rather brief and not very great pressure against the posterior perineum. The latter, encountering the infant's brow and face, thus presses the chin further toward the chest as it forces the occiput forward. Such a slight nudge usually suffices to reduce the excessive tension on the greatly stretched soft parts, caused by the unfavorable position of the head, so that no tear results during its birth. The brief pressure must be applied, of course, in the interval between labor contractions . . . and repeated frequently with the flat of the hand. In the course of a few intervals between pains one thus succeeds in forcing the head through, up to the root of the nose, when delivery of the face can be left to nature.

If the perineum tears even slightly during birth of the head, delivery of the shoulders will usually enlarge the tear considerably. The ordinary method of supporting the perineum has never helped me prevent this . . . but I have encountered perineal lacerations only very rarely for several years.

Von Ritgen's prescription for perineal prophylaxis underwent considerable modification during the ensuing quarter century, his improved technique [6] favoring extension rather than flexion of the head. The application of von Ritgen's new procedure was restricted, moreover, to patients in whom a perineal laceration might otherwise be anticipated. His detailed description of the method explains his basis for selection:

When the occiput approaches the pubic arch and the largest circumference of the head has passed through the pelvic outlet, forcing the coccyx backward, making the posterior perineum about an inch broad, opening up the anus about an inch wide, and stretching out the anterior perineum from 2 to about 4 inches, the decision has to be made whether or not to permit completely unhampered birth of the largest circumference of the head through the introitus. If this exit can occur without threat of tearing the perineum, then the head and perineum should not be touched at all, so that the very rapidly ensuing rotation of the brow around the fulcrum of the neck at the lower border of the symphysis, and the simultaneous retraction of the perineum, can occur spontaneously without interference. The previously customary procedure of pressing the perineum forward and upward with the flat of the hand interferes with both of these processes and causes the perineal tear, for the pressure of the flat of the hand against the fetal head thins out the perineum further, even hindering its rapid retraction. Spontaneous delivery of the head should be allowed to occur, completely unhampered, if the entire external region of the introitus appears moist, warm, soft, and turgid at the onset of labor; if this preparation for birth progresses during labor; if the labia majora are greatly swollen; if the vaginal opening gapes widely; if the vaginal mucus becomes thicker and flows more abundantly; if the whole vagina dilates progressively; if the occiput becomes progressively more visible with the labor contractions and retracts markedly between them; if the stretching of the introitus is not very painful; and finally, if the perineum is rather thick and the transverse ligament remains rounded at its inner margin. But these phenomena rarely occur in primigravidas, especially the very young, the rather old, and the dark-skinned with tense ligaments.

In the absence of these manifestations the head should be held back; but excessive counterforce should not be applied against the expulsive contractions, for this might result in rupture of the vagina or even the uterus. It is all the more necessary to hold the head back, the broader, tenser, thinner, and smoother the perineum; especially if the latter presents the appearance of a glistening, thin, wet, almost transparent membrane over the head, and the transverse ligament becomes paper-thin, its inner border formed into a very sharp edge.

Von Ritgen's description of his technique, subsequently known as the Ritgen maneuver, followed:

The head cannot be held back with certainty by the flat of the hand; the procedure must be carried out instead by pressing against the occiput the tips of the thumb, index, and middle fingers, separated up to 2 inches, somewhat in the form of a triangle. As soon as delivery of the head appears imminent . . . and laceration of the perineum threatens, the three fingers should be kept constantly on the head, following all its movements, even if it recedes far back into the vagina after every contraction. During a contraction the head should be allowed to advance as far as possible without being delivered, up to the point of tearing the soft tissues. If there appears to be no danger of sudden birth of the head, the interval between contractions should be used for the diligent application of inunctions, both externally to the perineum and internally to the lower vagina; and after each inunction a warm emollient poultice should be held against the vaginal introitus. . . .

Returning to his technique for delivery of the head, von Ritgen continued:

With the three fingers of one hand against the occiput, holding the head back, the four fingers of the other hand are placed with their tips against the posterior perineum, behind the anal orifice, near the tip of the coccyx, and on either side of the median raphe. During the interval between contractions, preferably right after the cessation of a contraction, inward and upward pressure usually encounters the infant's chin, gliding it forward, while the three fingers on the occiput result in anterior extension of the head, which occurs slowly about the fulcrum of the neck, at the lower border of the pubic symphysis. Both hands are held motionless as soon as a contraction begins and until it is over. Immediately afterward the pressure is resumed against the chin. As the latter gradually advances, the external pressure on it must also advance, from the posterior perineum to the anal orifice and finally to the anterior perineum, until the chin is delivered across the transverse ligament. The external pressure should be applied somewhat laterally to the median raphe, so that one parietal boss can be delivered through the introitus before the other, this more effectively ensuring against a tear than when both bosses protrude through the introitus simultaneously.

The principles of von Ritgen's teaching, widely endorsed by subsequent generations of obstetricians, continue to find acceptance in modern practice. The Ritgen maneuver remains a valuable adjunct in vertex deliveries.

VON RITGEN'S LIFE

Ferdinand August Maria* Franz von Ritgen was born October 11, 1787, in Wulfen, duchy of Salm-Salm.[1,2] He received both his preliminary and medical education in Münster, then spent the years from 1808 to 1814 in various civil medical positions in Stadthagen and Medebach. During this period he developed a deep interest in obstetrics; and when only 27 years old, he was called to Giessen as professor of surgery and obstetrics and as director of the newly

* This is probably the correct form of the name, but Max appears in the place of Maria in several biographic references to von Ritgen.

built lying-in hospital. Here he remained and worked for the next 53 years.

When the new surgical clinic was completed in Giessen, von Ritgen was likewise made director of it, occupying this position from 1831 to 1837.

He later assumed the chair of psychiatry, to which he devoted himself with amazing energy and zeal. Even in the last winter of his life he began his lectures at 7 A.M., earlier than any other member of the faculty. In addition to his professorial duties von Ritgen found time during his long academic tenure to serve often as dean of the medical faculty, and twice as rector of the university.

Von Ritgen's literary activity encompassed a variety of topics. His obstetric text, *Handbuch der Niederen Geburtshülfe,* published in 1824, was revised in 1848 under the new title, *Lehr-und Handbuch der Geburtshülfe für Hebammen.* With Busch and Mende he founded and served as coeditor of the *Gemeinsame Deutsche Zeitschrift für Geburtskunde,* the first volume of which appeared in 1826. He remained a frequent contributor to this journal after its name was changed, first to *Neue Zeitschrift für Geburtskunde* and in 1853 to *Monatsschrift für Geburtskunde und Frauenkrankheiten.* His nonmedical writings embraced the fields of zoology, botany, philosophy, and astronomy; and for one of his publications, *Gemälde der organischen Natur in ihrer Verbreitung auf der Erde,* he was awarded a gold medal by the King of Prussia. In addition, he invented a number of instruments, including forceps, pelvimeters, a skull perforator, and a polyp snare.

The talents and contributions of the tireless von Ritgen received warm recognition. He held honorary memberships in countless scientific societies and an honorary doctorate of philosophy from the University of Giessen. He was given the honorary position of *Geheimer Medicinalrath* in 1830, was chosen to represent the city of Giessen in the second Chamber of the Estates from 1835 to 1841, and was elevated to the nobility by Grand Duke Ludwig II in 1840. After devoting the last decade of his life mainly to philosophic and astronomic studies, von Ritgen died on April 14, 1867.

REFERENCES

1. Birnbaum, K. F. J.: Ferdinand August Maria Franz von Ritgen. Nekrolog. *Monatschr. f. Geburtsk. u. Frauenkrankh.,* **29**:443–63, 1867.

2. Dohrn, R.: *Geschichte der Geburtshülfe der Neuzeit.* Part 1 (1840–1860). Franz Pietzcker, Tübingen, 1903, pp. 10–15.

3. Giffard, W.: *Cases in Midwifry. Revis'd and publish'd by Edward Hody, M.D.* Motte & Wotton, London, 1734, pp. 396–98, 415–16.

4. Harvie, J.: *Practical Directions, Shewing a Method of Preserving the Perinaeum in Birth, and Delivering the Placenta Without Violence.* D. Wilson & G. Nicol, London, 1767, p. 2.

5. Ritgen, F. von: Geburtshülfliche Erfahrungen und Bemerkungen. *Gemein. deutsch. Ztschr. f. Geburtsk.,* **3**:147–69, 1828.

6. Ritgen, F. von: Ueber sein Dammschutzverfahren. *Monatschr. f. Geburtsk. u. Frauenkrankh.,* **6**:321–47, 1855.

Edoardo Porro and   CHAPTER

Cesarean Hysterectomy*   *68*

Cesarean section, until the latter part of the nineteenth century, was regarded as one of the most hazardous of obstetric operations, to be undertaken only as a last resort. The operation was carried out 80 times in the United States before 1878, with a maternal mortality of 52.5 per cent. Not a single cesarean section was performed among the first thousand confinements in the Sloane Maternity Hospital from January 1, 1888, to October 1, 1890.[6] Abdominal hysterectomy, likewise, achieved medical respectability only in the closing decades of the last century. The earlier attitude toward this operation was epitomized editorially in the *London Medico-Chirurgical Review* of 1825:[4] "A more cruel, bloody, and ill-judged operation is not, we think, recorded in the annals of surgery. . . . We consider the extirpation of a uterus not previously protruded or inverted, one of the most cruel and unfeasible operations that ever was projected or executed by the head or hand of man." Before 1863 abdominal hysterectomy had proved fatal in seven eighths of the patients on whom it was attempted; only in three cases had it been performed successfully in the United States. Cesarean hysterectomy becomes something of a paradox, therefore, when viewed in historic perspective, for it evolved from efforts to circumvent the mortal danger of abdominal delivery by the addition to it of a similarly formidable procedure, uterine extirpation.

* This chapter originally published in *Surg., Gynec. & Obst.,* **106**:245–50, 1958; reprinted by permission. Copyright, 1958, by The Franklin H. Martin Memorial Foundation.
584

The history of cesarean hysterectomy dates back to 1768, exactly 100 years before it was first carried out in the human, when Joseph Cavallini successfully excised the pregnant uteri of dogs and sheep, proving that the organ was "not at all necessary to life," and speculated that a more fortunate generation would demonstrate that the womb "may be plucked out with impunity from the human body." The background of cesarean hysterectomy has been recorded by J. H. Young in his monograph on the history of cesarean section.[9] In 1809, Godofried P. Michaelis suggested that the great danger of cesarean section might be ameliorated by combining with it amputation of the uterus, but there is nothing to indicate that Michaelis ever made such an attempt himself. Similar thoughts were voiced by others. James Blundell, for example, in his obstetric lectures at Guy's Hospital stated in 1827:[2] "In speculative moments I have sometimes felt inclined to persuade myself, the dangers of the Caesarean operation might, perhaps, be considerably diminished by the total removal of the uterus." Blundell's efforts to test his hypothesis were limited to rabbits, however; others continued to experiment on bitches.

STORER'S OPERATION

The first cesarean hysterectomy on a woman was performed on July 21, 1868, by Horatio Robinson Storer. Storer was born in Boston in 1830, the son of David Humphreys Storer, successor to David Osgood as director of the Boston Lying-in Hospital.[5] After receiving his degree from the Harvard Medical School in 1853, young Storer went abroad to continue his training in Paris and London and to work with the great James Young Simpson in Edinburgh. Upon his return to Boston in 1855 he entered general practice; but, ever a nonconformist, he broke with prudish Bostonian tradition in 1862 by announcing himself a specialist in the diseases of women. He subsequently became the first American physician to teach gynecology as a separate subject. He was also the first surgeon to wear rubber gloves while operating. In 1866 Storer's sturdy independence resulted in his removal from the Harvard faculty. In this same year he performed the fourth successful abdominal hysterectomy in America, removing a myomatous uterus weighing 37 lb.[8]

Heartened by the happy outcome of this case, Storer was emboldened to resort to hysterectomy again, two years later, to stanch the hemorrhage from the uterus during a cesarean section. Storer had posted a milestone in obstetric history—but unwittingly, it would seem, for he did not even deem the event worthy of recording himself, and it remained for his assistant, G. H. Bixby, to report the case before the Boston Gynaecological Society.[1]

The patient, aged 37 years, consulted Storer on July 16, 1868, "for pregnancy complicated by a large obscure abdominal tumor." The tumor blocked the pelvis to such a degree that Storer predicted vaginal delivery of the infant would be impossible, even with craniotomy. He instructed the patient to notify Dr. Bixby at the onset of labor. Recalled Bixby:

Two days afterwards, . . . being out of town, I was telegraphed for, in great haste; from some mistake the message did not reach me for twenty-four hours. Upon my arrival . . . I found the patient suffering from slight pains, the water having passed off some hours previously. By vaginal examination I found the cervix dilated to the size of a dime-piece. Having got the finger past the point of obstruction by the tumor, there was not the least difficulty in detecting the foetal head, which presented still very high up, pressing upon the tumor from above. . . .

After consultation the next day among Professor D. H. Storer, Dr. H. R. Storer, a Dr. Warner, and Dr. Bixby, "it was decided to leave the case for some little time to the natural powers." Bixby continued:

I spent the night with the patient, during which she had . . . slight pains. Examination, however, revealed nothing new, and in the morning so completely in statu quo was the condition of everything, that I even doubted the fact of her being in labor at all. In the morning Dr. H. R. Storer saw the case again, and having satisfied himself that no progress whatever had been made, owing entirely to the presence of the tumor, and that this condition would continue, so far as any efforts on the part of nature were concerned, decided to proceed upon the following day to an abdominal section as the only possible chance of saving the mother's life.

July 21st . . . the patient was placed under the influence of chloroform, another examination made, and the following conclusions were definitely arrived at: 1st, that there was present, pregnancy complicated either by a fibro-cystic tumor of the uterus, or a multilocular ovarian cyst, with one of its appendages crowded down between the pelvis and the uterus; 2d, that even with mechanical interference the escape of the foetus per vias naturales was utterly impossible; 3d, that the space between the tumor and the pelvic wall, being less than one and a half inches, would not admit either of craniotomy, cephalotripsy, cranioclasm, or any other mechanical interference per vaginam; and 4th, that Caesarean section . . . was certainly indicated as the only resort, provided it were impossible to remove the tumor by abdominal section, and then proceed to a forced labor.

. . . Upon cutting through the peritoneum there presented a large, smooth, bluish-colored tumor, which might have been taken either for the impregnated uterus, a discolored cyst of the ovary, or a fibrous tumor. . . . Exploration with the hand within the abdomen established the existence of a fibro-cystic tumor of the left and lower anterior wall of the uterus, with an outgrowth nearly the size of the foetal head, originally pediculated, but now firmly adherent low down to the walls of the pelvis. On the right the uterus, with the foetal members plainly to be felt through its walls, was perceptible, but so retroflexed as to render it very difficult to cut into at this point.

An exploratory incision was now undertaken in the tumor situated at the left. Each stroke of the knife revealed a regular series of concentric layers of fibrous tissue, not unlike that of the uterus. After cutting down to the distance of about two inches, the scalpel glided suddenly into a cavity, filled with a thick, brown, semi-fluid, putrilaginous substance, evidently resulting from degeneration of the fibroid. The hemorrhage being already very profuse, and the danger from shock and exhaustion imminent, with a few rapid strokes of the knife, Dr. Storer extended his incision into the cavity of the uterus, and with all expedition removed a male child, weighing eight pounds; it being, as well as the placenta, in an advanced state of decomposition. . . . There was little time to be lost, for the hemorrhage from the incision into the vascular structure of the uterus, together with the open vessels at the site of the placental insertion . . . was perfectly frightful. It was apparent that the tumor in the uterine wall would necessarily prevent a perfect contraction of the organ, and thus render suppression of the hemorrhage impossible, contrary to what obtains in ordinary uncomplicated cases of Caesarean section.

With his usual self-possession, Dr. Storer decided to remove the whole mass as far as possible. . . . Accordingly, a large-sized trocar having been passed through the upper segment of the cervix uteri, and a metallic cord passed doubled through its canula, the whole was firmly tied in two parts. Fearing lest this constriction might not prove sufficient to check the hemorrhage from so vascular a part, especially the pedicle of the pelvic tumor, which was included in the ligature, the ecraseur with its chain outside the canula . . . was applied, and the mass slowly constricted. Having been removed, its stump was held by the ligature, and seared by the hot iron. Not feeling even then secure against a recurrence of hemorrhage, Dr. Storer applied his clamp-shield, which controlled the pedicle completely. Everything now being perfectly safe, without the least hemorrhage persisting, the abdomen was carefully cleansed of all coagula, and the wound brought together by ten deep silver sutures, which involved the peritoneum . . . The operation was commenced at half-past twelve M., and terminated at half-past three, P.M.

The patient recovered from the effects of the chloroform and "returned to consciousness in the happiest way, without complaining of the least pain or discomfort." The following day she began to fail, however, and succumbed on the third postoperative day. "It was a matter of surprise to all concerned," commented Bixby, "in view of the terrific character of the operation, that she should have survived it at all, and still more for so long a time."

PORRO'S OPERATION

Eight years elapsed before the next cesarean hysterectomy. In contrast to Storer's hasty decision to proceed with amputation of the puerperal uterus as a lifesaving hemostatic measure in a patient who had been in labor for three days, his three-hour operation, his apparent failure to appreciate the significance of his feat and his unconcern with its publication, and the fatal outcome to both mother and child, the operation performed by Edoardo Porro of Pavia, Italy, on May 21, 1876, was a carefully planned and rehearsed procedure carried out in 26 minutes under optimal conditions with survival of both patients. Porro, moreover, sensing the importance of his achievement, the first successful cesarean hysterectomy, publicized it in a report of 63 pages. The operation has since been known throughout the world as the Porro operation.

Until the time of Porro, cesarean section had suffered a particularly bleak

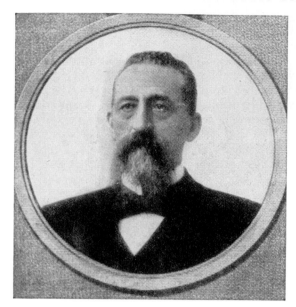

Fig. 68-1. Edoardo Porro (1842–1902).

record in Pavia, no woman ever having survived the operation in that city. On April 27, 1876, a 25-year-old primigravid dwarf, Julia Cavallini, was referred from the general hospital of Pavia to Porro's obstetric clinic in the university because of the suspicion of a malformed pelvis. The patient's surname, by coincidence, was the same as that of the experimenter who, a century earlier, had predicted that extirpation of the gravid uterus would one day be carried out safely in women. Between the ages of three and ten years the patient had suffered from rickets, and during this period was unable to support herself in the erect position without help. The resultant skeletal deformities were partially corrected in later years, and she became married to a teacher of dramatics. Her last menstrual period, a matter of some uncertainty, was recorded as mid-July, 1875.

She was 148 cm tall and presented the typical bony stigmas of rickets, including saber shins, knock-knees, bowlegs, enlarged joints, and scoliosis. The right iliac crest was 4 cm higher than the left. Obstetric examination revealed a normal intrauterine pregnancy at term, the vertex floating, and the fetal heart best heard in the left lower quadrant of the abdomen. The retropubic and subpubic arches were very narrow, the sacral promontory was very prominent and deviated to the right, and the pelvis narrowed transversely as well. The diagonal conjugate measured 7 cm. In addition, the superior strait was overhung by the spondylolisthesis of the lumbar vertebrae, which formed a sort of roof over the pelvic inlet.

"It was obvious," Porro wrote,[7] "that absolute disproportion existed and that cesarean section was mandatory." He therefore called a consultation with a group of his colleagues, gravely pointed out the impossibility of vaginal delivery or even embryotomy and that no alternative to cesarean section existed; and all solemnly concurred. Prolonged discussion followed concerning the location of the uterine incision and the methods for coping with the anticipated hemorrhage, some of the consultants even advocating inversion of the uterus after its evacuation, to be followed by vaginal hysterectomy. Tacit consent was finally given to Porro's proposed plan to amputate the uterus through the abdominal incision if serious hemorrhage were encountered after delivery of the infant.

The patient was admitted to the hospital in anticipation of labor, which began at 10 A.M., May 21, with rupture of the membranes. The patient's predicament was explained to her, but operation was deferred while she sought religious support. Recounted Porro:

I did not press the matter until 4 P.M. By now the pains were quite strong, and these alone sufficed to persuade the patient to accept our advice. . . . At 4:40 P.M. she was taken to the obstetric amphitheater, which had been heated to 18° C. Everything was in readiness. . . . To avoid confusion, all the assistants had been carefully instructed in advance, each as to his own duty. . . . At 4:42 P.M. the chloroform anesthesia was begun . . . and the amphitheater was rapidly filled with a large number of physicians and students. . . .

At 4:51 P.M. we began to cut through the abdominal wall, layer by layer, through a 12-cm incision in the linea alba. . . . After the peritoneal cavity was opened . . . the uterus was immediately incised, in the same direction and to the same extent as the abdominal incision. . . . Unable to deliver the fetal head with my right hand in the uterus, I finally reached up, grasped and delivered the right leg and thigh; the left leg, trunk, arms, and head followed immediately. We extracted a large [3300-gm] female infant, alive, healthy, well formed, and crying spontaneously. After tying and dividing the umbilical cord we proceeded to extract the placenta, which was removed intact, together with the major portion of its membranes. . . .

The uterus bled from its cut edges. We brought the organ out through the abdominal incision, and with our fingers we compressed the points that were bleeding most vigorously, but adequate hemostasis could not be obtained.

Attempts to control the bleeding by suture were also unsuccessful and finally abandoned. Narrated Porro:

It was providential that we had made all the preparations necessary for hysterectomy; otherwise the patient would surely have died.

Holding the uterus up out of the abdominal wound . . . we placed the strong wire snare of Cintrat at the level of the internal os and drew it very tight . . . winding it also around the left ovary, to hold the wire up and keep it from slipping down over the lower end of the cervix. . . . After we ascertained that the blood flow was completely shut off, we excised the uterus above the ligature . . . the constricted stump remaining within the ligature. . . . With the index finger of the right hand in the vagina, a large curved clamp was introduced through the left side of the cul-de-sac into the peritoneal cavity, the left hand serving as a guide. A 5-mm drainage tube was thus drawn down into the vagina from the peritoneal cavity.

We proceeded immediately with the peritoneal toilet. After removing two small blood clots and cleansing the uterine stump, we noticed a small ovarian cyst, the size of a small nut, attached by a long, thin pedicle to the part of the left ovary distal to the ligature. With a fine thread we excised this tumor distal to the ligature. . . . Suture of the abdominal wall was accomplished with a strong, pliable silver wire . . . only four sutures being necessary for perfect approximation.

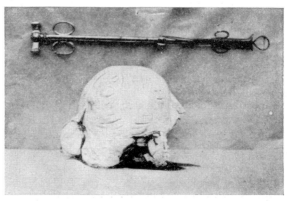

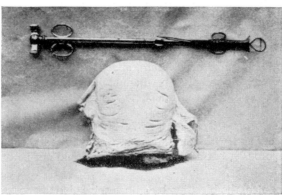

Fig. 68-2. Plate from Porro's paper,[7] showing anterior and posterior aspects of the excised uterus and adnexa, together with the snare of Cintrat.

The uterine stump was incorporated into the lower angle of the wound by means of the lowermost suture and painted with iron perchloride. The snare and handle were allowed to rest between the patient's legs. Thus was completed the first successful cesarean section in the city of Pavia and the first successful cesarean hysterectomy in history.

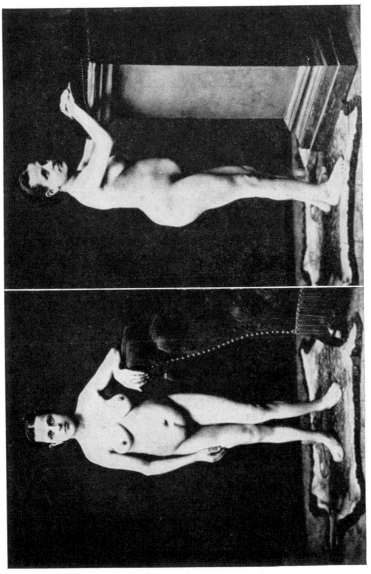

Fig. 68-3. Plate from Porro's paper,[7] showing Julia Cavallini after her convalescence from cesarean hysterectomy.

591

The patient's postoperative course was marked by vulvovaginitis, decubitus ulcers over the sacrum, suppuration at the lower end of the abdominal wound, and a urinary tract infection, but was characterized by Porro as "uneventful," for such trivia were completely overshadowed by the fact that the patient had indeed survived. The snare was removed with the gangrenous portion of the uterine stump on the fourth day after operation, and the sutures two days later. The vaginal drain was withdrawn the following week when Porro pronounced the abdominal wound "most beautiful and almost completely healed."

A long discussion concerning the morality of the operation was subsequently held with the Bishop of Pavia, who sanctioned the hysterectomy as a procedure for saving the patient's life. With this ecclesiastic backing, Porro stated before the Medical Congress of Turin: "I believe that the day is not far off in which medical science will pronounce its solemn verdict approving utero-ovarian amputation in every case of cesarean section." During the ensuing years the operation was indeed adopted in many centers as the standard procedure in cases of abdominal delivery, with a dramatic reduction in the maternal mortality resulting. Since Porro's day the indications for the operation have undergone much change, but cesarean hysterectomy continues to be known as the Porro section.

PORRO'S LIFE

Edoardo Porro, the son of an engineer, was born in Padua, September 17, 1842.[3] After obtaining his medical degree from the University of Pavia in 1866, he embarked on a course of postgraduate training at L'Ospedale Maggiore in Milan; but when the Austro-Prussian War broke out he forsook his studies and, together with his younger brother Paolo, volunteered in the fight for Italian unification under Garibaldi. In 1868 Porro returned to Milan as an assistant in the school of obstetrics in the provincial hospital of Santa Caterina, and three years later he was made director of the school. In response to a call from Pavia in 1875 Porro assumed the chair of obstetrics in the university, where he remained until 1882, when he achieved his major ambition, to head the School of Obstetrics of Milan. Here he spent the rest of his life, displaying a talent for hospital administration and helping to organize an anatomic institute and a surgical clinic. In addition to his professional activities he maintained an active interest in a liberal form of government, and in 1891 was elected to the Italian Senate. In 1902 Porro accidentally wounded his hand while operating on an infected patient. Never recovering from the sepsis that developed, he died on July 18. Porro's principal publications are listed in a 1902 issue of *Revue de Gynécologie* (Vol. 6, pp. 723–25).

REFERENCES

1. Bixby, G. H.: Extirpation of the puerperal uterus by abdominal section. *J. Gynaec. Soc. Boston*, 1:223–32, 1869.

2. Blundell, J.: Lectures on the theory and practice of midwifery, delivered at Guy's Hospital by Dr. Blundell. Lecture XXVII. Of the indication of the death of the foetus. *Lancet,* **2**:161–67, 1827–1828.

3. Castelli, G.: Edoardo Porro. *L'Ospedale Maggiore,* **26**:34–45, 1938.

4. Extirpation of the uterus. *London Med.-Chir. Rev.,* **3**:264–67, 1825.

5. Irving, F. C.: *Safe Deliverance.* Houghton Mifflin Co., Boston, 1942, pp. 104–19.

6. McLane, J. W.: The Sloane Maternity Hospital. Report on the first series of one thousand successive confinements from January 1st, 1888, to October 1st, 1890. *Am. J. Obst.,* **24**:385–418, 1891.

7. Porro, E.: Dell' amputazione utero-ovarica come complemento di taglio cesareo. *Ann. univ. med. e chir.,* **237**:289–351, 1876.

8. Storer, H. R.: Successful removal of the uterus and both ovaries by abdominal section; the tumor, fibro-cystic, weighing thirty-seven pounds. *Am. J. M. Sc.,* **51**(n.s.):110–39, 1866.

9. Young, J. H.: *Caesarean Section. The History and Development of the Operation from Earliest Times.* H. K. Lewis & Co., Ltd., London, 1944, pp. 93–107.

Wilhelm Latzko and Extraperitoneal Cesarean Section

Cesarean section without pain was made possible by Simpson's introduction of anesthesia into obstetrics in 1847,[11] and the dreaded prospect of uncontrollable bleeding was eliminated by Sänger's description in 1882 of a method for precise coaptation of the uterine wound edges with sutures.[10] A spectacular decline in the previously prohibitive cesarean section mortality resulted from the application of these great boons to operative obstetrics, but their benefits failed to extend any significant measure of relief to the neglected or infected patient delivered by the abdominal route. Death from peritonitis remained her almost certain fate.

In contrast to the aseptic technique of twentieth-century obstetrics and the specific antibacterial agents available for prophylaxis and treatment, understanding as well as effective therapy of infection remained beyond the reach of the early-nineteenth-century practitioner. His bumbling efforts to prevent or overcome inflammation after cesarean section are well exemplified by the measures outlined in Dewees' *Compendious System of Midwifery,*[3] probably the outstanding American text of its day. Wrote Dewees:

This must be attempted by a strict antiphlogistic regimen, confining the patient to barley water, thin gruel, tapioca, rennet whey, &c.—forbidding, in the most earnest manner, all stimulating drinks, meats, broths, &c.; in a word, every thing animal, or spirituous, unless some contraindications may exist, or arise. . . . With

594

the same object in view, Baudelocque recommends the same plan; but he unfortunately, in his enumeration of the antiphlogistic articles, reckons veal and chicken broth, both, or either of which, I would most positively forbid. He also recommends, that the patient should suckle her child if it be living; if not, to have the breast drawn by glasses or puppies.

Among the special operations designed to circumvent or reduce the hazard of postoperative peritonitis were cesarean hysterectomy and division of the pelvic brim by symphysiotomy or pubiotomy, which have been discussed previously. Another procedure aimed at eliminating this forbidding specter in patients requiring abdominal delivery was extraperitoneal cesarean section, which has been practiced for over a century and by a variety of approaches and techniques, each associated with the name of its principal proponent. The possibility of extracting the fetus through the maternal abdomen without opening the peritoneal cavity was first conceived in 1820 by Ferdinand von Ritgen, stimulated by the success of Abernethy and Cooper in extraperitoneal ligation of the external iliac artery for aneurysm.

The plan of the operation, as later described by von Ritgen,[8] was carefully laid out in advance:

(1) The obstetrician would station himself at the patient's right side, insert a male catheter, press the bladder with it toward the left, and then give it to an assistant to hold. Another assistant, standing at the left of the patient's chest, places one hand below the umbilicus, the other to the left of it, and draws the uterus toward him, as a result of which the skin in the region of the incision is put on a stretch. (2) An elliptical incision is now made in the skin, from the region of the iliac crest almost to the pubic symphysis. . . . (3) The skin incision is followed by a similar incision through the muscle, carried out with great care not to injure the peritoneum. The transected arteries, as the epigastric, abdominal, and circumflex iliac . . . are ligated immediately [the modern type of hemostat had not yet been invented]. (4) The cellular tissue that covers the peritoneum inferiorly can now be separated with the finger or scalpel handle, the wound edges spread, and the abdominal cavity undermined, to permit an approach behind the walls of the vagina. (5) At this point the operator inserts a bladder sound into the vagina so that the tip elevates the vaginal wall above the middle of the right innominate line. At the same time the assistant holding the uterus draws it sharply away from the ilium and pubis, so that as much as possible of the lower part of the vagina is brought forward. (6) The operator now presses the tip of the bladder sound through the vaginal wall, protecting the neighboring parts from injury with the index finger, middle finger, and thumb. (7) After the point has penetrated, a blunt-pointed knife is led into the groove and the vagina divided toward the urethra, which must not be injured. The sound is then removed and the incision continued, over the right index finger, as far as possible toward the rectum without injuring it. (8) If this incision has left a 2- to 3-inch rim of vaginal membrane hanging from the right half of the cervix, this can now be divided up to the edge of the uterus with scissors. (9) A napkin soaked in warm oil is now placed over the

wound and the emergence of the child through it awaited. During this time the uterus must constantly be drawn sharply upward and to the left. . . . (10) After delivery of the child the wound is cleansed and then closed with sutures for the skin and muscles and adhesive-plaster strips. The vaginal wound is to be left alone initially, and later merely moistened with hemlock injections.

The uterine arteries and veins obviously must be divided when the vaginal vault is incised. I do not attach great significance to this, however, for the arteries of this region are only of such strength that they soon stop bleeding spontaneously when completely transected. As to the divided veins, I would rely with confidence on pressure from the presenting fetal head, the retraction of the uterus after delivery of the child, and tamponade with a sponge to combat all danger from this source.

Von Ritgen's first opportunity to try out his new operation came on October 1, 1821. The patient, 37-year-old Joan Peter, "a short, very delicately built person with dark eyes and hair," had had three successful pregnancies previously. A prolonged illness in 1819 led to a severe disturbance in her nutrition, resulting in profound weakness, confinement to bed toward the end of the following year, and ultimately the development of osteomalacia. The patient later conceived again, despite the warning of her physician. When summoned to her aid at the calculated end of her present pregnancy, he found her pelvis severely distorted and contracted, "but the bones were not sufficiently soft to permit the use of forceps"[!] The same physician, von Ritgen noted, "had recently delivered with forceps two children whose mothers suffered from even higher degrees of pelvic contraction, but their bones were so pliable that they gave with the head grasped by the forceps, allowing delivery." Deciding on cesarean section in the present case, the physician turned to von Ritgen, who later wrote:

I betook myself immediately . . . to the patient, where we found the necessary number of assistants. . . . I found her very emaciated, with a small, rapid pulse but afebrile. Complaining of great weakness, she was completely resigned to the pain and the possible outcome of the operation, and wished only that the child be saved. Her labor pains had begun during the forenoon of the preceding day, subsided toward evening, resumed during the night, and grown stronger up until five o'clock of the present morning, since which time they recurred at intervals of five to eight minutes.

Von Ritgen's examination confirmed the distortion of the pelvis and vertebrae previously observed by his colleague:

The uterus lay with the fundus deviated toward the patient's left, the cervix toward her right side. The cervix, 2½ inches dilated, felt soft and edematous. The head presented in R.O.P., with the left parietal bone lying over the caved-in right pubic bone of the mother. The sacral promontory was very easily palpable and the head rather high, its engagement prevented by the projection of the last two lumbar vertebrae. . . .

I wished to postpone the operation until complete dilatation, so as to be able to deliver the child quickly after the incision was made; but the patient's great weakness would not permit any further delay. After her bladder and bowel were emptied and she received a dose of opium, the operation was begun about 10 A.M. The patient was placed supine on a firm table covered with a mattress, a large sheet of oilcloth, and a pillow. . . .

I made the incision on the right side, through the skin and muscle, according to the previously described plan. The divided arteries of the lower abdominal wall were ligated and the vaginal wall exposed on the right side, where the cellular tissue could be separated easily with the finger tips. I inserted the handle of my wooden pelvimeter into the vagina, and by pushing the head of this instrument against the vaginal vault, elevated the latter. . . . After transferring the pelvimeter to the first assistant, I incised the vaginal vault in its elevated position and enlarged the opening . . . almost to the urethra, until the incision was 1½ inches long. The bleeding from the divided vessels of the vaginal vault was negligible and stopped spontaneously.

I then proceeded to extend the incision another 1½ inches posteriorly; but scarcely was this done when one torrent of blood gushed into the wound and another out of the vagina. Without delay I pressed a sponge, soaked in cold water, into the wound, and this stopped the bleeding completely. I awaited a uterine contraction, but this was weaker than the previous ones and failed to propel the child forward perceptibly. I then decided to incise the cervix with the next contraction and to extract the child's head; but when I removed the sponge, the blood raged forth again so violently that I had to abandon this idea and push the sponge back into the vaginal wound at once. The decision was therefore made to leave the delivery of the child to nature if possible. . . . The next half hour was devoted to reviving the patient with wine, cinnamon drops, and the like, and to stimulation of the uterine contractions; but these stopped completely, and the patient's strength sank very low. The fetus still showed active movements, and immediate intervention became imperative in order to salvage it at least. Symphysiotomy could have been performed easily, with the anticipation of much give at the sacroiliac articulations because of the softening of the bones; but this would have involved the point where the sponge was stanching the hemorrhage and still would not have permitted immediate delivery of the child. Renewed bleeding from the vaginal wound was just enough to contraindicate podalic version and extraction. While we were deliberating over the procedure to use, the patient lapsed into unconsciousness. . . . As soon as she regained consciousness, I quickly seized the knife, made an ordinary cesarean incision, and in a few moments extracted a vigorous male infant.

The sponge was then removed and the wound closed without suture of the uterus. The child survived, but the mother died on the third postoperative day, to the surprise of none.

Von Ritgen's attempt at extraperitoneal abdominal section thus ended in failure: not only with loss of the patient, but with abandonment of the planned procedure. It must be noted, moreover, that the operation he had outlined and sought to execute entailed incision of the vagina rather than the uterus. Properly speaking, therefore, it must be called an abdominal elytrotomy rather than a cesarean section. The former term was applied by L. A. Baudelocque [1] to a similar operation later described by him.

The earliest published reference to extraperitoneal section of the uterus proper appears in a letter dated September 28, 1824, from W. E. Horner, adjunct professor of anatomy in the University of Pennsylvania, to W. P. Dewees, reproduced in the latter's textbook.[3] Wrote Horner:

The Caesarean operation, as commonly performed, puts into such danger the life of the mother, that it is still a desideratum to ascertain some modification of it, which may diminish its fatality, and thereby inspire the profession with more confidence and promptness in undertaking it. Several changes in it have been proposed from the time of its first adoption. . . . They all involve the necessity of cutting into the cavity of the peritoneum, on which circumstances, it is generally conceded, the great danger of the operation depends.

This operation has been a frequent subject of conversations which I have held with our common friend, Dr. Physick, and I have been as often instructed by the views which he has taken of it. More than two years ago, it being then a matter of particular inquiry with me, I was struck by the following proposition of his in regard to it, which made a very strong impression on me, and the justness of which I have ever since been extremely anxious to verify by dissection. It is well known to anatomists, that but a very small portion of the upper anterior part of the vagina, in the unimpregnated state, is covered by peritoneum, and that the portion of peritoneum which lies upon the forepart of the cervix uteri and vagina is connected to them by a long, loose, cellular tissue, which allows the peritoneum, in the distentions of the urinary bladder, to be separated still farther up from the vagina.

It has not been equally remarked, that this peritoneal covering of the vagina is of a very fugitive character, and that in the moderate distentions of the bladder, the peritoneum leaves completely the vagina, and applies itself to the bladder. It is also true, that if the distention of the bladder be much increased, the peritoneum even leaves the anterior face of the cervix uteri; and its reflexion to the bladder departs thence at the lower part of the *body* itself of the uterus. . . .

Dr. Physick, founding his ideas upon a similar observation made in early life, during the dissection of a pregnant woman, proposes, that in the Caesarean operation, a horizontal section be made of the parietes of the abdomen, just above the pubes. That the peritoneum be stripped from the upper fundus of the bladder, by dissecting through the connecting cellular substance, which will bring the operation to that portion of the cervix uteri where the peritoneum goes to the bladder. The incision being continued through this portion of the uterus, will open its cavity with sufficient freedom for the extraction of the fetus. All of which the Doctor supposes may be done by a careful operation, without cutting through the peritoneum.

It is evident, that if this be a practicable operation, it will diminish immensely the tendency to peritoneal inflammation, and will, in fact, put it on a foundation of danger very closely allied to the taking up of the external iliac artery, near its origin, by turning aside the peritoneum. . . .

Knowing the value which you . . . put upon the suggestions of a person whose mind is so remarkable for its professional sagacity and resources, I have thought that even a proposition not yet confirmed by actual experience of its success, would not be an unacceptable addition to the fund of information you are about to communicate to the public.

For reasons no longer clear a half century elapsed before any effort was made to put Physick's suggested procedure into practice. In February, 1870, T. Gaillard Thomas,[13] apparently unaware that a similar operation had been proposed almost 50 years before, performed an extraperitoneal cesarean section experimentally on a patient who had died of eclampsia, undelivered, near the end of the ninth month. A month later Thomas [14] attempted the operation on a woman desperately ill with pneumonia at the end of the seventh month, but probably had little expectation of saving either mother or child, both of whom succumbed. In 1874 Alexander Skene recorded another unsuccessful resort to extraperitoneal cesarean section, carried out after a failed attempt to deliver the child by craniotomy. A happy outcome to the operation was achieved for the first time two years later, when Skene [12] delivered a living, 10-lb infant to a 31-year-old rachitic patient whose diagonal conjugate measured 2¾ in. and who had lost three infants previously in attempted vaginal deliveries.

LATZKO'S OPERATION

Modifications of the extraperitoneal approach were proposed by Frank and Sellheim; but the operation was performed only sporadically until 1909, when Latzko [7] reported only two maternal deaths among 30 patients operated on by a technique he had recently perfected, and no infant loss attributable to the operation itself. Heightened interest in the procedure was stimulated by Küstner's superb record,[5] three years later, of 72 such sections with no mortality from infection and only one maternal death in all, this being charged to the anesthetic. The Latzko operation's principal difference from the approach suggested by Physick almost a century earlier lay in the lateral displacement of the bladder and peritoneum in the former, in contrast to the separation of the peritoneum from the dome of the bladder and the downward displacement of this organ recommended by Physick. Since the second decade of the present century the Latzko procedure has remained the most popular type of extraperitoneal cesarean section, although the operation's nomenclature has become complicated by a recent spate of minor modifications.

Latzko presented a report of his first operation, performed on April 26, 1908, before the Viennese Medical Society the following week. The patient,

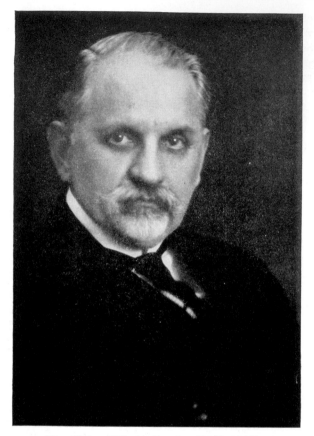

Fig. 69-1. Wilhelm Latzko (1863–1945).

a primigravida, had been in good labor for 18 hours, with her membranes ruptured for 20 hours. The fetus lay in L.O.A., and the cervix was dilated 4 cm. Reported Latzko: [6]

The pelvis was flat, the conjugata vera reduced to 8 cm. The large caput and the overriding of the cranial bones attested the strength of the labor.

After four hours of expectant waiting the situation remained unaltered. . . . It was clear that with the existing pelvic relations delivery of an intact infant was most probably not to be anticipated. But I did not want to abandon at the outset the hope of obtaining a living child. A choice had to be made, therefore, between enlarging the pelvis, by symphysiotomy or pubiotomy, or cesarean section. I decided on the last, but not by classic cesarean section . . . but sought instead a method that would permit opening the uterus extraperitoneally with technical simplicity. My procedure was as follows:

After filling the bladder with 150 cc of fluid, I made a longitudinal incision through the linea alba down to the peritoneum, separated the rectus muscles, bluntly dissected the flaccid bladder from the cervix, and held it to the right with an abdominal retractor. Below the bladder separation and above the loose serosa sufficient room was provided to divide the cervix and lower uterine segment longitudinally. After delivery of a 3600-gm fetus and the placenta the uterine incision was sutured. The mobilized bladder fell back into position spontaneously and the normal anatomic relations were restored by closure of the abdominal wall in layers.

In his definitive account and evaluation of this extraperitoneal procedure a year later [7] Latzko focused his critical attention on pubiotomy and destructive operations on the fetus, the alternative procedures employed in the management of dystocia resulting from disproportion. The advantages of extraperitoneal cesarean section were, as Latzko listed them:

1. It is independent of the degree of disproportion. This advantage is shared with the classic operation, but modern requirements for asepsis limit the latter to the relatively few aseptic cases.

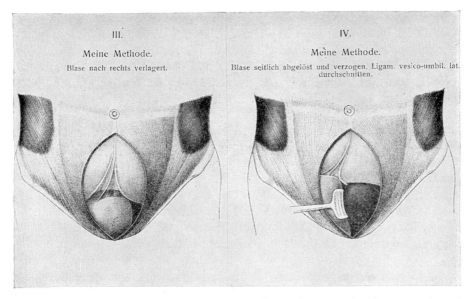

Fig. 69-2. Illustrations from Latzko's paper,[7] showing steps in his extraperitoneal cesarean section. (Reproduced by permission of *Wiener Klinische Wochenschrift.*)

2. It is an operation of delivery, not a preliminary one like splitting the pelvis, and can therefore be carried out at any stage of labor as soon as maternal or fetal indications arise.

3. It allows the forces of labor the greatest latitude, and is thus a conservative operation in the broadest sense. Among 100 cases of classic cesarean section for various indications there are always a number in which spontaneous delivery probably would have occurred with a longer period of waiting. With extraperitoneal cesarean section we can await the indication until the very last moment, so that we never run the risk of performing it unnecessarily.

4. It permits complete control of its technique at all times, in contrast with operations for splitting the pelvis.

5. It is associated with less danger of injury to adjacent structures than is splitting the pelvis.

6. Producing a simple, soft-tissue wound, it is probably less dangerous than pubiotomy, with its complicated bone fracture. . . .

The antibiotics of the mid-twentieth century and the excellent safety record of the low cervical cesarean section, together with the increasing rarity of neglected cases of dystocia, have combined to reduce the importance of the extraperitoneal cesarean section in modern practice. Indeed, in many large obstetric centers this operation is no longer found necessary. Some obstetricians still resort to it, however, not only for infected patients but as the cesarean section of choice.

LATZKO'S LIFE

Wilhelm Latzko was born in Vienna, March 3, 1863.[2,4,9] After graduating in medicine from the University of Vienna in 1886 he trained in surgery under Professor Albert and in obstetrics and gynecology under Breisky. In 1902 Latzko was made director of gynecology at the Wiedner Krankenhaus, where he was succeeded later by Joseph Halban after accepting a similar appointment in the Bettina-Pavillon of the Elisabeth-Spital. He also held the title of extraordinary professor of obstetrics and gynecology in the university. In 1927 he gave a series of lectures at the medical faculty in Buenos Aires, and returned to Argentina in 1939, because of Nazi oppression, prior to settling in New York. He served as consultant to the Margaret Hague Hospital in Jersey City and the Beth Israel Hospital in New York, where he died at the age of 81, February 11, 1945, of cirrhosis and primary carcinoma of the liver. Autopsy revealed no evidence of the intestinal neoplasm for which he had undergone operation 15 years before.

Latzko was a man of many parts. In addition to his professional duties in Vienna, he served temporarily as editor of the weekly newspaper, *Wiener Sonn-und Montags Zeitung,* following the death of his father-in-law. He also assumed the management of an electric-light-bulb factory, another of the family enterprises. He mastered the Spanish language on short notice before his 1927 visit to Argentina, and gave all his lectures there in that tongue. He found his principal source of relaxation in music and excelled at the piano. For many years Latzko's chief professional interest lay in gynecologic urology, and he contributed chapters on this subject to Lichtenberg's *Handbuch der Urologie* and the Halban-Seitz *Biologie und Pathologie des Weibes.* Latzko's name is also associated eponymically with his procedure for the cure of vesicovaginal fistula.

REFERENCES

1. Baudelocque, L. A.: *Opération Césarienne. Élytrotomie ou section du vagin, précédée, ou non, de la ligature, ou de la compression de l'artère iliaque interne.* Paris, 1844.
2. Deaths: William Francis Latzko. *J.A.M.A.,* **127**:942, 1945.
3. Dewees, W. P.: *A Compendious System of Midwifery, Chiefly Designed to Facilitate the Inquiries of Those Who May Be Pursuing this Branch of Study,* 4th ed. Carey & Lea, Philadelphia, 1830, pp. 580–84.
4. Kagan, S. R.: *Jewish Medicine.* Medico-Historical Press, Boston, 1952, p. 481.
5. Küstner, O.: Uber den extraperitonealen Kaiserschnitt. *München. med. Wchnschr.,* **59**:2321–22, 1912.
6. Latzko, W.: *In* Vorhandl. ärztl. Gesellsch. u. Kongressberichte. *Wien. klin. Wchnschr.,* **21**:737–39, 1908.
7. Latzko, W.: Der extraperitoneale Kaiserschnitt, seine Geschichte, seine Technik und seine Indikationen. *Wien. klin. Wchnschr.,* **22**:477–82, 1909.
8. Ritgen, F. A. von: Geschichte eines mit ungünstigem Erfolge verrichteten Bauchscheidenschnittes und Folgerungen daraus. *Heidelberg klin. Ann.,* **1**:263–76, 1825.
9. Rojas, D. A.: Palabras del Senor Presidente con motivo del fallecimiento del miembro honarario extranjero. *Bol. Soc. de obst. y ginec. de Buenos Aires,* **24**:97–99, 1945.
10. Sänger, M.: *Der Kaiserschnitt bei Uterusfibromen nebst vergleichender Methodik der Sectio Caesarea und der Porro-Operation.* W. Engelmann, Leipzig, 1882.
11. Simpson, J. Y.: Notes on the employment of the inhalation of sulphuric ether in the practice of midwifery. *Month. J. M. Sc.,* **7** (Part 2):721–28, 1847.
12. Skene, A. J. C.: Gastro-elytrotomy successfully performed. *Am. J. Obst.,* **8**:636–39, 1876.
13. Thomas, T. G.: Gastro-elytrotomy; a substitute for the caesarean section. —A paper read before the Yonkers Medical Association. *Am. J. Obst.,* **3**:125–39, 1871.
14. Thomas, T. G.: Laparo-elytrotomy: A substitute for the caesarean section. *Am. J. Obst.,* **11**:225–47, 1878.

Vasili Vasilievich Stroganov*
and His Eclamptic Regimen †

CHAPTER

70

Satisfactory treatment of disease presupposes knowledge of its cause. So long as eclampsia remains "the disease of theories," its etiology undiscovered, management of this dramatic disorder of pregnancy must be empiric. Efforts to control its convulsions have included such drastic and diverse measures as cold compresses, hot packs and pilocarpine to induce sweating, chloroform, purging, blistering, bloodletting, leeching, accouchement forcé, and cesarean section.

A case report from Thomas Willis' *Essay of the Pathology of the Brain and Nervous Stock,*[9] published in 1684, exemplifies some of the seventeenth-century methods of coping with convulsions in pregnancy. Willis wrote:

Instituting Curatory intentions, according to this kind of *Aetiology,* I order'd to have blood taken from this sick Lady, at what time she most grievously laboured, out of the *Saphena vein,* and within two days, to be given her a gentle Cathartick, and that to be reiterated, once or twice in a week: Also on other days, Morning and Evening, I gave her spirits of Harts-horn, and at other hours, twice or thrice

---

* Transliterated from the Cyrillic into the Latin alphabet, Stroganov is sometimes spelled *Stroganoff* or *Stroganow*; Vasili appears also as *Vasilii, Vasily, Wasili,* and, in its Anglicized form, *Basil.*

† This chapter originally published in *Obst. & Gynec.,* 11:234–39, 1958; reprinted by permission. Copyright © 1958, by the American College of Obstetricians and Gynecologists.

in a day, of the *Powder of Pearls*, and *Crabs-eyes*, with a Dose of the following Julup: Take of the *water of Snails*, and of *Worms magisterial* each three Ounces, of *Saxifrage* and *black-Cherries* each four Ounces, of *Hysterical water* two Ounces, of the *syrrop of Corrals* an Ounce and a half, of the tincture of Costor one Dram, mingle them: The bath of sweet herbs was frequently used; when necessity urged, she took *Opiats* always with good success: *Vesicatories* were applied to the inward part of either thigh, also to the hinder part of her neck; also *Fomentations, Oyntments, Clisters, Cupping-glasses, Sneezing-Powders,* with many other manner of administrations were prescribed, according to the exigencies of the symptoms.

Artificial termination of pregnancy was then recommended for many years as the crux of therapy for antepartal eclampsia, and hastening of delivery for convulsions occurring during labor, for what could have been more logical than to remove, as quickly as possible, the *sine qua non* of the disease? The somber experience of astute observers, however, led them to repeated protest against the shocking mortality associated with forceful and traumatic efforts at delivery of the convulsing parturient. A conservative approach to eclampsia was clearly recommended by Denman as early as the eighteenth century, but the wisdom of his teaching has had to be relearned, unfortunately, by several subsequent generations of obstetricians. Wrote Denman: [2]

Some writers have recommended the speedy delivery of the patient, as the most eligible, and only effectual method of removing puerperal convulsions; but others have insisted that the labour should be uninterrupted.

From the histories of all the cases of puerperal convulsions which have been recorded, it appears, that a greater number have died of those who were delivered by art, than when the labours were resigned to nature.

As far as my experience enables me to judge, we ought not to attempt to deliver women with convulsions before some progress is made in the labour.

The voice of conservatism was raised again in 1823 by Dewees, in an effort to stem the tide of traumatic intervention. Dewees pleaded: [3]

[Should we find] that there is no change made in the os tincae, nor any evidence of uterine contraction—in a word, not a symptom of labour . . . then, should we attempt delivery by forcing the mouth of the uterus, as some direct, we should inevitably destroy our patient; delivery in this case is not to be thought of, because there is no effort of nature for this object; and where this effort does not manifest itself, it were madness, nay, I had like to have said, *murderous* to attempt it. Our whole duty in this case consists in proper medical treatment. . . .

Denman in England and Dewees in America were two of the most highly respected figures in obstetrics, and their teachings carried great influence. With the birth of anesthesia in the mid-nineteenth century, however, obstetric surgery assumed new license; and the admonitions of conservatism were promptly forgotten by the new generation of obstetricians in their treatment of eclampsia. Accouchement forcé again began to flourish and the maternal mortality to soar. In a report on the experience with eclampsia in the Boston Lying-in Hospital, Green [4] noted in 1892 that six of the ten patients died in whom labor had been induced during the preceding eight years. Others began to report equally bad results with other types of operative intervention.

Again, therefore, in 1896, the earlier warnings against active interference in eclampsia were renewed, together with a plea for conservative management. From the Rotunda in Dublin Tweedy preached: [8]

It is an unfortunate fact that the surgical treatment is growing in favour day by day, and this is not surprising, for not only has it the sanction of great names, but it also affords the medical attendant much satisfaction, substituting as it does an active mode of treatment for inactivity with apparent impotence. I cannot but think, however, that it is unsound in theory and disastrous in practice.

. . . We should pause before inducing labour, knowing as we do that the danger of the disease is enormously increased by the multiplicity of the fits, and that the fits are easily induced by reflex stimulation. Thus a vaginal examination, abdominal palpation, massage of the kidneys, cold blasts of air, but worst of all, and above all, the dilatation of the cervix, have been observed over and over again to increase the frequency and severity of the attacks.

Tweedy's program of sedation became the basis for modern conservative management:

Let me now turn to the method of treating eclampsia that has been pursued in that institution [the Rotunda Hospital] for upwards of three years. . . . I allude to the hypodermic injection of large doses of morphin. Beginning with the injection of ½ grain, this is followed in two hours by ¼ grain, and so on gradually, until either the symptoms are alleviated or until 2 grains have been given in twenty-four hours. If, in spite of this treatment, labour sets in, forceps are applied to hasten delivery so soon as the os will safely admit their application; but it is held that manual dilatation of the cervix, which in reality means a bursting of that structure, is not a justifiable proceeding.

STROGANOV'S METHOD

At the dawn of the twentieth century the maternal mortality from eclampsia varied between 20 and 30 per cent in most clinics. Forced labor remained the vogue in most quarters. Suddenly, tremendous impetus was given to the newly revived conservatism by a dramatic report from Russia. Stroganov, in 1899, gave a preliminary accounting of 45 cases treated by his new method, and the following year read his first definitive report (Fig. 70-2),[7] before the obstetric section of the thirteenth international congress in Paris, encompassing 92 cases of eclampsia treated over a three-year period with

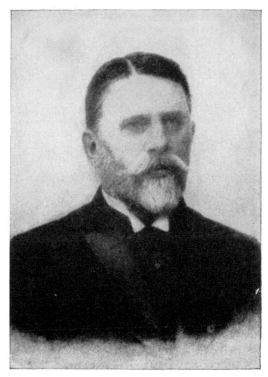

Fig. 70-1. Vasili Vasilievich Stroganov (1857–1938). (Courtesy of USSR Ministry of Health.)

an unprecedented maternal mortality of only 5.4 per cent. This paper revolutionized the treatment of eclampsia, and the "Stroganov regimen" was quickly adopted, with modifications, throughout the world. Stroganov himself continued to make minor changes in therapeutic detail during the ensuing decades, but the principles of his treatment have remained largely unaltered.

The low mortality reported by Stroganov was all the more impressive because the clientele of his clinics included the worst and most neglected cases of eclampsia. Indeed, of the five deaths, two occurred in patients admitted in coma after 20 convulsions at home, and another as a result of puerperal sepsis. In only two of the 92 cases, therefore, was his treatment charged with failure. Subsequent Russian experience [6] confirmed the value of Stroganov's regimen. Twelve hospitals in Leningrad treated 400 cases of eclampsia by the Stroganov method exclusively during the years 1932 and 1933, and obtained a maternal mortality of 4 per cent without resorting to cesarean section in a single case. By 1935 Stroganov was able to report on 1113 cases treated under his supervision, with a 3.7 per cent mortality. The infants in this series shared with their mothers in the benefits of conservative management, the uncorrected fetal mortality declining to the gratifying low of 20 per cent.

Stroganov directed his therapeutic efforts at support of the patient's circulatory, respiratory, and renal functions; but some of the measures he employed, such as the rectal instillation of saline solution, have received no endorsement or have actually been contraindicated by more recent studies of the pathologic physiology of pregnancy toxemia. He wrote: [7]

Another excellent agent for regulating the heart's activity is digitalis. When the pulse was over 110–120 beats per minute, I often prescribed digitalis until the rate was lowered, preparing 180 gm of an infusion of 0.5 to 0.6 gm of digitalis leaves and giving 6 tablespoons in 24 hours, by mouth if the patient was conscious and by rectum if comatose.

. . . During and after each attack all measures should be taken to prevent or reduce as much as possible the entry of mucus and food into the larynx and trachea. The mucus is usually removed from the mouth by a finger wrapped in a cloth or by a pair of tongs, and if a great quantity of mucus is present and cannot be reached the patient is placed on her right side during the attack so that the fluid can drain out more easily by itself. To improve the oxygenation of the heart it is very important to have the patient breathe oxygen as soon as respiratory movement begins and until the cyanosis disappears. It is just as important to see to the proper activity of the lungs after the attack. The movements of the thoracic cage should not be restricted by any kind of heavy object lying on it, nor by an uncomfortable position of the patient. If the patient is very sick I consider it important that even her hands not lie on her breasts and that her chest not press against any resistant object, even a pillow or heavy blanket. In severe cases, if much mucus is present in the respiratory passages and tends to collect in the lungs, the patient's position should be changed from time to time. The supine position is preferred by most patients, but for optimal pulmonary function and to facilitate the drainage of fluids from the respiratory passages, the patient should be turned from side to side every one to one-and-a-half hours. . . .

In the face of frank or impending pulmonary edema, with impaired gaseous exchange within the lungs, Stroganov recommended dry cupping over the chest and back or actual bleeding, but admitted that he had not found occasion to resort to the latter in his 92 cases. He stressed the gravity of convulsions.

The most important objective in the treatment of eclampsia is elimination of the convulsions . . . which disrupt the functions of the heart, lungs, kidneys, and liver. The oftener the attacks occur, the more disastrous their effects. After nine or ten attacks a woman, previously in the bloom of health, may be at the brink of the grave. The best results in eclampsia depend on the prevention or reduction in frequency of these convulsions. For this purpose I regard the systematic, prophylactic use of morphine and chloral hydrate as a comparatively innocuous measure. Experience has long shown that two sedatives, acting concurrently, are more effective than one, even if given in larger dose. In eclampsia, moreover, an effect is neces-

CXVII. Изъ Петербургскаго Клиническаго Повивальнаго Института.

Къ лѣченію эклампсіи.

Проф. В. В. Строганова.

(Докладъ, читанный въ акушерскомъ отдѣлѣ XIII Международнаго Съѣзда въ Paris'ѣ.)

Какъ извѣстно, и до настоящаго времени предсказаніе при эклампсіи далеко неблагопріятно: 20—30% смертности встрѣчается во многихъ клиникахъ Европы. Способы лѣченія этой болѣзни далеко еще не общепризнаны и очень часто не подтверждены большимъ числомъ наблюденій. Въ этомъ я вижу естественное слѣдствіе нашего незнакомства съ патогенезомъ данной болѣзни; безъ знанія патогенеза лѣченіе не можетъ быть научно обоснованнымъ и должно быть исключительно эмпирическое. Такъ, въ настоящее время одни предлагаютъ для лѣченія этой тяжелой болѣзни большіе пріемы морфія, другіе—хлоралъ-гидратъ, американскую чемерицу (veratrum viride), кровопусканія, потогонныя, ускоренное родоразрѣшеніе; и, наконецъ, въ послѣднее время многіе совѣтуютъ введеніе физіологическаго раствора поваренной соли. Даже и наиболѣе испытанные и распространенные способы лѣченія, къ каковымъ я отношу примѣненіе большихъ пріемовъ морфія и хлоралъ-гидрата, подвергаются сомнѣнію въ послѣднее время, какъ это видно, напр., изъ работъ Gürich'а[1], отвергающаго благодѣтельное вліяніе морфія, и Fehling'а[2], относящагося подобнымъ-же образомъ и къ хлоралъ-гидрату.

Въ нижеслѣдующемъ я опишу способъ, который я примѣнялъ въ теченіи 3 послѣднихъ лѣтъ, и, прежде всего, остановлюсь на результатахъ его. Съ апрѣля 1897 года по май 1900 года, въ учрежденіяхъ, гдѣ проводился нижеописанный способъ лѣченія, было 90 случаевъ эклампсіи, а именно: въ Клиническомъ Повивальномъ Институтѣ 61, въ завѣдуемомъ мною Петербургскомъ Городскомъ Родильномъ Пріютѣ имени проф. Красовскаго (бывшемъ Александро-Невскомъ) 11, въ Петербургскомъ Родовспомогательномъ Заведеніи (съ 20/II 1900 по 10/V 1900 г., когда я консультативно принималъ участіе въ лѣченіи эклампсіи въ этомъ учрежденіи) 18; наконецъ 2 случая этой болѣзни я наблюдалъ въ частной практикѣ, при содѣйствіи съ другими врачами. Такимъ образомъ, въ общей сложности, за это время я имѣю 92 случая эклампсіи. Прежде всего, остановлюсь на смертности матерей. Изъ 92 умерли 5, т. е., 5,4%. Если мы примемъ во вниманіе, что Клиническій Повивальный Институтъ и Петербургское Родовспомогательное Заведеніе служатъ мѣстами, куда врачи преимущественно направляютъ тяжелые случаи эклампсіи не только изъ частной практики, но даже и изъ клиникъ, то приведенная цифра пріобрѣтаетъ особенный интересъ. Подробный разборъ отдѣльныхъ случаевъ смерти повышаетъ этотъ интересъ еще болѣе. Въ самомъ дѣлѣ, 3 смертельные исхода получились при слѣдующихъ обстоятельствахъ.

I. № 1255, 1899 г. Смерть отъ воспаленія легкихъ, на 8-й день послѣ прекращенія эклампсическихъ приступовъ.—Больная поступила въ Повивальный Институтъ послѣ 20 приступовъ эклампсіи на дому, въ крайне тяжеломъ, коматозномъ состояніи. Въ Институтѣ она имѣла лишь одинъ приступъ, быстро оправилась; на слѣдующій день, имѣя уже нормальную температуру и пульсъ, она пришла въ сознаніе. Но въ тотъ-же день произошло рѣзкое повышеніе температуры и съ признаками воспаленія легкаго. Смерть на другой день. Вскрытіе, произведенное проф. Н. П. Ивановскимъ, подтвердило прижизненное распознаваніе.

II. № 55, 1900 г. Повивальный Институтъ. Больная доставлена изъ Клинической Больницы. Смерть черезъ 4 часа послѣ поступленія.—Поступила въ Институтъ уже умиравшей, послѣ 20 приступовъ на дому и въ дорогѣ. Дыханіе дѣлалось возможнымъ лишь при боковомъ положеніи больной и при оттягиваніи нижней челюсти вверхъ и впередъ, какъ при глубокой хлороформной асфиксіи. Языкъ чрезвычайно увеличенъ. Тотчасъ приготовлено было все для кесарскаго сѣченія на мертвой, въ виду или остановившагося сердцебіенія плода. Въ Институтѣ былъ лишь одинъ приступъ, тотчасъ по поступленіи. Смерть черезъ 4 часа. Кесарское сѣченіе. Извлеченіе живаго плода, который, перенеся тяжелую эклампсію, умеръ черезъ 10 дней.

III. № 666, 1900 г. Петербургское Родовспомогательное Заведеніе. Легкій случай эклампсіи. Гнилокровное заболѣваніе на 20-й день послѣ родовъ и эклампсіи. Смерть черезъ 7 дней отъ гнойнаго воспаленія брюшины.—Единственный аутохтонный (т. е., развившійся въ учрежденіи) изъ кончившихся смертью. Больная имѣла лишь 6 приступовъ средней силы. Затѣмъ эклампсія прекратилась. Въ послѣродовомъ времени эндометритъ. Лихорадочная температура прекратилась на 10 день. На 20-й вновь поднятіе температуры, гнилостное пораженіе влагалища, перешедшее на матку и брюшную полость. Смерть на 27 день послѣ родовъ.

Ясно, что 3 приведенные случая должны быть выдѣлены въ особый рядъ, такъ какъ смерть въ нихъ произошла или вслѣдствіе осложненія постороннимъ случайнымъ заболѣваніемъ, или вслѣдствіе того, что больная уже при поступленіи находилась въ безнадежномъ состояніи.

Но и остальные 2 случая смерти представляли серьезныя осложненія эклампсіи уже и при поступленіи больныхъ въ учрежденіе. Прежде всего, слѣдуетъ отмѣтить, что оба они были внѣшніе.

Больная № 155, 1900 г. (IV случай) поступила въ Повивальный Институтъ съ явленіями начавшагося отека легкихъ, въ крайне тяжеломъ состояніи, послѣ 8 приступовъ эклампсіи на дому, въ присутствіи врача. Тотчасъ по поступленіи былъ еще 9 приступъ. Предупреждающее лѣченіе морфіемъ и хлоралъ-гидратомъ, 3-й и послѣдній приступъ въ Институтѣ. Роды на концу слѣдующаго дня. Значительное улучшеніе, но затѣмъ ухудшеніе и смерть отъ нараставшаго паралича сердца.

V. № 1377, Петербургское Родовспомогательное Заведеніе. Больная прибыла съ приступомъ тяжелой эклампсіи. 4 года назадъ ей была произведена тиреоидэктомія. Не смотря на предупреждающее лѣченіе морфіемъ и хлоралъ-гидратомъ, приступы продолжались. Поэтому произведено прободаніе мертваго плода при родахъ, открытомъ на 3 пальца. Прекращеніе эклампсіи. Сильнѣйшее послѣродовое кровотеченіе вслѣдствіе атоніи матки. Смерть на 4-й день послѣ родовъ и эклампсіи, при явленіяхъ нараставшаго паралича сердца.

Такимъ образомъ только въ этихъ двухъ случаяхъ можно видѣть, что лѣченіе эклампсіи не сопровождалось успѣхомъ; но мы видѣли, въ какомъ тяжеломъ состояніи находились эти больныя въ началѣ лѣченія и какія осложненія наблюдались у нихъ потомъ.

Перехожу къ вопросу о дѣйствіи примѣнявшагося лѣченія въ остальныхъ случаяхъ эклампсіи. При этомъ я могу только отмѣтить въ высокой степени благопріятное вліяніе его. Такъ, у одной больной, которая имѣла 31 приступъ въ теченіи 4 дней и которую считали уже умиравшей, послѣ примѣненія предложеннаго мною лѣченія былъ только одинъ слабый приступъ, и затѣмъ наступило медленное выздоровленіе. Больная № 159, 1900 г., Повивальнаго Института имѣла 10 приступовъ на дому и лишь 1 въ Институтѣ, куда прибыла съ явленіями уже начавшагося отека легкихъ; выздоровленіе.

Чтобы точнѣе показать вліяніе предлагаемаго лѣченія на число приступовъ, приведу таблицы всѣхъ случаевъ, бывшихъ въ послѣдніе 3 года въ Повивальномъ Институтѣ, а для сравненія и таблицы случаевъ эклампсіи въ другихъ родовспомогательныхъ заведеніяхъ Петербурга за тоже время, данныя о которыхъ мнѣ удалось получить.

Такъ, въ Клиническомъ Повивальномъ Институтѣ въ 1897—1898 учебномъ году, среднимъ числомъ, наблюдалось въ стѣнахъ учрежденія у каждой эклампсической больной по 2,9 приступа. (См. таблицу I-ую), въ 1898—1899 году по 3,3 (см. таблицу II-ую), и, наконецъ, въ 1899—1900 го-

Таблица I-я. Случаи эклампсіи въ Повивальномъ Институтѣ въ 1897—1898 учебномъ году (А—развившіеся въ Институтѣ, а Е—внѣ Института).

	№		Число приступовъ внѣ Института	Число приступовъ въ Институтѣ		№		Число приступовъ внѣ Института	Число приступовъ въ Институтѣ
1	№ 882	A	0	5	11	436	E	1	0
2	1036	A	0	3	12	451	A	0	1
3	1145	A	0	1	13	580	E	1	4
4	1364	A	0	1	14	597	A	0	?
5	1371	A	0	1	15	600	A	0	?
6	1422	A	0	15	16	208	A	0	1
7	1457	A	0	1	17	703	A	0	4
					18	719	A	0	1
	1898.							11	+ 49
8	52	A	3	5					
9	336	A	0	1		49:17 = 2,9			
10	355	E	6	4					

[1] Lothar Gürich, Der Wert des Morphins bei der Behandlung der puerperalen Eklampsie.

[2] H. Fehling, Volkmann's Sammlung klinischer Vorträge, № 248: Die Pathogenese und Behandlung der Eklampsie im Lichte der heutigen Anschauung.

Fig. 70-2. First page of Stroganov's report [7] on his new method of treating eclampsia.

sary both on the sensory centers and the convulsive center. The best agent for the former is morphine; for the latter, chloral hydrate. . . . By means of the two remedies together convulsive attacks can usually be stopped for 24 to 48 hours. In the milder cases the patient regains consciousness after 24 hours, the urinary output increases, and its albumin concentration falls off sharply. In cases of severe headache or prolonged coma, the morphine–chloral hydrate sedation should be continued, especially if labor has not stopped. . . . In practice I employ the following schedule of treatment for eclampsia of moderate severity: Immediately after the first attack or upon the arrival of the patient in the hospital I inject 0.015 gm of morphine hydrochloride subcutaneously. An hour later, or sooner if the patient is restless, the injection is repeated, even in the absence of another attack. Two hours after the second injection, or earlier if an attack threatens, I administer 2 to 3 gm of chloral hydrate per rectum. I repeat the rectal instillation four hours later, either in the same dosage or, if the patient has quieted, in a slightly smaller one. . . . I repeat this after six and again after eight hours.

In the more severe cases . . . the medication should be given at more frequent intervals. . . . Under this treatment the patient usually falls into a deep sleep, which is very desirable and which obviates the need for further sedative therapy. . . .

Obviously, eclamptic patients should be protected from all stimuli—visual, auditory, mechanical, chemical, and, when consciousness returns, psychologic. All manipulations of the sexual organs, even catheterization of the bladder, should be performed under chloroform anesthesia. Despite the use of such large amounts of sedatives, labor usually proceeds normally.

Delivery of the infant is another important part of the treatment, for in 50 to 60 per cent of the cases the convulsions stop after the end of labor. . . . Therefore, as soon as delivery appeared to present no danger to mother or child, it was carried out immediately under chloroform anesthesia. . . . In none of my 92 cases was induction of labor done for eclampsia. . . . Medical treatment, stopping convulsions and improving the condition of the patient . . . eliminated the need for forceful methods, which are dangerous for both mother and child.

STROGANOV'S LIFE

Vasili Vasilievich Stroganov was born December 29, 1857, in Viaz'ma, Russia.[1,5] He began the study of medicine at the Voenno-Meditsinskaya Akademiya in 1880 and during his student days served also as a substitute physician in the rural areas near his birthplace. After graduation he acted for a period as the district doctor in Nezhinsk; but soon becoming interested in obstetrics, went in 1885 to the Povival'nyi Institut, the central governmental research institute for obstetrics and gynecology, where he was made professor in 1897. His dissertation on the bacteriology of the female genital tract during the various periods of life was published in 1893; and in the same year he was also appointed to the staff of the lying-in hospital, Aleksandro-Nevskii Rodil'nyi Dom. In 1896 Stroganov assumed an additional teaching responsibility, at the Institut Dlya Usovershenstvovaniya Vrachei. It is estimated that he taught a total of 4000 midwives, 10,000 medical students, and 7000 physicians, at least 15 of whom subsequently assumed important positions as professors of obstetrics. He wrote 150 medical articles and three books, the best known of which, on the prophylactic treatment of eclampsia, went into three Russian editions as well as translations into English and French.[6] His other main works included a volume on the principal complications of pregnancy and labor, and a book on practical obstetric problems, which enjoyed the popularity of four editions. He was elected to honorary membership in countless medical societies, in Ireland, Scotland, Belgium, and Yugoslavia, as well as in Russia. The Belgian Obstetrical and Gynecological Society awarded him a prize of 12,000 francs for outstanding work in his specialty, but he promptly presented this honorarium to anti-Fascist organizations in Spain and China. Stroganov was recognized as one of the first medical scientists in the world to protest against German atrocities preceding World War II. He died September 24, 1938, in his eighty-first year. The Russian Ministry of Health has created a prize of 10,000 rubles, named in Stroganov's honor, for the best work on eclampsia.

REFERENCES

1. Bublichenko, L. I.: Vasilii Vasil'evich Stroganov. *Akusherstvo i Ginekol.*, **1**:10–11, 1939.
2. Denman, T.: *Aphorisms on the Application and Use of Forceps and Vectis; on Preternatural Labours, on Labours Attended with Hemorrhage, and with Convulsions,* 4th ed. Johnson, London, 1793, pp. 102–3.
3. Dewees, W. P.: *Essays on Various Subjects Connected with Midwifery.* Carey & Lea, Philadelphia, 1823, pp. 169–70.
4. Green, C. M.: Puerperal eclampsia: The experience of the Boston Lying-in Hospital during the last eight years. *Am. J. Obst.*, **28**:18–44, 1893.
5. Kvater, E. I.: Vasilii Vasil'evich Stroganov kak uchenyi i vrach. *Sovet. med.*, **11–12**:92, 1938.
6. Stroganoff, B.: *Traitement de l'Éclampsie: Technique Actuelle du Traitement Prophylactique.* Masson & Cie, Paris, 1935.
7. Stroganov, V. V.: K" Lecheniyu Eklampsii. *Vrach. delo*, **21**:1137–40, 1900.
8. Tweedy, E. H.: Eclampsia. *Tr. Roy. Acad. Med. Ireland*, **14**:272–84, 1896.
9. Willis, T.: *An Essay of the Pathology of the Brain and Nervous Stock: in Which Convulsive Diseases are Treated of.* Translated from the Latin by S. P. T. Dring, J. Leigh, & C. Harper, London, 1684, p. 76.

Carl Siegmund Credé, Placental Expression, and the Prevention of Neonatal Ophthalmia*

CHAPTER

71

Expulsion of the placenta, the denouement to the birth act, varies like the latter from a simple, rapid process to a tedious, delayed effort that may tax the skill and judgment of the obstetrician and the patience of the parturient and her family. Harried by the fear of uterine bleeding that may result from retention of the afterbirth, doctors and midwives alike have resorted to a variety of techniques, often forceful, to expedite the delivery of that organ. Most textbooks of the early-nineteenth century advocated a waiting period of five to ten minutes after the birth of the infant for separation of the placenta. Combined external and internal palpation then disclosed its location; if already in the vagina it was delivered with the assistance of the intravaginal fingers and traction on the cord. This method, while simple enough when carried out by the expert, was dangerous in the hands of the inexperienced or the impatient, leading occasionally to avulsion of the cord, laceration and incomplete removal of the placenta, injuries to the cervix and lower uterine segment, and even inversion of the uterus.

EXPRESSION OF THE PLACENTA

Carl Credé sought to eliminate these hazards in 1854, substituting for vaginal extraction of the placenta its abdominal expression by a method

* This chapter originally published in *Obst. & Gynec.*, **10**:335–39, 1957; reprinted by permission. Copyright © 1957, by the American College of Obstetricians and Gynecologists.

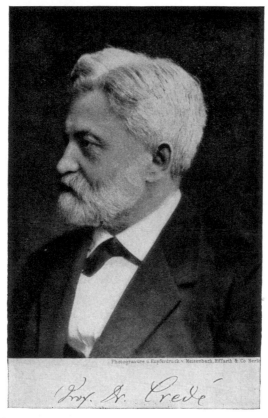

Fig. 71-1. Carl Siegmund Franz Credé (1819–1892).

with which his name has since been associated. Credé pointed out the dangers of a prolonged third stage and outlined his method of placental expression in the following words: [2]

In most cases the placenta is expressed from the uterus by spontaneous postpartum contractions after about a quarter hour. Even if the third stage lasts a long time it is not necessarily harmful to the parturient. . . . However, hemorrhage can occur at any moment; and the longer the time elapsed after birth of the child the more difficult is artificial removal of the placenta from the uterine cavity, should this become necessary. . . . In order not to leave the parturient too long in an agitated state of worry over the final stage of labor, and at the same time not to keep the physician needlessly from other important professional duties . . . it is quite proper and legitimate to expedite artificially the desultory process of nature. The intervention necessary to bring forth the separated placenta from the maternal birth canal is so slight that it is inconsequential in comparison to the hazards of delayed spontaneous expulsion. The simplest and most natural method of artificial delivery of the placenta consists in stimulation and augmentation of the lazy uterine contractions. A single vigorous contraction of the uterus brings the whole process to a speedy termination. In a countless number of cases without exception, I have succeeded in producing an artificial and strong contraction a quarter to half hour after birth of the child, by means of massage of the fundus and body of the uterus through the abdominal wall, gently at first and then progressively more vigorously. As soon as it reached the peak of its contraction, I grasped the whole uterus with my entire hand, so that the fundus lay in my palm with my five fingers surrounding the corpus, and then exerted gentle pressure. Under my fingers I always felt the placenta glide out of the uterus, and indeed this usually occurred with such force that the placenta appeared immediately at the external genitalia, or at least in the lower vagina. The patient experienced no more discomfort from the manual grasp than from the pain that accompanies the firm uterine contraction. Moreover it is unnecessary to disturb her by inserting the finger or hand into the sensitive genital organs in order to remove the placenta by forceful pulling and tugging.

In his subsequent teaching,[3] Credé emphasized the importance of selecting the proper moment for the application of pressure, only at the height of a contraction, and the futility of pressure on the relaxed organ.

Apparently unbeknown to Credé was the fact that a similar method of placental expression had been used many years earlier by Samuel Bard and by John Harvie. Bard, author of the first textbook of obstetrics published in America,[1] wrote in 1807, in his instructions to the midwife for delivering the placenta:

If, on the contrary, she cannot reach the root of the string, let her examine the patient's belly; she probably will find the womb soft and flaccid, resting on the lower side, or perhaps hanging a little over the pubes; by taking it in the hollow of her hand, compressing it moderately, raising it up towards its natural position, and at the same time rubbing the surface briskly with the hand, she will soon perceive the womb to contract in size, and to assume the form of a ball of considerable firmness; after this, a very few pains will probably deliver the placenta. . . .

Even earlier, in 1767, John Harvie, a nephew by marriage of William Smellie, had written: [7]

There is another safe method of assisting nature in the delivery of the *placenta,* and which, for these five or six years last past, I have found to answer generally very well in practice. As soon as the child is committed to the care of the nurse, let the accoucheur apply his hand upon the belly of the woman, which is then very loose, and he will readily feel the contracting *uterus:* then having placed the flat of the hand over it, let him, by a light and gentle pressure, bring it downwards, or towards the *pubes,* and he will feel the uterus sensibly contracting, and often will feel it so reduced in size, as to be certain that the *placenta* is expelled. By this method we will seldom have anything to do afterwards, but to help it through the *os externum,* if even so much remains undone.

Historians have not overlooked Harvie's and Bard's priority in advocating abdominal expression of the placenta by means of the contracted uterus, but the procedure still retains its popular designation as the *Credé maneuver*.

PREVENTION OF OPHTHALMIA NEONATORUM

The name of Credé is also associated eponymically with one of the most important advances in obstetric practice of the nineteenth century, the prevention of gonococcal ophthalmia in the newborn. As early as 1854 Credé had recognized inflammatory lesions of the mother's lower genital tract as the source of this scourge, the commonest cause of blindness in infants, for in his *Klinische Vorträge* [2] he wrote:

At the same time, the effect on the fetus must not be overlooked; for during the act of birth the infant's eyelids are coated with the corrosive mucus, which then becomes continuous with the conjunctiva and thus becomes the most frequent cause of blennorrhea.

It was not until a quarter century later, however, that Credé hit upon an effective method of prophylaxis, his first definitive paper on the subject appearing in 1881.[4] The following quotations are taken from it:

Eye inflammations in the newborn in general occur less often in the upper classes, most often in the proletariat; in the lying-in hospitals they are associated with a rapidly progressive and very serious disturbance. Therefore, in order to test further the method of prophylaxis recommended by me, I direct my attention at the very outset to those colleagues who work in lying-in hospitals or obstetric clinics and, like me, frequently see diseases.

Probably shared by most obstetricians will be my view that the exceedingly common catarrhal conditions and inflammations of the vagina result from gonorrhea, and that the infectiousness of the discharge continues long after the specific gonorrheal manifestations have disappeared; indeed that infection is still present in the maternal vagina, even in cases where almost no discharge is any longer to be found, if an eye inflammation develops within the first few days after birth.

In the Leipzig Lying-in Hospital the possibility of transmission of infectious material from another infant with infected eyes can be completely excluded, for every child with infected eyes is removed with its mother to the infirmary, which is completely isolated from the section for postpartum patients. Furthermore, the puerperae can scarcely infect the infants by means of their fingers, which might be contaminated with lochia, because the infants always lie so far away from the mothers in their beds that the mothers cannot reach them, only coming in contact with the infants when they are put to the breast by the attendants.

I thus came to the conclusion . . . that, almost without exception, the affected infants in my institution become infected only through direct transfer of the vaginal discharge into their eyes during the act of birth. . . .

For a long time I occupied myself with the important problem of finding ways and means for preventing the illness ruinous to so many eyes, for best getting at the infecting discharge.

My first efforts included the most meticulous management and as thorough a cleansing as possible of the vagina of the pregnant and parturient patients. The results, however, were meager, not satisfactory. The eye infections declined in number, but they did not disappear. I then began disinfecting the infant's eyes themselves, and henceforth the results became surprisingly favorable. . . .

In October, 1879, I made the first experiment with prophylactic instillations into the eyes of the newborn immediately after birth, using a solution of borax (1:60), which I considered the mildest, least caustic agent. At first this was done only to the infants of affected mothers, in whom vaginal irrigations had also been carried out during the entire labor. But this procedure too did not lead to the desired goal; and from December, 1879, instead of the borax I used solutions of silver nitrate (1:40), which was squirted into the eyes immediately after birth. Before the instillation the eyes were carefully washed with a solution of salicylic acid (2:100). The infants of affected mothers treated in this manner remained well; while other infants who had not been treated prophylactically, because we did not consider their mothers to be affected, continued to get sick. . . .

From June 1, 1880, on, all eyes without exception were disinfected immediately after birth with a weak solution of silver nitrate (1:50). However, the solution was no longer squirted in, but only a few drops of it were instilled, by means of a small glass tube, into each eye, previously cleansed as before and gently held open by an assistant. The eyes were then soothed for 24 hours with linen compresses soaked in salicylic solution (2:100). The repeated vaginal douches were then given up entirely. . . . All the infants treated in this manner remained spared from eye inflammations, even of the slightest degree, although many of the mothers showed vaginal blennorrhea and trachomatous proliferations. . . .

Credé closed his case with the following tabular presentation of the incidence of ophthalmia neonatorum in his hospital during the recent years preceding and in the six months following the routine application of his new method of prophylaxis:

Years	No. of Births	Cases of Ophthalmia	Per Cent
1874	323	45	13.6
1875	287	37	12.9
1876	367	29	9.1
1877	360	30	8.3
1878	353	35	9.8
1879	389	36	9.2
1880 to May 31	187	14	7.6
1880 June 1 to Dec. 8	200	1*	0.5

* In this case the eyes were not disinfected; therefore the true incidence should be considered 0.0 per cent.

Later in the same year (1881), Credé published a supplementary report [5] of 400 new cases, 300 of which were treated by a simplified technique, again without a single case of ophthalmia resulting. His final paragraph concluded with the prophetic words:

> A goal long striven for has been attained. Now all infants born in lying-in hospitals are sure to be protected . . . this prophylactic measure cannot fail to blaze a trail for itself in private practice. May this soon come about!

CREDÉ'S LIFE

Carl Siegmund Franz Credé was born on December 23, 1819, in Berlin, Germany, where his father, a French immigrant, held a high position in the Ministry of Health and Education.[6,8,9] After attending the Friedrich-Wilhelm Gymnasium, young Credé entered the study of medicine at the University of Berlin, but spent one semester in Heidelberg, where he met the illustrious Naegele. Graduation at age 22 was followed by visits to the clinics in Belgium, Paris, Vienna, and Italy, after which Credé returned to Berlin with the hope of obtaining a position in the surgical clinic. Finding no opening at the time, he accepted an assistantship in obstetrics under Professor von Busch and remained at this post for the next five years.

In 1849 Credé qualified as an independent lecturer in obstetrics. His first class began with only four students but rapidly increased in size as his teaching ability became recognized. Three years later, in 1852, he was appointed director of the School for Midwives in Berlin and chief physician to the Charité Hospital. Here he established a gynecology department, the first separate and exclusive department of its kind in continental Europe. In 1856 Credé was called to Leipzig to fill the chair of obstetrics vacated by the death of Jörg. Remaining here for the rest of his professional life, he continued to demonstrate an unusual talent for organization and administration until poor health forced his retirement in 1887. His illness proved painful and lingering, and he finally died of prostatic cancer on March 14, 1892.

With von Busch, von Ritgen, and von Siebold, Credé served as coeditor of the *Monatsschrift für Geburtskunde,* and when this was succeeded by the *Archiv für Gynäkologie,* Credé served as its editor for 39 years, initially as coeditor with Spiegelberg, and alone after the latter's death. Among the distinguished obstetricians trained by Credé were Ahlfeld, Fehling, Leopold, and Sänger. Credé was the first to introduce the cephalotribe into Germany, but this was soon replaced by the cranioclast. His principal literary works were his three books: the two-volume *Klinische Vorträge über Geburtshülfe* (1854); his *Lehrbuch der Hebammenkunst* (1875), which went through five editions; and his *Gesunde und Kranke Wöchnerinnen* (1886), which warned against unnecessary internal examinations as a cause of puerperal infection. Credé's most enduring contribution to posterity was his method of eradicating gonococcal ophthalmia, the commonest cause of blindness in children.

REFERENCES

1. Bard, S.: *A Compendium of the Theory and Practice of Midwifery, Containing Practical Instructions for the Management of Women During Pregnancy, in Labor, and in Child-Bed; Calculated to Correct the Errors, and to Improve the Practice, of Midwives; As well as to Serve as an Introduction to the Study of this Art, for Students and Young Practitioners.* Collins & Perkins, New York, 1807, p. 129.
2. Credé, C. S. F.: *Klinische Vorträge über Geburtshülfe.* Hirschwald, Berlin, 1854, pp. 160, 599–600.
3. Credé, C. S. F.: *In* Versammlung deutscher Naturforscher und Aerzte in Königsberg im Jahre 1860. Verhandlungen der Section für Gynäkologie. Sept. 17 meeting. *Monatschr. f. Geburtsk. u. Frauenk.,* **16**:337–42, 1860.
4. Credé, C. S. F.: Die Verhütung der Augenentzündung der Neugeborenen. *Arch. f. Gynäk.,* **17**:50–53, 1881.
5. Credé, C. S. F.: Die Verhütung der Augenentzündung der Neugeborenen. *Arch. f. Gynäk.,* **18**:367–70, 1881.
6. Findley, P.: *Priests of Lucina. The Story of Obstetrics.* Little, Brown & Co., Boston, 1939, pp. 258–62.
7. Harvie, J.: *Practical Directions, Shewing a Method of Preserving the Perinaeum in Birth, and Delivering the Placenta Without Violence.* D. Wilson & G. Nicol, London, 1767, pp. 45–46.
8. Leopold, G.: Carl Siegmund Franz Credé. Gedächtnissrede gesprochen in der gynäkologischen Gesellschaft in Dresden am 14 April 1892. *Arch. f. Gynäk.,* **42**:193–213, 1892.
9. Simpson, A. R.: Presidential address. *Tr. Edinburgh Obst. Soc.,* **18**:5–13, 1893.

Max Madlener, Ralph Pomeroy, Frederick Irving, and Tubal Sterilization

CHAPTER

72

"It has always seemed to me that one of the opprobia of medicine is . . . to advise the patient not to become pregnant again, and at the same time be morally certain that within a few months she will return in the same condition." This lament, uttered by J. W. Williams in 1921,[14] has since been voiced with decreasing frequency as obstetricians have assumed a role of greater responsibility for the social welfare of their patients. Limitation of reproduction has taken its place alongside the treatment of infertility as a proper function of the physician. Insurance against conception may be just as important to the fertile woman as the construction of an artificial vagina to the patient born without one, in permitting enjoyment of a normal sex life. Dickinson and Gamble [4] have defined the field for sterilization as including "all those who because of heredity and physical condition are totally unfit to have children, as well as those parents for whom another child would be very unwise, or an actual danger, and who lack intelligence or persistence to use other means of control."

Termination of woman's reproduction is accomplished most simply and effectively, and with least disturbance of other functions, by bilateral occlusion of the fallopian tubes. It is usually carried out following therapeutic abortion, at hysterotomy or cesarean section, or very soon after vaginal delivery. Under these conditions the operation is technically simple, can be performed in a few minutes, increases the period of hospitalization scarcely if at all, and eliminates the danger of a new conception soon after the patient's return home.

Sterilization by division of the fallopian tubes was first recommended by Blundell [3] in the early-nineteenth century, as a means of preventing the hazards of dystocia in women with markedly contracted pelves. He wrote:

If the pelvis be contracted in so high a degree that parturition, by the natural passages, is impossible, I need scarcely tell you, that the shortest way to avoid the necessity of the operation [cesarean section], would be by abstinence altogether from intercourse with the other sex. The most solid resolution, however, may sometimes thaw; and when a woman is married, she may be placed under those circumstances in which it is not very easy to adhere to this advice, her life perhaps falling a sacrifice to her neglect. My friend Dr. Hull, of Manchester, once transmitted me the case of a woman whose pelvis was contracted in a high degree; she knew her situation, remained in a state of abstinence many years, but afterwards became pregnant and died. Now is there any mode in which, when the obstruction of the pelvis is insuperable, the formation of a foetus may be prevented? In my opinion, there is; for if a woman were in that condition, in which delivery could not take place by the natural passage, provided she distrusted the circumstances in which she was placed, I would advise an incision of an inch in length in the linea alba above the symphysis pubis; I would advise further, that the fallopian tube on either side should be drawn up to this aperture; and lastly, I would advise, that a portion of the tube should be removed, an operation easily performed, when the woman would, for ever after, be sterile.

In the optimistic hope that a woman undergoing cesarean section might survive the operation, Blundell further advised:

To preclude the possibility, therefore of a second need for the incisions, before closing the abdomen, the operator, I conceive, ought to remove a portion, say one line, of the fallopian tube, right and left, so as to intercept its calibre—the larger blood-vessels being avoided. Mere division of the tube might be sufficient to produce sterility, but the further removal of a portion of the canal appears to be the surer practice. I recommend this precaution, therefore, as an improvement of the operation.

It is doubtful that tubal sterilization was actually carried out until May 22, 1880, when S. S. Lungren, of Toledo, Ohio, performed a secondary cesarean section on a patient with a contracted pelvis. In his case report,[10] published the following year, Lungren tersely noted:

It was at first intended to remove the ovaries with Smith's pile clamp and the actual cautery, but in consideration of the danger of hemorrhage jeopardizing the operation, the Fallopian tubes were tied instead with a strong silk ligature about one inch from their uterine attachment.

The hazy understanding of utero-ovarian physiology that prevailed in Lungren's day is betrayed by this interesting footnote to his article:

As it was a question of some interest what would be the result of menstruation in this case, after tying the Fallopian tubes, the solution was fortunately determined in so far as it could be, in so short a time as has already elapsed since the operation. Eight weeks after, she had a discharge identical with the menstrual in appearance, lasting for five days. . . . Four weeks after, she menstruated again.

A rash of techniques for tubal sterilization broke out during the next few decades; but each operation was marred by a disturbing proportion of failures, resulting from the remarkable regenerative capacity of the endosalpinx and its tendency to re-establish the continuity of the tubal lumen or produce tuboperitoneal fistulas. Nürnberger's review [12] of the subject in 1917 listed 151 references, and by 1921 no less than 42 different procedures had been proposed.[5]

THE MADLENER STERILIZATION

One of the most popular of the sterilizing techniques was that devised by Max Madlener in 1910 and since known by his name. By 1919 he was able to report [11] on 89 patients subjected to his operation, 34 by laparotomy and 55 by anterior colpotomy. Three of the patients had died, but none of the survivors had conceived again. Madlener's technique was marked by its simplicity.

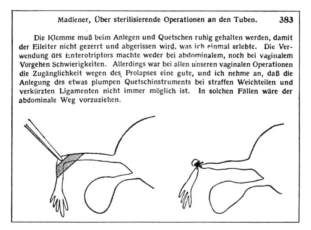

Madlener, Über sterilisierende Operationen an den Tuben. 383

Die Klemme muß beim Anlegen und Quetschen ruhig gehalten werden, damit der Eileiter nicht gezerrt und abgerissen wird, was ich einmal erlebte. Die Verwendung des Enterotriptors machte weder bei abdominalem, noch bei vaginalem Vorgehen Schwierigkeiten. Allerdings war bei allen unseren vaginalen Operationen die Zugänglichkeit wegen des Prolapses eine gute, und ich nehme an, daß die Anlegung des etwas plumpen Quetschinstruments bei straffen Weichteilen und verkürzten Ligamenten nicht immer möglich ist. In solchen Fällen wäre der abdominale Weg vorzuziehen.

Fig. 72-1. Illustration from Madlener's paper,[11] showing his technique of tubal sterilization. (Reproduced by permission of *Zentralblatt für Gynäkologie*.)

He explained:

With a pickup forceps the operator grasps the tube where most mobile, thus not near the uterus but rather at or distal to its midportion. The tube is elevated, to angulate at approximately 90°. Then, with the other hand, one applies the crushing clamp to the tube just under the tip of the forceps. The part of the tube running to and from the forceps is thus encountered obliquely, and at the same time a small knuckle of the mesosalpinx is crushed with it. With an assistant holding the pickup forceps one now applies the jaws of the crushing forceps, which are compressed by closing the fist tightly, so that the tissue is surely crushed paper thin. After the clamp is removed, and while the tube is still held in the forceps, a thin thread ligature is placed in the groove. Small hematomas occasionally occur at the edge of the groove, but these are of no importance.

Although he had encountered no failures, Madlener insisted:

I am not so prejudiced that I regard the procedure used by me as absolutely certain. I believe, however, that re-establishment of the tubal lumen with regeneration of the tubal epithelium is not to be feared after this crushing. In my opinion the only danger lies in the possibility of tearing the tubal serosa and in the resultant formation of a tuboperitoneal fistula. This danger is slight, however, if one handles the instruments carefully and avoids sharp-edged instruments.

MADLENER'S LIFE

Max Madlener is known primarily as a general surgeon rather than a gynecologist. He was born in Memmingen, Germany, January 12, 1868.[13] After studying in Munich, Berlin, and Kiel he served for several years as assistant in surgery to Angerer and in gynecology to Amann before settling down to practice in Kempten in 1896. Four years later he was put in charge of the regional hospital there and in 1912 was made its medical director, a position he held until his retirement in 1947. He died suddenly of a stroke on May 17, 1951, at the age of 83. In addition to his technique for tubal sterilization, Madlener achieved renown for his studies on the pathogenesis, prophylaxis, and treatment of goiter, his subtotal gastrectomies for stomach ulcer, and his intestinal resections for carcinoma of the large bowel.

THE POMEROY STERILIZATION

In contrast to Madlener's satisfactory experience with his procedure, in the hands of others it soon led to a considerable number of failures, usually traceable to the very complication he had warned against, tuboperitoneal fistula formation. As a result, the Madlener technique has largely been supplanted in the United States by a more certain method of tubal sterilization devised by Ralph Pomeroy. Curiously, the Pomeroy technique was never presented to the medical public by its originator. Only after Pomeroy's death was his operation described by his associates, Bishop and Nelms,[2] at a meeting of the New York State Medical Society on June 6, 1929. Reporting on 100 consecutive cases with no known failures, the authors stated:

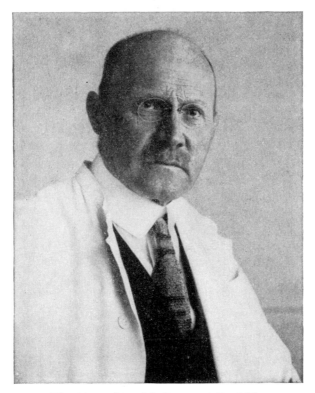

Fig. 72-2. Max Madlener (1868–1951).

Any surgical procedure should exhibit three principles which we will align alliteratively: Simplicity, Safety, Security. We can easily demonstrate to you that the procedure which we present is *simple*. It would seem also as though it must be accepted as one which is as *safe* as any invasion of the peritoneal cavity. As to *surety*, we will state that there is no known case of ours that has become pregnant. . . .

The method we are advocating we first saw in the hands of the late Ralph Pomeroy who made no claim for originality but stated that he had never seen it done. Its simplicity lies in the fact that it is nothing more or less than that a loop in the loose, middle portion of the tube is ligated with *absorbable* suture material and resected. It takes but a few seconds during a laparotomy and usually no longer by vagina. . . . As to safety . . . the vessels that are apt to be involved are ligated before section, so there ought to be only a few drops of blood loss. . . . As to surety . . . the first critical thought is that we use absorbable suture material . . . our practice having been to utilize a double strand of No. 1 chromic catgut. No absorption occurs until there is no fear of bleeding and when it does the two cut ends draw apart. . . . During this period the plastic exudate of the peritoneum has been thrown out and becomes organized, and here is the secret of the process. Nature throws over a barrier of new peritoneum and it becomes a perma-

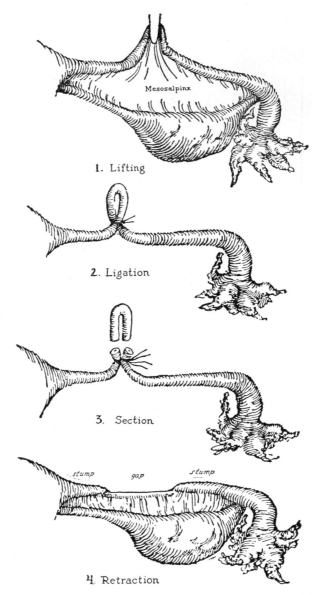

1. Lifting

Mesosalpinx

2. Ligation

3. Section

stump　　gap　　stump

4. Retraction

Fig. 72-3. Technique of Pomeroy sterilization. (Reproduced from Dickinson, R. L., and Gamble, C. J.: *Human Sterilization. Techniques of Permanent Conception Control.* Waverly Press, Baltimore, 1950.)

624

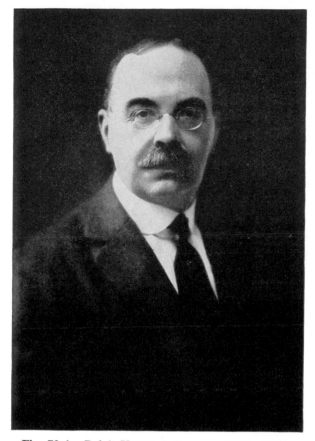

Fig. 72-4. Ralph Hayward Pomeroy (1867–1925).

nent one with no chance, we feel confident, of fistula formation. . . . We definitely do *not* crush the tube first . . . for the crushed tissue may open a way for fistula formation.

POMEROY'S LIFE

Ralph Hayward Pomeroy was born in New York City, January 12, 1867, the ninth-generation descendant of Eltweed Pomeroy, who settled in Dorchester, Massachusetts, in 1630.[1,9] He received his B.A. from Wesleyan University, Middletown, Connecticut, in 1887 and graduated from Long Island College Hospital two years later. After an internship at Charity Hospital, later known as City Hospital, he was made instructor in obstetrics in his alma mater, where he was promoted to the rank of associate professor in 1912. He was one of the founders of the Williamsburg Hospital in Brooklyn, and served as consulting obstetrician to the Kings County Hospital and several

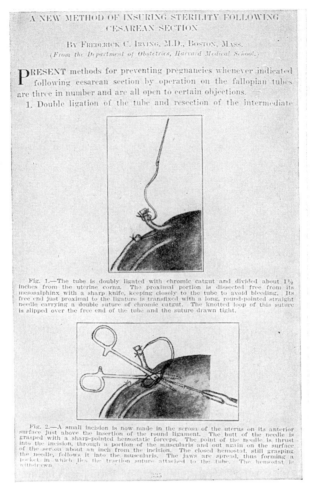

A NEW METHOD OF INSURING STERILITY FOLLOWING
CESAREAN SECTION

By FREDERICK C. IRVING, M.D., BOSTON, MASS.

(From the Department of Obstetrics, Harvard Medical School.)

PRESENT methods for preventing pregnancies whenever indicated following cesarean section by operation on the fallopian tubes are three in number and are all open to certain objections.

1. Double ligation of the tube and resection of the intermediate

Fig. 1.—The tube is doubly ligated with chromic catgut and divided about 1½ inches from the uterine cornu. The proximal portion is dissected free from its mesosalphinx with a sharp knife, keeping closely to the tube to avoid bleeding. Its free end just proximal to the ligature is transfixed with a long, round-pointed straight needle carrying a double suture of chromic catgut. The knotted loop of this suture is slipped over the free end of the tube and the suture drawn tight.

Fig. 2.—A small incision is now made in the serosa of the uterus on its anterior surface just above the insertion of the round ligament. The butt of the needle is grasped with a sharp-pointed hemostatic forceps. The point of the needle is thrust into the incision, through a portion of the muscularis and out again on the surface of the serosa about an inch from the incision. The closed hemostat, still grasping the needle, follows it into the muscularis. The jaws are spread, thus forming a pocket in which lies the traction suture attached to the tube. The hemostat is withdrawn.

Fig. 72-5. First page of Irving's original paper,[7] showing his method of tubal sterilization. (Reproduced by permission of *American Journal of Obstetrics and Gynecology.*)

other Brooklyn hospitals. He was chosen president of the Kings County Medical Society in 1916 and was the only man elected twice to the presidency of the New York Obstetrical Society. He was also a fellow of the American Gynecological Society. Pomeroy died August 22, 1925. In addition to his sterilization operation, his name is associated with a technique for rotating the head from a posterior position by manipulation of the anterior shoulder.

THE IRVING STERILIZATION

More certain to produce permanent sterilization than either the Madlener or Pomeroy techniques, and hence preferred by many American obstetricians,

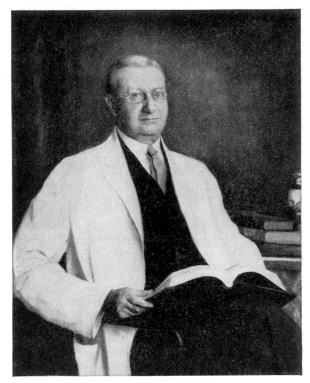

Fig. 72 6.   Frederick Carpenter Irving (1883–1957).

is the somewhat more intricate procedure proposed by Irving.[6,7] Introduced in 1924, Irving's method was redescribed with minor improvements in 1950, when 814 cases were reported without a single failure. As Irving detailed his modified technique: [8]

One and one-half inches from its cornual insertion, the tube is elevated in the bite of a clamp. The mesosalpinx below this point is pierced by a hemostat in a bloodless area. The distal portion of the tube is ligated with No. 1 chromic catgut. Proximal to this a double suture ligature of the same material, mounted on a half-curved, round-pointed needle and knotted about three inches from its ends, is tied about the tube which is divided between the two ligatures. . . . A stab wound is made in the myometrium at the proximal end of the tube. A sharp-pointed hemostat is plunged into the uterine wall through this stab wound as far as its lock and its tips spread, thus making a pit. A grooved director is inserted in this pit as far as it will go and the half-curved needle on a needle holder is passed along the director to the extreme depth of the pit and is brought out on the surface of the uterus. . . . The director is removed. Traction on the suture ligature causes the tube to enter the pit for approximately three-quarters of an inch. . . . One strand of the double suture ligature is cut, a cross-stitch is made in this superficial portion of the uterine wall, and the free ends are tied, thus anchoring the tube deeply in the myometrium. . . . The small wound at the point of entrance of the tube is closed with a figure-of-eight suture of chromic catgut, thus completing the operation. . . . The distal portion of the divided tube is not treated in any way; it is not necessary to bury its cut end in the broad ligament.

IRVING'S LIFE

Frederick Carpenter Irving was born in Gouverneur, New York, May 30, 1883. After obtaining his preparatory education at the Phillips Exeter Academy in New Hampshire, he received his A.B. degree from Harvard College in 1906 and his M.D. from the Harvard Medical School four years later. His postgraduate training consisted of a year as house pupil in the Massachusetts General Hospital and a similar period as house physician in the Boston Lying-in Hospital. During World War I he served in France and Italy with the U. S. Army Medical Corps. In 1931 Irving was appointed professor of obstetrics in the Harvard Medical School and subsequently obstetrician-in-chief to the Boston Lying-in Hospital, positions he held until 1947. In 1951 he retired to Belleair, Florida, where he died December 24, 1957. He served as president of the American Gynecological Society in 1951. Irving's popular writings and speeches are characterized by his knowledge of the classics and Greek mythology. His books include *A Textbook of Obstetrics* (1936), *Safe Deliverance* (1942), and *Outline of Abnormal Obstetrics* (1943). An obstetric forceps of Irving's design is also named for him.

REFERENCES

1. Bishop, E.: Ralph Hayward Pomeroy: An appreciation. *Brooklyn Hosp. J.,* **5**:67–72, 1947.
2. Bishop, E., and Nelms, W. F.: A simple method of tubal sterilization. *New York State J. Med.,* **30**:214–16, 1930.
3. Blundell, J.: *The Principles and Practice of Obstetricy.* Ed. by T. Castle. Duff Green, Washington, 1834, pp. 352, 360.
4. Dickinson, R. L., and Gamble, C. J.: *Human Sterilization. Techniques of Permanent Conception Control.* Waverly Press, Baltimore, 1950.
5. Flatau, W. S.: Sterilisierung durch Knotung der Tube. *Zentralbl. f. Gynäk.,* **45**:467–69, 1921.
6. Fox, F. H.: A comparison of the Irving and Pomeroy methods of tubal sterilization. *Surg., Gynec. & Obst.,* **71**:462–68, 1940.
7. Irving, F. C.: A new method of insuring sterility following cesarean section. *Am. J. Obst. & Gynec.,* **8**:335–37, 1924.
8. Irving, F. C.: Tubal sterilization. *Am. J. Obst. & Gynec.,* **60**:1101–9, 1950.
9. Kosmak, G. W.: Ralph Hayward Pomeroy, M.D., 1867–1925. *Tr. Am. Gynec. Soc.,* **51**:302–5, 1926.
10. Lungren, S. S.: A case of cesarean section twice successfully performed on the

same patient, with remarks on the time, indications, and details of the operation. *Am. J. Obst.*, **14**:78–94, 1881.

11. Madlener, M.: Über sterilisierende Operationen an den Tuben. *Zentralbl. f. Gynäk.*, **43**:380–84, 1919.

12. Nürnberger, L.: Die sterilisierenden Operationen an den Tuben und ihre Fehlschläge. *Samml. klin. Vortr.*, N.F. No. 731–34, 33–114, 1917 (Gynäk. No. 258–261).

13. Schindler, C.: Max Madlener. *München. med. Wchnschr.*, **85** (Part 1):65–66, 1938.

14. Williams, J. W.: The problem of effecting sterilization in association with various obstetrical procedures. *Am. J. Obst. & Gynec.*, **1**:783–93, 1921.

Johannes Pfannenstiel and the Pfannenstiel Incision

Access to the pelvic viscera in gynecologic operations may be gained by either of two main types of incision: the midline or longitudinal, extending from the pubic symphysis to the umbilicus; and the transverse, a gently curvilinear incision placed in the skin fold slightly above the mons veneris. The latter variety, gratifying to most patients because of its cosmetic superiority over the former, differs from the midline incision in other respects as well, such as exposure and healing characteristics, according to the particular method of division and reapproximation of the abdominal layers beneath the skin.

Some operators incise only the skin and subcutaneous tissues transversely, dividing the fascia, separating the rectus muscles, and cutting the peritoneum in the midline. Others divide all these layers transversely. The majority of gynecologists who employ the transverse incision for laparotomy follow the technique described by Pfannenstiel in 1900.[4]

PFANNENSTIEL'S TECHNIQUE

The transverse suprapubic incision of the skin had been recommended shortly before by Rapin[5] and by Küstner.[2] Pfannenstiel sought to retain the cosmetic advantages of Küstner's incision, while reducing the hazard of subsequent hernia formation. After using his own incision in 51 cases he reported:[4]

630

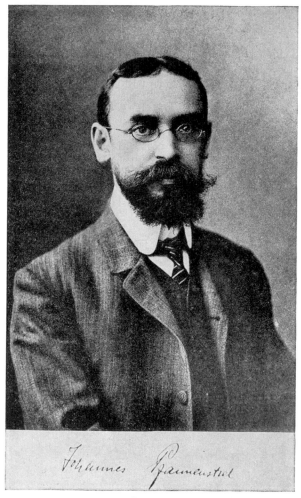

Fig. 73-1. Hermann Johannes Pfannenstiel (1862–1909).

[It] appears to give absolutely certain protection against hernias. This method, which I would designate as the suprapubic transverse fascial incision, is a modification of Küstner's suprapubic transverse incision. It is clear that the latter type of incision prevents hernia no more and no less than the longitudinal incision through the entire abdominal wall, as we now know that hernia occurs in the course of defective healing of the fascia, and that a good union of the overlying skin guarantees no protection against hernia. . . . I therefore cut through not only the skin but also the entire fascial layer, and only then, after separating the fascia toward the umbilicus, did I divide the muscle layer and peritoneum longitudinally, in order thus to maintain the complete integrity of the aponeurosis along the extent of the longitudinal incision of the abdomen. My expectation was confirmed, namely to thus obtain an absolutely firm scar. Although this method provides other significant advantages also, I do not wish to recommend it yet to my colleagues, for I am quite convinced that an ultimate verdict will only be possible after years.

The Pfannenstiel incision, in the words of the author, is carried out as follows:

A slightly arched incision is made at the upper border of the hair growth, in the fold which the panniculus of obese persons forms over the pubic symphysis (Fig. 4) [Fig. 73–2]. This is carried through the subcutaneous fat and should be about 8-10-12 cm long, depending upon the purpose of the operation. It thus extends from one superficial epigastric artery to the other, occasionally farther out

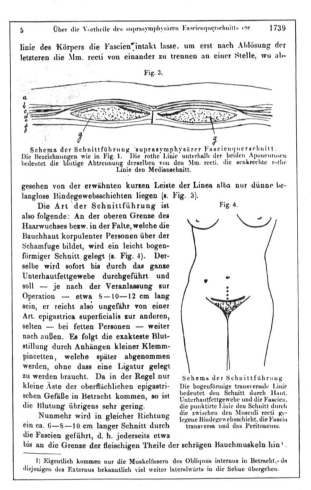

5   Über die Vortheile des suprasymphysären Fascienquerschnitts etc   1739

linie des Körpers die Fascien intakt lasse, um erst nach Ablösung der letzteren die Mm. recti von einander zu trennen an einer Stelle, wo ab-

Fig. 3.

Schema der Schnittführung 'suprasymphysärer Fascienquerschnitt. Die Bezeichnungen wie in Fig. 1. Die rothe Linie unterhalb der beiden Aponeurosen bedeutet die blutige Abtrennung derselben von den Mm. recti, die senkrechte rothe Linie den Medianschnitt.

gesehen von der erwähnten kurzen Leiste der Linea alba nur dünne belanglose Bindegewebsschichten liegen (s. Fig. 3).

Die Art der Schnittführung ist also folgende: An der oberen Grenze des Haarwuchses bezw. in der Falte, welche die Bauchhaut korpulenter Personen über der Schamfuge bildet, wird ein leicht bogenförmiger Schnitt gelegt (s. Fig. 4). Derselbe wird sofort bis durch das ganze Unterhautfettgewebe durchgeführt und soll — je nach der Veranlassung zur Operation — etwa 8—10—12 cm lang sein, er reicht also ungefähr von einer Art. epigastrica superficialis zur anderen, selten — bei fetten Personen — weiter nach außen. Es folgt die exakteste Blutstillung durch Anhängen kleiner Klemmpincetten, welche später abgenommen werden, ohne dass eine Ligatur gelegt zu werden braucht. Da in der Regel nur kleine Äste der oberflächlichen epigastrischen Gefäße in Betracht kommen, so ist die Blutung übrigens sehr gering.

Nunmehr wird in gleicher Richtung ein ca. 6—8—10 cm langer Schnitt durch die Fascien geführt, d. h. jederseits etwa bis an die Grenze der fleischigen Theile der schrägen Bauchmuskeln hin[1].

Fig. 4.

Schema der Schnittführung. Die bogenförmige transversale Linie bedeutet den Schnitt durch Haut, Unterhautfettgewebe und die Fascien, die punktirte Linie den Schnitt durch die zwischen den Musculi recti gelegene Bindegewebsschicht, die Fascia transversa und das Peritoneum.

1) Eigentlich kommen nur die Muskelfasern des Obliquus internus in Betracht, da diejenigen des Externus bekanntlich viel weiter lateralwärts in die Sehne übergehen.

Fig. 73-2. Page from Pfannenstiel's paper,[4] with illustrations showing the location and extent of his incision.

in fat individuals. The most meticulous hemostasis follows by means of small clamps, which are removed later without requiring a ligature. Since only small branches of the superficial epigastric vessels come into the field, as a rule, the bleeding is very slight anyway.

An incision about 6-8-10 cm long is now made through the fascia in the same direction, i.e., up to the edge of the fleshy part of the oblique abdominal muscles on either side. In the process several layers are divided simultaneously: (1) the very thin and inconstant superficial fascia, and (2) both of the aforementioned aponeuroses. If lengthening of the incision is necessary for any reason, this can be carried out laterally, into the muscle; indeed, this can be done without danger, since the direction of the muscle fibers coincides with that of the incision. There is almost no bleeding at all from the fascial incision.

Now the aponeurotic plate is separated from the underlying layer, whereupon the pyramidalis muscles are immediately exposed. These are highly variable in size, often surprisingly well developed in delicate individuals and vice versa. Occasionally the pyramidalis muscle is completely lacking, as is also known to the anatomists. . . . The freeing of the tendon plate is carried out upward about 6 cm. The separation from both sides of the midline is easily accomplished in this way; only occasionally does one need to use scissors. The tendinous ridge of the linea alba, on the other hand, must be divided with a scalpel. The pyramidalis muscles, whose upper insertion is to be found in the linea alba, thus lose their attachment and usually retract back toward the symphysis.

Next, the longitudinal incision follows, while the fascia is retracted upward. The two rectus muscles are separated from each other, partly by blunt and partly by sharp dissection, down to the thin transversalis fascia. The latter is then picked up and cut through . . . together with the properitoneal fatty tissue and peritoneum. Of course, the fascial incision must be utilized as widely as possible, both upward and downward, in order to provide exposure, and one can safely go right down to the symphysis.

Suture of the abdominal wall follows naturally from the type of incision, resulting in at least three, usually four, layers. The peritoneum is sewed first, with a continuous suture. Then the recti are likewise united, usually with a few continuous stitches, whereupon the upper angles of the pyramidalis muscles are attached to the recti at points corresponding to the original insertions. I have repeatedly omitted this last suture . . . because the muscles also fall together satisfactorily without it, and this has not appeared detrimental to later healing. The second row of sutures, on the other hand, is absolutely essential; otherwise a gaping separation of the muscles occurs. . . . Through-and-through sutures are then placed through the skin, with careful inclusion of the underlying tissue (rectus muscles) to prevent pocket formation. . . . These sutures, three to five in number, are not tied immediately, but the third layer, the fascial suture, is placed first, with the most meticulous coaptation of the edges. . . . Finally, only the tying of the previously placed skin sutures (fourth layer) remains. If the wound edges are thereby well approximated, it is seldom necessary to add more than one or two intermediary sutures.

Pfannenstiel's report encompassed 51 cases. About three fourths of the patients had pelvic inflammatory disease. The other pathologic findings included uterine myomas, retroversion, ectopic pregnancy, and ovarian tumors, one of which was the size of a man's head. Through his transverse incision Pfannenstiel carried out a variety of procedures, including subtotal hysterectomy, suspension of the uterus, and excision of the adnexa. There was no mortality, no incisional hernias developed, and the surgical exposure proved entirely satisfactory. Wrote Pfannenstiel:

The operative field with the transverse incision often provides a better view than with the usual longitudinal incision for laparotomy. Because of its low position the incision leads directly to the proper operative field much more easily and surely than does the longitudinal incision. The abdominal muscles can be retracted as far laterally as the transverse incision extends through the fascia, for they are freed from their covering aponeurosis; whereas with the traditional longitudinal incision the tense ligamentous layer makes lateral retraction difficult. With lax musculature the suprapubic transverse incision substantially facilitates all surgical intervention in the lateral parts of the pelvis.

Prevention of incisional hernia was Pfannenstiel's principal objective, and much of his discussion centered on this problem. He stated:

The favorable results of my incision clearly show that separation of the rectus muscles cannot occur. With the traditional longitudinal incision every hole in the fascia must eventually lead to a cleft in the muscle also, since the fascia grows together with its underlying bed, the rectus muscle; and the transversus abdominis muscles, by dragging on the fascia, also draw the recti apart and in this way provide a locus minoris resistentiae for the intra-abdominal pressure. Quite different with the transverse fascial incision: here also the fascia grows together with the underlying muscle; however, since the aponeuroses are not divided in the direction of the muscle but form instead much more of an intact protective plate, diastasis of the recti cannot occur, even with increased intra-abdominal pressure and with faulty union of the muscles in the midline.

Of the cosmetic advantages of the transverse incision Pfannenstiel wrote:

Although the aesthetic point of view, considered objectively, does not seem so important, still it is valued highly enough by the laity to deserve consideration. Related to this is the fact that the patient, understandably, considers the low transverse incision as less ominous than the median . . . and reconciles herself to the former as readily as to a vaginal operation.

Pfannenstiel clearly recognized the limitations of exposure provided by his incision, despite his earlier protestations to the contrary. In his own words:

The longitudinal incision remains indicated for large tumors just as in all cases in which exposure of the entire pelvis appears in advance to be necessary, as, for example, in cases of known carcinoma of the uterus and ovaries, or of large abscesses of the tubes, which should be removed intact. The suprapubic transverse incision should be used only in cases where a smaller opening of the abdomen suffices for carrying out all the necessary procedures in a thorough and conservative manner. It should supplant vaginal celiotomy where this has proved inadequate . . . and is indicated principally for procedures on the internal genitalia which permit conservation of the uterus.

PFANNENSTIEL'S LIFE

Hermann Johannes Pfannenstiel was born June 28, 1862, in Berlin, where his father was a bank director.[1] He studied at the University of Berlin, receiving his medical degree in 1885. After brief periods of gynecologic study with von Rabenau in Berlin and Pauly in Posen, Pfannenstiel was appointed assistant in the Breslau Frauenklinik, under the direction of Fritsch. Here the aspiring young gynecologist established many happy and profitable professional associations, which included the illustrious Heidenhain, Mikulicz, Ponfick, Born, and Lubarsch. In 1896 he assumed direction of the gynecology division of the Hospital of the Elizabethan Sisters, and in the same year was named coeditor of the *Archiv für Gynäkologie*. His practice thrived, but Pfannenstiel yearned for a completely academic career. An invitation to the chair of obstetrics and gynecology in the University of Giessen in 1902 was therefore accepted with enthusiasm; and with this post he took over both the Universitäts-Frauenklinik and the school for midwives.

Here he carried out major administrative changes during the next five years, organized a program of maternal and child hygiene for the Grand Duchy of Hessen, and acquired a new wing for his clinic. In 1907, as the building was nearing completion, he was called to Kiel, as successor to Werth. Pfannenstiel had helped found the Northwest German Obstetrical and Gynecological Society, and now reorganized the Medical Society of Kiel. His career was abruptly cut short when he pricked his finger during an operation, the resulting infection causing his death on July 3, 1909, only a few days after his forty-seventh birthday.

Pfannenstiel's principal field of interest was gynecologic tumors, especially ovarian neoplasms and parovarian cysts. His 1890 thesis, *Ueber die Pseudomucine der cystischen Ovarialgeschwülste,* was followed by papers on the genesis of ciliated epithelial cysts, the histogenesis of teratomas, and, perhaps most important, his study of papillary tumors of the ovary, "Ueber die papillären Geschwülste des Eierstocks." [3] While in Breslau, Pfannenstiel carried out studies on the implantation of the fertilized ovum, which served as the basis for his monograph, *Ueber die Eieinbettung und Placentarentwicklung,* published in von Winckel's textbook of obstetrics, but Pfannenstiel made the mistake of believing that the syncytium was of maternal origin.

The abundant clinical material available to Pfannenstiel in Giessen and Kiel provided excellent opportunity for the development and evaluation of surgical procedures. His efforts to cope with the contracted pelvis in obstetrics led him, in stepwise fashion, from the induction of premature labor, to pubiotomy, and finally to cesarean section. In gynecologic surgery he contributed to the technique of plastic operations for uterine prolapse; but his name is best remembered in association with his transverse suprapubic approach to the pelvis, the "Pfannenstiel incision."

REFERENCES

1. Kroemer, P.: Hermann Johannes Pfannenstiel. *Arch. f. Gynäk.*, **89**:I–VII, 1909.
2. Küstner, O.: Der suprasymphysäre Kreuzschnitt, eine Methode der Coeliotomie bei wenig umfänglichen Affektionen der weiblichen Beckenorgane. *Monatschr. f. Geburtsh. u. Gynäk.*, **4**:197–98, 1896.
3. Pfannenstiel, J.: Ueber die papillären Geschwülste des Eierstocks. Anatomische und klinische Untersuchungen zur Klärung der Frage ihrer Malignität. *Arch. f. Gynäk.*, **48**:507–605, 1895.
4. Pfannenstiel, J.: Über die Vorteile des suprasymphysären Fascienquerschnitts für die gynäkologischen Koliotomien, zugleich ein Beitrag zu der Indikationsstellung der Operationswege. *Samml. klin. Vortr.* (Neue Folge), Gynäk. No. 68–98, 1897–1900 (Klin. Vortr., N.F. No. 268, Gynäk. No. 97, Feb., 1900).
5. Rapin: [Discussion at Internat. Gynec. Cong., Geneva, Sept. 4, 1896.] *Centralbl. f. Gynäk.*, **20**:1016, 1896.

Arnold Sturmdorf and His Tracheloplasty

CHAPTER

74

Amputation has long ranked as one of the principal methods of treating hypertrophy, prolapse, laceration, and chronic inflammation of the uterine cervix and still comprises an important part of certain vaginal plastic procedures. A cardinal feature of the modern operation consists in carefully covering the freshened margins of the residual cervical stump with mobilized flaps of the vaginal membrane. "In the old method of amputation," however, according to J. Marion Sims,[3] "the suppuration continued for five or six weeks, and sometimes longer, before the parts were entirely cicatrized," for no effort was made to fashion an epithelial covering for the new external os.

The first cervical amputation in which the vaginal membrane was used as a stump covering was reported by Sims in 1861. The patient, aged 46, had suffered from procidentia for 15 years. Pessaries having proved unsatisfactory, she finally sought surgical relief from her discomfort. Wrote Sims: [3]

When she was fully under the influence of ether, Dr. Pratt, the House Physician, informed me that the ecraseur was broken, hence there was no alternative but to amputate by the cutting process. For this purpose I used scissors, expecting the hemorrhage to be less than by the knife. I removed about five-eighths of an inch of the cervix, cutting at right angles and within half an inch of the vaginal insertion. On beginning the operation, I intended to leave the cut surface to heal by the granulating process, which usually takes five or six weeks, but while sponging the wound and waiting for the hemorrhage to cease, I discovered that the stump could be covered over with healthy vaginal tissue, in the same manner

637

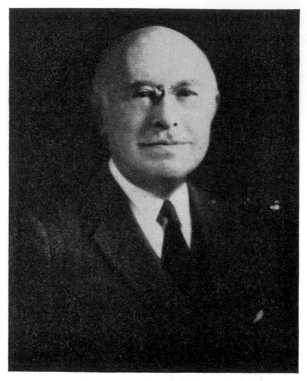

Fig. 74-1. Arnold Sturmdorf (1862–1934).

that a stump of an arm or a leg is covered with skin after amputation by the circular method. This was done by passing four sutures of silver wire . . . through the anterior and posterior borders of the wound, which when tightly drawn, brought its edges into apposition in a straight line across the middle of the stump, covering it completely, but leaving a small central opening for the os, just over the outlet of the cervical canal. . . . The sutures were removed at the end of a week, the parts having healed entirely by the first intention.

Following Sims's publication cervical amputation found new favor among gynecologists, and was soon supplemented in the late-nineteenth and early-twentieth centuries by the more conservative methods of trachelorrhaphy devised by Emmet, Schroeder, Kelly, and Sturmdorf. The lacerated or inflamed cervix assumed a prominence almost equal to that of the retroverted uterus as a presumed cause of female complaints.

STURMDORF'S TECHNIQUE

In an address before the Medical Society of the County of New York on October 25, 1915, Arnold Sturmdorf [4] distinguished clearly between the clinical significance of cervical lacerations themselves and that of the commonly associated infection. He said:

If we recall that it is not the cervical laceration as such, but its consequences, which we attempt to prevent or cure by operation, the enumerated post-operative derangements make it conspicuously evident that the prevalent methods of cervix amputation, while surgically successful, not only fail to restore normal functions in a large proportion of cases, but are capable of inciting the identical disturbances for the relief of which the operation was instituted. That it is not the tear in the cervix, but the induced complications which bring the patient to the operating table, is amply demonstrated by the countless women who bear cleft cervices presenting ununited cicatricial edges, unproductive of any symptoms whatsoever; and it follows as a self-evident deduction that the limitations of trachelorrhaphy like the indications for cervix amputations must be governed by the nature and degree of existing concomitants, not by the extent of the cervical injury. A single tear may initiate the most serious train of complications in one patient, while a more extensive multiple injury may prove perfectly innocuous in another.

The dominating fundamental factor that establishes the morbidity of a cervical lesion is the *incidence of infection*. . . . The objective and subjective features presented in this chronic stage of the condition are simply and graphically depicted in every textbook, but the nature and significance of the intermediate pathologic phases in the morbid chain that link cause and effects are obscured by a haze of standardized misconceptions and fallacious dogma. Thus the theory of reflex neuroses from alleged "pinching of the cervical nerves by scar-tissue in the angles of laceration" is almost but not quite obsolete; yet equally absurd is the accepted statement that the relative sterility of women with lacerated cervices is due to a cicatricial stenosis of the cervical canal, for it is obvious that an os which affords egress to billions of blood-cells during every menstruation, will certainly give ingress to an active spermatozoid, the thickest part of which measures less than half the diameter of a single red blood-corpuscle.*

Sturmdorf visualized the cervix as the primary focus in many cases of ascending lymphangitis involving the myometrium and uterine adnexa. "It follows as an obvious corollary," he wrote, "that the indications for, and limitations of, trachelorrhaphy or cervix amputation respectively, must be governed by their relative efficacy in the elimination of the infectious cervical focus and the restoration of normal uterine functions." The tracheloplastic technique devised by him has since been known as the Sturmdorf procedure, and his ingenious method of covering the cervical stump with vaginal membrane as the Sturmdorf suture.

The steps of the operation, as described by its originator, include:

1. Outlining and free mobilization of an ample circular flap from the vaginal coat of the cervix.

2. Complete excision of the entire cervical mucosa to the internal os, *with preservation of its peripheral muscular layers*.

3. Sutural coaptation of the vaginal cuff to the denuded cervical cavity.

* By permission of *Surgery, Gynecology and Obstetrics*.

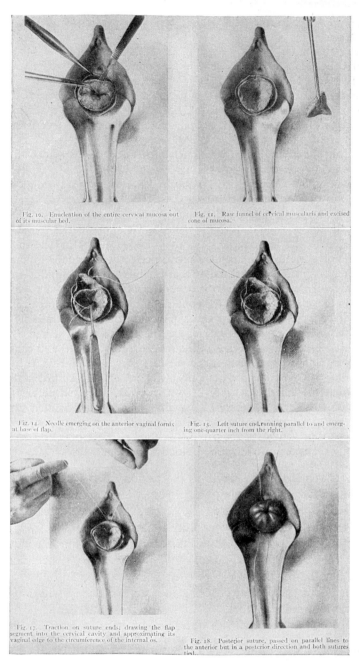

Fig. 10. Enucleation of the entire cervical mucosa out of its muscular bed.

Fig. 11. Raw funnel of cervical muscularis and excised cone of mucosa.

Fig. 14. Needle emerging on the anterior vaginal fornix at base of flap.

Fig. 15. Left suture end running parallel to and emerging one-quarter inch from the right.

Fig. 17. Traction on suture ends; drawing the flap segment into the cervical cavity and approximating its vaginal edge to the circumference of the internal os.

Fig. 18. Posterior suture, passed on parallel lines to the anterior but in a posterior direction and both sutures tied.

Fig. 74-2. Illustrations from Sturmdorf's paper.[4] (By permission of *Surgery, Gynecology and Obstetrics*.)

The main object in the first step is the formation of an ample mobile cuff of vaginal mucosa. With this in view, the outlining incision is carried around the cervix, closely skirting the demarcating border between its healthy vaginal sheath and the diseased mucosa, running parallel to the indented line at the lacerated points. The edge of vaginal covering thus outlined is freely mobilized by blunt dissection from its underlying tissues, completely around the entire cervix, up to the level of the internal os, exposing the circular arteries as for high amputation. In very extensive lesions it becomes necessary to brush the lower pole of the bladder from its uterine and vaginal attachments for a sufficient distance upward.

The pouting everted cervical mucosa is now circumcised and cored out of its muscular bed as a hollow cone, leaving a raw funnel-shaped cavity.

Trimming the loose vaginal cuff to serve as an accurate lining to the interior of this muscular funnel, its retention in this position is secured in the following manner: Beginning with the anterior segment of the circular flap, a long strand of heavy silkworm gut is passed on its vaginal surface, transversely through the free border of its central tip one-eighth of an inch from the edge, like a mattress suture, the entrance and exit of the strand embracing a quarter inch of tissue.

The right free end of the suture is now carried into the cervical cavity to a point just above the internal os, where piercing all the tissues in a direction forward, upward, and to the *right,* emerges from the vaginal surface at the base of the flap.

The left free suture end after reaching the same point above the internal os, passes in the same manner forward, upward, and to the *left,* so that the two free ends, diverging in their transit, reappear on the surface of the anterior vaginal fornix, about one-fourth inch apart, where they are left loose for the time. The suture course for the posterior flap segment runs parallel to the above, but in a posterior direction, its free ends emerging on the surface of the posterior vaginal fornix. Now by tightening each individual set of suture ends, we draw the flap segments into the cervix, line its whole cavity with vaginal mucosa, the edge of which is thus approximated to the circumference of the internal os, where it is retained in apposition as long as desired. In most cases no further suturing is necessary or desirable, but should either lateral edge gape, an additional chromic stitch may be introduced. The sutures are left long to facilitate their removal. . . .

The specific features of the operative method thus outlined effect the complete elimination of the infectious focus by extirpation of the diseased cervical mucosa; preserve the normal arrangement, contour, and functions of the cervical musculature; obviate the mechanical difficulty; and secure the permanency of accurate sutural coaptation of flap to stump.*

Sturmdorf's operation was predicated upon the concept, then gaining in popularity, that a multitude of human ills were traceable to foci of infection, such as the tonsils, gallbladder, appendix, and cervix. Although this interpretation of disease now claims few adherents, Sturmdorf's technique remains the tracheloplastic method preferred by most gynecologists.

* By permission of *Surgery, Gynecology and Obstetrics.*

STURMDORF'S LIFE

Arnold Sturmdorf, born in Vienna, August 26, 1862,[1,2] migrated to New York as a youth. He showed great aptitude for mathematics and taught this subject before deciding on a medical career and while pursuing his studies at Columbia University's College of Physicians and Surgeons, from which he graduated in 1886. Subsequently he was appointed associate surgeon to the Woman's Hospital, attending gynecologist and professor of gynecology at the New York Polyclinic (1909 to 1916), and consultant to several other hospitals in Manhattan and Brooklyn. Although especially interested in gynecology, he practiced general surgery as well, and pioneered in developing the operation of perineal prostatectomy. His principal literary effort, *Gynoplastic Technology,* was published in 1919. Sturmdorf was almost as well known for his musical as for his medical interests. An excellent violinist, he played with several string quartets in New York. Most of New York's operatic stars were his personal friends. He died of coronary occlusion, March 13, 1934.

REFERENCES

1. Deaths. Arnold Sturmdorf. *J.A.M.A.,* **103**:1871, 1934.
2. Kagan, S. R.: *Jewish Medicine.* Medico-Historical Press, Boston, 1952, p. 481.
3. Sims, J. M.: Amputation of the cervix uteri. *Tr. M. Soc. State of New York,* 367–71, 1861.
4. Sturmdorf, A.: Tracheloplastic methods and results. A clinical study based upon the physiology of the mesometrium. *Surg., Gynec. & Obst.,* **22**:93–104, 1916; also *Am. J. Obst.,* **73**:325–31, 1916.

John Webster, John Baldy, and the Baldy-Webster Suspension*

The second half of the last century ushered in an era that has been characterized as "the dark ages of operative furor" in the treatment of uterine retroversion, then the commonest gynecologic disease. The leading gynecologists of the period regarded retrodisplacement of the uterus as a frequent cause of a large variety of complaints in women. The importance imputed to retroversion is abundantly evident in the textbooks of the day. In the narrative volume *Clinical Notes on Uterine Surgery,*[12] published in 1866, J. Marion Sims tells the following story:

> [A lady] was riding on a pony in the suburbs of the city of Montgomery, Alabama, where I then resided. It took fright and suddenly jumped from under her— she fell, striking her pelvis on the ground. I saw her soon afterwards; her sufferings were very severe. Besides the contusions from the fall, she complained of rectal and vesical tenesmus. On examination, I found a complete retroversion of the uterus. . . .

Equally impressive is Sir James Young Simpson's introduction to his lecture on retroversion, which appears in his *Clinical Lectures on the Diseases of Women:* [11]

* This chapter originally published under the title "John Clarence Webster, John Montgomery Baldy, and Their Operation for Uterine Retroversion" in *Surg., Gynec. & Obst.,* **102**:377–80, 1956; reprinted by permission. Copyright, 1956, by The Franklin H. Martin Memorial Foundation.

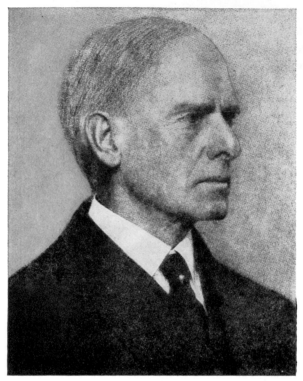

Fig. 75-1. John Clarence Webster (1863–1950). (Reproduced from *Proc. Inst. Med. Chicago,* **18**:175, 1950.)

A patient who came to my house the other day remarked that she had come walking, and added that it was the first time she had walked out of doors for 3 years. Such an incident is of not infrequent occurrence. The lady I refer to talked with another, with whose sister she was acquainted, and that sister had for about fifteen years been unable to walk; and I wish to teach you today what it was that prevented these ladies, as it prevents others, from walking, and to teach you also how you may relieve their symptoms and rectify their malady.

Against such a background of authoritative teaching a large number and variety of surgical procedures were developed for the cure of retroversion, and the operations were practiced with abandon indeed. "The round ligaments were folded, ligated, plicated, shirred, plaited, planted, transplanted, replanted, drawn over, above, and through the broad ligaments and fastened to the back of the uterus," as stated by Fluhmann.[7] Mr. Alexander of Liverpool, the inventor of a well-known and one of the first suspension operations, having been asked by a group of visiting surgeons in 1911 to demonstrate it, stated that he sent one of his four assistants into the north, one into the east, one into the west, and one into the south of Liverpool but that each returned after diligent search with the report that in all of that great city he had been unable to find one woman who had not already had the Alexander operation for suspension of the uterus.[5]

Suspension operations for the primary purpose of correcting uterine retroposition have fallen greatly in popularity in the past several decades and are now carried out almost exclusively as incidental procedures in conjunction with myomectomy, tubal plastic operations, and the conservative surgical therapy of pelvic inflammatory disease and endometriosis. Among the best known of the suspension procedures developed in America, and still performed occasionally today, is the Baldy-Webster operation.

The operation consists of drawing a limb or knuckle of each round ligament behind the uterus through a perforation made in the broad ligament, and suturing the round ligaments posterior to the corpus, thereby supporting the latter in an anterior position. This principle was probably carried out in 1900 or earlier by a Dr. Andrews of Chicago, according to Baldy,[4] but the first description of the operation was published in 1901 by Webster.[13] This report was a model of brevity, the entire text and an illustration comprising but one column of one page in *The Journal of the American Medical Association* (Fig. 75-2).

WEBSTER'S LIFE

John Clarence Webster was born in Shediac, New Brunswick, Canada, October 21, 1863, and died there on March 16, 1950.[6,8,9] He studied medicine at Edinburgh, where he won the gold medal for his thesis, first prize for research in 1894 and 1896, and a total of 14 prizes and awards between the years 1883, when he received his degree of doctor of medicine, and 1896, when he returned to Canada to become associated with McGill University and the Royal Victoria Hospital. For six years following his graduation at Edinburgh he worked as assistant to Sir Alexander Simpson, professor of midwifery. In 1899, Webster was called to Chicago to the chair of obstetrics and gynecology at Rush Medical College, where he remained until 1919, when he returned to his native Canada because of poor health. While in Chicago the Websters began a collection of Oriental *objets d'art,* which subsequently became one of the most famous in the world, containing an outstanding section of Japanese prints. After returning to Shediac, Webster developed a deep interest in Canadian history and devoted himself to its study and to the collection of historic mementos. The Webster Collection of Canadiana was the second largest in existence when donated to the New Brunswick Museum. Webster was responsible for establishing a number of history museums and the restoration of several others. In recognition of this interest he was appointed to

RETROVERSION OF THE UTERUS. 913

A SATISFACTORY OPERATION FOR CERTAIN CASES OF RETROVERSION OF THE UTERUS.

J. CLARENCE WEBSTER, M.D.
Professor of Obstetrics and Gynecology, Rush Medical College, affiliated with the University of Chicago; Obstetrician and Gynecologist, Presbyterian Hospital.
CHICAGO.

During the past year I have carried out the following procedure in a number of cases where operative interference has been deemed advisable for retroversion of the uterus.

The patient being in the Trendelenburg position, the abdomen is opened, adhesions are separated and other pathologic conditions, which may be present, attended to. The fundus of the uterus is elevated and pushed forward. A small hole is then made through the broad ligament on one side under the utero-ovarian ligament near the uterus. Through it a pair of forceps is passed from behind in order to grasp the round ligament about an inch from its uterine end. The latter is then pulled through the broad ligament in a double fold. It is carried across the back of the uterus a short distance above the utero-sacral ligaments and is then stitched in this

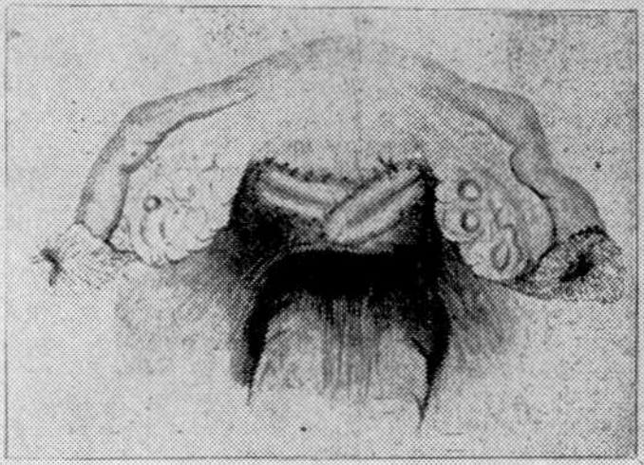

Diagram representing the round ligaments doubled up, drawn through the broad ligaments and stitched to the posterior surface of the uterus above the utero-sacral ligaments.

position with chromic catgut. A similar procedure is carried out on the other side, the second round ligament being stitched to the back of the uterus above or below the first one or crossing it. The amount of overlapping of the round ligaments depends upon their length and laxity.

Each ligament is also stitched to the edge of the hole in the broad ligament. As a result of this operation, the round ligaments are much shortened and through their new attachment to the posterior and lower part of the uterus, act both in elevating the uterus as a whole and in preventing it from returning to its retroverted position. The ovaries are also elevated. No raw surface is produced on which adhesions can form. No new ligament is formed to act as a possible cause of intestinal obstruction and of trouble in pregnancy and labor. The normal range of uterine movements is not materially altered. There is no possibility of any interference with pregnancy and labor.

The operation can be performed equally well by vaginal section. It seems, therefore, to me to be more advantageous than the other operative procedures commonly employed in the treatment of retroversion of the uterus.

Fig. 75-2. Webster's original paper [13] on the surgical treatment of uterine retroversion. (Reproduced by permission of *The Journal of the American Medical Association.*)

the Historic Sites and Monuments Board of Canada and served for a period as chairman. His withdrawal from practice proved far from a retirement.

BALDY'S SUSPENSION OPERATION

Baldy's association with the Baldy-Webster operation appears to be based upon the vigor of his writings and his bold personality rather than upon his contribution to the development of the operation itself. His first description of his suspension operation, in which the round ligaments were divided, differed significantly from the procedure described earlier by Webster. Wrote Baldy in 1902: [1]

The following operation, which I have devised after much thinking and experimenting, retains every advantage of [Webster's] operation and does away with all its disadvantages.

The round ligament on each side of the uterus is picked up and a ligature thrown about it close to the uterus, so placed as to secure the artery. The round ligaments are then severed close to the ligatures. This leaves the uterine ends of the ligaments ligated and the other ends free and bleeding. The bleeding is controlled by a fine ligature to each vessel or by sutures which fasten them in the next step of the operation. A pair of forceps is now made to perforate the broad ligament from its posterior aspect (at the point at which the round ligament is cut on the anterior surface), and the cut end (the pelvic end) of the round ligament is grasped in the bite of the forceps . . . and pulled through the hole in the broad ligament (made by the forceps in perforating) until it protrudes on the posterior side of the broad ligament. The opposite side is treated in a similar manner. The cut ends of the round ligaments are now attached by means of sutures to the cornua of the uterus directly back of the original point of attachment of the normally attached round ligament. . . . The point of attachment may be higher or lower than this, as the surgeon may find necessary to accomplish the result. If necessay as much of the round ligament is cut off, before suturing it to the uterus, as is necessary to take up any slack and give the proper amount of tension and support to the uterus. This ends the operation. The suture is a continuous one and may be either chromicized gut or silk. The effect of this procedure is to draw the fundus of the uterus upward and forward into a perfect position.

Baldy later modified his technique,[2,3] so that the operation ultimately became almost identical to the procedure originally devised by Webster, but nowhere in Baldy's writings is any indication to be found of modesty toward his own work or of diplomacy in his expressed views of the work of others. The opening paragraph of his 1902 paper reads:

Alexander's operation is of course a thing of the past except in the hands of a few—a very few. It will die altogether, like all transitional operations, in the future. Hysterorrhaphy, ventrosuspension, or whatever else one cares to call this class of operations, will most probably follow in its footsteps shortly.

In his later evaluation of the operation,[2,3] Baldy wrote:

I have performed it almost constantly . . . modifying it here and there at times as apparent difficulties arose and as it seemed necessary to overcome certain objections and certain faults in results; and I find at the present time a completed technic which is, I think, perfect.

In 1915 he stated: [4]

> The one point in the operation . . . which I hold superior to all other operations is the fact that when the operation is performed not only is the uterus itself put in a proper position but the ovaries are also replaced and held up at a proper level without any extra manipulation. I do not hold that this is done better than in any other operation because there is no other operation in which it is done at all. . . .

Overlooked by subsequent generations of gynecologists, but far greater to his credit than the operation with which his name is associated, is the dissenting voice raised by John Baldy in protest against the promiscuous practice of uterine suspension. As early as 1909 he wrote: [2]

> Retrodisplacements of the uterus are mostly coincidental with other lesions, and where such is the case the symptoms almost universally come from the associated disease. . . ."The treatment of retrodisplacements" is then a misnomer; it should be "the treatment of conditions in connection with which retrodisplacements of the uterus occur as an incident."

Baldy's fearless remarks at a symposium on the surgical treatment of retroversion of the uterus, sponsored by the Philadelphia Medical Society, December 9, 1914, may not have endeared him to his colleagues but left no doubt as to his feelings. The other members of the symposium included John G. Clarke, Howard A. Kelly, Barton Cooke Hirst, Edwin B. Cragin, J. Wesley Bovée, D. Tod Gilliam, J. Clarence Webster, and E. E. Montgomery. Baldy, the concluding speaker, stated:

> I am not at all sure that I am justified in taking part in a meeting of this character holding the views I do on the subject. In my opinion nine-tenths of the operations performed on women for retrodisplacements are uncalled for. . . .
> As to the number of operations performed for this condition under any circumstances, Dr. Cragin is such an old and warm friend that I would hate to tell him what I thought of him for doing two hundred retrodisplacement operations in a single year. In order not to be too personal to Dr. Cragin I would like to include in that remark all the speakers of the evening who are sitting on the platform with me.
> . . . It looks to me as though the possible number of retrodisplacement operations performed in this country is limited only by the number of females in existence.

BALDY'S LIFE

John Montgomery Baldy was born in Danville, Pennsylvania, on June 16, 1860.[10] He studied medicine at the University of Pennsylvania, graduating in

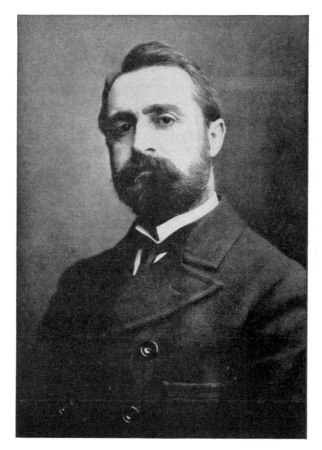

Fig. 75-3. John Montgomery Baldy (1860–1934). (Courtesy of American Gynecological Society.)

1884, and after an internship at the Philadelphia Hospital, engaged in general practice in Scranton for a few years. He then returned to Philadelphia for special study in gynecology and in 1891 was appointed professor of gynecology at the Old Philadelphia Polyclinic Hospital, later becoming surgeon-in-chief at the Gynecean Hospital. He was one of the first advocates of the radical surgical treatment of pelvic inflammatory disease. His most important literary product was *The American Textbook of Gynecology,* which he edited. In 1908 he served as president of the American Gynecological Society.

Baldy was greatly interested in raising the standards of medical training, and was appointed in 1912 as president of the Pennsylvania Bureau of Medical Education and Licensure. He inaugurated the state's requirement of a year's internship for eligibility for medical licensure examination and established minimum standards for all hospitals employing interns. He later served as the state commissioner of welfare for two years, before his retirement in 1923. He died of a self-inflicted bullet wound at his home in Devon on December 12, 1934.

REFERENCES

1. Baldy, J. M.: A new operation for retrodisplacement. *Am. J. Obst.*, **45**:650–54, 1902.
2. Baldy, J. M.: Treatment of uterine retrodisplacements. *Surg., Gynec. & Obst.*, **8**:421–34, 1909.
3. Baldy, J. M.: Operation for retrodisplacement of the uterus. *J.A.M.A.*, **56**:481–84, 1911.
4. Baldy, J. M.: The surgical treatment of retroversion of the uterus. *Surg., Gynec. & Obst.*, **20**:614–15, 1915.
5. Clarke, J. G.: The operative treatment of retroversion of the uterus. *Surg., Gynec. & Obst.*, **20**:597–98, 1915.
6. Davis, C. H.: John Clarence Webster, 1863–1950. *Gynec. Tr.*, **73**:263–65, 1950.
7. Fluhmann, C. F.: The rise and fall of suspension operations for uterine retrodisplacement. *Bull. Johns Hopkins Hosp.*, **96**:59–70, 1955.
8. Heaney, N. S.: John Clarence Webster, 1863–1950. *Proc. Inst. Med. Chicago*, **18**:174–76, 1950.
9. Priest, F. O.: Dr. John Clarence Webster. *Canad. M.A.J.*, **64**:351–53, 1951.
10. Schumann, E. A.: John Montgomery Baldy, 1860–1934. *Gynec. Tr.*, **60**:339–42, 1935.
11. Simpson, J. Y.: *Clinical Lectures on the Diseases of Women*. Adam & Charles Black, Edinburgh, 1872, p. 764.
12. Sims, J. M.: *Clinical Notes on Uterine Surgery*. William Wood & Co., New York, 1866, p. 15.
13. Webster, J. C.: A satisfactory operation for certain cases of retroversion of the uterus. *J.A.M.A.*, **37**:913, 1901.

Léon Le Fort and the | CHAPTER

Le Fort Operation* | *76*

At a meeting of the Académie Royale de Médecine in Paris in April, 1825, a new procedure was described for the surgical cure of uterine prolapse, the report being recorded soon thereafter by the following brief note in the proceedings of the meeting: [1] "M. Baudelocque, au nom d'une commission, lit un rapport sur un Mémoire de M. Girardin, relatif à un nouveau procédé pour la cure radicale de la descente de l'utérus. Ce procédé consiste à provoquer l'oblitération de l'orifice du vagin."

The "M. Girardin" mentioned in this note was probably Nicolas Vincent Auguste Gérardin, who was born in 1790 and died in 1868, but he never published anything on the subject. Ten years later, however, at the August 25 meeting of the Académie Royale de Médecine in 1835, the same Gérardin spoke up [2] to assert French priority in the invention of this new operation for the cure of uterine prolapse, if not priority in its actual performance, thus implying that he had merely suggested the principle of treatment originally rather than having actually performed the operation himself.

The idea of partially occluding the vaginal introitus in order to restrain the sagging uterus found expression during the next half century in a number of operations designed by Simon, Spiegelberg, Hegar, and others.[3,6,7] Common to all was the principle of removing part of the vaginal membrane, approximating

* This chapter originally published under the title "Léon Le Fort and His Operation for Uterine Prolapse" in *Surg., Gynec. & Obst.,* **104**:121–24, 1957; reprinted by permission. Copyright, 1957, by The Franklin H. Martin Memorial Foundation.

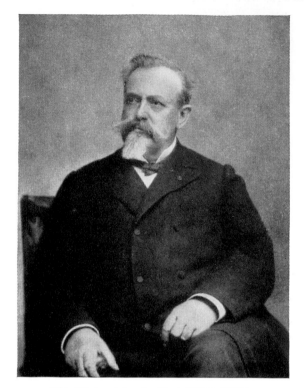

Fig. 76-1. Léon Le Fort (1829–1893).

and suturing together the partially denuded anterior and posterior walls, this procedure usually being combined with perineorrhaphy. In 1877 Léon Le Fort[5] redescribed the principle of partial colpocleisis and reported his own modification of the vaginal plastic operation that has been known ever since as the Le Fort operation. Despite its disadvantages of interfering with the vagina's coital function and rendering the uterus subsequently inaccessible by vaginal approach, the simplicity and safety of the operation still commend it for the correction of uterine prolapse in the elderly and poor-risk patient.

LE FORT'S OPERATION FOR UTERINE PROLAPSE

Le Fort took note of the previously published operations but expressed his dissatisfaction with them as the stimulus for his own improvisations. He wrote:

Procedures less dangerous and easily performed but ineffective, or else effective but hard to perform . . . carrying dangers for the patient, such were the alternatives offered me by surgery when, on November 10, 1876, there consulted me at the Beaujon Hospital a woman of 48 years, a laundress by trade, suffering from complete prolapse of the uterus. The illness seemed to date back six months.

The patient had had three children, the youngest 11 years old, all deliveries being normal. Menstruation was always regular. In May, 1876, she noticed at the vulva a tumor, which appeared intermittently at first, at intervals of approximately 15 days. . . .

In October the tumor began to appear every day, acquiring the size it possessed at the time of operation. Finally, eight days before the patient was hospitalized, reduction of the mass became impossible and pain set in, accompanied by a sensation of heaviness. . . .

The patient asked to be relieved of her infirmity and preferred any kind of operation to the need of wearing a bandage. I therefore had to ask myself what procedure I could use and, as I have just stated, the standard operations seemed unsatisfactory to me. Careful examination of the mechanism by which prolapse occurs suggested to me the principle of the operation that I subsequently performed with complete success. In the case of my patient, as in almost all women who find themselves in this condition, it is not the uterus that protrudes from the vulva primarily, nor is it the uterus that pulls down the anterior and then the posterior wall of the vagina. What is usually noticed first is a cystocele, the protrusion of the anterior vaginal wall outside the vulva. As the cystocele becomes progressively more prominent the uterus finally arrives at and beyond the vulva, as if pulled down by the prolapse of the vesicovaginal septum. The part of this septum nearest the vulva protrudes first, the rest following as a sort of unfolding; and the same effect is produced on the posterior wall, the mucosa of which usually slides over the rectal mucosa, which retains almost its normal position. As the uterus descends, the parts of the anterior and posterior vaginal walls, which are in contact when the uterus is in its normal position, separate more and more from each other as they protrude outside the vulva to allow passage of the deepest parts of the vagina, and finally the uterus.

Evidently, if one could keep the vaginal walls in contact with each other, thus preventing one of them from going forward and the other backward, he could prevent prolapse completely. This is what I sought to do, striving to make the contact intimate and permanent and to restore the anterior and posterior vaginal walls to the same level in reuniting them by suture.

Cognizant of the disadvantages of too extensive a reduction of the vagina, Le Fort carefully limited his dissection.

To thus suture these walls at a certain height entailed closing up the vagina; but the very numerous cases of septate vagina collected in my thesis of 1863 on congenital abnormalities of the uterus and vagina showed that even a complete vertical closure of the vagina scarcely hinders delivery and does not interfere with coitus at all. So in order to cure prolapse I only needed to perform partial dissection and partial closure.

This is not all. In vaginal plastic operations one operates after replacing the uterus, thus in the depths of the vagina, and . . . the operation is long, laborious, and more difficult and tiresome than an operation for vesicovaginal fistula. In my method, on the contrary . . . everything can be done externally and with great ease. Here is how it is done:

Without trying to reduce the uterus, which was completely outside the vulva, and with the patient in the dorsal decubitus position, I first made four incisions in the anterior wall of the vagina, delimiting a flap of mucosa, which I raised, giving me a dissected area about 6 cm long and 2 cm wide and extending to the part nearest the vulva. . . . Then, lifting the prolapsed uterus toward the abdomen in order to bring the posterior aspect of the mass into view, I carried out a dissection of it similar to that which I had made on the anterior wall. . . . This done, I partially replaced the uterus, enough to bring together the uterine edges of these two dissected surfaces, and I applied three sutures to the transverse edges, reuniting the anterior and posterior vaginal walls in linear fashion. I then proceeded to reunite the lateral edges, passing a silver thread . . . through the edge of the anterior dissected surface . . . then the corresponding edge of the posterior dissected surface on each side. . . . Tightening these sutures served to reduce the prolapse of the uterus by bringing the opposing walls of the vagina together. This reduction was effected as the sutures were placed, and when the two edges of the dissected surfaces were reunited in their entire extent, the reduction was complete. . . .

Le Fort carefully left the wire sutures long, to facilitate their later removal. He wrote:

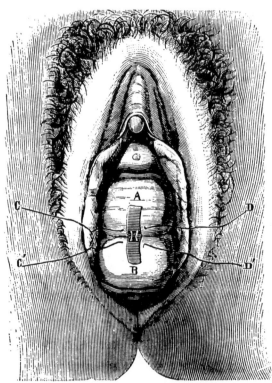

Fig. 76-2. An illustration from Le Fort's paper,[5] showing a stage in the operation of partial colpocleisis.

After ten days I began to remove the sutures. The therapeutic result was perfect; the uterus was supported perfectly, and when I had the patient cough and strain while squatting, there was no suggestion of any protrusion from the vulva; their wasn't even any appreciable pouting.

The second stage of the operation was carried out later:

I could have thus limited my intervention, and I would have done so if I had wished to sacrifice the patient's interests to my desire to show . . . the happy result of the operation. But the fourchette was so lax and so wide that I feared to see the result compromised later by the absence of support at the side of the vulva. I therefore completed the operation with a dissection at the fourchette and neighboring parts. . . . I did the suturing in two layers according to my method . . . and when the patient was discharged . . . the reunion was complete and definitive in its whole extent and along the entire surface of the dissection. . . . The perineal floor, reconstructed by the second operation, gives support to the vaginal walls and prevents any tendency to their protrusion. . . . The patient, relieved of all pain and discomfort, was able to perform strenuous work and carry heavy loads, and obtained from the operation all the benefit she could possibly hope for.

LE FORT'S LIFE

Léon Le Fort was born in Lille, France, December 5, 1829.[4] At the age of 17 years, he entered the business of his father, a clothing merchant, but was permitted to return to his studies a year later, after his aversion for the business began to affect his health. He entered the College de Lille in 1848, but was soon called to military duty in the national guard of the province, which he served with great distinction. Inspired by the campaign of Paris, he decided to follow a military career as had his grandfather, who gained renown in the siege of Lille in 1792. Although Le Fort's father was unsympathetic to a military future for his son, he wisely refrained from rigid opposition to it, proposing in compromise that Léon enter the army's sanitary corps.

By the time the military hospitals of instruction were closed and the students dismissed in 1850, Le Fort had developed sufficient interest in medicine to pursue its study in civil life. A violent defender of civil liberties, he participated in the citizens' revolt against the *coup d'état* of December, 1851, and narrowly escaped being taken prisoner. He then settled down to the serious study of medicine in Paris, where he served as intern in 1852. In 1858 he received an appointment as aide in anatomy after publishing a distinguished thesis on the structure of the human lung. In this work he called attention to direct communications between the bronchial and pulmonary blood vessels, anastomoses with which his name is still associated. He later became interested in methods for resecting the knee and hip, and published valuable papers on the subject, pointing out the importance of surgical hygiene.

Like his contemporary, Tarnier, Le Fort became engrossed in the concept of contagion before the birth of the science of bacteriology, basing his concepts entirely on statistical reasoning. In 1865 he carried out a large-scale statistical investigation of 1,823,093 births in England, Ireland, Holland, Belgium, Germany, Austria-Hungary, Russia, Sweden, and Switzerland, comparing the results in home deliveries with those conducted in hospitals; but his conclusions, based on the doctrine of contagion, were so contrary to existing ideas that the director of hospital administration, under whose sponsorship the study was undertaken, refused to publish Le Fort's report. Applying the principles of asepsis to his surgical service in the Hospital Cochin in 1867, he performed seven leg and thigh amputations during the next two years without a single death, whereas the mortality from this type of operation had been as high as 65.7 per cent in the rest of Paris.

Le Fort's professional interests encompassed many fields, including medical administration, military medicine, public health, and demography. He published papers on congenital malformations of the uterus and vagina, abdominal and vaginal hysterectomy, chloroform anesthesia, and numerous plastic procedures, including skin grafting, perineorrhaphy, and correction of exstrophy of the bladder. He ligated the common carotid to cure pulsatile exophthalmos and was the first in France to perform nephrectomy for ureteral fistula. In 1873 he was called to the chair of surgery in Paris, replacing Denonvilliers, and in 1875 he was elected president of the Societé de Chirurgie.

Ever ready to defend the rights of the individual, Le Fort demanded justice for women accused of prostitution, in a historic debate on the public prophylaxis of syphilis before the Académie Royale de Médecine in 1888. "Je respecte la loi," he declaimed, "je hais l'arbitraire. Pour protéger la santé publique, je demande une loi! Pour protéger une femme qui peut être injustement accusée, je demande des juges."

Le Fort maintained a country home in Menestreau, where he was chosen mayor of the community. It was here that he pursued his principal avocations, the rearing and care of birds and fish. He died October 19, 1893, at the age of 63.

REFERENCES

1. Académie Royale de Médecine proceedings. *Arch. gén. de méd.*, **8**:132, 1825.
2. Académie Royale de Médecine proceedings. *Gaz. méd.*, **3**(n.s.):558, 1835.
3. Hegar, A.: Ueber Operationen bei Prolapsus. *Arch. f. Gynäk.*, **6**:319–20, 1874.
4. Jaccoud, S.: *Léon Le Fort, 1829–1893. Éloge prononcé a l'Académie de Médecine dans la séance annuelle du 10 Décembre 1907.* Masson & Cie, Paris.
5. Le Fort, L.: Nouveau procédé pour la guérison du prolapsus utérin. *Bull. gén. de thérap.*, **92**:337–44, 1877.

6. Simon, G.: *Mittheilungen aus der Chirurgischen Klinik des Rostocker Krankenhauses während der Jahre 1861–1865. II. Abtheilung. Beiträge zur Plastischen Chirurgie, vorzugsweise zu den Plastischen Operationen an den Wandungen der zugängigen Körperhöhlen.* Carl Reichenecker, Prague, 1868, pp. 275–93.

7. Spiegelberg, O.: Zur Entstehung und Behandlung des Vorfalls der Scheide und Gebärmutter. *Berl. klin. Wchnschr.,* **9**:249–50, 262–64, 1872.

Thomas James Watkins and the Watkins Interposition

CHAPTER 77

Most gynecologists view the uterus as an organ of reproduction exclusively. Some regard menstruation as a separate, although related uterine function, acknowledging that its value may be entirely psychologic. A dwindling minority still cling to the belief in the organ's endocrine action, particularly on the ovaries and mammary glands. Practically all agree that after the menopause the uterus serves no known function but looms only as a potential liability. Scarcely ever is the uterus thought of as a prosthesis. Yet it has been used precisely for this purpose in the surgical treatment of uterine prolapse associated with cystocele since the latter part of the nineteenth century. Indeed, during the first decades of the present century the interposition operation, usually known as the Watkins interposition, which employs the uterine fundus as an obturator for the defective anterior pelvic diaphragm and a buttress for the base of the bladder, was one of the most popular of the vaginal plastic procedures. Wrote Watkins,[13] in agreement with the Manchester school:

I do not believe it advisable to remove the uterus in any case of prolapse unless it is the seat of disease which indicates its extirpation as I believe as good, or better results can be obtained by other means with less danger to life, with less danger of complications and with less suffering after the operation.

The origins of the interposition operation go back to 1886, when von Rabenau [9] reported on a new method for curing retroversion. After amputating part of the cervix, chiefly the anterior lip, and separating the bladder from the uterus, he delivered the fundus through the anterior cul-de-sac and sutured the anterior surface of the uterus to the anterior wall of the vagina. Two years later Sänger [10] suggested that the uterine corpus might be sutured to the un-opened anterior vaginal wall, an operation that was carried out forthwith by Schücking [11] with the aid of a special needle and holder that he introduced into the endometrial cavity. A similar procedure, which he called vaginal hys-teropexy, was soon reported by Törngren,[12] in which the corpus was sutured to the anterior wall of the vagina by means of a long needle that penetrated the walls of both vagina and uterus and followed the intrauterine guide especially designed for the purpose. These blind operations lacked appeal, however, and neither Schücking nor Törngren received any published endorsement of his work. The principle of vaginal fixation for the retroverted uterus had taken hold, nonetheless, and was firmly established by Mackenrodt's numerous publications [8] and by Dührssen's meticulously detailed report of 207 per-sonally performed operations, published in 1894.[4]

The European contributions to the transposition operation during the ensuing five years are well summarized and clearly illustrated in the Döderlein-Krönig *Operative Gynäkologie*.[3] W. A. Freund,[5] who had previously used the uterine fundus as a plug in the repair of vaginal fistulas, reported a similar technique in 1896 for the correction of uterine prolapse. After delivering the fundus into the vagina through the posterior cul-de-sac, he sutured the anterior wall of the uterus to the posterior wall of the vagina and the posterior wall of the uterus to the anterior wall of the vagina. In the dome of the fundus, which was now the dependent, presenting part of the uterus, occluding the vagina, he made an artificial opening for drainage. In 1900 Fritsch [6] modified Freund's operation, delivering the uterus anteriorly and suturing its posterior surface to the denuded anterior vaginal wall but covering the uterus with flaps from the posterior vaginal wall.

Wertheim, in the April 8, 1899, issue of the *Centralblatt für Gynäkologie*,[15] made the first clear reference to the use of the uterine fundus as a supportive platform for the bladder. He stated:

The body of the uterus appeared to me, because of its size and shape, to be very well suited to act like a sort of ball against the cystocele, and the acute anteversion and deployment of the uterus necessarily resulting from the operation must oppose the prolapse of the vagina in a salutary manner.

Wertheim delivered the corpus anteriorly, sutured its posterior surface to the denuded anterior vaginal wall, leaving the dome and anterior wall of the uterus exposed within the vagina. Schauta's operation differed from Wertheim's only in covering all of the uterus with the anterior vaginal membrane, except for a small area on the fundus.

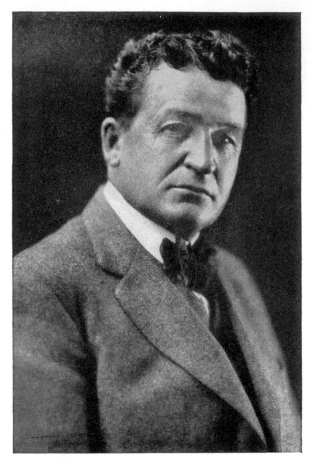

Fig. 77-1. Thomas James Watkins (1863–1925). (Courtesy of American Gynecological Society.)

WATKINS' OPERATION

The interposition operation best known to American gynecologists was first performed by T. J. Watkins on January 29, 1898. His report was presented before the Chicago Gynecological Society on September 15, 1899, and appeared in print before the end of the year,[13] the same year in which Wertheim's paper was published. Since then many have quibbled over the question of priority. It would appear that Wertheim was the first to clearly state the mechanical principle of the interposition operation in its simultaneous correction of cystocele and prolapse but that Watkins published the first description of the interposition operation as we now know it. Schauta later claimed that he had been using an almost identical procedure since 1889.

Watkins' patient was a Mrs. J.T.A., aged 58.

[She] dated her illness from birth of last child, which occurred 22 years before. Her suffering had increased since the menopause, which occurred four years previously. She suffered much distress from "bearing-down" pains, backache, and pain in the inguinal regions on walking and standing. A protrusion at the vulvar orifice mechanically interfered with walking and sitting. She also suffered from leucorrhoea and vesical irritability. Examination revealed a large cystocele and rectocele. The uterus was atrophied, retroverted, and prolapsed to the second degree.

After the patient was prepared for operation, in the words of Watkins:

The uterus was curetted and separated from the vagina by a circular incision. The bladder was separated from the uterus by blunt dissection and the peritoneal cavity opened in front of the uterus. The anterior wall of the uterus was grasped by bullet forceps and the organ anteverted. About two inches of the upper portion of the anterior vaginal wall was now sutured to the upper border of the broad ligaments lateral to the uterus, and to the fundus of the uterus with silkworm-gut sutures. The posterior vaginal wall was incised, longitudinally in the medium line from the cervix downward, about one inch so as to allow the cervix to be displaced upward and backward. The wound in front of the cervix was now closed by silkworm-gut sutures inserted transversely, that is, parallel to the line of incision anterior to the cervix. The operation had at this stage lengthened the anterior vaginal wall, obliterated the cystocele, and forced the cervix upward and backward into its normal location. One silkworm-gut suture secured the cervix in the angle of the incision in the posterior vaginal wall. Emmet's perineorrhaphy was made to correct the prolapse and displacement of the posterior vaginal wall. The sutures were removed at the end of four weeks when the union was found to be perfect. The vagina was about normal length, the uterus anteverted and the vaginal walls free from prolapse. . . . The result was much better than any I have seen follow other operations for like conditions.

Watkins recognized, as had his European colleagues, the limitations of the operation:

The operation is not adapted to cases during the child-bearing period on account of the danger of complications to gestation and labor. [When performed during the reproductive age it should always be accompanied by tubal sterilization.] This operation, however, is adapted to the most difficult cases of uterine prolapse and cystocele as these usually occur after the menopause as the result of senile atrophy.

With increasing experience Watkins made minor modifications in his original operation, but its three principles, which he enunciated in 1906 in a second, well-illustrated paper,[14] remained unchanged:

1. The bladder is supported by and rests upon the posterior wall of the uterus.
2. The uterus is elevated in the pelvis by being tipped forward—in fact, its position is changed about 180°. The twist produced in the broad ligaments by the

change in the position of the uterus perceptibly shortens them. This twisting of the broad ligaments is the chief factor in correcting the uterine prolapse. 3. The tendency for the uterus and bladder to prolapse, following the operation, are antagonistic, as any sagging of the bladder increases the anterior displacement of the uterus, and any prolapse of the uterus elevates the bladder-wall.*

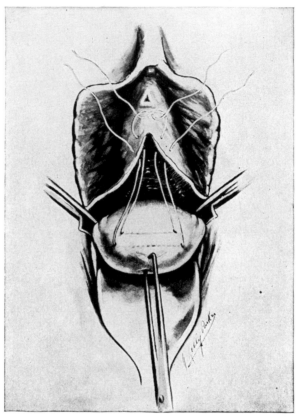

Fig. 77-2. Illustration from Watkins' 1906 paper,[14] showing a step in his operation. (By permission of *Surgery, Gynecology and Obstetrics.*)

The interposition operation has undergone further modification in the hands of Watkins' followers, who have usually amputated the cervix as part of the procedure. This eliminates the risk of subsequent cervical cancer, but pathologic changes can still occur in the body of the uterus. Access to the endometrial cavity then becomes exceedingly difficult. Chiefly because of this hazard in postmenopausal patients and the incompatibility between the operation and later pregnancy in younger women, the interposition procedure gradually became less popular among gynecologists, and by the middle of the twentieth century had largely been supplanted by the Manchester opera-

* By permission of *Surgery, Gynecology and Obstetrics.*

tion and vaginal hysterectomy combined with anterior colporrhaphy. In the Sloane Hospital for Women, for example, not a single interposition operation was performed in 1956 among 1758 gynecologic operations, including 143 for uterine prolapse. The operation has not been completely abandoned, however, for some gynecologists continue to regard it as the procedure of choice

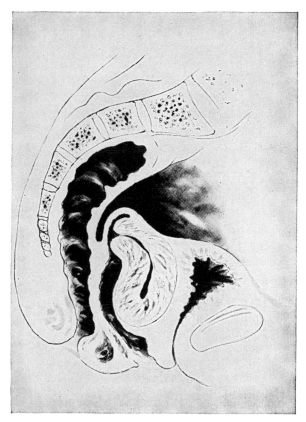

Fig. 77-3. Another illustration from Watkins' 1906 paper,[14] showing the position of the interposed uterus at the completion of his operation. (By permission of *Surgery, Gynecology and Obstetrics.*)

in an occasional case of uterine descensus with large cystocele and small corpus, especially in the elderly or poor-risk patient. It offers a rapid and simple method of compensating for the relaxed supports without sacrificing the coital function of the vagina.

WATKINS' LIFE

Thomas James Watkins was born July 6, 1863, on a farm near Utica, New York, where his early youth was spent in "toil and drudgery." [1,2,7] After working his way through preparatory school he attended the medical department of the University of Michigan from 1880 to 1883, when he transferred to Bellevue Hospital Medical College in New York City, obtaining his M.D. there in 1886. He subsequently interned at the Utica City Hospital, St. Peter's Hospital in Brooklyn, and the Woman's Hospital in New York where, under Emmet, he developed an interest in vaginal plastic surgery. In 1889 Watkins moved to Chicago, and for the next 34 years served on the faculty of Northwestern University, being promoted to professor of gynecology in 1916. He also served as attending gynecologist to the St. Luke's, Wesley, and Mercy Hospitals in Chicago. He helped found the American College of Surgeons, was elected president of the American Gynecological Society for 1915, and chairman of the American Medical Association's Section on Obstetrics, Gynecology and Abdominal Surgery for 1919. He died of a heart attack on April 1, 1925.

REFERENCES

1. Curtis, A. H.: Thomas J. Watkins, M.D., F.A.C.S. *Surg., Gynec. & Obst.,* **40**:712–13, 1925.
2. Deaths: Thomas James Watkins. *J.A.M.A.,* **84**:1065, 1925.
3. Döderlein, A., and Krönig, B.: *Operative Gynäkologie,* 3rd ed. Georg Thieme, Leipzig, 1912, pp. 276–90.
4. Dührssen, A.: Ueber die operative Heilung der mobilen und fixirten Retroflexio uteri auf vaginalem Wege an der Hand von 207 eigenen Operationsfällen, mit besonderer Berücksichtigung der Dauerfolge. *Arch. f. Gynäk.,* **47**:284–448, 1894.
5. Freund, W. A.: Abstract of report to the Naturforscherversammlung in Frankfurt a. M. *Centralbl. f. Gynäk.,* **20**:1009–10, 1896.
6. Fritsch, H.: Prolapsoperation. *Centralbl. f. Gynäk.,* **24**:49–53, 1900.
7. Kosmak, G. W.: Thomas J. Watkins, M.D. *Am. J. Obst. & Gynec.,* **9**:593–94, 1925.
8. Mackenrodt, H.: Alwin Mackenrodt. *Zentralbl. f. Gynäk.,* **50**:1042–50, 1926.
9. Rabenau, F. von: Ueber eine neue operative Behandlung der Retroflexio uteri. *Berl. klin. Wchnschr.,* **23**:284–86, 1886.
10. Sänger, M.: Über operative Behandlung der Retroversio-flexio uteri. *Centralbl. f. Gynäk.,* **12**:34–43, 1888.
11. Schücking, A.: Die vaginale Ligatur des Uterus und ihre Anwendung bei Retroflexio und Prolapsus uteri. *Centralbl. f. Gynäk.,* **12**:682–86, 1888.
12. Törngren, A.: Nouvelle manière de pratiquer l'hystéropexie vaginale. *Arch. de Tocol. et de Gynéc.,* **18**:34–43, 1891.
13. Watkins, T. J.: The treatment of cystocele and uterine prolapse after the menopause. *Am. Gynaec. & Obst. J.,* **15**:420–23, 1899.
14. Watkins, T. J.: Treatment of cases of extensive cystocele and uterine prolapse. *Surg., Gynec. & Obst.,* **2**:659–67, 1906.
15. Wertheim, E.: Zur plastischen Verwendung des Uterus bei Prolapsen. *Centralbl. f. Gynäk.,* **23**:369–72, 1899.

Karl Schuchardt and the Schuchardt Incision

CHAPTER

78

Gynecologists remain divided over the preferred surgical approach to the pelvic viscera. For all but the simplest intrapelvic procedures the majority favor abdominal laparotomy; but an impressive and authoritative group of pelvic surgeons still regard the vaginal approach as superior for a variety of gynecologic operations, including hysterectomy. The latter school evolved from the urgent search by nineteenth-century gynecologists for an alternate method of treating uterine cancer; for in the days before anesthesia and asepsis, hysterectomy by the abdominal route carried with it a staggering mortality.

Langenbeck's account [5] of an abdominal hysterectomy, performed in 1825 for advanced cervical cancer, vividly illustrates the surgery of that era, when speed took precedence over hemostasis. He reported:

> Standing at the left side of the patient, I cut through the skin and linea alba from the pubic symphysis to approximately 2 inches below the umbilicus. With several strokes of the finger I then separated the wound edges. . . . I was helped in [finding the correct place to open the peritoneum] by the tip of the catheter pushed up [by an assistant] sufficiently firmly against the apex of the bladder to elevate the latter. Remote from this point I grasped the peritoneum with forceps at the upper part of the incision, held it up in a point, and cut off the tip. In the resultant opening I inserted a grooved director, and with it as a guide, dilated the opening enough to insert my index finger. With it I elevated the peritoneum and split it up and down. . . . I now inserted my left hand into the abdominal

665

cavity, grasped the uterine fundus, drew it up as far as I could, and alongside my hand . . . I advanced a pair of long scissors with short blades and blunt tips. I then cut the right broad ligament, which could easily be felt on a stretch . . . close to the uterus. . . . I could then bring the uterus up even more with my left hand and thus put the vagina on a stretch. I now grasped the uterus closer to the vagina, into which a wooden sound had been inserted so that I could be absolutely sure of its position, directed the scissors against the taut vagina, and cut through it below the hard tumor growing out from it. I was then able to pull the uterus so far out of the abdominal cavity that I could separate it from the left broad ligament with a scalpel. . . . The abdominal wound was closed with adhesive plaster and a sponge placed in the vagina. Only seven minutes were required for completion of the operation[!] [The patient died the following day.]

In an effort to circumvent the hazards of abdominal hysterectomy, Langenbeck resorted to the vaginal approach for his next patient with uterine cancer, in one of the earliest attempts to excise the nonprolapsed uterus through the vagina. This operation, although doomed to failure likewise, embodied a notable advance in vaginal surgery. To improve exposure and provide access to the vaginal vault Langenbeck began with a deep relaxing incision into the perineal body, the forerunner of the Schuchardt incision. He wrote:

After emptying the urinary bladder with a catheter I cut through the posterior commissure of the labia majora, but the incision stopped short of entering the rectum. This [perineal incision] is essential, for otherwise the hand cannot be brought to the place where the vagina must be separated from the uterus; and because otherwise, after this separation, one cannot reach up to the fundus with his hand. . . . After this incision was made I was able to insert my whole left hand, which it was impossible to do previously, because the space between the pubic arch and the posterior commissure was too narrow.

Even after Freund's epochal complete abdominal hysterectomy in 1878 [2,3] the appalling mortality from this operation discouraged most surgeons, who therefore persisted in their efforts to find a safer approach to the pelvic contents. Cervical amputation had long been recognized as inadequate treatment for cancer, and the urgent necessity of complete hysterectomy led to a variety of novel but short-lived operations, including a posterior, sacral approach.[8] For more than 50 years little or no use was made of Langenbeck's relaxing incision of the perineum. Only with the renewed and successful efforts of late-nineteenth-century gynecologists to revive vaginal hysterectomy was the value of preliminary perineotomy rediscovered.

On April 2, 1881, Olshausen,[7] operating on a 61-year-old nullipara with uterine cancer, facilitated his approach to the pelvis by first making two lateral incisions in the perineum. Within the next decade other operations were being carried out with greater frequency per vaginam, including myomectomy and ovariectomy. In his report on these procedures in 1890 Leopold [6] advised that "if the vagina is too narrow it should be split by longitudinal lateral incisions, deep enough so that a broad posterior retractor can be inserted easily. These longitudinal incisions approach each other as they extend internally, and merge with the vaginal vault incision that is made in circumcising the cervix."

As their newly acquired skill in vaginal surgery increased, gynecologists recognized fewer contraindications to a vaginal attack on the pelvic viscera. Adequate exposure became the primary desideratum. The two major obstacles to vaginal hysterectomy, Dührssen [1] wrote in 1891, were a marked contracture of the vagina, as from senile involution, and a significant increase in uterine size. Each of these barriers was readily surmountable by appropriate incision of the perineum and vagina.

Dührssen recounted his experience with the first type of problem in a postmenopausal virgin with corpus cancer:

After grasping the cervix with a tenaculum and pulling it down, I first tried to pass a suture around the base of the ligaments on either side, in order to make the operative field more accessible by means of these traction sutures and to facilitate circumcision of the portio. This procedure was found to be impossible, however, because of the very narrow and rigid vagina. I therefore divided the vaginal tube, the levator ani, and the constrictor cunni on the right side by means of an incision (Scheidendammincision) and was then able to perform total hysterectomy very easily.

In a second patient, with fibroids, the size of the uterus required multiple incisions of the posterior vaginal wall before the organ could be delivered. Dührssen explained:

The direction of the incision, which after repair has a length of 6–7 cm in the vagina and on the perineum, is midway between the ischial tuberosity and the anus. I prefer this deep unilateral incision as basically superior to the more superficial bilateral incisions of Leopold, because repair of the former is faster and its end result better cosmetically and probably functionally as well. With the unilateral incision the vulva is intact after healing is complete, only a fine scar remaining in the perineum. With bilateral incisions, on the other hand, a defect in the vulva always persists, favoring leucorrhea and possibly the development of prolapse also.

SCHUCHARDT'S MEDIOLATERAL INCISION

On November 21, 1893, Karl Schuchardt [9] was confronted with a large, ulcerating cervical cancer that had extended onto the vagina and into the left parametrium, limiting the mobility of the uterus. In his earnest efforts to effect a cure of the stricken, 35-year-old mother of eight, Schuchardt under-

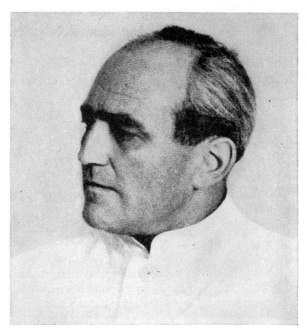

Fig. 78-1. Karl August Schuchardt (1856–1901). (Courtesy of National Library of Medicine, Washington, D. C.)

took a critical evaluation of the available methods of surgical treatment. The sacral approach had found favor in cases of uterine cancer with fixation of the parametria and broad ligaments, as it had for extirpation of the rectum for malignant tumors of this organ. Reasoned Schuchardt:

> The sacral method of hysterectomy has not only extended our limits of operability, in that patients can thereby be completely cured who were previously considered inoperable, but it has above all opened an approach through which the uterus and its adnexa are far more readily accessible to surgical treatment than before. Vaginal hysterectomy, by the very nature of the operation, must be carried out blindly in a very large measure. The progressively placed mass ligatures and even the prior clamping have a somewhat unsurgical character, whereas with the sacral approach one can grasp each vessel nicely and ligate it individually, and examine the parts to be removed more precisely and differentiate the diseased from the healthy.
>
> It seems obvious that further advance of the limits of surgical treatment of uterine cancer can come about only if we can apply to the uterus also the same principles that have been proved correct in the treatment of cancer of other parts of the body. No one would think today of excising a cancer of the lip or breast without simultaneously investigating carefully the immediate and remote surrounding areas of the primary cancer and the associated lymph nodes. The standard axillary dissection in breast cancer, for example, has developed from this

theoretically sound requirement. The treatment of uterine cancer, despite such apparently favorable results from vaginal hysterectomy, has not, for a long time, stood on as high a plane as the surgical treatment of cancer of other parts of the body. In the former case the operator usually contents himself with removal of the primarily diseased organ without regard for the further extension of the cancer into the lymphatic channels. The peculiar technique of vaginal hysterectomy makes it impossible to recognize, much less remove, cancerous growths in the parametria that were not palpable preoperatively. Indeed, everyone knows how difficult is palpation of small cancerous nodes in the axilla, for example, in cases of breast cancer, and how easily they are discovered as soon as the axilla is opened for dissection. Thus even the most experienced finger will probably not encounter small carcinomatous parametrial infiltrations that would be discovered in operative procedures that expose the broad ligaments adequately.

The fact that the sacral method, which until now has been the only one to provide such exposure, is more serious and dangerous, clearly stands in the way of its general adoption. Resection of part of the sacrum and the coccyx and transection of the sacrosciatic ligaments are unquestionably formidable procedures, even if they do not weaken the pelvic floor. Even osteoplastic resection of the sacrum scarcely contributes to making the operation less mutilating. . . . In addition to the difficulty of the operation, a long period of wound healing follows, which usually requires packing and secondary closure in the cases that run a satisfactory course. This has led to application of the sacral approach only to very bad cases of uterine cancer with tumorous infiltration of both broad ligaments and therefore no longer operable by the [usual] vaginal route. Methods must therefore be sought that combine the advantages of the sacral approach, namely precision of operation and accessibility of the broad ligaments, with the relative safety and rapid convalescence offered by vaginal hysterectomy.

With his objective thus defined, but ignoring, perhaps unwittingly, the previous efforts of others to augment vaginal exposure, Schuchardt proceeded to describe his preliminary division of the perineum:

[It is accomplished] without any bony operation and without transection of the sacrospinous or sacrotuberous ligament or the levator ani, in order to make more accessible from below a uterus whose mobility is limited by cancerous infiltration of the parametrium. With the patient in the lithotomy position and her buttocks elevated, a large, essentially sagittal incision is made, somewhat convex externally, beginning between the middle and posterior third of the labium majus on the side of the involved parametrium, extending posteriorly toward the sacrum, and stopping two fingerbreadths from the anus. The wound is deepened only in the fatty tissue of the ischiorectal fossa, leaving the funnel of the levator ani muscle, the rectum behind it, and the sacral ligaments intact. Internally the side wall of the vagina is opened into the ischiorectal fossa and the vagina divided in its lateral aspect by a long incision extending up to the cervix. There thus results a suprisingly free view of all the structures under consideration, and removal of the uterus as well as the cancerous nodes in the broad ligament on this side can be carried out with the greatest certainty and ease. . . .

Further experience must teach whether division of the vaginal tube can also be carried out bilaterally. Perhaps in such a case, in the presence of carcinomatous infiltrations in both broad ligaments, the skin incisions do not need to be quite so large as with unilateral involvement of the parametrium.

Modern medical authors may well marvel at the speed of nineteenth-century publication. Schuchardt performed his operation on November 21, 1893; yet his report appeared in print in the *Centralblatt für Chirurgie* that same year!

Mediolateral incision of the perineum, whether or not carried deep into the ischiorectal fossa as advocated by Schuchardt, has since been known as the Schuchardt incision. The gynecologic counterpart of the obstetric episiotomy, it constitutes an invaluable adjunct whenever increased exposure of the vaginal vault is required, as in the repair of certain vaginal fistulas, as well as in radical vaginal hysterectomy for uterine cancer.

SCHUCHARDT'S LIFE

Karl August Schuchardt was born in 1856 in Göttingen, Germany, where his father served as a governmental physician.[4] Young Schuchardt studied medicine in the universities of Jena, Strassburg, and Göttingen, graduating from the last in 1878, and devoted the next eight years to specialized training, first in pathology under Ponfick, and then in surgery under Volkmann. After practicing in Halle for four years, he was made an official in the state hospital in Stettin and was ultimately appointed director of its surgical division and professor in the university. His writings embraced a wide variety of surgical topics, including tuberculous fistulas of the rectum, tumors of the larynx, bladder, breast, and uterus, appendicitis, and gastric ulcer. He also published a comprehensive treatise on diseases of the bones and joints. Schuchardt died on October 28, 1901, at the age of 45, of sepsis resulting from an accidental needle prick received while operating.

REFERENCES

1. Dührssen, A.: Bemerkungen zur Technik der vaginalen Totalexstirpation des Uterus. *Charité-Ann.* (Berlin), **16**:513–22, 1891.
2. Freund, W. A.: Eine neue Methode der Exstirpation des ganzen Uterus. *Samml. klin. Vortr.*, No. 133. Gynäk. No. 41, 911–24, 1878.
3. Freund, W. A.: Zu meiner Methode der totalen Uterus-Exstirpation. *Centralbl. f. Gynäk.*, **2**:265–69, 1878.
4. Gerdeck, W.: Nekrolog. Karl Schuchardt. *Deutsche med. Wchnschr.*, **27**:883, 1901.
5. Langenbeck, C. J. M.: Beschreibung zweier, vom Herausgeber verrichteten, Exstirpation krebshafter, nicht vorgefallener Gebärmutter. In Langenbeck, C. J. M. (ed.): *Neue Bibliothek für die Chirurgie und Ophthalmologie.* Hahn, Hannover, 1828, Vol. 4, pp. 698–728.

6. Leopold, G.: Die operative Behandlung der Uterusmyome durch vaginale Enucleation, Castration, Myomotomie und vaginale Totalexstirpation. *Arch. f. Gynäk.*, **38**:1–80, 1890.

7. Olshausen, R.: Ueber Totalexstirpation des Uterus nach zehn eigenen Fällen. *Berl. klin. Wchnschr.*, **18**:497–501, 518–21, 1881.

8. Ricci, J. V.: *One Hundred Years of Gynaecology, 1800–1900.* Blakiston Co., Philadelphia, 1945, pp. 178–79.

9. Schuchardt, K.: Eine neue Methode der Gebärmutterexstirpation. *Centralbl. f. Chir.*, **20**:1121–26, 1893.

Ernst Wertheim and the

Wertheim Operation *

CHAPTER

79

Carcinoma of the uterine cervix provides one of the few examples in medical history of a method of treatment, once discarded by the majority of the profession, later being reclaimed. Radical hysterectomy, abandoned by most American gynecologists after the advent of radiotherapy in the early part of the present century, has enjoyed an impressive resurgence during the last decade and now bids fair to take a place of equal importance along with irradiation techniques in the treatment of cervical cancer. Whereas earlier generations of gynecologists concerned themselves with the relative merits of the radical abdominal versus the radical vaginal operation, the primary therapeutic choice now lies between surgery and irradiation.

Suggestions that the cancerous uterus might be surgically extirpated were first made by Wrisberg and by Osiander toward the close of the eighteenth century.[7] It was not until almost a century later, however, in 1878, that Freund [2,3] performed the abdominal operation on which the modern radical hysterectomy for cervical cancer is based; and only in 1895 that Ries, one of Freund's students, first suggested dissection of the pelvic lymph nodes in conjunction with this operation.[8] Abdominal hysterectomy was soon taken up by a number of gynecologists in their somber efforts to combat the disease.

* This chapter originally published under the title "Ernst Wertheim and His Operation for Uterine Cancer" in *Cancer*, **9**:859–65, 1956; reprinted by permission. Copyright © 1956, by the American Cancer Society, Inc.

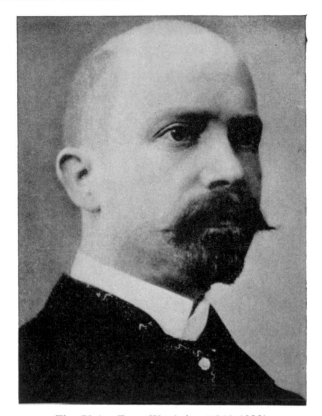

Fig. 79-1. Ernst Wertheim (1864–1920).

WERTHEIM'S HYSTERECTOMY

Foremost among them was Ernst Wertheim, who devoted himself relentlessly to the development of the operation, acquired a vast experience with it, and popularized it to the extent that the procedure soon became known as the Wertheim operation—a designation it still retains although the procedure has been greatly modified during the ensuing 50 years.

Wertheim first performed his operation in 1898 and, in the decade from 1900 to 1910, published a score of papers and discussions [10-28] dealing with various aspects of the problem, his writings on the subject culminating in a monograph, published in 1911, entitled *Die erweiterte abdominale Operation bei Carcinoma colli Uteri*,[29] based on 500 cases. The futility of cervical amputation, founded on the erroneous concept that carcinoma of this organ was slow to invade the parametrium, had already been demonstrated, as Wertheim, arguing for a bolder approach, pointed out in his introduction:

As the hopes that had been placed in partial removal of the uterus as a substitute for total hysterectomy . . . were not destined to be fulfilled, even in carefully selected cases, the teaching lost validity that carcinoma of the uterus is exceptional and that it proceeds beyond the bounds of the uterus only late in its development; and the realization began to mature that one had to strive to remove as much as possible of the surrounding tissue together with the primary tumor in order to achieve better results, as is the case with operative procedures for cancer of other organs.

Then, as now, the parametrium was the objective of the operation and the ureter its bête noire. Wrote Wertheim:

It was a priori clear that methodical treatment of the ureters was indispensable to a so-called extended operation. Extensive removal of parametrial tissue for a successful approach to advanced cases was associated with the greatest danger to the ureters, unless preliminary safeguard was taken, as is obvious from operative experience as well as from the topographic anatomy.

At first I sought to achieve this safeguarding of the ureters by retaining the hitherto predominant vaginal hysterectomy, by catheterizing the ureters preoperatively, and by leaving the catheters in place during the operation in order to make sure of the ureters while we accomplished the widest possible removal of the parametrium from the pelvic wall. . . . The amount of parametrial tissue thus removed did not satisfy us, however, and . . . the blood loss was still quite heavy if very much parametrium was removed.

It thus came about that we trusted more and more in the idea of the abdominal approach. The resulting view and accessibility of the ureters in their course through this region is incomparable and can be achieved in no other way. This approach provides the further advantage that the other surroundings of the uterus are also most accessible and can be dealt with precisely in relation to the spread of the carcinoma.

The previous experience of others in exposing the ureters at hysterectomy was meager and conflicting. Wertheim therefore embarked on this surgical venture "only with great care and under strict control."

After a few cases, however, we had the feeling that our approach was correct. Exposure of the ureters succeeded easily; the insight that we gained into the method of spread of the carcinoma proved surprisingly instructive; removal of the surrounding tissue and the regional lymphatics became very extensive; and, the greatest achievement of all in our opinion, the operation could be performed in cases so advanced that, according to the prevailing views, they were considered as absolutely inoperable by the vaginal approach. Although the mortality was disturbingly high at first, we had the confident conviction that we could succeed in reducing it.

The pathologic findings encouraged Wertheim to continue. He wrote:

The correctness of our procedure was proved to us by histologic examination of the extirpated organs. These showed the teaching to be false that cervical cancer transgresses the bounds of the uterus only late, for in a considerable number of apparently early cases the carcinoma had already sent its offshoots and advance guards to the parametrium and regional lymph nodes. This had not been shown previously by histologic examinations of this sort; for everything that was known at that time about the spread of cervical cancer was based on cases in which the illness had proved fatal, that is, on far advanced cases, long inoperable.

Under the caption of indications for the operation, Wertheim wrote:

The extended abdominal operation demonstrated, at the outset, that the entire surroundings of the diseased uterus can be extirpated, and this knowledge has broadened the indications for the operation. Whereas infiltration of the parametrium with fixation of the uterus so that the organ could not be pulled down . . . was a contraindication to the vaginal operation, with our operation we can attack cases with parametrial infiltration and feel confident that fixed organs, such as the bladder, rectum, and ureters, can be freed and the diseased uterus removed completely, even in advanced cases of carcinoma.

We therefore gradually broadened the indications for operation. Before the year 1898, 15 operations were done among 100 patients with uterine cancer who presented themselves at the Vienna Clinic. With the aid of the extended abdominal operation this number soon rose to 30 per cent; with our increasing experience it rose to 50 per cent; and in the last two years it has been 61.9 per cent. . . .

Since it is impossible to determine the extent of spread of the disease by examination, one must consider every operation for carcinoma of the uterus as an exploratory laparotomy. Only after the abdomen is opened is it possible to say whether the operation can be completed or not. Laparotomy provides the opportunity of seeing the condition of the lymph nodes, the ureters, the bladder, and the rectum. The eye can see, the fingers can palpate, and, if this is not enough, the peritoneum can be opened up without the operation losing its exploratory character. Even dissection of the ureters and loosening of the bladder or rectum do not prejudice the situation, for the incised peritoneum can be resutured and closed. This is an advantage over the vaginal method, in which one often becomes aware of the uselessness of the procedure at a stage of the operation when turning back is no longer possible.

. . . We first palpate the regional lymph nodes. If enlarged lymph-node tumors are present, an attempt is made to remove them. If this proves impossible, the operation is abandoned and the abdomen closed. . . . Next comes investigation of the ureters. If the ureters are dilated, showing themselves through the peritoneum, then they must be dissected; for the dilatation simply indicates that the carcinoma is compressing them, and only by dissection, particularly of their vesical portion, can one determine whether it is possible to liberate them. After this the bladder and rectum are investigated. Bladder fixation is usually revealed by the formation of a collar and a wrinkled appearance of the peritoneum over the affected area. . . . If the bladder is already invaded by the carcinoma, then loosening it . . . is of no avail; resection is the only thing left.

Wertheim presented a chronologic listing of the 500 patients operated on from November 16, 1898, to October 29, 1909, with a tabulation of the

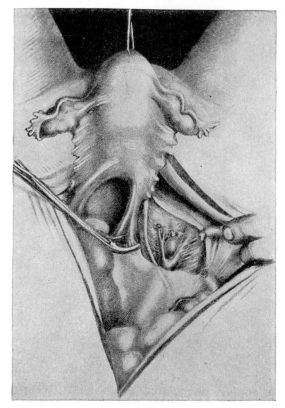

Fig. 79-2. An illustration from Wertheim's monograph,[29] showing a stage of his operation. (Reproduced by permission of Urban & Schwarzenberg, Munich.)

cardinal clinical and pathologic details and the follow-up data. He gave a detailed description of the operative technique, dealing minutely with the many problems associated with the operation.

Considering first the prevention of infection from the primary carcinomatous focus, Wertheim wrote:

The great mortality that followed the ordinary abdominal uterine extirpation was caused principally by septic infection. In uterine carcinoma this danger is particularly great because pathogenic organisms are invariably present in large numbers in the carcinomatous focus. . . .

We had originally hoped to solve this problem by cleansing the primary focus of the cancer by means of the curette and Paquelin cautery, but this procedure did not prove effective (4 of our 23 patients died of peritonitis). It then occurred to us . . . not to open the vagina at all from the abdominal side, but to leave the liberated organs attached to the vaginal tube and remove them from below after the peritoneum had been sutured and the abdominal wound closed.

This would have made it impossible for infection to occur from the primary focus, but in severing the vagina according to this method we find much bleeding from the paravaginal tissues, which is difficult to control because of inadequate visualization. . . . We now sever the vaginal tube from above after all the organs have been liberated, but with the additional precaution of clamping off the vagina first and severing it below the clamp. . . .

We invariably carry out this preparation [excochleation and Paquelin cauterization of the primary tumor] immediately preoperatively. If it be done several days before the operation an inflammatory reaction often occurs as a result of organisms being squeezed out during the excochleation. In spite of the most careful preparation and antiseptic tamponade, a new discharge will soon issue from the carcinoma, with the multiplication of bacteria. If a tampon of very strong antiseptic is used (10 per cent zinc chloride or formalin, for example) it may severely damage the tissues, and this has an unfavorable effect on the patient's postoperative recovery. . . . We fill the vagina with 1 per cent sublimated gauze.

We are not completely satisfied even with all these precautions, because during the manipulation of the uterus incidental to the operation . . . infective particles may still be expressed from the carcinoma. Before the vagina is opened and immediately after the clamps have been applied, the sublimated gauze is removed. . . . The vagina is then opened sufficiently for us to push enough sterile gauze through to again cleanse the vagina and remove every bit of fluid that may have collected. One cannot guard too carefully against possible infection from the primary focus. . . . It is absolutely essential that the vaginal tube be opened only as the last step in the operation.

Discussing care of the wound, Wertheim stated:

The best way to drain the peritoneum after gynecologic operations is through the vagina. This holds true after complete hysterectomy. . . . We resort to peritoneal drainage only when indicated as in other laparotomies—namely, after pus is spilled, when large raw areas are left, or where there is danger from bowel perforation.

We consider it wise to drain in cases where the entire pelvis has been laid bare, where large masses of parametrium and paravaginal tissue, and perhaps lymph nodes, have been removed, and where relatively large dead spaces have been created. We drain the pelvis after peritonization in such cases, to prevent the accumulation of blood or serum. The possible presence of streptococci in the dissected connective tissues increases the need for drainage.

. . . The chief consideration is to prevent contamination of the operative field from particles of the primary focus, which is infected with hemolytic streptococci in about half the cases.

Wertheim next considered the problem of hemostasis:

The control of bleeding is the most difficult problem associated with the radical abdominal operation. This problem does not result, as has been thought, from the extirpation of the regional lymph nodes, but from the removal of the parametrium. The more thoroughly the latter is removed the nearer one gets to the pelvic floor and the more difficult it is to avoid the adjacent veins of the pelvic fascia, which bleed more or less, and the control of which is by no means easy. For this reason . . . we carried out prophylactic ligation of the hypogastric arteries after the thirteenth case but were disappointed in our expectations. . . . Despite hypogastric ligation the uterine artery, on being cut, spurted as vigorously as though no ligature had been applied, and we therefore soon discontinued this practice.

From the ninety-seventh case on we availed ourselves of the so-called parametrium clamps . . . of which three or four suffice for each side. These clamps, applied against the pelvic floor, on the roots of the parametrium, prevent bleeding from individual points. Because of their curves, the clamps are easily replaced by ligatures. The use of these clamps provides certain protection against air embolism. . . .

A lengthy and detailed discussion was devoted to management of the ureters and the prevention and treatment of ureterovaginal fistulas. Wertheim wrote:

Liberation of the ureters is a necessary step in the radical abdominal operation.

It is usually easy to locate the ureters. The pelvic portion of the ureter is often visible through the peritoneum, and to reach it and free it from the connective tissue one needs only to split the peritoneum in the appropriate place. If the subperitoneal fat is thick or the parametrium thickened, the ureters will not be seen; they can be reached readily, nevertheless, by splitting the peritoneum. . . . Sometimes the ureter will reveal itself by its peristalsis. . . .

We have never catheterized the ureters preoperatively and allowed the catheter to remain in situ during the operation. This is superfluous and inadvisable, in our opinion, for it does not leave the ureteral mucosa undamaged.

To reach the vesical portion of the ureter easily, liberate the parametrium as well as the uterine vessels and proceed in the following manner: The index finger is forced along the ureter through the parametrium until the finger tip is visible near the bladder, the latter organ already having been freed from the uterus. The index finger being under the part of the parametrium that contains the uterine vessels, these vessels can now be clamped and tied off at leisure. . . . It is usually easy to force the index finger under the parametrium. The uterine vein is torn occasionally, but this accident is of no great moment. Only when the parametrium is infiltrated with carcinoma is difficulty encountered in forcing the finger through. . . .

After the parametrium is separated, the vesical part of the ureter is easily reached, either by a few snips of the scissors or a little teasing of the tissues. Liberation of the bladder itself now becomes a relatively easy matter. . . .

In advanced cases it is very difficult to free the vesical part of the ureter; and in a few instances it literally has to be dug out. At first we did not expect the ureter to be free of carcinoma in these advanced cases, and we deliberated on the advisability of resection. Histologic examination of these ureters, however, taught us the extraordinary resistance these organs have to carcinomatous invasion . . . and this was further corroborated, for we can show brilliant results even in very advanced cases.

. . . There is no doubt in our minds that the cause of ureteral fistula is necrosis of the wall of the ureter from interference with its nutrition, resulting from isolation of the ureter itself. Opinions differ as to the manner in which isolation of the ureter leads to necrosis. Preservation of the vessels leading to the ureters is only of minor importance; it is more important to preserve the sheath of the ureter. . . . If we notice that the wall of the ureter has been injured we carry out immediate resection.

One of the most important differences between Wertheim's procedure and the modern operation for cervical cancer is revealed in Wertheim's attitude toward the regional lymphatics. He wrote:

This question has been attacked from various points. In opposition to the view that removal of the entire lymphatic system is the foremost requirement is the fact that this is neither possible nor necessary. Even if one admits that in a few cases carcinomatous metastases may be found in nodes slightly enlarged, say to the size of a pea, it is still a fact that carcinoma is never found in the spindle-shaped nodes normally present in the pelvis, as well as in some that have become enlarged into a chainlike formation.

Reliance only on palpation of the various regions is inadequate for making sure that no enlarged regional lymph nodes are overlooked. It is necessary to split the peritoneum and expose the vessels, so that one can palpate between and under them and pick up the cellular and fatty structures between the fingers. Only in this way can one avoid leaving enlarged lymph nodes behind.

It was our aim at first to free the lymph nodes and include them with the removal of the parametrium. . . . Theoretically this method offers an advantage, for the lymph vessels are also included with the removal of the nodes. Experience proved, however, that these lymph nodes tear away during the operative manipulations; so we arrived at the practice of extirpating the lymph nodes at the close of the operation. Only in those advanced cases of carcinoma where inspection and palpation show the lymph nodes to be enlarged and fixed do we begin the operation with the removal of the lymph nodes, and if we find it impossible to extirpate them the operation is abandoned. . . .

In searching for enlarged nodes we proceed in the following order: First we search along the common iliac; then we follow the external iliac to the internal abdominal ring. The index finger is then advanced into the obturator foramen, in order to reach the triangle between the external iliac and hypogastric, and when enlarged nodes are found in this space the obturator nerve is dissected entirely free. In some cases this nerve is completely surrounded by diseased nodes, but the nerve can almost always be freed from them. Only in one case did we have to resect it. We complete the search in the sacral region.

The greatest caution must be exercised where the carcinomatous nodes have become fixed to the iliac vessels. . . . Injury to the iliac veins is a most unpleasant occurrence. . . .

The conclusions to Wertheim's treatise portray his continuing efforts to establish the superiority of the abdominal to the vaginal operation:

It cleared up so much that could not be explained by the vaginal operation, and one began to understand why the vaginal operation was inadequate to achieve success in such a large number of cases. . . . Our knowledge of the behavior of the regional lymphatics and parametrium, of the mode of spread of the carcinoma, and of what might be expected from a surgical operation, was put on a secure basis for the first time by the extended abdominal operation.

. . . There is no doubt that the indications for the vaginal operation for uterine cancer had been too conservative. . . . Most gynecologists went so far as to reject operation in cases where the parametrium was only slightly infiltrated and the mobility of the uterus only slightly limited! Histologic examinations of the parametria widely excised in the extended abdominal operation showed that not every infiltration is invariably carcinomatous; and that rather stiff and infiltrated parametria are often free of carcinoma, while, contrariwise, parametria that feel quite supple on clinical examination may be carcinomatous or may have transmitted the carcinoma to the regional lymph nodes.

We are convinced that simple vaginal hysterectomy, had it utilized this knowledge, would surely have improved its end result. Many a patient has undoubtedly been sent away who could have been helped even by a simple vaginal hysterectomy, and it appears altogether possible that attention to this fact might have succeeded in raising the absolute performance of this operation somewhat beyond the present limits. . . .

Wertheim realized the futility of surgery for many patients with cervical cancer, and with the priceless wisdom of the seasoned surgeon he counseled, in conclusion, against the unbridled extension of the operation. He wrote:

Not in the progressively wider extension of the indications but in the most precise possible execution of the operation do we see the possibility of a further improvement of the end results. The precision of execution can be achieved without an increase in the operative mortality, while an extension of the indications is scarcely possible without it. . . .

Modern surgical experience continues to demonstrate the validity of this principle.

WERTHEIM'S LIFE

Ernst Wertheim, one of Austria's most renowned gynecologists, was born in 1864 in Graz, where his father was a chemist.[1,4,5,6,9] After completing his early education and medical training there, young Wertheim worked for a period in Prague as assistant to Schauta. When the latter was invited to Vienna in 1891, to be head of the I Universitäts-Frauenklinik, Wertheim went along with him and continued to serve as Schauta's assistant until 1897. Wertheim was then made chief of the II Universitäts-Frauenklinik, a position he filled with the greatest distinction for the next 13 years, during which time physicians from all over the world were attracted to his clinic, to witness the work of this master surgeon.

Wertheim also held an appointment at the Cancer Hospital, which had been endowed by one of the Rothschilds in memory of his wife, who had died of mammary cancer. This hospital, devoted primarily to gynecologic cancer, was equipped with the most modern laboratories and facilities, and it was here that Wertheim developed the operation that bears his name. It is said that he performed more than 1300 such operations and that not a single patient was lost to follow-up! In 80 of these cases he carried out histologic study of the parametrium and lymph nodes, examining the prodigious total of 40,000 serial sections. An automobile accident in 1913 resulted in a fracture of the base of his skull, leaving him with permanently impaired hearing.

Wertheim's name is associated with two other major achievements: his work on the gonococcus, and his contributions to the understanding and cure of uterine prolapse. Early in his professional career he developed a method for culturing the gonococcus and followed this up with fundamental observations on the bacteriology of the organism and its method of propagation in human tissues. Although best remembered today for his abdominal hysterectomies, Wertheim showed consummate skill as a vaginal operator as well and became known for his vaginal plastic procedures and vaginal operations for uterine suspension. His *Die operative Behandlung des Prolapses* [30] enjoyed an excellent reception. Wertheim was one of the leading advocates of the vaginal approach to the pelvic viscera. Together with Micholitsch he published an atlas on vaginal operations, describing the removal of the uterine adnexa and even large myomas by this route.[31] Although rubber gloves had been part of the surgeon's accouterment for a number of years, Wertheim spurned them, stating to his students: "Das sicherste Mittel, Infektionen zu vermeiden, ist gut zu operieren."

In 1906 Wertheim came to the United States on a lecture tour. With Bumm he served during his last years as editor of the *Archiv für Gynäkologie*. He was notoriously brusque in manner, but those close to him ascribed this to his conscious efforts to conceal the depression that plagued him so frequently. He found his principal source of relaxation in deer hunting and athletic sports. He was an excellent skier and had the reputation of being one of the best skaters in Vienna. On one occasion he made a balloon trip over the Alps. Wertheim died on February 15, 1920, at the age of 56.

REFERENCES

1. Anon: Professor Wertheim. [Obituary.] *Brit. M. J.*, **1**:455 56, 1920.
2. Freund, W. A.: Eine neue Methode der Exstirpation des ganzen Uterus. *Samml. klin. Vort.*, No. 133. Gynäk. No. 41, 911–24, 1878.

3. Freund, W. A.: Zu meiner Methode der totalen Uterus-Exstirpation. *Centralbl. f. Gynäk.,* **2**:265–69, 1878.

4. Halban, J.: Professor Dr. Ernst Wertheim. [Obituary.] *Wien. med. Wchnschr.,* **70**:409–12, 1920.

5. Kermauner, F.: Ernst Wertheim. [Obituary.] *Wien. klin. Wchnschr.,* **33**:183–85, 1920.

6. Latzko, W.: Professor Dr. Ernst Wertheim. [Obituary.] *Wien. med. Wchnschr.,* **70**:545–49, 1920.

7. Ricci, J. V.: *The Genealogy of Gynaecology,* 2nd ed. Blakiston Co., Philadelphia, 1950, p. 394.

8. Ries, E.: Eine neue Operationsmethode des Uteruscarcinoms. *Ztschr. f. Geburtsh. u. Gynäk.,* **32**:266–74, 1895.

9. Weibel, W.: Ernst Wertheim. [Obituary.] *Zentralbl. f. Gynäk.,* **44**:281–85, 1920.

10. Wertheim, E.: Zur Frage der Radicaloperation beim Uteruskrebs. *Arch. f. Gynäk.,* **61**:627–68, Pl. X-XIX, 1900.

11. Wertheim, E.: Beitrag zur Frage der Radicaloperation beim Uteruskrebs. *Wien. klin. Wchnschr.,* **13**:1101–5, disc. 1119–23, 1178–80, 1900; Schlusswort, pp. 1178–80.

12. Wertheim, E.: Diskussion: [Waldstein: Endresultate der operativen Behandlung des Gebärmutterkrebses mit Krankenvorstellung.] *Centralbl. f. Gynäk.,* **24**:674–75, 1900.

13. Wertheim, E.: Abdominale Totalexstirpation der Vagina. *Centralbl. f. Gynäk.,* **24**:1393–96, 1900.

14. Wertheim, E.: Über die Radikaloperation bei Carcinoma uteri. *Verhandl. d. deutsch. Gesellsch. f. Gynäk.,* **9**[1901]:161–67, 1901.

15. Wertheim, E.: Kurzer Bericht über eine 3. Serie von 30 Uteruskrebsoperationen. *Centralbl. f. Gynäk.,* **26**:249–52, 1902.

16. Wertheim, E.: Ein neuer Beitrag zur Frage der Radikaloperation beim Uteruskrebs. *Arch. f. Gynäk.,* **65**:1–39, Pl. I-VI, 1902.

17. Wertheim, E.: Traitement chirurgical du cancer de l'utérus. *Rev. de gynéc. et de chir. abdom.,* **6**:843–52, disc. 925–34, 1902.

18. Wertheim, E.: Zur Kenntnis der regionären Lymphdrüsen beim Uteruskarzinom. *Centralbl. f. Gynäk.,* **27**:105–10, 1903.

19. Wertheim, E.: A discussion on the diagnosis and treatment of cancer of the uterus. *Brit. M. J.,* **2**:689–95, disc. 695–704, 1905.

20. Wertheim, E.: Carcinom der Gebärmutter. *Verhandl. d. deutsch. Gesellsch. f. Gynäk.,* **11**[1905]:469–75, 1906.

21. [Wertheim, E.]: Diskussion zur Carcinomtherapie. *Verhandl. d. deutsch. Gesellsch. f. Gynäk.,* **11**[1905]:516–17, 1906.

22. Wertheim, E.: Ueberblick über die Leistungen der erweiterten abdominalen Operation beim Gebärmutterkrebs. *Wien. klin. Wchnschr.,* **19**:787–88, 1906.

23. Wertheim, E.: The radical abdominal operation in carcinoma of the cervix uteri. *Surg., Gynec. & Obst.,* **4**:1–10, disc. 101–13, 1907.

24. Wertheim, E.: Bericht über die Erfolge der erweiterten abdominalen Uteruskrebsoperation. *Verhandl. d. deutsch. Gesellsch. f. Gynäk.,* **12**[1907]:722–23, 1908.

25. Wertheim, E.: [Discussion of] Traitement du cancer des organes génitaux de la femme. *Soc. internat. de Chir.,* Cong. 2 [1908], **1**:541–44, 1908.

26. Wertheim, E.: Die Leistungen der erweiterten abdominalen Uteruskrebs-operation. *Zentralbl. f. Gynäk.,* **32**:175–78, 1908.

27. Wertheim, [E.]: Gynäkologie und Urologie. *Ztschr. f. Urol.* (Beihft.: Verhandl. d. deutsch. Gesellsch. f. Urol., 2. Kong.), **3**:56–65, disc. 64–94, 1909; Schlusswort, pp. 92–93. Also abstr.: Urologie und Gynäkologie. *Ztschr. f. Urol.,* **3**:564, disc. 564–65, 1909.

28. Wertheim, E.: Die Spätresultate der erweiterten abdominalen Uteruskrebs-operation. *Compt.-rend., Cong. internat. de med.* [1909 (Sect. 8)]:473–78, 1910. Also transl.: Résultats éloignés de l'opération abdominale élargie dans le cancer de l'utérus. *Ann. de gynéc. et d'obst.,* [1909]:637–41, 1909.

29. Wertheim, E.: *Die erweiterte abdominale Operation bei Carcinoma colli Uteri (auf Grund von 500 Fällen).* Urban & Schwarzenberg, Berlin, 1911.

30. Wertheim, E.: *Die operative Behandlung des Prolapses mittelst Interposition und Suspension des Uterus.* J. Springer, Berlin, 1919.

31. Wertheim, E., and Micholitsch, [H.]: *Die Technik der Vaginalen Bauchhöhlen-Operationen.* S. Hirzel, Leipzig, 1906.

Index